Clinical
OBSTETRICS AND
GYNAECOLOGY

Dedication

This book is dedicated to the millions of women worldwide who will suffer disability, lose their babies, or lose their lives through the want of adequate reproductive healthcare.

Commissioning Editor: Ellen Green

Project Development Manager: Janice Urquhart

Project Manager: Frances Affleck

Designer: Sarah Russell

Clinical
OBSTETRICS AND
GYNAECOLOGY

Edited by

James Drife MD FRCOG FRCPEd FRCSEd HonFCOGSA

Professor of Obstetrics and Gynaecology, University of Leeds;
Honorary Consultant Obstetrician and Gynaecologist,
The Leeds Teaching Hospitals NHS Trust, Leeds, UK

Brian A. Magowan MRCOG, DCH

Consultant Obstetrician and Gynaecologist,
Borders General Hospital,
Melrose, UK

Illustrated by Ian Ramsden

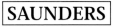

An Imprint of Elsevier Science

Edinburgh • London • New York • Oxford • Philadelphia • St Louis • Sydney • Toronto 2004

SAUNDERS
An imprint of Elsevier Limited

First published 2004

ISBN 0702017752

British Library Cataloguing in Publication Data
A catalogue record for this book is available from the British Library

Library of Congress Cataloging in Publication Data
A catalog record for this book is available from the Library of Congress

Notice
Medical knowledge is constantly changing. Standard safety precautions must be followed, but as new research and clinical experience broaden our knowledge, changes in treatment and drug therapy may become necessary or appropriate. Readers are advised to check the most current product information provided by the manufacturer of each drug to be administered to verify the recommended dose, the method and duration of administration, and contraindications. It is the responsibility of the practitioner, relying on experience and knowledge of the patient, to determine dosages and the best treatment for each individual patient. Neither the Publisher nor the editors and contributors assume any liability for any injury and/or damage to persons or property arising from this publication.

The Publisher

 ELSEVIER SCIENCE

your source for books, journals and multimedia in the health sciences

www.elsevierhealth.com

The
publisher's
policy is to use
**paper manufactured
from sustainable forests**

Printed in China

Preface

To witness the joy of a new birth is a thrill that is never lost, and the subsequent bond between the professionals, the parents and the baby is a powerful one. Such a profound psychological, social and cultural event is vividly fixed in the parents' minds and, when everything goes well, it is truly marvellous experience.

For a physiological process, however, pregnancy is surprisingly hazardous. Worldwide, over half a million women die every year from pregnancy-related causes and many of these lives could be saved with the most basic of healthcare provision. Even with the best medical care, however, lives are still lost and there is the temptation in affluent countries to over-medicalize normal pregnancy, perhaps interfering when there are no real problems. Such interference serves to increase the risk of harm. Obstetrics therefore faces two challenges: how to provide more effective care in countries with limited resources and how to make our interventions more appropriate in the affluent world.

The speciality, however, is even wider than this. Obstetrics and gynaecology includes a whole range of medical practice, from psychosexual problems to radical cancer surgery. One couple in seven has a problem with subfertility, and the subject of contraception affects most people at some time in their lives. Many of medicine's most taxing ethical dilemmas are also concentrated in our specialty and it is this overall diversity that makes our clinical practice so fascinating and challenging.

There have been some spectacular innovations over recent decades but just as impressive are the steady advances throughout each clinical area – even while this book has been in preparation. No individual can keep up with all of these and we are grateful to our colleagues with specialised knowledge who wrote the first drafts of many of these chapters. We have tried to achieve uniformity of style and the responsibility for the final version is ours.

We hope that, as well as summarising current knowledge in the specialty, this book will help inspire some readers. New ideas from fresh and interested people are always needed. The public is demanding ever higher standards from doctors in general and obstetricians in particular, and we are privileged to be a part of a speciality in which the clinical stakes are high. The challenges are more than matched by the rewards.

Finally, we would like to acknowledge our debt to *Clinical Medicine* by Kumar and Clark, whose original book set new standards for medical texts, and in terms of writing style and presentation helped to inspire the writing of this book.

J. D.
B. M.

Contributors and Advisers

Dr Margaret Balls
Senior Clinical Medical Officer, Contraception and Sexual Health, Burmantofts Health Centre, Leeds, UK

Dr Christopher P. Bennett
Department of Clinical Genetics, St James's University Hospital, Leeds, UK

The late **Mr D. Bromham**
Formerly Senior Lecturer in Obstetrics and Gynaecology, St James's University Hospital Academic Unit of Obstetrics and Gynaecology, Leeds, UK

Dr Peter Buchan
Formerly Consultant in Obstetrics and Gynaecology, Borders General Hospital, Melrose, UK

Mr E. John Buxton
Consultant Gynaecological Surgeon and Oncologist, BUPA Hospital Leeds, Leeds, UK

Dr Sharon Cameron
Lecturer in Reproductive Medicine, The Simpson Centre for Reproductive Health, The Royal Infirmary of Edinburgh, Edinburgh, UK

Dr Mark Chadwick
Senior Houses Officer, Basic surgical Trainee, Torquay Hospital, Torquay, UK

Professor Hilary Critchley
Professor of Reproductive Medicine, University of Edinburgh; Honorary Consultant Gynaecologist , Department of Obstetrics and Gynaecology, Centre for Reproductive Biology, The Royal Infirmary of Edinburgh, Edinburgh, UK

Dr Ian Currie
Consultant Obstetrician and Gynaecologist, Stoke Mandeville Hospital, Buckinghamshire, UK

Dr Peter Dear
Consultant Neonatal Paediatrician, Neonatal Intensive Care Unit, St James's University Hospital, Leeds, UK

Mr Martin DeBono
Consultant in Obstetrics and Gynaecology, Assisted Conception Unit, The Calderdale Royal Hospital, Halifax, UK

Dr Paul Dewart
Consultant Obstetrician and Gynaecologist, Honorary Senior Lecturer, St John's Hospital, Livingston, UK

Mr Ellis Downes
Consultant in Obstetrics and Gynaecology, Chase Farm Hospital, Enfield, UK

Professor James Drife
Academic Unit of Paediatrics and Obstetrics and Gynaecology, Leeds General Infirmary, Leeds, UK

Dr Colin Duncan
Clinical Lecturer in Reproductive Medicine, Department of Obstetrics and Gynaecology, The Simpson Centre for Reproductive Health, The Royal Infirmary of Edinburgh, UK

Mr David R. Fitzpatrick
MRC Senior Clinical Scientist, MRC Human Genetics Unit, Western General Hospital, Edinburgh, UK

Dr Michael Gannon
Consultant Obstetrician and Gynaecologist, Midland Regional Hospital, Mulingar, Eire

Mr Martin Griffiths-Jones
Consultant in Obstetrics and Gynaecology, St James's University Hospital, Leeds, UK

Dr Karl W. Hancock
Formerly Senior Lecturer in Obstetrics and Gynaecology, University of Leeds, Leeds, UK

Dr Henry C. Irving
Consultant Radiologist, Department of Radiology, St James's University Hospital, Leeds, UK

Mr Gerald J. Jarvis
Formerly Consultant Obstetrician and Gynaecologist, St James's University Hospital, Leeds, UK

Dr Nick Johnson
Consultant Obstetrician and Gynaecologist, Royal United Hospital, Bath, UK

Mrs Christine Landon
Consultant Gynaecologist and Urogynaecologist, Leeds General Infirmary, Leeds, UK

Mr Geoffrey Lane
Consultant Gynaecological Oncologist, St James's University Hospital, Leeds, UK

Dr I. Laing
Consultant Neonatologist, Neonatal Unit, Simpson Centre for Reproductive Health, The Royal Infirmary of Edinburgh, Edinburgh, UK

Contributors and Advisers

Dr Hamish MacDonald
Formerly Consultant Obstetrician and Gynaecologist, St James's University Hospital, Leeds, UK

Mr Ronald MacDonald
Formerly Consultant Obstetrician and Gynaecologist, Leeds General Infirmary, Leeds, UK

Dr Rosemary MacDonald
Formerly Consultant Anaesthetist, St James's University Hospital, Leeds and Postgraduate Dean, Yorkshire, UK

Dr Brian Magowan
Consultant Obstetrician and Gynaecologist, Borders General Hospital, Melrose, UK

Mr Gerald Mason
Consultant in Feto-Maternal Medicine, Leeds General Infirmary, Leeds, UK

Dr Eric Monteiro
Consultant in Genitourinary Medicine, Leeds General Infirmary, Leeds, UK

Dr Philip Myerscough
Honorary Fellow, Department of Obstetrics and Gynaecology, University of Edinburgh, Edinburgh, UK

Dr J. Onwude
Consultant Gynaecologist Springfield Hospital, Chelmsford, UK

Mr A. J. Rutherford
Consultant in Reproductive Medicine and Gynaecological Surgery, Assisted Conception Unit, Leeds General Infirmary, Leeds, UK

Professor James S. Scott
Formerly Dean of the Faculty of Medicine and Professor of Obstetrics and Gynaecology, University of Leeds, Leeds, UK

Professor J. Thornton
Professor of Obstetrics and Gynaecology, Academic Division of Obstetrics and Gynaecology, Nottingham City Hospital, Nottingham, UK

Dr Graeme Walker
Specialist Registrar in Obstetrics and Gynaecology, The Simpson Centre for Reproductive Health, The Royal Infirmary of Edinburgh, Edinburgh, UK

Dr M. A. Waugh
Consultant in Genitourinary Medicine, Department of Genitourinary Medicine, Leeds General Infirmary, Leeds, UK

Dr Janet Wilson
Consultant Physician in Genitourinary Medicine, Centre for Reproductive Health, Leeds General Infirmary, Leeds, UK

Contents

Fundamentals

1

Women's health in the 21st century

Introduction

Obstetrics and gynaecology is a specialty concerned with women's health issues and many of these issues are about having children. Depending on your viewpoint, the specialty can be seen as the study of the creation of new life, or as the study of gene survival and evolution. Such important subjects cannot simply be considered in terms of physiology and pathology, but must take into account the way in which the reproductive process affects individuals and society, and the way in which it interacts with culture and religion. Some insight into this is essential to a clinical understanding of this specialty.

Only a few aspects of this vast subject can be touched on in this chapter. We will begin by considering the different roles that men and women may have in society, and explore how attitudes to reproduction vary throughout the world. Next, some key worldwide problems will be outlined including violence, rape, prostitution, and female genital mutilation. Finally there is a short section entitled 'Women as patients' looking at how these issues affect healthcare for women.

Women and men in a changing world

Sexual dimorphism

Men are usually physically bigger and stronger than women, and this physical power has the potential for abuse. We, the editors, strongly support the ancient Greek view that 'women's nature is different from that of men but not of any lesser or greater value'. Both should be held with equal respect in any society. If anything, physical vulnerability demands that even greater respect is required, and failure to demonstrate such respect should not be tolerated.

Cultural attitudes

Early civilizations were not all male-dominated. In Babylon and ancient Egypt women were financially independent and in Sparta women owned two-thirds of the land. Female warriors were numerous among the Celts: Queen Boadicea was not a unique figure. In the Greek city states, however, decisions were taken by adult male citizens, and the Roman senate consisted entirely of men. From the time of the Roman empire until the 20th century, legislative bodies throughout the world have often been exclusively male.

A number of practices reflect an underlying attitude that, at times in the past, women have been viewed as second-class citizens. The Sultan of the Ottoman Empire, for example, disposed of unwanted wives by sewing them into weighted sacks and throwing them into the Bosporus. Pre-18th century 'witch hunts' in Europe led to the death of old, single women by hanging or burning, and prostitutes were occasionally punished by death as late as the 17th century. Another extreme example of abuse is suttee – the practice in which a widow is burned, voluntarily or otherwise, on her husband's funeral pyre – which has been followed by the ancient Egyptians, the Scandinavians, the Chinese, and peoples of Asia and Africa.

Historical perceptions of a male-dominated world, however, may in part be related to the fact that many historians have been male and may have recorded a biased view of history. Closer scrutiny reveals that women have very capably held dominant roles in many societies. The Greek philosopher Plato said 'that man and women with the same natural ability should receive the same education and training and to the same kind of work.' Many rulers in ancient Egypt, starting with the Cleopatras, were women.

Despite this, however, there are many parts of the world in which women are still treated as second-class citizens. They have less money, less influence, more restrictions and, often, a much greater workload than men. Importantly, they may be seen as having a lower priority for healthcare, particularly when young or when having their first (and often most hazardous) pregnancy.

Religion

Very early religions involved goddess-worship. Shrines to the 'Great Goddess' have been found in numerous places in Europe, Africa, Asia and Australia. In the modern monotheistic religions, however – Judaism, Buddhism, Christianity, Islam – God is thought of as male. His prophets were male and even today the priests are almost all male. This has profound effects on religious teaching, ranging from Old Testament attitudes to menstruation (see below), to Muslim restrictions on women's dress and contemporary Roman Catholic views on contraception.

Feminism

'Feminism,' which means different things to different people, has evolved over the past 200 years. Latterly, women's movements have proliferated in many countries and the United Nations declared 1975 as International Women's Year. The aims of 'feminism' now vary from country to country: in some the goals are very basic, such as abolishing the custom of buying a bride; and in other countries the goals include attacking stereotyping and ensuring equality of opportunity in institutions which still have a male-dominated ethos.

Education

Physical differences between the sexes have been used to limit women's education and employment. The American historian Harold Speert quotes a popular book from 1874:

A girl cannot spend more than four, or, in occasional instances, five hours of force daily upon her duties, and leave sufficient margin for the general physical growth that she must make. If she puts as much force into her brain education as a boy, the brain or the special apparatus will suffer.

Few would accept this view today, but women in many societies are offered less education than men. It is relevant to note that in the Indian state of Kerala, where female literacy rates are high, the rate of maternal mortality is very low.

Employment

Worldwide

Manual work, particularly in agricultural communities, has been shared by men and women over the centuries. Women labourers helped build pyramids in Egypt and temples in Greece. Women tend to be the main burden bearers in Africa and still work as navvies in the Far East.

Household work has been the responsibility of the woman in all societies. This may involve childcare, growing crops, making clothes, cooking, making bread, and even butchering and brewing. In many less affluent countries, women often have a very much greater workload than their husbands.

The UK

With the industrial revolution in the 18th century, women began working in factories and even in coal mines, and during the First and Second World Wars, women often undertook munitions or other 'men's work'. Many of these were married women.

Of the current British workforce of 27.3 million people, 12.1 million (44%) are female, of whom 40% are in part-time jobs. Girls tend to leave school with better qualifications than boys but women are less likely than men to achieve managerial or professional jobs. The average gross hourly earning (excluding overtime) for a woman in 2001 was 81.6% of the average earned by her male counterpart.

Attitudes to reproduction

Menarche

In some primitive cultures the menarche is a public event celebrated by the whole tribe. In Western society, however, it is generally secret. According to Havelock Ellis in 1896 about half of American schoolgirls had either no advance knowledge or only vague knowledge at the time of their first menses, and things were probably much the same 50 years later. Reverend Chad Varah founded the charity the Samaritans in 1953 after officiating at the funeral of a girl who had committed suicide after experiencing her first menses. Simone de Beauvoir, in *The Second Sex* in 1949, distinguished between a girl's reactions to puberty and to the menarche:

She is proud of becoming a woman and watches the maturing of her bosom with satisfaction, padding her dress with handkerchiefs and taking pride in it before her elders; she does not yet grasp the significance of what is taking place in her. Her first menstruation reveals this meaning, and her feelings of shame appear. … All the evidence agrees in showing that whether the child has been forewarned or not, the event always seems to her repugnant and humiliating.

In 1970 Germaine Greer was more graphic in *The Female Eunuch*:

The arrival of menarche is more significant than any birthday, but in the Anglo-Saxon households it is ignored and carefully concealed from general awareness. For six months while I was waiting for my first menstruation I toted a paper bag with diapers and pins in my school satchel. When it finally came, I suffered agonies lest anyone should guess or smell it or anything. My diapers were made of harsh towelling, and I used to creep into the laundry and crouch over a bucket of foul clouts, hoping that my brother would not catch me at my revolting labours. It is not surprising that well-bred, dainty little girls find it difficult to adapt to menstruation, when our society does no more than explain it and leave them to get on with it.

Many sex education programmes now aim to prepare girls as well as possible for menarche, emphasizing if possible, the positive symbolism rather than these feelings of shame.

Attitudes to menstruation

The word 'menstrual' is derived from the Latin words for 'moon' and 'month'. The menstrual cycle is almost uniquely human, occurring in only a few other species such as Old World monkeys and anthropoid apes. Reproductive cycles in other mammalian species include an annual cycle in the sheep, and oestrus cycles in dogs and cats. The fact the menstrual cycle does not occur in domestic or farm animals may have added to its mystery in the eyes of our ancestors. In primitive tribes,

adult females spent much of their time either pregnant or lactating, and the appearance of unexplained vaginal bleeding may have been frightening.

Myths and taboos have been attached to menstruation in many cultures. In some 'primitive' societies menstruating women were segregated in special 'menstrual huts'. In ancient China menstrual blood was not allowed to touch the ground for fear of offending the Earth spirit and in ancient Egypt, ritual cleansing baths were mandatory at the end of menstruation. Hindu teaching according to the Parsi sage Zoroaster was that: 'A woman in her courses is not to gaze upon the sacred fire, sit in water, behold the sun or hold conversation with a man.' Chapter 15 of the Book of Leviticus prescribes the cleansing that a woman must undertake at the end of her 'discharge of blood', which appears to have been regarded in the same way as discharges due to disease. The Roman historian Pliny, in an infamous diatribe, attributed numerous noxious qualities to menstrual blood, calling it, for example, 'a fatal poison … causing fruit to fall from branches and dulling razors'.

During the Victorian era, middle and upper class women in the UK and America were regarded as delicate, and this attitude underlay the advice given about menstruation. Speert quotes a book published in many editions from the late 19th century until 1928:

Rest is just as important during menstruation as cleanliness, if not more so. … It is an outrage that many delicate, weak girls and women must stay on their feet all day or work on a machine when they should be at home in bed or lying down on a couch. … there should be as much rest as possible. For delicate and sensitive girls it is always best to stay away from school during the first and second days … It is best that dancing, bicycle riding, horseback riding, rowing, and other athletic exercises be given up altogether during the means. Automobile riding and railroad and carriage travel prove injurious in some instances.

In 1876, however, one of the first women to graduate in medicine in the USA, Mary Putnam Jacobi, published a report 'The Question of Rest for Women during Menstruation', which questioned the idea that menstruation was an affliction that weakened women. She performed experiments showing that muscular strength did not change during the monthly cycle, and she conducted a survey which suggested that a significant proportion did not suffer pain, discomfort or weakness at all during menstruation.

Sanitary protection

Rags or pieces of linen are commonly used as sanitary protection in many parts of the world, and these are often washed and used again. In 1921, disposable sanitary towels were marketed in the USA under the brand name Kotex, and the idea of internal tampons was patented in 1937 when the Tampax company was founded. Use of disposable protection did not spread around the world until after the Second World War. In the UK, television advertising of sanitary protection was banned entirely until 1979 and only gained acceptance in the mid-1980s as public attitudes altered. Surveys by the Independent Broadcasting Authority at the time commented: 'A broad picture of increasing acceptance of the advertising over the period emerged. Nevertheless it is recognised that a minority, mainly of older women, remain opposed to it.'

Attitudes to sex

Attitudes to sex vary throughout the world. The average age at first intercourse worldwide is 18 years, ranging from 16–17 in America and many European countries to 20–22 years in the Far East. Of those who are sexually active, the average number of sexual partners is 7. The variation, however, is wide – from an average of 14 in America, 10 in Japan, and 8 in the UK to 4 in Nigeria, 3 in India and 2 in China.

The question of whether sex education encourages earlier sexual activity is a controversial one. It is pertinent, however, that while The Netherlands has a very high level of sex education and accessibility to sexual health clinics, it has a very low teenage pregnancy rate. Patients are offered the choice between their family practitioner and family orientated clinics and, as in Sweden, doctors are forbidden to disclose any information to the parents of teenagers. In the UK, on the other hand, there has been active opposition to some sex education in schools, and many sex-obsessed quarters of the media have fuelled this repressive atmosphere with stories of sexual scandal and the view that 'the innocent must remain innocent'. Such views are also prevalent in America, with many sex education programmes being directed only at 'disaster prevention', and with little emphasis on love or relationships.

Homosexuality

Modern attitudes towards homosexuality are underpinned by religious, legal and medical views. Before the Middle Ages, homosexual acts appear to have been widely tolerated or ignored by the Christian church throughout Europe. Beginning in the later 12th century, however, hostility toward homosexuality began to take root, and eventually spread throughout European religious and secular institutions. Religious teachings became enforced into legal sanctions, with statutes described in Latin or such oblique phrases as 'wickedness not to be named'.

The medical world debated whether homosexuality was a medical condition, and views ranged from that of Richard von Kraft-Ebing who believed that it was a 'degenerative sickness' to Sigmund Freud's view that we are all innately bisexual, and that we become homosexual or bisexual depending on our experiences. Most would now agree that our sexuality is, to a large part, inborn. The diagnosis of 'homosexuality' was removed completely as a psychiatric diagnosis in 1986.

Current worldwide problems

Abortion and infanticide of females

The birth of a son is more valued than the birth of a daughter in some societies and the practice of killing unwanted female babies at birth has been widespread, particularly in China and India. The practice is condemned in the Koran, Book 81: 'When the infant girl, buried alive, is asked for what crime she was thus slain.' In some countries, it is not uncommon for a termination to be requested if an ultrasound scan reveals a female fetus.

Violence and rape

Physical violence against women can take the form of physical or sexual abuse. In some cultures, violence against women is accepted and societal norms blame the woman for the violence perpetrated against her. These attitudes may also occasionally be held by healthcare workers, sometimes resulting in an inadequate or inappropriate response to women who seek help. In most other cultures, where violence against women is not considered to be acceptable, there is still a surprisingly large problem.

Around 1 in 4 women worldwide will suffer from domestic violence at some stage in their lives and, in many countries, statistics suggest that more than 50% of women who are murdered are killed by their intimate partner. In other studies, more than 95% of women who are raped already know their assailant. Violence against women can have both short- and long-term health consequences including sexually transmitted infections, and unwanted pregnancies which may in turn lead to unsafe abortions. Women living with partners may not feel able to make their own decisions about contraceptive issues, or even about staying or leaving the relationship, and the psychological implications are immense: victims of rape are eleven times more likely to experience clinical depression, and are also at greater risk of drug- and alcohol-related problems, and even suicide.

It is important that we bear these issues in mind when meeting patients. A history of such problems is unlikely to be volunteered spontaneously and considerable tact may be required to explore these areas.

Prostitution

Prostitution is, of course, not new. The Greeks, in the 4th century BC, saw prostitution as greed on the part of women. By the first century AD the Romans, under the emperor Caligula, established a series of brothels with a proportion of the profits coming to the state, and even in the 4th century AD it was perfectly acceptable, even expected, for a man to have sex with prostitutes in addition to his wife. In the 6th century AD, however, Christianity swept through the Roman world, changing the codes of morality, and chastity was perceived as a virtue for both women and men. Prostitution moved from being a public service to a religious crime against women.

These views were further supported by the rise of feminist movements in the 19th century in Europe. In addition to the exploitation mentioned above, women in the 21st century become prostitutes for other reasons: poverty, drugs, susceptibility to pressure from friends, and, not uncommonly, following a history of sexual abuse.

The UN estimates that around 4 million women are currently being trafficked as part of the sex industry. These women are usually from particularly poor countries and they may find themselves socially abandoned. They are lured with promises of legitimate work but sold into a prostitution network, often in more affluent areas or countries.

Female genital mutilation

'Female circumcision', now known as female genital mutilation, varies from Sunna (excision of the prepuce of the clitoris) to the more extensive excision of the clitoris, the labia majora and the labia minora. It is carried out because of custom and tradition: it predates Islam and is not part of this religion. The age at which the operation is carried out varies from birth to just before marriage, but it is most commonly performed at around 7 years of age. Anaesthesia is rarely used.

Although such procedures are against the law in the UK, over 100 million women have been subjected to this practice worldwide, particularly in a geographical band from the Horn of Africa to Nigeria. In Somalia and Ethiopia over 90% of girls are believed to have been mutilated in this way.

Sexually transmitted infections (STIs)

The World Health Organization estimates that 40 million adults are living with HIV/AIDS and that almost half of these are women. Most live in developing countries, with two-thirds estimated to be in Africa and one-quarter in Asia. There are also estimated to be a third of a billion cases of STIs worldwide, many of which are associated with long-term morbidity, particularly in women. Such infections are the commonest worldwide cause of infertility.

Women as patients

Worldwide

Of the world's three billion women, over 80% live in developing countries or very poor countries, and over

the last 50 years, while the health of children throughout the world has improved, there has been little change in the overall health of women.

The World Bank has recognized that female reproductive problems are the most important health issues facing adults in the developing world. 'Reproductive health' has been defined as 'a condition in which the reproductive process is accomplished in a state of complete physical, mental and social well-being'. Most of the world's women fall far short of this ideal.

The number of maternal deaths worldwide is over 500 000 per year, with almost all of these occurring in developing countries. Many of these are due to complications of termination of pregnancy, usually carried out by unskilled hands, and often illegally. Improved access to contraception has the potential to make a difference in this area; more than 580 million couples are now using contraception but 100 million women, mostly in developing countries, are not, in spite of an expressed desire to do so.

Gender equality is seen as an important factor in limiting population growth, as this will allow women access to contraceptive services. Women and their reproductive needs should be at the top of the international health agenda. Equality means far more than achieving the right to reproductive health but it seems clear that reproductive health cannot be fully achieved without considerable improvements in the status of women.

UK

Women in the UK are more likely than men to consult their GP. At the extremes of life, when consultation rates are highest, the sex ratio is equal, but between the ages of 16 and 44 the average number of consultations per person per year is 3 for males and 5 for females. Women are also more likely to attend hospital as inpatients or outpatients and are also more likely to report acute sickness.

Although life-threatening conditions occur in obstetrics and gynaecology, in developed countries such as the UK most patients in antenatal and gynaecology clinics are not acutely ill. They may be being screened for disease, for example, or may be requesting sterilization, fertility treatment or help with menopausal symptoms. Pregnant women in particular may not like being referred to as 'patients'. Healthy people are more questioning than sick people, and women attending gynaecology or antenatal clinics may already be well informed about their conditions.

Conclusion

Decisions about what is 'normal' or 'abnormal' and even what is 'ethical' or 'unethical' may depend on a woman's cultural and religious background, age and personal experience. Sterilization of a healthy human being, for example, was regarded as unethical in the UK until the 1960s but is now a common procedure, though it still remains unacceptable in some countries. Presenting symptoms may also be influenced by the way a woman views her role in society: the menopause is welcomed in some parts of the world and treated as a disorder in others. Attitudes to woman's health issues, and indeed to broader gender issues, are constantly changing in all countries, and change can sometimes occur surprisingly quickly. Doctors who remain unaware of such changes may alienate some of their patients and will provide less than optimal care.

Key points

- Reproductive health is more than just the study of physiology and pathology: it involves a more holistic picture about how an individual is influenced by her society, culture and religion. Doctors providing reproductive healthcare must be aware of these issues.

- As men are usually physically more powerful than women, there is the potential for abuse. This can involve violence, rape, prostitution and female genital mutilation. Beside our duty to treat individual patients, we also have a more global duty to speak out and act against such abuses throughout the world.

2 Obstetrics and gynaecology: a brief historical overview

Introduction

Obstetrics is as old as humankind itself. Gynaecology, however, could be argued to date back to ancient fertility symbols, such as the 'Venus de Willendorf' found in western Europe between 22 000 and 24 000 BC. While it is tempting to consider the history of obstetrics and gynaecology together, they cannot be separated from developments in other branches of medicine, including those of the Mesopotamians, Egyptians, Greeks, Romans and Chinese. The influence of Hippocrates (c.460–377 BC), for example, the first person to deliver medicine from superstition and sorcery, was profound. In the same way, the discovery of the circulation by William Harvey (1578–1657), the identification of infective agents by Anton van Leeuwenhoek (1632–1723), the anatomical descriptions of Leonardo da Vinci (1452–1519), and the pathological work of Battista Morgagni (1682–1771) and Rudolph Virchow (1821–1902) signalled quantum leaps throughout all medical fields.

Only the faintest historical sketch of the history of obstetrics and gynaecology can be drawn here, but without considering history at all we are liable to see ourselves at the pinnacle of medical refinement, rather than as part of a much more humbling developmental continuum. A few key developments are outlined below.

Gynaecology

One of the earliest works to discuss gynaecological remedies was the Ebers Papyrus, an Egyptian text dating from before 1200 BC. It contained, amongst other compendia, treatments for prolapse of the uterus, instructions on how to carry out an abortion and remedies for a variety of vulval complaints. Both Aristotle (384–322 BC) and Hippocrates (see above) knew about the existence of the ovaries, uterus, vagina and vulva, and it was Aristotle who was the first to document that intercourse was necessary for pregnancy to occur. He believed, however, that semen and menstrual blood mixed in the uterus to form a fetus, and it was a Roman physician, Claudius Galen (AD 129–200), who first suggested that the ovaries were involved. He suggested that there was a mixing of the male semen with 'female semen' from the ovaries, and that while the fetal viscerae were derived from the mother, it was the father who contributed the brain.

Fundamentals

By the middle ages, it was thought that the 'egg' contained a miniature, but fully formed, human being – the preformation theory. This belief was countered with the argument that the miniature human being would also have to contain its own miniature human being and so forth ad infinitum, and the theory was replaced with the concept of epigenesis – that new structures arise in the course of development. With the discovery of spermatozoa by van Leeuwenhoek (see above), the realization of their significance by Rudolph Kölliker in 1841 and the identification of ova by Karl Ernst von Baer in 1827, the true nature of the reproductive process became clear. In 1978, a baby girl called Louise Brown became the first child to be born as the result of in vitro fertilization, a process developed by Patrick Steptoe and Robert Edwards in England.

Gynaecological surgery

Gynaecology is divided into many subspecialties and the history of each is a book in itself. Gynaecological surgery will be considered further. It is likely that the very earliest gynaecological operations were female circumcisions, or ceremonial infibulations. It is also likely that abortions have been practised from very early times, but details about these are very limited indeed. The first abdominal surgery carried out for any reason was carried out for gynaecological pathology. Robert Houston (1678–1734) practising in Glasgow in 1701 operated at a local farm on a Margaret Miller, a 58-year-old woman with a very rapidly growing ovarian tumour that was pressing on her abdominal organs to the point where she had great difficulty in breathing. He opened the abdominal wall using a sharpened trocar made of pinewood and bored through the thick wall of the cyst, emptying it of a 'jelly-like substance like glue, which contained steatoceous and atheromatous tissue with hydatids'. He stitched up the abdomen, covering the wound with a compress and a cloth soaked in French brandy. Mrs Miller made a complete recovery.

It was in America, however, that the first ovarian cyst was actually removed. Ephraim McDowall (1771–1830) was asked to see a Mrs Jane Todd Crawford in 1809 at her home in Kentucky. Her ovarian tumour was so large that it was again difficult for her to breathe, and it was making her life a misery. She came to see him riding on a horse, resting the tumour on the horn of her saddle. On Christmas day of that year, also auspiciously a Sunday, McDowall began the operation. There was no anaesthesia, no antisepsis and only one assistant, and throughout the operation Mrs Crawford recited the Psalms. He made an 9-inch left-sided paramedian incision, emptied the cyst, delivered the tumour (which weighed 22 lb) and closed the abdominal cavity. The operation took only 25 minutes and Mrs Crawford recovered to eventually outlive the surgeon who had performed her operation.

The operation of ovariotomy became more accepted as the 19th century progressed, particularly with the development of specific blood vessel clamps by Thomas Spencer Wells (1818–1897), in Hertfordshire (Fig. 2.1). Importantly, however, it was the work of Joseph Lister (1827–1912), who advocated the use of carbolic acid to prevent infection during surgery, and Louis Pasteur (1822–1895), the father of modern bacteriology, who made the process of abdominal surgery significantly safer.

It is probable that the first hysterectomy was performed accidentally, in Milan in 1812, when a GB Poletta, intending to amputate a woman's cervix vaginally, found to his surprise he had removed the entire uterus as well. The patient died 3 days later from peritonitis. He had been assisted by a DB Monteggia, who performed the first deliberate vaginal hysterectomy in 1822. The first abdominal procedure was probably carried out by Charles Clay in 1863 in Great Britain, and abdominal hysterectomy gained popularity for the treatment of large fibroids and for intrapartum transverse lie with arm prolapse. By the last quarter of the 19th century abdominal and vaginal hysterectomies were being performed with equal enthusiasm for fibroids but it was WE Fothergill in Manchester who pioneered prolapse surgery, without hysterectomy, much as the operations are performed today.

Amongst the large number of surgeons who pioneered gynaecological surgery, three warrant particular

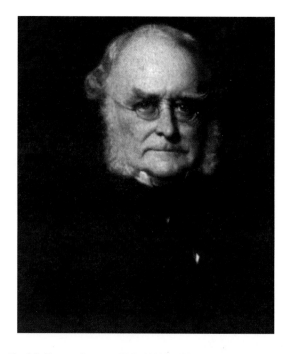

Fig. 2.1 **Thomas Spencer Wells (1818–1897), who developed specific blood vessel clamps.** (Reproduced with permission.)

mention. The first is the American James Marion Sims (1813–1883) who invented the operation of vaginal fistula repair (Fig. 2.2). A key to his success with this operation was in the idea of placing the woman in the prone position, an idea he had had after correcting an acute retroversion in an obese lady who had fallen from a horse. By bending a pewter spoon to an angle of 90° he was able to retract the posterior vaginal wall, and he eventually identified silver wire as the most suitable suture material for the repair. He travelled to New York, London and Paris and met both Spencer Wells (see above) and Sir James Young Simpson (see below).

The second surgeon to mention is Ernst Wertheim (1864–1920), who was born in Austria. Near the end of the 19th century there was no effective cure for carcinoma of the cervix and it was Wertheim's opinion that, although cervical cancer appeared to be a local disease, radical excision was required to obtain any true hope of cure. His operation involved dissection of the ureters throughout their length to enable excision of the parametrium and lymph nodes. Although operating at a time when there were no trained anaesthetists and no blood transfusion, he achieved a remarkably high survival rate and by the time of his death had carried out the operation 1300 times. Marie Curie isolated radium in 1911 and, shortly afterwards, radiation treatment was use for cancer therapies. Wertheim felt that this new treatment affected the role of his own operation which

he believe had 'toppled and collapsed in an instance'. It is now appreciated the Wertheim hysterectomy is superior to radiation treatment for early-stage disease.

William Francis Victor Bonney (1872–1953), an Englishman, is felt by many to have been the greatest operative gynaecological surgeon of all time. He himself carried out more than 500 Wertheim's operations, but also taught the art of conservative surgery including both the removal of fibroids with reconstruction of the uterus, and ovarian cystectomy with reconstruction of the ovary. He designed many of the instruments used in gynaecological surgery today and was also a skilled gastrointestinal and urological surgeon. His beautifully illustrated textbook on gynaecological surgery, with many of the illustrations drawn by himself, is still of relevance today.

More recently, there have been major developments in laparoscopic surgery. Laparoscopy was first used in humans in 1910 when Jacobaeus, from Sweden, used the technique to visualize the viscera in patients with ascites. Following technical developments, including the development of the cold light by Fourestiere in Paris in 1943, intra-abdominal surgery became possible and the operation of female sterilization was described. Much of this pioneering work was by the same Patrick Steptoe of IVF fame mentioned above. It is now possible, though not always appropriate, to perform the most major gynaecological operations laparoscopically.

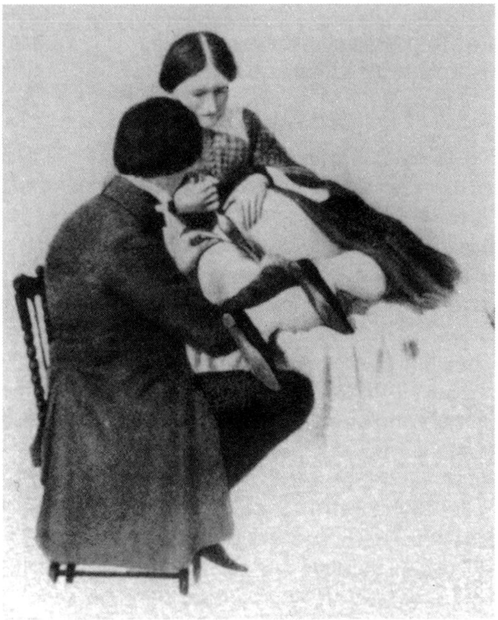

Obstetrics

Obstetrix was the Latin word for midwife. It is thought to derive from *obstare* (to 'stand before'), because the attendant stood in front of the woman to receive the baby. Only in the 20th century did the subject taught in medical schools change its name from 'midwifery' to 'obstetrics', perhaps because a Latin name seemed more academic than the Anglo-Saxon, derived from *mid*, 'with', and *wyf*, 'woman'. The history of obstetrics is inextricably linked with the history of midwifery and indeed the first successful caesarean section in the British Isles was performed by an Irish midwife, Mary Donally, in 1738.

The earliest birth attendants were women and in ancient mythology, goddesses (not gods) were present at deliveries. Prehistoric figures and ancient Egyptian drawings show women giving birth in the sitting or squatting position, and birthing stools and midwives are also mentioned in the Old Testament. The writings of Hippocrates in the fifth century BC include a description of normal birth.

The Renaissance

Soranus of Ephesus (AD 98–138) described antenatal care, labour, and the management of malpresentation by

Fig. 2.2 **James Marion Sims (1813–1883) who invented the operation of vaginal fistula repair.** Seen operating on a vesico-vaginal fistula. (Reproduced with permission.)

internal version and breech extraction. He advised that during labour a woman should be nursed in bed until delivery was imminent, and then moved to the birthing chair, when the midwife would sit opposite her, encouraging her to push, before receiving the baby on to papyrus or cloth.

The first obstetric pamphlets were printed in Latin or in German in the latter part of the 15th century but had little clinical impact. In 1513, however, an obstetric textbook by Eucharius Rosslin, an apothecary from Freiburg, appeared. *Der Schwangern Frauen und Hebamen Rosengarten*, known as 'the Rosengarten', was translated into Dutch in 1516 and reprinted many times in Dutch and German over subsequent decades. In 1532 his son published a Latin translation of the book, which became the forerunner to *De Conceptu et Generatione Hominis*, a Latin text published in 1554 by Jacob Rueff (1500–1558), a surgeon and obstetrician in Zurich. Rueff's practical experience of obstetrics improved Rosslin's original text but the subject matter was similar to that of Soranus. Rueff described toothed forceps for extracting a dead baby (such instruments were already known in Arabia) and recommended internal and external manipulation to achieve footling presentation.

For well over 1000 years, obstetricians had managed obstructed labour by converting the presentation to a footling breech and delivering the baby by traction. Delivery of the aftercoming head, Rueff wrote, could be facilitated by pressure on the maternal abdomen. If this seems crude to us nowadays, we should remember that in the long era before caesarean section the main risk of obstructed labour was death of the mother. The obstetrician would only be summoned once the midwife realized that problems were developing, and often by that stage the baby would be dead. (The stethoscope was not invented until the 19th century, so it was not possible to monitor the fetal condition.)

It has been suggested that the popularity of Rosslin's and Rueff's textbooks led to tension between doctors and midwives because doctors – barred as men from attending normal childbirth – could now learn midwifery from the printed page. If this was the reason for the emergence of the 'man-midwife', it took some time to happen. The immediate effect of the rediscovery of ancient learning seems to have been on the teaching of midwifery. During the 16th century the great French military surgeon Ambroise Pare (1510–1590) founded a school for midwives in Paris. Pare wrote about podalic version and breech extraction and about caesarean section, which he is said to have either performed or supervised not only after the death of the mother but also, at least twice, on living women. One of Pare's pupil midwives went on to attend the French court and one of the babies she delivered – a girl named Henrietta Maria – became Queen of England at the age of 16 when she married King Charles I in 1625.

17th century

It was not until the 17th century that 'accoucheurs' (male midwives) became fashionable in France and in 1663 a surgeon attended a mistress of Louis XIV. The best known of the French accoucheurs was Francois Mauriceau (1637–1709), whose name is familiar to today's obstetricians by reason of the so-called 'Mauriceau–Smellie–Veit manoeuvre' for dealing with the aftercoming head in a breech delivery. This manoeuvre – almost second nature to 20th-century obstetricians – involves turning the baby to face posteriorly and inserting a finger in its mouth to maintain flexion of its head. It had in fact been described several years before Mauriceau's birth by another French accoucheur, Guillemeau (1550–1612). In the tradition of medical giants, Mauriceau reproduced Guillemeau's description without any acknowledgement. Mauriceau had experienced obstetric tragedy on a personal level. His sister suffered an antepartum haemorrhage due to placenta praevia and none of the doctors called to see her dared to attempt treatment, which of course involved internal version and breech extraction. Mauriceau delivered her himself but she died nonetheless.

In 1668 Mauriceau published his celebrated text, *Traité des Maladies des Femmes Grosses*, which was translated into several languages and went through many editions. He was indeed an innovator. He pioneered primary suturing of the perineum after delivery, 'cleansing … with red wine then applying three or four stitches'. He introduced the practice of delivering women in bed rather than on a stool. Nevertheless he remained steadfastly opposed to caesarean section, on the understandable grounds that it was almost invariably fatal to the mother.

'Man-midwifery' reached Britain in the 17th century but remained less fashionable than in France. The most famous practitioners in this country were the Chamberlen family. William Chamberlen, a French Huguenot refugee, had fled to England in 1569 and one of his sons, Peter (1575–1628), moved to London and became surgeon to the Queen, attending the wives of both James I and Charles I in childbirth. Thus Henrietta Maria, herself delivered by a pupil of Ambroise Pare, was attended by another of medicine's immortals. Peter Chamberlen, however, fell out with professional colleagues, including William Harvey, and was arrested in 1612. It was probably Peter who developed the obstetric forceps which famously remained the Chamberlens' family secret for the best part of a century.

Peter's eldest son, also called Peter (1601–1683), became a doctor and in turn his eldest son, Hugh Chamberlen (1630–c.1720) carried on the family tradition. Hugh was a close contemporary of Mauriceau and in fact translated Mauriceau's treatise on midwifery into English. Nevertheless there was some rivalry between the two. Hugh offered the secret of the forceps

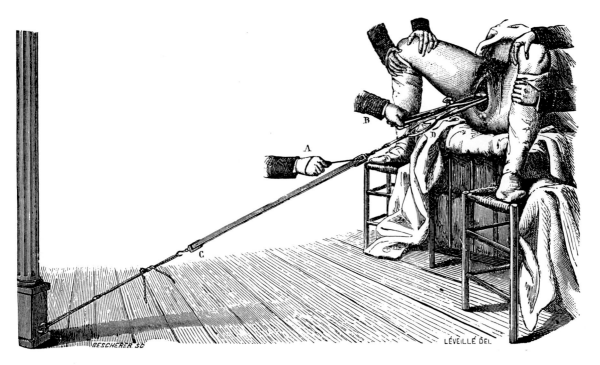

Fig. 2.3 **Delore's method of axis traction using pulleys and cords attached to the axis traction rod handle of Tarnier's forceps.** (Reproduced with permission from the Royal College of Surgeons of England.)

to the French government in 1670 but seems to have finally divulged it to a Dutchman, Roger Roonhuysen, in 1693, after which the forceps monopoly remained with the Roonhuysen family in Amsterdam for another 60 years. During this time, rather inevitably, the secret was slowly leaked. There have been numerous modifications to the original design (Fig. 2.3).

The Chamberlen forceps were designed with a cephalic curve to fit around the baby's head but lacked the pelvic curve characteristic of the modern forceps. As long as they remained a secret, the skills of Chamberlens, who carried out deliveries under a sheet or blanket, must have seemed almost magical. Despite becoming public knowledge, however, the forceps remained controversial. Initially their use was confined to some man-midwives who lived near the Chamberlens in Essex and to a few skilled specialists. Such a specialist was William Smellie (1697–1763), who led the way in establishing obstetrics as an academic discipline in Britain in the 18th century.

18th century

A Scotsman, Smellie was born in Lanarkshire and practised there for some years before enrolling to study medicine at Glasgow University. In 1738 he went to London for training in obstetrics. The first British school of midwifery had been founded in London in 1725 and the first Chair of midwifery in Edinburgh 1 year

later. In 1739 Smellie went to Paris for further obstetric training but, dissatisfied with the teaching there, he returned to London and began giving midwifery courses of his own. His advertisements stated that a 2-year course of lectures cost 20 guineas, and that 'The Men and Women are taught at different hours'.

Among Smellie's contributions were improvements to the forceps. He added the pelvic curve and adopted the 'English lock', which allowed the blades to be inserted separately into the vagina and then brought together. Again, these ideas were occurring to several practitioners around the same time. The 'English lock' may have been discovered by Edmund Chapman, a man-midwife of Essex, after he lost the screw of the Chamberlen forceps in the bedclothes of one of his patients. Smellie was a great teacher, and laid down rules for using the forceps which are remarkably similar to those still taught today. He published his landmark *Treatise on the Theory and Practice of Midwifery* in 1752.

Smellie is famous as 'the master of British midwifery'. His reputation is not merely national and he has been described as one of the most important obstetricians of all times and countries. He was a man of humanity and common sense but was 'sadly lacking in the social graces, and a poor conversationalist'. He was violently opposed by some London midwives, one of whom, Elizabeth Nihell – herself trained at the Hôtel-Dieu in Paris and the author of a *Treatise on the Art of Midwifery* – memorably called him 'a great horse

God-mother of a he-midwife'. Smellie returned to the relative peace and quiet of Lanark in 1759.

By the latter part of the 18th century accoucheurs were fashionable in England. William Hunter (1718–1783) was another Scotsman who graduated from Glasgow University and then studied in Edinburgh before coming to London to join Smellie, who was 21 years his senior. Hunter, the older brother of the famous surgeon John, was more skilled than Smellie in the manners of polite society and at the age of 30 became Surgeon Accoucheur to the Middlesex Hospital. At 44 he was made consultant to Queen Charlotte and at 50 he was elected to the Royal Society. He is perhaps most famous for his *Atlas of the Human Gravid Uterus*.

Hunter exemplifies the development of obstetrics in Britain towards the end of the 18th century. Although he knew about forceps he took pride in using them rarely and commented that his had rust on them. He praised the virtues of conservative management. Nevertheless he was one of the first obstetricians to enter the field of normal labour, which had hitherto been the prerogative of female midwives, and this led inevitably to tension. When Queen Charlotte was delivered in 1762 of the future King George IV, the midwife, Mrs Draper, was inside the room and Hunter was kept outside in case of emergencies. Eventually he persuaded the Queen to be rid of Mrs Draper so that he himself could conduct the delivery.

Not all Royal pregnancies had such a happy outcome. The dangers of leaving things to nature were illustrated by the tragic death in childbirth of Princess Charlotte, George IV's only child. In 1817, at the age of 21, Charlotte went into labour with her first baby, afterwards found to be a boy weighing 9 lb. Labour began more than 2 weeks after the due date and lasted for 50 hours. The baby was stillborn, the placenta was removed with difficulty and 6 hours later Charlotte herself died. Forceps had been kept in readiness but were never used and indeed may not have improved the outcome. Nevertheless the obstetrician, Sir Richard Croft, was widely criticized and shot himself a few days later. King George was left without an heir, and the throne passed first to his brother and then to his niece, who became Queen Victoria.

19th century

At the start of the 19th century childbirth was still dangerous and it remained so, despite several advances, until well into the 20th century. Among the poor, rickets caused pelvic deformities. Maternal death affected all social classes, and across England and Wales 1 in 200 pregnancies ended in the death of the mother. In maternity hospitals, however, the death rate was often much higher than this. 'Lying-in' hospitals had been founded in cities such as London and Dublin in the middle of the 18th century, with trained midwives and

accoucheurs to attend the poor. From an early stage, however, they were subject to frequent epidemics of puerperal fever, during which the maternal death rate might reach between 2 and 8 per 100 deliveries – around 10 times the rate outside hospital.

The contagious nature of puerperal fever had been recognized by Alexander Gordon, years ahead of his time, at the end of the 18th century. Gordon graduated from Aberdeen University in 1775 and served as a naval surgeon before studying midwifery in London and returning to Aberdeen in 1785 as probably the only accoucheur in the city. Aberdeen experienced an epidemic of puerperal fever from 1789–1792, and Gordon published his *Treatise on the Epidemic of Puerperal Fever in Aberdeen* in 1795. He realized that the disease was transmitted from one case to another by doctors and midwives, and that there was a close relationship between puerperal fever and erysipelas (later found to be caused by the streptococcus). Movingly, he wrote: 'It is a disagreeable declaration for me to mention, that I myself was the means of carrying the infection to a great number of women.' Gordon also argued that the disease could be cured by venesection, an opinion that was accepted and widely quoted at the time, unlike his first conclusion, that the disease was contagious, which was ignored until it was rediscovered many years later.

Eventually others reached the same conclusion, including Oliver Wendell Holmes (1809–1894), the American doctor and writer. In Boston in 1843 Holmes read an eloquent paper ('There is no tone deep enough for regret, and no voice loud enough for warning') emphasizing the doctor's role as vector of infection, and proposing that a doctor involved in active obstetrics should never take any active part in post-mortem examination of cases of puerperal fever.

Four years later, his Hungarian contemporary Ignaz Semmelweiss (1818–1865), working in Vienna, was shocked by the death of an admired professor whose finger had been cut during an autopsy on an infected case. Semmelweiss, who was struggling to understand the fearsome death rate in his obstetric unit, concluded that cadaveric material caused infection, and he made his students wash their hands in chlorinated lime between the post-mortem room and the labour ward. Within months during 1847 he reduced deaths in his unit to a level similar to that in the neighbouring midwife-led unit, where staff did not attend post-mortems.

The views of both Holmes and Semmelweiss were initially disbelieved. Semmelweiss, in particular, was ridiculed and he returned to his native Budapest. His monumental book *Die Aetiologie, der Begriff, und die Prophylaxis der Kindbettfiebers*, was finally published in 1861 but, despite his careful observations, was rambling and discursive. Unlike Holmes, he did not live to see the day in 1879 when Louis Pasteur identified the streptococcus as the cause of puerperal fever.

Meanwhile in Britain, 'midwifery' had become a compulsory subject for medical students in 1833 in Scotland and 1866 in England. James Young Simpson (1811–1870) was appointed Professor of Midwifery in Edinburgh in 1840. Simpson refined the obstetric forceps, producing a design that is still in use today, and also experimented with a vacuum extractor. In 1847, the year he was appointed physician to the Queen in Scotland (at the age of 36), he experimented with chloroform. Ether anaesthesia had been discovered in January of that year. Simpson and three friends first inhaled chloroform on 4 November 1847. Four days later he administered it to a patient, a Mrs Carstairs, who was so grateful that she named her baby girl 'Anaesthesia'. He reported the case to the Medico-Chirurgical Society of Edinburgh on 10 November 1847. Three weeks later, at the Society's meeting on 1 December, he was praising chloroform in glowing terms: 'All of us, I most sincerely believe, are called upon to employ it by every principle of true humanity, as well as by every principle of true religion.'

Nonetheless, Simpson met strong opposition from doctors and clergy, who quoted the book of Genesis: 'In sorrow shalt thou bring forth children'. In 1853, however, John Snow administered chloroform to Queen Victoria during the birth of her eighth child. Chloroform became widely accepted in obstetric practice and Simpson became a baronet in 1866, choosing as the inscription on his coat of arms 'Victo dolore' (pain conquered).

Among his many publications, Simpson recognized the contagiousness of puerperal fever almost at the same time as Semmelweiss. He did not, however, recognize the importance of the work of Joseph Lister (1827–1912), who began his experiments on antisepsis while Professor of Surgery in Glasgow in the 1860s. Lister moved to Edinburgh in 1869 and may have been present when the city was brought to a halt by Simpson's funeral in 1870. Listerian antisepsis, which involved the use of a carbolic acid spray, had spectacularly reduced deaths from sepsis in general surgery and was first introduced into obstetrics in 1870 in Basel, Switzerland, by Johann Bischoff, an obstetrician who had visited Lister in Glasgow. Deaths from puerperal fever in Bischoff's hospital fell dramatically. By the 1880s Listerian antisepsis was adopted by most British and American lying-in hospitals, but at the end of that decade modern asepsis was replacing the antiseptic spray.

The developments of asepsis and anaesthesia in the 19th century paved the way for the introduction of caesarean section. The name 'caesarean' is probably derived, not from Julius Caesar, but from the Latin *caedere*, to cut. The Roman law *Lex Caesare* stated that a woman who died in late pregnancy should be delivered soon after her death, and if the baby died they should be buried separately.

Caesarean section

The first caesarean section of modern times is attributed to a Swiss sow-gelder, Jacob Nufer, who in 1500 gained permission from the authorities to operate on his wife after she had been in labour for several days. She subsequently had five successful vaginal deliveries, leading some to doubt the authenticity of the story. After Nufer, the first caesarean sections with survival of the mother were performed in Ireland by Mary Donally in 1738; in England by Dr James Barlow in 1793; and in America by Dr John Richmond in 1827. The 'first' in the British Empire outside the British Isles was performed in South Africa before 1821 by James Miranda Barry, an Edinburgh graduate who masqueraded successfully as a man from 1809 until her death in 1865, though in fact caesarean sections had been performed in Africa by indigenous healers for many years.

All these operations, however, were performed without anaesthesia. In the mid-19th century death rates remained high and caesarean section was often combined with hysterectomy. In the 1880s, with the advent of asepsis, a conservative operation was developed and the 'classical' operation – a vertical incision in the upper part of the uterus – became more frequently used. This incision does not heal well, however, and in 1906 the modern 'lower segment' operation was introduced, a technique which carries less risk of subsequent rupture.

Instrumental delivery

The 20th century also saw developments in the technique of instrumental delivery. Although numerous obstetricians had tried to achieve fame by making minor changes to Simpson's design, almost all forceps required the baby's head to be facing the mother's back and there was no effective way of dealing with deep transverse arrest. In 1916 Christian Kielland, a Norwegian obstetrician, designed 'rotational' forceps for use when the head is in other positions. Use of these forceps safely requires considerable experience, and these skills still complement the use of vacuum extractors today. The modern vacuum extractor (or ventouse) was invented by Tage Malmström of Sweden in the 1950s. It may cause less maternal trauma than forceps but it is less reliable at achieving delivery. It was initially slow to gain acceptance in Britain but eventually became popular in the 1990s.

The obstetric forceps have remained controversial throughout their history, and in the 20th century a major reason was that they were used too readily and sometimes without the necessary skill. At the end of the 19th century and during the first decades of the 20th, obstetrics formed a major part of general practice, and in the interests of efficiency a busy GP would often apply the forceps rather than waiting for a normal delivery.

In response to a plea for conservatism in the *British Medical Journal* of 1906, several GPs wrote attacking elaborate aseptic precautions as unnecessary and normal delivery as impossible for 'civilized' women. One GP wrote: 'I use chloroform and the forceps in every possible case, and have done so for many years.' This epidemic of unnecessary intervention was one of the reasons why the maternal mortality rate in Britain in 1935 was the same as it had been at the beginning of Queen Victoria's reign.

Maternal mortality

Pregnancy has always carried a risk to the mother's life. The Taj Mahal commemorates a queen who died having her twelfth child in 1635. Thomas Jefferson, the US president, lost his wife after a delivery in 1782, Charlotte Bronte died of hyperemesis gravidarum in 1855 and, in 1865, Isabella Maysom ('Mrs Beeton') died at the age of 29 after her fourth delivery. The 19th century maternal mortality rate of 1:200 still applied in the 1930s.

Britain's maternal mortality rate, however, began to fall dramatically in 1935, with the introduction of sulphonamides. Until then, despite asepsis, nothing could be done for women who contracted puerperal fever. John Williams, a respected American obstetrician, commenting on suggested remedies at a meeting in 1925, said: 'If you have a virulent organism and a non-resistant woman, death is the almost universal outcome, no matter what you do, and there is no use deceiving ourselves.' In the 1930s the overall death rate from puerperal fever in Queen Charlotte's Hospital, London, was 25%.

The breakthrough came with the synthesis in Germany of the antibacterial dye Prontosil. This was the result of a systematic search and the theory that a substance active against bacteria might be based on a dye because dyes adhere strongly to organic matter. Gerhardt Domagk (1895–1964), working for the German firm Bayer, tested Prontosil, a sulphonamide, on infected mice with dramatic effect in 1932 and published his results in 1935 after the patents were secure. He was awarded the Nobel Prize for Medicine in 1939, though he did not receive it until 1947.

Supplies of Prontosil reached London in 1936 and were tested on mice by Leonard Colebrook (1883–1967), a graduate of St Mary's Hospital, London, who had initially worked with Alexander Fleming and had begun research on puerperal fever in the 1920s after the wife of a close friend died of the disease. Colebrook then used Prontosil, with some misgivings, on a desperately ill woman in Queen Charlotte's Hospital. 'She was watched at intervals through the night by staff "in the oddest assortment of nightwear". The next morning her temperature had fallen from 104°F to normal.' In the first trial of 38 patients, the mortality was 8%, compared to 26.3% just before the drug was introduced.

Sulphonamides in the form of 'M&B' (manufactured by May and Baker) transformed the treatment of puerperal fever and were followed shortly by penicillin and later by other antibiotics. The effect on the national maternal mortality rate was spectacular and deaths from this cause almost disappeared. Later in fact, in the 3 years 1982–1984, not a single death was recorded from infection after normal delivery, although nowadays a few cases occur each year from this cause.

This success against infection was followed by efforts focused on other causes, such as the introduction of safe blood transfusion and the use of ergometrine and oxytocin for the prevention of postpartum haemorrhage. More recently, improvements in obstetric anaesthesia, including widespread use of epidurals and the exclusion of junior anaesthetic trainees from the labour ward, have reduced anaesthetic deaths to almost zero. Deaths from thromboembolism have been reduced, first by ending the practice of prolonged bed rest after delivery, and more recently by improved thromboprophylaxis for women at high risk. The maternal mortality rate in Britain is now around 1 in 10 000.

In developing countries, however, maternal mortality is still a major problem. In some parts of Africa beyond the reach of obstetric services the maternal mortality rate, even today, is as high as 1%. Across the globe, one woman dies of pregnancy every minute of every day. The causes are sepsis, haemorrhage, hypertensive disease and unsafe abortion – the same causes that were common in Britain 70 years ago.

The safety of the fetus

In the second half of the 20th century attention in the developed world shifted from the mother to the fetus. Two developments allowed this to happen. Fetal monitoring in labour became possible by detecting the fetal electrocardiogram and by sampling fetal scalp blood. These techniques were pioneered by Edward Hon, born in China but working in California, Roberto Caldeyro-Barcia of Montevideo, and Erich Saling of Berlin. Their major papers were published in the early 1960s.

The other, more important, development was obstetric ultrasound, which was developed by Ian Donald, an obstetrician, and Tom Brown, an engineer, working in the Queen Mother's Hospital in Glasgow. Donald (1910–1987) graduated BA from the University of Cape Town and obtained his medical degree from the University of London, moving to the Regius Chair in Glasgow in 1954. Medical ultrasound was developed from the method used to detect submarines during the Second World War, and at first required the pregnant patient to be immersed in a bath of water. Then it was realized that water-soluble jelly transmitted ultrasound waves. Donald and Brown's first paper, with John Macvicar, was published in *The Lancet* in 1958. The next 40 years saw remarkable developments of the technique, which led to the development of the specialty of fetal medicine and went on to transform other medical specialties.

Despite improvements in the safety of late pregnancy for the fetus, childbirth is still about 100 times more dangerous for the baby than for the mother. The UK perinatal mortality rate (the number of stillbirths and early neonatal deaths), having been 7% in 1935, was 0.8% in 1990.

Women in medicine

Medicine has attracted many women, but their entry into medicine has only recently become more straightforward. The Roman historian Hyginus records that the women of Athens – too modest to see male doctors – were fast dying out in childbirth. In 300 BC a young Athenian maiden called Agnodike, wishing to resolve the problem, cut off her hair, dressed up as a man and went to Alexandria where she studied medicine and midwifery under Herophilus, a famous doctor. On her return to Athens, still disguised as a man, she set up a practice and in order to put her reluctant patients at their ease, would lift up her cloak and reveal her true sex. She became so popular among female patients, however, that the male doctors – jealous of her success and eager to protect their profession – had her prosecuted on a charge of corrupting men's wives.

In 1220 the University of Paris introduced statutes to debar women from admission to its medical school and in 1485 the king of France issued a decree withdrawing women's right to work as surgeons. Between 1389 and 1497 in Frankfurt there were 15 licensed women doctors in practice, and in the 15th century German women were presenting theses at medical schools. In Italy some universities disbarred women from attending but the University of Bologna had a female professor of medicine in the 14th century, as well as a woman pathologist.

The first woman to practise medicine in the UK in modern times was Elizabeth Blackwell (1821–1910). Born in Bristol, she emigrated with her family to the United States when she was 11. Her father died 6 years later, leaving a widow and nine children. Elizabeth graduated in New York State in 1849, becoming the first woman doctor in the United States. She went on to La Maternité, Paris and St Bartholomew's Hospital in London and became the first woman on the UK Medical Register in 1859. She became Professor of Gynaecology in the London School of Medicine for Women in 1874.

Elizabeth Garrett (1836–1917), the first woman medical graduate in the UK, graduated in 1865. It is said that when asked why she wanted to be a doctor instead of a nurse like any other woman, she replied: 'I should naturally prefer £1000 to £20 a year.' She was made a visiting physician to the East London Hospital in 1870 and received the degree of MD from the University of Paris.

Until the 1960s most British medical schools imposed a limit on the proportion of female medical students. Nowadays in all British medical schools over 50% of graduates are female. There is evidence that patients of both sexes are more satisfied by consultation with female doctors than with male doctors. Women patients in general prefer women doctors, not only for gynaecological but for other consultations.

Women in obstetrics and gynaecology

Figures from the Royal College of Obstetricians and Gynaecologists show that, in the year 2001, women made up 66% of career senior house officers, 48% of specialist registrars and 22% of consultant obstetricians and gynaecologists in the UK. In 1995 the proportion of women consultants was 12%.

Recent changes

With the safety of childbirth now generally taken for granted in many affluent countries, the main issue for maternity care at present is the quality of the birth experience for the woman and her partner. Services are encouraged to provide choice, including home or hospital delivery, epidurals or waterbirths. With the increased safety of obstetric anaesthesia, a few women are choosing caesarean section and the caesarean section rate is rising in many countries. In Britain it was less than 3% in the 1950s and over 20% in 2000. In Rio de Janeiro it is around 90% and some people fear that this is the future for Britain. In the USA, however, it reached a peak in the 1980s at around 40% (among private patients) before falling to around 25%. Many obstetricians expect the rate in Britain to plateau around 20–25%, with caesarean section replacing difficult vaginal delivery but not easy labour.

What of the future? Over the next decade or two, the most noticeable change in British obstetrics will be the feminization of the specialty. Almost every one of the pioneers named in this brief historical summary has been male. A small number of men have trained to become midwives. The gender difference between the medical and midwifery professions, present since the time of Hippocrates, is about to disappear.

Medical ethics

Introduction

Obstetricians and gynaecologists probably face more ethical dilemmas than most specialists. All doctors occasionally have to decide about problems such as euthanasia, obtaining consent when autonomy is impaired, and truth telling when a bad outcome is foreseen. Only our specialty regularly deals with requests for prenatal diagnosis, abortion, assisted conception and contraception. These are particularly difficult moral problems because of the people and issues involved.

Consider, for example, surrogate motherhood. The commissioning parents, the surrogate parents, the baby, and the other children of both families, all have a direct interest. Treatment may be expensive and matters of life and death and sexuality are involved, leading to public and religious interest. It is hardly surprising that opinions are strongly held and often divided. This chapter indicates some of the ways in which thoughtful people may move forward (Box 3.1).

In the first part of the chapter some of the concepts of moral philosophy will be discussed in general terms. In the second half two real moral dilemmas – surrogacy and abortion – will be discussed in more detail, to provide examples of moral philosophy in practice.

General concepts

Definitions

Philosophy is the critical study of knowledge, in particular that knowledge which we obtain by introspection, rather than by experiment. The Ancient Greeks used the word in a general sense to include all of science as well, but in those days the experimental sciences formed only a tiny part of academic activity. Today we

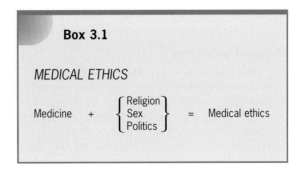

Box 3.1

MEDICAL ETHICS

Medicine   +   { Religion / Sex / Politics }   =   Medical ethics usually exclude mainstream experimental science and most of medical science, leaving only contemplative knowledge for philosophy.

One of the main techniques of philosophy is the use of analogies to clarify our thinking. We may for example try to imagine an analogous situation where we have no personal involvement, or a situation where only one aspect of the problem is varied to see whether it is that aspect which is really affecting our views. We call these exercises thought experiments.

Moral philosophy is the philosophy of right and wrong, good and bad – what ought and ought not to be done. Ethics is another word for the same thing. Medical ethics is the critical analysis of the concepts, beliefs and arguments underlying those medical decisions with a moral component.

There are three possible ways to decide whether an action is right. First by asking if it is legal. This is a very low standard. Many actions such as deceiving your sexual partner about an affair are morally wrong but not illegal. The law restricts itself to public wrongdoing and to rules which are enforceable. Doctors will wish to do better than to simply keep on the right side of the law and they usually follow stricter rules, in the form of a professional ethical code.

We can therefore also judge the rightness of an action by whether it conforms to our professional code. This is a higher standard than the criminal law but still hardly adequate for most of us.

Professional codes often provide little guidance in contentious areas, and ultimately both law and ethical codes derive their authority from people's conclusions about what actions are morally right before God, or their consciences. Moral philosophy helps us think clearly at this level.

Fundamental principles of ethics

All moral authorities provide numerous principles, or rules, for moral guidance, such as Moses' Ten Commandments. Some rules are specifically religious, but the remainder can usually be reduced to the three fundamental principles of autonomy, beneficence and justice. Although other principles could be selected, few people will disagree with these three, and they are a good starting point for newcomers to moral philosophy.

The three rules are as follows:

'Respect autonomy'

The word autonomy means literally 'self-governance'. Individuals act autonomously when they themselves control their thoughts and actions. While we must, where possible, respect the freedom of fully autonomous individuals there is dispute as to how we should treat individuals with reduced autonomy. For example it would be wrong to force adults to undergo moral, or any other, education against their will, even for their own good, but we are happy to force children to go to school.

'Maximize beneficence'

Beneficence means 'the doing of good for others'. It is a particularly important principle for doctors, who have a special obligation to do good, even sometimes acting against their own interests. Difficulties arise not only when the doctor's self-interest conflicts with doing good, but also when the doctor and patient disagree about what is good. If antibiotics will cure a sore throat and the patient wants to take them, the correct course is clear. However, if the doctor believes that they will do more harm than good but the patient still wants them, should the doctor maximize beneficence by refusing to prescribe, or respect autonomy and hand them over?

'Act justly'

While we may all think we know how to act justly, there is much philosophical debate about the principles of justice. This is reflected in the mainstream political debate between 'right' and 'left' in society. Two extreme definitions of justice emphasize fairness and entitlement respectively. Socialists tend to argue that a system of resource allocation is just if the results are fair. Fairness need not of course mean equality. The most prominent modern philosopher in this area is John Rawls of Harvard, who uses the thought experiment of 'deciding from behind a veil of ignorance' (see Box 3.2). We will

---

Box 3.2

DECIDING FROM BEHIND A VEIL OF IGNORANCE (JOHN RAWLS)

Imagine a community of, for example, men and women, intellectuals and dunces, athletes and weaklings, doctors, bank clerks and coal miners, deciding how to allocate its resources. The members should ask themselves what system they would choose as if they did not know to what class they would belong. They would not select an unjust system because they would not know whether they would be the beneficiaries or victims of it. Rawls argues that people behind this veil of ignorance would choose to maximize the welfare of the least well-off group, and only permit inequalities which benefited that group. This method is supposed to provide philosophical support, for example, for the justice of redistributive taxation.

see later, in the abortion decision, that modification of the veil of ignorance can be a powerful tool for moral decision-making.

Libertarians, on the other hand, usually argue that, while it would be nice to do away with inequalities, it is unjust to take something from its rightful owner. They claim that we should decide whether someone is entitled to own something – a seashell for example – not by enquiring how many seashells everyone else has, but rather by asking how the seashell came to be owned in the first place.

If the answer is that it was picked up on the seashore where it belonged to no one and where there were plenty left, or that someone else picked it up and freely sold or gave it on, the ownership is just. Rightful ownership is defined by how it came about historically, not by how much other people may have. The most prominent modern philosopher supporting this view is Robert Nozick, also of Harvard (Box 3.3).

What if these principles conflict?

Often there is a conflict between the principles, autonomy, beneficence and justice, and one or other must take precedence. The various philosophical and religious codes and systems which have been advanced to resolve these difficulties fall into two main classes: consequentialist and deontological.

Consequentialist systems are those that judge morality by results. They are sometimes parodied by the phrase: 'the end justifies the means'. The most developed consequentialist system of ethics is utilitarianism. In its classical form a single scale of utility is recognized, with happiness at one end and suffering at the other. All outcomes can in theory be placed on this scale and we should select the course of action which maximizes utility.

There are many complications. For example, different utilitarians have argued that we should aim to maximize total utility, average utility or the utility of the least well-off individual. In a further refinement, Rawls (see above) aims to maximize the utility of the least well-off group of people.

The principles of autonomy and justice are incorporated by sophisticated utilitarians, who argue (1) that happiness is not simply pleasure but rather the satisfaction of autonomous preferences, and (2) that the widespread concern with fairness results in just actions being the only ones which also maximize utility.

The problems of how to measure utility or happiness are considerable, but in principle solvable, by looking at how much people will pay to have or avoid a certain outcome, or how they will choose between bets.

Deontological arguments Although most religious systems of ethics are deontological the word comes from the Greek *deon*, duty, not from the Latin *deus*, god. A deontological argument is one which claims to contain its own justification within itself without reference to its consequences.

Most religions have moral codes, such as the Ten Commandments, which we are to obey without reference to the consequences, and which are justified by their supposed divine origin. Arguments of the form that people have an absolute right not to be killed, that women have a right to do what they like with their own bodies, or that we must always tell the truth are, unless justified by consequentialist arguments, also deontological.

The most famous non-religious deontological theory is the supreme moral law which Immanuel Kant believed that all rational agents must recognize. Kant formulated his principle in different ways: 'Act only on that maxim that you can at the same time will should be a universal moral law' and 'No person should be treated merely as a means, but always also as an end in themselves'. The first formulation is more familiar to us from Jesus' Sermon on the Mount: 'Do unto others as you would they do unto you'. It is sometimes called 'The Golden Rule' or the principle of 'universalizability' and is recognized by many as an important component of utilitarianism. Nevertheless, utilitarians would not accept that people cannot be used as a means to an end, if the end is important or valuable enough.

In Box 3.3, Nozick argues deontologically that we have a duty to respect property, while in Box 3.2, Rawls (although he will not admit it) is a utilitarian who judges justice by its results.

Box 3.3

IF AN INEQUALITY ARISES JUSTLY CAN IT EVER BE UNJUST? (ROBERT NOZICK)

Consider a community of 1000 people each with £100 disposable cash. One of them is Wilt Chamberlain, a star basketball player. Each of the other 999 people voluntarily spends £10 to watch him play and he ends up with £10 000 while the others sink into poverty with £90 each.

If the initial distribution was just, is the present distribution just? What if the inequality had resulted from everyone gambling £10, and one person winning £10 000? If we believe that the unequal distributions are unjust and devise a system of reallocation (taxation?) we are also restricting freedom to exploit talents or to gamble.

Some other principles

'Primum non nocere'

'Above all do no harm'. This commonly heard phrase seems to imply that doctors have a primary duty to avoid harm, and that it takes precedence over doing good. While it is obviously true that in general we should avoid harm, a moment's thought will show that we cannot make 'avoiding harm' take precedence over 'doing good'. Vaccination, surgery and most drug treatments cause, or at least risk, some harm for the sake of greater benefit. The principle may have some limited scope, if it is argued that doctors only have a duty to do good for their patients, but have a duty not to do harm to everyone. The avoidance of harm thus has a wider scope than doing good, but it does not follow that it should necessarily take precedence when the two principles conflict.

The 'acts and omissions' doctrine

Though shalt not kill but needs't not strive
Officiously to keep alive.

Clough

Clough's couplet was written as a satirical description of doctors' behaviour, but is sometimes elevated to the status of a moral principle by doctors who believe there is a moral difference between actively killing, and passively allowing a person to die. The distinction has never stood up to close examination, and philosophers are constantly trying to steer doctors away from it.

First, the distinction is often merely semantic and it is not difficult to rephrase an active killing in such a way as to make it an omission. For example a patient on a ventilator may be actively killed by switching off the ventilator, or passively killed by failing to re-plug it in after temporarily unplugging it to change the fuse. The former is an act, the latter an omission – but where is the moral difference?

The idea of a moral difference between acts and omissions often seems attractive because most examples of active killing with which we are familiar are morally wrong, or at least bad acts which it would be better had they not occurred – such as murder, accidents and killing in war. In contrast most examples of 'letting die' are perpetrated by good doctors with the best intentions and good consequences – such as letting pneumonia be the 'old man's friend', or not operating to close a large neural tube defect in a neonate. The difference, however, is not in the act or the omission, but in the morally relevant facts of the case, such as whether the victim wanted to die, whether the intent was to relieve suffering or gain an inheritance, etc. (Box 3.4).

The double standard that most doctors have about active and passive euthanasia may have adverse consequences. A decision not to treat a patient may be made by a single doctor acting alone who may not be in full possession of all the facts and may have bad motives. Far from a rapid pain-free death, withholding treatment may cause continued suffering and a delayed and slow death. In contrast we demand considerable safeguards against error or bad intent before active killing, and if we permit it, ensure that the result is rapid, pain-free and certain. It is not so obvious why active killing is regarded by most doctors with such horror.

The doctrine of 'double effect'

This was first articulated by Thomas Aquinas and has been developed in great detail by Roman Catholic theologians to describe circumstances where it is morally permissible to cause evil in the pursuit of good. A classic example of its use is by Catholic doctors who are opposed to abortion, but nevertheless justify operating to remove an ectopic pregnancy. Non-Catholics may feel it has little relevance to them, but they should be aware of it.

The principle in its full form states that an action with both good and bad effects is permissible if:

1. the action is good in itself
2. the intention is solely to produce the good effect
3. the good effect is not produced through the bad effect
4. there is sufficient reason to permit the bad effect.

The last of these conditions is uncontroversial but the other three cause difficulties:

- The first would prevent telling lies to achieve a good end.
- The second seems to be self-deceiving if not actually hypocritical. If we know that a bad result will follow from our action, how can we honestly say that we do not intend it?

> **Box 3.4**
>
> ### ACTS AND OMISSIONS
>
> A man stands to gain a large inheritance if his baby brother dies. One day he enters the boy's bathroom with the intent of drowning him and making it look like an accident. As he enters, the little boy slips on the soap, bangs his head, slips unconscious under the water, and drowns. The older brother only has to put out his hand to save him, but instead stands by to ensure that he really is dead, and then leaves the room. Is the omission to save him morally any different from the intended act of drowning him?

- The third condition seems to rule out amputation for tumour where the good aim of saving the patient is achieved through the bad effect of removing the limb.

Nevertheless the doctrine does remind us that intent is morally important. If we intended good, and bad resulted, we are morally less culpable than if we actually intended to cause the same harm.

'Slippery slopes'

It is frequently claimed that we should not do a certain action because we would, by so doing, place ourselves on a 'slippery slope' and in future be unable to restrain ourselves from another action which is clearly morally wrong. For example, some people argue that a law which allows abortion for so-called 'serious' indications such as rape, risk to the mother's life, or severe fetal abnormality, puts doctors on a slippery slope that makes it difficult for them to resist doing abortions for apparently less 'serious' reasons such as unplanned pregnancy.

The argument is superficially attractive but, like the doctrine of 'double effect', it is less convincing when examined closely. If it means anything, it means that an action (A) that is morally right can be made wrong simply because there is some other action (B) that is morally wrong – and we are afraid that if we perform action A we may be unable to restrain ourselves from doing action B. We are to believe that on a scale of superficially similar actions where one end of the scale is 'morally right' and the other end 'morally wrong' we should draw the line not where right actions become wrong, but at some point further towards the 'right' end. We will thus do some wrongs by omitting to do some right actions.

The argument is nonsense if we can decide for other reasons where the line should actually be drawn. It is usually used simply as a debating point by people who wish to discredit an opponent's argument by allying it to a more extreme position. As philosophers we should beware of such tricks.

'Natural law'

An instinctive reaction to many reproductive technologies is: 'It's unnatural and therefore it's wrong'. The Roman Catholic prohibition on artificial contraception rests heavily on the argument that 'natural' intercourse is associated with a chance of conception and artificial contraception by breaking this link is wrong. It is hard for doctors to use this argument because their whole profession is dedicated to interfering with 'Nature'.

It is also incorrect to apply 'natural law' to contraception. The majority of acts of coitus in primitive or 'natural' societies are not fertile because of the contraceptive effects of breast-feeding. Many evolutionary biologists believe that the high sexuality of *Homo sapiens*

has evolved not simply because it maximizes the chance of conception but that it maintains pair bonds which are important because of the prolonged development of human children.

Specific examples

In this part we provide two practical examples of philosophical argument on a medical dilemma. The first, surrogacy, is fairly easy, but the second is perhaps the most difficult and contentious dilemma in moral philosophy – abortion.

Surrogacy

There are two types of surrogate parenthood:

- 'Full surrogacy' is the term used when an infertile couple (the commissioning parents) provide their own sperm and ovum to be fertilized in vitro and transferred to the surrogate mother who carries the baby to maturity and hands it over after delivery.
- 'Partial surrogacy' is more common, and describes the situation where the surrogate's own egg is used and she conceives as a result of artificial insemination by the commissioning father. The baby that the surrogate carries is genetically hers but she plans to hand it over at delivery.

Is a doctor morally justified in assisting at partial surrogacy?

One way to proceed is to list all the individuals involved and then to ask ourselves whether for each of them the doctor who helps with surrogacy is maximizing beneficence, respecting autonomy and acting justly. Using a crude shorthand one result of such thinking is shown in Table 3.1.

It is good for the resulting fetus that the surrogacy takes place since otherwise it would never exist. Even if it is in some way disturbing to be a surrogate child it is surely better than to never have existed. It must be little worse than being adopted or poor, for example, and even most severely handicapped people are glad to have existed.

If the various other people in Table 3.1 are dealt with in turn it soon becomes clear that the only people significantly wronged by surrogacy are members of disadvantaged groups who may feel discriminated against. This type of argument has led us and most philosophers to argue for the permissibility of surrogacy. The case against it is likely to rest on arguments from 'natural law', or on hypothetical harms which may result.

Abortion

Most people learn at a very young age that killing humans is wrong, and if they consider the matter at all,

Table 3.1
The ethics of surrogacy

	Autonomy	Beneficence	Justice
The surrogate mother	+	+ or −	+
Her partner	+	+ or −	+
The commissioning mother	+	+	+
Her partner	++	+	+
The surrogate baby	++	+	+
The existing children of the surrogate mother	0	−	0
The existing children of the commissioning parents	0	+ or −	0
The doctor(s)	+	+	+
Other people in society especially the poor	0	0	0 or −

+   The provision of surrogacy follows this principle
−   The provision of surrogacy will break this principle
0   The provision of surrogacy is neutral with regard to this principle
+ or −   The effect of providing surrogacy on this principle is either unclear or disputed

they feel that killing an unborn fetus is particularly wrong, because the child is both innocent and defence-less. Nevertheless, most societies tolerate abortion. Since only a minority of these women undergo more than one abortion, it has been estimated that in Britain at least 1 in 3 of the cohort of women entering puberty today will have an abortion during their lifetime.

The case against abortion

This can be stated as follows:

Proposition 1:   Killing innocent people is wrong.
Proposition 2:   The fetus is a person.
Therefore: The fetus should not be killed, and abortion is wrong.

BUT

Proposition 3:   People should be allowed to do as they like with their own bodies.
Proposition 4:   The mother is a person.
Therefore: The mother should be allowed to empty her uterus and have the abortion.

BUT

Proposition 5:   Where one person's right not to be unjustly killed conflicts with another person's right to do as she wishes with her own body, the right not to be unjustly killed take precedence.
Therefore: Abortion is wrong.

The case for abortion

There are three main lines of argument that claim to justify abortion. These are based on 'personhood', 'women's rights' and 'the Golden Rule'.

'Personhood' arguments

Although the fetus is a member of the species *Homo sapiens*, it is claimed that it is not a 'person' in the sense of an individual who may not be unjustly killed. A utilitarian would argue that the reason it is wrong to kill people is that they are conscious, they value their lives, and they would be deprived of their valuable future life by being killed.

However, the fetus is different from adult humans in morally important ways. It is neither conscious nor self-aware, and is deprived of nothing which it values by being killed. It therefore fails this test of 'personhood' and can be killed.

The importance of species   This argument can be buttressed by 'thought experiments', drawing analogies with other beings behaviourally similar to or even more developed than fetuses, such as some animals. If we are justified in killing animals for the relatively trivial reasons of preferring to eat meat or wear leather shoes, or for sport, why should we not kill fetuses for the more serious reasons of preventing the birth of a handicapped child or not forcing a woman to bear an unwanted pregnancy?

To permit the killing of animals but not fetuses would involve discrimination according to an arbitrary morally irrelevant criterion – membership of a species. Some philosophers have coined the word 'speciesism', analogous to 'racism' and 'sexism', for this sort of discrimination. A consequence of using the 'person' definition above is that killing higher animals such as gorillas and dolphins would also be wrong, if we believed that they were self-aware and valued their lives.

Many people have difficulties with this kind of argument since in the world as we know it, only one species, *Homo sapiens*, is a serious contender for 'personhood'. The arbitrariness of defining personhood as membership of the human species, is not immediately obvious.

Philosophers, however, have offered a number of thought experiments to draw attention to the problem. Imagine that one day we meet creatures from outer space. How should we decide whether to have them for dinner in one sense or the other? Most of us would use behaviour, rather than membership of our species, or appeal to divine revelation, to decide, especially if we remember that the alien may also be deciding whether it is morally permissible to eat us. Similar decisions may one day have to be made about computers that behave intelligently and apparently value their existence.

The difference between fetus and neonate The above line of reasoning appears to lead to the counterintuitive conclusion that not only may fetuses be killed but so also may newborn babies and the mentally handicapped, who also fail this test of personhood. Some philosophers have gone so far as to argue that infanticide is indeed sometimes permissible, although its side-effects, such as the offence caused to other persons, mean that it would rarely be permitted in practice. On this view the personhood of a newborn infant is a social construct which society does not choose to bestow on unborn fetuses.

There have been societies, such as the Spartans, whose members withheld personhood from newborns, and there are other societies – those which do not permit abortion – who bestow it on unborn fetuses. The arbitrary nature of such a social construct is disquieting to many, but it is surely no more arbitrary than membership of a species, or the possession of a soul indicated by religious revelation.

'Women's rights' arguments

The other point at which pro-abortionists engage the pro-life lobby is at Proposition 5. They argue that even if the fetus is to be regarded as a person who may not normally be unjustly killed, the mother should not be forced to carry it for 9 months against her will. It may be kind of her to do so, but she should be allowed to escape the burden. We do not expect people to give even a pint of blood against their will to save other people's lives.

This line of argument has been put most forcefully by the American philosopher Judith Jarvis Thompson in a famous thought experiment. She drew an analogy with forcing someone to give aid to a paradigm person, in her example a famous violinist. The analogy was with pregnancy resulting from rape, but it can easily be modified to include other cases of unwanted pregnancy (see Box 3.5).

Thompson's intuition and that of many women (and men) is that, while it would be kind of you to stay connected, strong personal reasons such as career and family needs would justify disconnection. Moreover, disconnection would still be justified if your behaviour had to some extent led to your kidnap. For example, you might have been well aware that the music lovers

---

Box 3.5

'THE FAMOUS VIOLINIST'

Imagine that a world-famous violinist develops a fatal kidney disease. He will die unless he is connected to the circulation of another person, but the disease is self-limiting, and after 9 months he will recover to full health. Unfortunately, he has a rare blood group and no-one with that group is willing to be connected. A group of music lovers search the world for a suitable person, and find you. You may not agree to their proposal, so they kidnap, anaesthetize and connect you to the violinist's circulation. When you wake up they explain what has happened; you are outraged and demand to be disconnected. They remind you that you only need to stay connected for 9 months and that without you the violinist will die. Must you remain connected?

---

were searching for a person to kidnap, but nevertheless persisted in going home by a secluded route because you wanted the pleasure of viewing the sunset. By analogy, taking sexual pleasure does not commit you to bearing the unwanted pregnancies which occasionally result. Anyone who wishes to understand the strength of feeling of a woman bearing an unwanted pregnancy should read Thompson's forceful paper.

This argument is strongly disputed. Many individuals maintain that their intuitions are different from Thompson's; you should remain connected, and (by analogy) the rape victim should bear the child. Moreover, neither 'women's rights' nor 'personhood' arguments carry much force with the parents of an abnormal child who want a baby but are considering abortion because of the handicap. They do not see the fetus as a 'non-person' who can be killed like an animal, and they want to bear a baby. Why do they want the abortion and how can they justify it?

'Golden Rule' arguments

Both the above arguments have rested heavily on deontological claims, either that the fetus does or does not have a fundamental right not to be unjustly killed, or that a woman has fundamental rights to do as she likes with her own body.

Even pro-abortionists usually recognize that abortion is a problem, not just because of things intrinsic to the fetus at the time the abortion is done (for reasons given above), but because of the potential of the fetus to become a human person. This 'potentiality' argument is usually dismissed on two grounds. Firstly, we do not normally treat things according to their potential state, but rather according to their actual state. I cannot treat you as if you were dead although you are inevitably going to be in that state one day. More seriously, it is imagined that acceptance of the 'potentiality' argument would commit us to treating sperms and eggs as potential people, and maximizing fertility at all costs.

This need not always be the case if we are utilitarians. Although it is not clear whether utility is maximized by permitting or forbidding abortion in general, a consensus may be possible for fetal handicap. The argument is based on the Golden Rule and makes use of a variation on the veil of ignorance (Box 3.6).

Box 3.6

ABORTION AND THE GOLDEN RULE

'We should do as we are glad was done to us.'

If we are glad that we were not aborted, we should not abort the fetus. If there were only one fetus/potential person to consider, that would be the end of the matter and abortion would be wrong. However, if we take 'potentiality' seriously, there is not just the fetus of this present pregnancy to consider, but also all the other potential babies which this mother may have if her present pregnancy is ended. These other future people may later be glad that the abortion took place.

Consider a woman carrying an abnormal fetus who plans a particular family size. There are two potential people to consider – the abnormal fetus and the 'replacement' fetus which will exist only if the abortion is done. The abnormal fetus would wish that the abortion does not happen. However, the replacement fetus will wish the opposite, that the abortion is done. We can resolve the conflict by our thought experiment, by asking what we would choose if we were forced to live through both potential people's lives. If we chose no abortion, we would have one handicapped life and one non-life (the replacement fetus will not be conceived because its mother will be busy caring for her handicapped child). If we chose the abortion, we would have one non-life (the abortion) and one healthy life (that of the replacement fetus). Surely, even from this 'potential person' perspective, we would choose that the abortion takes place. Consistency, and the Golden Rule, indicate that we should act as we would wish done to ourselves, and choose the abortion.

The argument from the Golden Rule has good philosophical reasons to support it. It appeals to a principle, with which anyone can agree, rather than to intuitions which often conflict. Those of us who wonder if our intuitions are indeed correct can use this principle against which to test them.

At a practical level it captures the feelings of parents of a handicapped fetus much better than the 'personhood' and 'women's rights' arguments. They love and want to bear their baby, and if they kill it they will grieve severely. They will frequently say that they are acting in the child's interest to avoid a life of suffering.

If the abnormality is relatively mild, outside observers who consider only the present abnormal child, may find the parents' attitude hard to accept, since the child is still likely to have a life of more value than no life at all. Only a few abnormalities are so severe that it can be confidently said that no life would be better than an, albeit imperfect, affected life.

However, parents usually see clearly the choice between the perfect child of their dreams, which they will still probably bear if they undergo the abortion, and the handicapped child they are carrying. If both these potential people are considered, it is not difficult to support the abortion even from the fetus's perspective.

Key points

- Ethical principles can be considered in three main rules: autonomy (respecting the freedom of individuals), beneficence (the doing of good for others) and justice (acting fairly).

- If these principles conflict, difficulties can be resolved using 'consequentialist' arguments (the end justifies the means) or deontological arguments (which claim to contain their own justification without reference to their consequences).

- Other important principles are 'primum non nocere' (above all do no harm), the 'acts and omissions' doctrine which proposes that there is a difference between actively killing and passively allowing to die, and the doctrine of 'double effect' where it may be permissible to cause evil in the pursuit of good.

4

Clinical genetics and molecular biology

The origin of life

The time between the formation of the earth 4500 million years ago and the point where there appeared to have been a huge increase in the diversity of animals around 500 million years ago is termed the Precambrian. To speak of 'the Precambrian' as a single unified time period is misleading, for it makes up roughly seven-eighths of the Earth's 4500 million year history and it contains the most important events in biological history. The Earth formed, the first tectonic plates developed, the atmosphere became enriched in oxygen and life began.

The oldest fossils known, nearly 3500 million years old, come from the Precambrian and are fossils of bacteria-like organisms. These organisms were pro-karyotes, single-celled organisms that lack a membrane-bound nucleus and usually lack membrane-bound organelles (like mitochondria or chloroplasts). Eukaryotes appeared later. These more complex cells have a membrane-bound nucleus and, although very diverse, still share fundamental characteristics of cellular organization, biochemistry, and molecular biology. The eukaryotes were able to cluster together to form larger organisms – all animals, plants, fungi, and protists.

There must have been a point when there was no life and then another point when there was life. There must have been a first earthly life form, which gave rise to daughter organisms who in turn further divided and so forth until there were huge numbers of life forms which were then able to evolve into different species. All these organisms must have originated from one initial organism, a sort of biological equivalent of the universe's highly compressed primordial state at the time of the big bang. This first hypothetical organism has been called LUCA, the last universal common ancestor.

Chains of nucleic acids probably joined at random, forming a chemical with the property of replication. These chains became contained within structures which they used for transport, the earliest 'organisms' – LUCA. In reality, LUCA was either a bacteria- or protozoa-like organism, probably living deep under-ground in hot igneous rocks, and there was probably a huge dynamic colony of these short-lived organisms rather than one specific individual. It is from this 'society' of organisms that we are descended, and it is from these early nucleic acid chains that our own genome is derived.

The sequence of the human genome, the complete set of human genes, was first published in 2001 after a highly charged competition between a public project (The International Human Sequencing Consortium) and a private company (Celera Genomics). The gene sequence is not a list of ordered instructions put together in a logical manner but a relatively random jumble of DNA sequences surrounded by masses of junk DNA. Some sections are repeated over and over again for no obvious reason and there are numerous other 'parasitic' segments of DNA 'hitching' a free ride. There are also sequences that code for something quite specific but are switched off and inactivated. The genome lacks any logical order because, instead of being designed in a logical way, it has evolved over perhaps 50 billion copyings.

There appear to be about 26 000–31 000 protein-coding genes in the human genome compared with 6000 for a yeast cell, 13 000 for a fly, 18 000 for a worm and 26 000 for a plant. Indeed only 94 of 1278 protein families in our genome appear to be specific to vertebrates. We have barely begun to realize the potential of this new information for both good and, much more importantly, for harm. To understand the role of this DNA, and its implication for inherited disease, it is necessary to examine the structure of genes more closely.

Genes and DNA

A gene is a hereditary factor that can be passed from parents to their offspring. Clinical genetics is the study of such factors and the diseases that they cause. We now know that human genes consist of deoxyribonucleic acid (DNA). This is a long-chain molecule made up of four different nucleotide bases: adenine, thymine, guanine and cytosine (ATGC for short). Each three-base sequence (a codon) corresponds to a particular amino acid, so that a series of bases code for a polypeptide or a protein, with either a structural or enzymatic role. At the molecular level, genes consist of the sequence of DNA that acts as the unit controlling the formation of a single peptide or protein. Some DNA sequences control protein synthesis, some provide the amino acid sequence and, as noted above, some appear inactive.

Chromosomes

DNA is packaged in the cell nucleus in large units called chromosomes and, at certain stages of the cell cycle, these chromosomes can be visible under the light microscope. The number varies between species, but the human has 46: 22 pairs of similar chromosomes (autosomes) which do not vary between the sexes, and two sex chromosomes which do. The two chromosomes in a pair are called homologous chromosomes. They carry the same genes in the same order, but are inherited

from different parents. Females carry two X chromosomes, and males one X and a smaller Y chromosome. The karyotype is the chromosomal complement of an individual. It is conventionally written as the total number of chromosomes followed by a list of the sex chromosomes. The normal male karyotype is thus 46XY and the normal female 46XX.

During somatic growth, cells divide by a process of mitosis which involves initially doubling the number of chromosomes so that, after division, each cell inherits a full complement, exactly the same as the parent cell. In contrast, gametes (sperm and eggs) are produced by the process of meiosis, which involves two cell divisions, but only one chromosome duplication. This means that the final gamete contains only one chromosome from each homologous pair. At fertilization the full complement is restored.

An important process occurs during meiosis 1, the first meiotic cell division. After doubling into two sister chromatids during interphase each chromosome pairs with its homologue. A crossover (chiasma) forms between two of the four homologous chromatids resulting in the exchange of a variable amount of chromosomal material and a corresponding shifting of genes from each chromosome to its homologue.

Abnormalities in chromosome number

Problems in meiosis or fertilization may result in a range of abnormal chromosome complements. For example an additional set of chromosomes, polyploidy, usually results from the fertilization of one egg by two sperm. A triploid conceptus will have the karyotype 69XXX, 69XXY or 69XYY, and such pregnancies usually miscarry spontaneously. If the pregnancy persists into the second trimester the fetus will typically be severely growth restricted, with multiple congenital abnormalities, and the placenta may show cystic changes typical of a hydatidiform mole (p. 285).

Aneuploidy

Aneuploidy is the addition or absence of a single chromosome (autosome or sex chromosome). Among live-borns the commonest aneuploidies are trisomy (one extra) of the autosomes 13, 18 or 21, and a range of extra or missing sex chromosomes. Trisomy 21 (Down's syndrome) is the most common aneuploidy in live-borns, affecting approximately 1 in 600 births. Affected individuals usually have a range of physical abnormalities and severe mental handicap, but often survive into adulthood (p. 341). Trisomy 13 (Patau's syndrome) and trisomy 18 (Edward's syndrome) are usually associated with multiple congenital abnormalities, and death in the new-born period (p. 342).

A missing chromosome is called monosomy. Only monosomy X (45X or Turner's syndrome) is compatible with viability. Monosomy X is one of the sex chromosome aneuploidies and others include 47XXX, 47XXY, and 47XYY. Affected individuals may have genital abnormalities and reduced fertility but generally have little or no mental retardation, or other serious phenotypic abnormalities.

Pregnancies with other types of aneuploidy usually miscarry spontaneously, typically in the first trimester, and about half of first trimester miscarriages are thought to occur for this reason. Monosomy X is the most common single chromosome abnormality found in those miscarriages which are analysed. Live births of 45X fetuses amount to only a few per cent of the 45X conceptions that occur, whereas trisomy 21 fetuses, in contrast, usually survive to delivery with only about one-third miscarrying spontaneously.

Causes of aneuploidy

Aneuploidy is usually caused by meiotic non-dysjunction in the egg rather than in the sperm, and is more common with advancing maternal age. Mono-somy X is an exception. It is usually caused by mitotic loss of a paternal sex chromosome post-fertilization, is not affected by maternal age, and may even be more common in younger women.

Mosaicism

If non-dysjunction occurs during mitosis of a normal zygote, or if some cells from a trisomic zygote lose the extra chromosome early in development, a fetus may develop with both a normal and abnormal cell lines. This is mosaicism. It occurs in about 2% of Down's syndrome fetuses and in a variable proportion of those with Turner's syndrome. In general the clinical abnormalities of mosaic fetuses are less severe than those of the full abnormality. Some aneuploidies (e.g. trisomy 8) are lethal in the pure form and only occur among live-borns as mosaics.

Other abnormalities

A marker chromosome is an extra piece of chromosome material of unidentified origin. Usually the marker consists of inactive DNA, or it is balanced by a corresponding missing piece of chromosomal material elsewhere, such that the individual is phenotypically normal. Occasionally there is trisomy of a piece of active DNA, and mental or physical abnormalities occur.

Structural chromosome abnormalities

Chromosome breaks and abnormal DNA repair cause a range of structural abnormalities which may cause problems directly, or be passed on down the germ cell line and cause later imbalances during meiosis. These include deletions, insertions, inversions, duplications, and translocations. Translocations may be reciprocal or Robertsonian. Reciprocal translocations occur when a piece of one chromosome has become separated and is attached to another chromosome. If the chromosome from which the extra piece came is missing the corresponding piece, the total quantity of chromosomal material is unchanged and the translocation is said to be balanced. If, however, there is extra material on one chromosome with no balancing missing piece on another, the individual will be trisomic for the translocated piece. Similarly, if a piece is missing without a balancing extra piece elsewhere, the individual will be monosomic for the missing piece. Such unbalanced translocations are usually associated with mental or physical abnormality.

Robertsonian translocations involve the acrocentric chromosomes 13, 14, 15, 21 or 22. The inactive short arms of the involved chromosomes are lost and the long arms become joined at the centromere. A carrier of a Robertsonian translocation only has 45 chromosomes, but the total quantity of active genetic material is unchanged, and the phenotype is normal. The most important Robertsonian translocation is that between chromosome 14 and 21. A female with such a transloca-tion has a 45XX t(14:21) karyotype. The possible out-comes for her offspring depend on the chromosomal complement that is passed to the egg during meiosis. For simplicity we assume the offspring are female.

1. If she passes only her normal 14 and 21 chromosomes into the egg the resulting fetus will have a normal karyotype.
2. If she passes on only the double translocated chromosome the fetus would carry the same balanced translocation as her.
3. If she passes on the double (14:21) chromosome as well as a normal 21 chromosome, the karyotype after fertilization will be 46XX +21 t(14:21), and the baby will be affected with Down's syndrome.
4. Similarly if she passes on the double (14:21) chromosome as well as the normal 14 chromosome the fetus will have trisomy 14. Such pregnancies usually miscarry.
5. If she passes on an egg with the missing 14 or 21 chromosome, not balanced by the extra translocated chromosome, the offspring will be monosomic for 14 or 21 respectively. Such pregnancies also usually miscarry.

Although the risk of any one egg receiving each of the possible chromosome complements is approximately equal, the risk of having a live-born baby with Down's syndrome depends also on the relative chance of such eggs being fertilized, and on the risk of spontaneous miscarriage with each translocation. The risk of un-balanced outcome is lower if the father carries the translocation, presumably because unbalanced sperm have reduced fertilizing ability. The risk of Down's

Fundamentals

syndrome for a mother with a balanced 14:21 transloca-tion is about 10%, but it is only about 2% if the father carries the same translocation. For other translocations special tables of risks may be consulted.

Balanced rearrangements such as a translocation do not usually matter, since the total chromosome complement is unchanged. However, rearrangements occurring for the first time in a family (de novo) are sometimes an exception. In about 5% of such cases a piece of chromosome is lost when the rearrangement first occurs. This may not be detectable under the microscope, but if it involves any genes, as it usually will, it will probably cause mental handicap or physical abnormality. If apparently balanced rearrangements are detected in a fetus by prenatal testing, the first step in investigation is to check the parental karyotype. If a parent carries the same balanced rearrangement the fetus is not at increased risk of phenotypic abnormality. If neither parent has the rearrangement the risk of abnormality in the child is about 5%.

Single gene abnormalities

In general genes consist of a piece of DNA coding for a single protein. An example is the gene for cystic fibrosis, located near the middle of the long arm of chromosome 7. The particular site of a gene on the chromosome is called the locus of the gene. Since all normal individuals carry two versions of each homologous chromosome they also carry two copies of each gene. Alternative forms of a gene are called alleles. The terms gene and allele are sometimes used interchangeably although usually only one is correct. Most genes can exist in more than two alleles, but within one individual there can only be two alleles, since there are only two copies of the gene. The cystic fibrosis gene exists as a normal allele, and as a large number of abnormal alleles, each caused by a different mutation of the bases making up the gene. The commonest mutation of the cystic fibrosis gene is a deletion of three bases which should code for a phenylalanine amino acid at position 508 in the CF protein. This mutation or abnormal allele is called delta F508 (delta for deletion, F for phenylalanine!). This mutation accounts for 70% of abnormal CF mutations worldwide, although this varies between 50–85% in different populations. All other CF mutations are com-paratively rare, for example the G542X mutation which accounts for about 4% of mutations in Scotland. Over 400 abnormal CF mutations have been described.

The genotype is the allelic composition of the individ-ual, and the phenotype is what is actually seen. A pheno-type is said to be dominant if it is expressed when the individual has only one copy of the corresponding allele, and recessive if it is only expressed when the individual has two copies of the allele. Cystic fibrosis is a recessive phenotype. The genotypes and phenotypes for cystic fibrosis are shown in Table 4.1. The genotype is said

Table 4.1
Genotypes and corresponding phenotypes for a recessive condition, cystic fibrosis

Genotype	Phenotype
N/N (two copies of the normal allele)	Unaffected by CF
N/F508 (one normal allele and one CF F508 allele)	Unaffected by CF
F508/F508 (two copies of the CF F508 allele)	Affected by CF
F508/G542X (one copy each of two different CF mutations)*	Affected by CF

* Note that different mutation combinations can cause the same disease. However, sometimes different mutation combinations are associated with more or less severe phenotypes.

to be heterozygous if the individual carries two different alleles and homozygous if it carries two identical ones.

An example of a dominant phenotype is Huntington's disease. This is a rare neurodegenerative disorder causing choreiform (jerky) movements, dementia and death in young and middle-aged adults (mean age of onset 38). The gene is located near the tip of the short arm of chromosome 4. The phenotype is dominant because it appears if individuals carry only one copy of the abnormal HD allele (Table 4.2).

A special situation applies to the phenotypes of genes located on the X chromosome. An example is Duchenne muscular dystrophy (DMD). Women who possess an abnormal dystrophin gene usually also possess a normal one on their other X chromosome, and are therefore not affected by the disease. However, half their children will inherit the abnormal gene. Since boys have only one X chromosome, those boys who inherit the abnormal gene will not have a corresponding normal one, and will be affected. They usually die in childhood without having children. Sons who inherit the normal DMD allele will not be affected and will not pass on the disease. Daughters who inherit the abnormal allele will also inherit a normal allele from their fathers and will be unaffected by the disease. However, they will pass on the abnormal allele to half their sons who will be affected, and half their daughters who will be carriers. This pattern of inheritance is called X-linked or sex-linked inheritance (Table 4.3).

Table 4.2
Genotypes and corresponding phenotypes for a dominant condition, Huntington's disease

Genotype	Phenotype
N/N (two copies of the normal allele)	Unaffected by Huntington's disease
N/HD (one normal allele and one HD allele)	Affected

Table 4.3
Genotypes and corresponding phenotypes for an X-linked condition, Duchenne muscular dystrophy

Genotype	Phenotype
Normal X/normal X	Unaffected female
Normal X/Y	Unaffected male
DMD X/normal X	Unaffected carrier female
DMD X/Y	Affected male

Pedigrees

Geneticists need to know the interrelationships of individuals, and this is documented by drawing a pedigree, or family tree. The symbols used are fairly standard (Fig. 4.1). Often the mode of inheritance of a phenotype can be inferred from the pedigree. Figure 4.2 is an example of a large pedigree from a family carrying an allele for a dominant phenotype, familial hypercholesterolaemia. Dominant inheritance has the following features:

- All affected individuals have at least one affected parent.
- Males and females are affected in about equal numbers.
- Both males and females transmit the trait.
- Matings of heterozygous affected individuals with unaffected individuals produce approximately $^1/_2$ affected, and $^1/_2$ unaffected, offspring.

Figure 4.3 is a pedigree from a recessive phenotype, cystic fibrosis. Recessive inheritance has the following features:

- Most affected individuals have two unaffected parents.
- The trait is expressed in both sexes and transmitted by either sex to both male and female offspring in approximately equal numbers.
- Matings between unaffected heterozygotes yield about $^3/_4$ unaffected offspring and $^1/_4$ affected offspring.

Figure 4.4 is a pedigree for an X-linked phenotype, Duchenne muscular dystrophy. X-linked inheritance has the following features:

- Many more males than females are affected.
- Father-to-son transmission is never seen.
- Among the sons of carrier mothers about half are affected and half unaffected.
- All the daughters of a mating between a carrier mother and an unaffected male will be unaffected, but about half will be carriers.

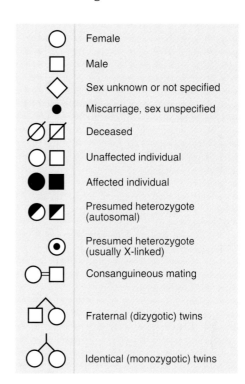

Fig. 4.1 **Some of the symbols used for drawing pedigrees.**

Figure 4.5 shows another X-linked pedigree, that of some of the descendants of Queen Victoria. The affected individuals had haemophilia. The X-linkage can be inferred from the excess of males, lack of father-to-son transmission and the existence of unaffected carrier females.

There are a large number of inherited human phenotypes. Nearly 2000 have been proven to be autosomal dominant, over 600 autosomal recessive and about 150 X-linked (Box 4.1). Table 4.4 lists some of the common

---

Box 4.1

A RULE OF THUMB FOR DECIDING IF A DISORDER IS LIKELY TO BE RECESSIVE OR DOMINANT

Almost all disorders caused by enzyme deficiencies are recessive. Most disorders caused by defects in non-enzymatic (i.e. structural) proteins are inherited as dominants. The reason seems to be that although heterozygotes make only half as much of the normal gene product as homozygous unaffected individuals, this is usually enough to get the job done in the case of enzyme reactions. However, in the case of structural proteins the abnormal gene product often actively interferes with normal cell function.

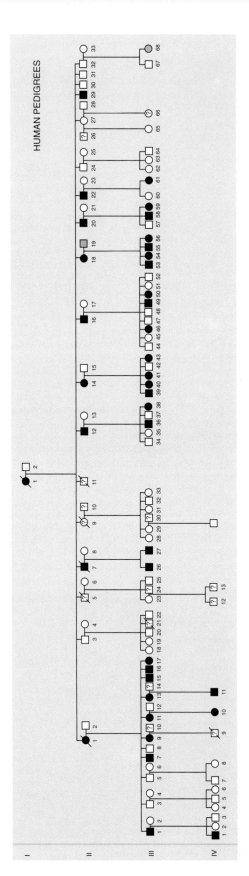

HUMAN PEDIGREES

Fig. 4.2 **An example of an autosomal dominant phenotype.** A large pedigree of familial hypercholesterolaemia.

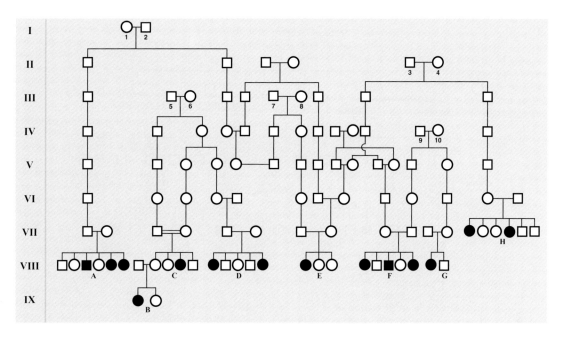

Fig. 4.3 **An example of an autosomal recessive phenotype.** A large pedigree of cystic fibrosis.

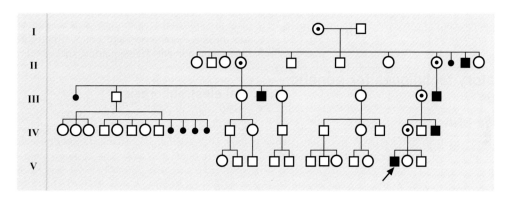

Fig. 4.4 **An example of an X-linked phenotype in which affected males do not reproduce.** A large pedigree of Duchenne muscular dystrophy.

Table 4.4
Some autosomal dominant phenotypes and the chromosomal locations of their genes

Name	Description	Site
Hereditary angioneurotic oedema	Allergy-caused itching and swelling	11p
Malignant hyperpyrexia	Abnormal response to anaesthesia	19q
Marfan's syndrome	Tall, loose joints, eye and heart defects	15q
Myotonic dystrophy	Difficulty in relaxing contracted muscles, muscle wasting, cataracts, mental retardation	19q
Neurofibromatosis	Multiple tumours of peripheral and central nervous system	17q
Retinoblastoma	Tumours of the retina of the eye and predisposition to bone cancer	13q

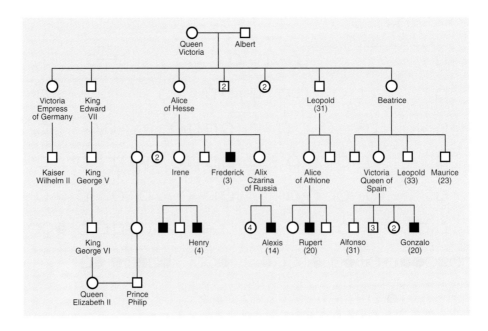

Fig. 4.5 **A famous family affected with an X-linked condition, haemophilia.**

autosomal dominant phenotypes and their locations, Table 4.5 some common recessive ones and Table 4.6 some that are X-linked.

Laboratory techniques for genetic analysis

Obtaining DNA

It is relatively easy to extract DNA from any tissue containing nucleated cells, because it is remarkably resistant to breakdown by heat, trauma or chemicals. You just mince the tissue up, add a detergent to break up the cell membranes, and remove the proteins with an organic solvent. The remaining sticky stuff is DNA.

Gel electrophoresis

DNA molecules are negatively charged and will move towards the positive pole of a gel electrophoresis apparatus. They can then be visualized by adding a fluorescent dye that binds to DNA. The distance each molecule

Table 4.5
Some autosomal recessive phenotypes and the chromosomal locations of their genes

Name	Description	Site
Albinism	Absence of melanin in eyes, hair and skin	11q
Alpha$_1$-antitrypsin deficiency	Lack of protease inhibitor causing lung and liver disease	14q
Cystic fibrosis	Chest infections and malabsorption	7q
Friedreich's ataxia	Cerebellar degeneration	9q
Alpha thalassaemia	Defects in alpha chain of haemoglobin, variable anaemia	16p
Phenylketonuria	Mental deterioration	12q
Sickle cell disease	Anaemia, liver, bone and spleen damage	11p
Beta thalassaemia	Defects in beta chain of haemoglobin, anaemia, bone, liver and spleen damage	11p
Tay–Sachs disease	Developmental retardation, paralysis and early death	15q
Wilson's disease	Defects in copper metabolism, liver damage	13q

Table 4.6
Some X-linked phenotypes and the chromosomal location of their genes

Name	Description	Site
Colour blindness	Colour blindness	Xq
Duchenne muscular dystrophy	Muscle damage and death in teens	Xp
G6PD deficiency (favism)	Haemolytic anaemia caused by certain drugs	Xq
Haemophilia	Abnormal haemostasis	Xq
Lesch–Nyhan syndrome	Defect in purine metabolism, mental retardation, cerebral palsy, self-mutilation	Xq
Ornithine transcarboxylase (OTC) deficiency	Excess ammonia in blood, mental deterioration	Xp
Testicular feminization (androgen insensitivity)	XY individuals with testes, female external genitalia, normal breasts and blind vagina	Xq
X-linked mental retardation with fragile site	Mental retardation, large testes, ears and jaw	Xq

travels is inversely proportional to its size. By adding DNA of known size to one channel of the gel, it is possible to measure the size of the pieces of DNA in a particular preparation. DNA tends to wash off electrophoresis gel, so for further analysis it is usually transferred onto special nitrocellulose paper to which it sticks firmly. This process is called Southern blotting.

Electrophoresis of whole DNA molecules is not very revealing. We learn more by first digesting the DNA with one or more restriction enzymes. These are enzymes that cut DNA at specific points. Sometimes a mutation of an important gene is associated with the presence or absence of a particular restriction site. If so, the mutation can be detected simply by looking for the particular restriction site. An example is sickle cell disease, which is caused by a single point mutation in the beta-globin gene. The mutation consists of a substitution of A for T in the sixth codon of the gene. This changes the codon from CTC coding for glutamic acid, to CAC which codes for valine. The sequence, including the adjacent codons, changes from GGA<u>CTC</u>CTC to GGA<u>CAC</u>CTC. The restriction enzyme MstII cuts DNA at sequences GGACTCC. It will thus cut the normal sequence but not the mutated sequence. If DNA from a homozygous sickle cell sufferer is digested with MstII and separated by gel electrophoresis, a fragment will be produced which is 1.35 kb rather than the normal 1.15 kb fragment. A heterozygote will produce one 1.15 kb and one 1.35 kb fragment. To put it another way the sickle cell mutation causes loss of an MstII cleavage site.

Recombination

Many other DNA analysis procedures make use of the phenomenon of recombination. DNA is double stranded, with each base on one strand paired with the opposite one on the other, according to the scheme A–T and C–G. This makes one strand complementary to the other. If double-stranded DNA is heated the two strands will separate, but when later cooled they will recombine correctly. If a piece of DNA corresponding to a known gene, sometimes loosely called a 'gene probe', is incubated with a DNA sample, it will hybridize with the sample DNA so long as it can find its complementary sequence. By labelling the gene probe with a radioactive or fluorescent marker the gene can be identified in a DNA electrophoresis band. Abnormal genes can also be located in histological or cytological preparations by this technique which is known as 'in situ hybridization'.

Gene linkage

Imagine two genes, say one for blue or brown eyes, and one for straight or curly hair. If they were on different chromosomes there would be no relationship between the inheritance of either phenotype. It would be random whether a particular eye colour allele, and particular hair curliness allele, went into the same or different gametes. Similarly if the genes were far apart on the same chromosome there would be no relationship between their inheritance, because a crossover would often occur between them. However, if they were close together on the same chromosome they would tend to be inherited together. This is linkage. Imagine that brown eyes and curly hair were dominant, and one parent, say the father, had single copies of both alleles. If he passed on the brown eye allele to a child he would almost certainly pass on the curly hair allele as well. If a child was born with brown eyes we could predict that it would also have curly hair. Note that the inheritance of brown eyes and curly hair together would only apply to that particular family. In other families brown eyes might be inherited with straight hair. Establishing which alleles are inherited together in a particular family is establishing the phase of the linkage.

Occasionally a crossover occurs even between genes that are close together. On that occasion the alleles will not be inherited together. By studying many individuals within a family and large numbers of families, and recording how often this occurs it is possible to measure the degree of linkage between genes. This is related to the physical distance between the genes.

The eye colour and hair curliness example is imaginary. A real example is colour blindness and haemophilia, the genes for which lie close to each other on the X chromosome. In those rare families which have individuals with colour blindness and haemophilia, the two conditions will tend to be inherited together, or inherited separately, depending on the phase in the family.

There are too few obvious phenotypic features linked to important disease genes to be of any clinical use in diagnosis. However, there are many silent mutations in non-coding regions of DNA some of which cause a change in restriction enzyme site. These are called restriction fragment polymorphisms. If they are linked to an important gene they are called restriction fragment linked polymorphisms (RFLPs). In the same way as we could use the presence of brown eyes to predict inheritance of the curly hair gene, we can use the presence of a linked polymorphism to predict inheritance of a particular allele of the linked gene. Note that we must first know the phase of the polymorphism/mutation in that particular family. This usually means that we must test some affected family members. Linkage analysis is no use for population screening.

The polymerase chain reaction

No assay technique is sufficiently sensitive to detect a single copy of any abnormal DNA sequence directly, and typically many thousands of copies are required before a labelled probe will be detectable. The polymerase chain reaction (PCR) enables the production of sufficient DNA from the very smallest piece of DNA using the enzyme DNA polymerase. This enzyme copies DNA. Two short polynucleotide sequences (primers) are used to trick the enzyme into only copying the region of DNA between the primers. By repeating the copying process over many PCR cycles, large quantities of the sequence between the primers are synthesized. Identifying and making primer sequences either side of interesting pieces of DNA is now a multimillion-dollar business.

PCR has many uses. If only small quantities of fetal DNA are available from a chorionic villus or amniocentesis sample, there is no longer a need to culture the cells before analysis. Instead PCR is used to amplify the gene to be tested. Viral and bacterial infections can often be detected without culture by amplifying their gene sequences. Experimentally, it is now possible to amplify DNA obtained from biopsy of human embryos, fertilized in vitro, for pre-implantation diagnosis, and to amplify fetal DNA present in the maternal circulation, for non-invasive prenatal diagnosis.

DNA fingerprinting

Some regions of DNA appear to have no function and differ widely between people. Within these regions, certain sequences of DNA are repeated in tandem and the number of these repetitive sequences varies between individuals, giving them their name – variable number tandem repeats (VNTRs). By cutting DNA with restriction enzymes, the resulting fragments will vary in size between individuals. If these are separated on a gel and identified with probes that hybridize to the VNTRs, a pattern of bands will appear. There is sufficient variation in the population to make the chance of two individuals (apart from identical twins) having the same pattern, extremely small. This has many uses in forensic medicine. It is also useful for paternity testing, and in prenatal diagnosis, for ensuring that a supposed fetal sample is not maternal. For example a chorionic villus sample might indicate that the fetus was female and a carrier for cystic fibrosis, the same as the mother. Such a result is compatible with maternal contamination. We can confirm the fetal origin of the sample by DNA fingerprinting.

Key points

- A gene is a hereditary factor that can be passed from parents to their offspring. Clinical genetics is the study of such factors and the diseases that they cause.

- Aneuploidy is the addition or absence of a single chromosome, e.g. trisomy (one extra, like trisomy 13, 18 or 21), or monosomy (one less, like monosomy X). Triploidy is the presence of an extra complete haploid chromosomal set.

- Chromosome breaks and abnormal DNA repair may lead to deletions, insertions, inversions, duplications and translocations. These may cause problems directly, or be passed on down the germ cell line and cause later imbalances during meiosis.

- Single gene abnormalities account for a huge number of (often) rare disorders. Those inherited in an autosomal dominant fashion are usually compatible with survival to adulthood and include Huntington's disease, hereditary angioneurotic oedema, Marfan's syndrome, myotonic dystrophy and neurofibromatosis. Autosomal recessive disorders, such as cystic fibrosis, phenylketonuria and Tay–Sachs disease, not uncommonly present in childhood and may not be compatible with survival to reproductive age. The phenotypes of X-linked (or sex-linked) disorders, such as Duchenne muscular dystrophy, are much more severe in male offspring, with women acting as asymptomatic carriers.

Applications of statistics

Introduction

The science of statistics involves the collection, organization, analysis and interpretation of data. We use statistics to learn from experience. The elements of the subject are well covered in basic textbooks and are not repeated here. Instead we deal in this chapter with two particular problems:

1. the everyday difficulties of interpreting clinical tests, and
2. the more fundamental problem of identifying effective treatment from among all the possible interventions.

The latter problem has recently been eased for obstetricians because the best-quality research (that based on randomized controlled trials) has been collected, analysed systematically and regularly updated by a special unit in Oxford, UK, the National Perinatal Epidemiology Unit. Other groups are doing the same for gynaecology. The process is called meta-analysis. This textbook leans heavily on these formal analyses and the techniques are briefly described in this chapter.

Tests and their interpretation

What is a test?

Much of clinical medicine is concerned with prediction. After making a prediction, we can apply an effective treatment – if there is one. When we first meet a patient we are rarely if ever certain what the outcome will be and we have to carry out tests. A 'test' in the context of this chapter is any item of information that can help us. It includes items from the history, and observations from the clinical examination, as well as such things as laboratory blood tests and X-ray examinations.

Unfortunately tests are rarely perfect: some people with a positive result will not have the disease, and conversely some with a negative result will have it. This is why interpretation may be difficult.

Gold standards

Before we can describe how good a test is, we need to decide what outcome we wish it to predict. Ideally we would like there to be some outcome measure with which everyone can agree – a 'gold standard'. Examples might include:

- perinatal death
- multiple pregnancy
- Down's syndrome
- open neural tube defect.

Such diagnoses are unambiguous (although they may take some time to find out) and we can say for certain whether the test predicted the outcome correctly.

In practice, however, 'gold standards' are rare. Most tests have to be evaluated for their prediction of less important endpoints, such as low birth weight corrected for gestational age, or low Apgar scores. If our test is only validated against such less important endpoints, we must always remember that these are not what we are really interested in. We do not know for certain the relationship between these less important outcomes and the 'gold standards'.

Nevertheless, we will begin with gold standards, and consider first a test that is either positive or negative, and an outcome that is unambiguously present or absent. Tests are applied to populations, and for obstetricians the population is often pregnant women. Let us imagine 100 antenatal patients facing a test that is designed to predict whether the baby will live or die, and which can be either positive or negative. If we apply the test to all 100 women and then wait to see what happens, we might get a result like that illustrated in Figure 5.1.

This is the information that a scientist will have after completing research on a test. It is often called a two-by-two table. We can use such a table both to see how well the test performs, and to see what the risk of bad outcome is for an individual with a particular result.

Test performance

By counting vertically in Figure 5.1 we can see what proportion of the babies who did die (gold standard positive) were detected by the test (Fig. 5.2). This is the sensitivity or true positive rate (TPR). For this hypothetical test it is 90%. We can also see how many of the babies that lived were correctly predicted by the test (Fig. 5.3). This is the specificity or true negative rate (TNR) and for our hypothetical test it is 80%.

These test characteristics do not vary with the prevalence of the disease and are thus a stable measure of test performance. However, they do vary with the cut-off value at which we call a test 'positive' or 'negative'. We will look at both these effects below, but first let us look at the results in another way, to predict an individual patient's risk.

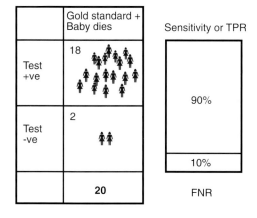

Fig. 5.2 **Sensitivity.** TPR, true positive rate; FNR, false negative rate.

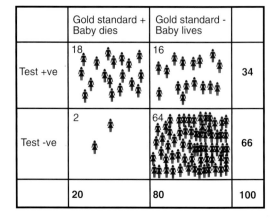

Fig. 5.1 **An imaginary test carried out on 100 antenatal patients designed to predict whether the baby will live or die.**

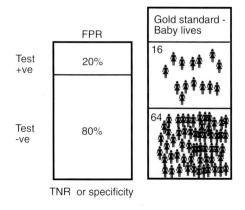

Fig. 5.3 **Specificity.** FPR, false positive rate; TNR, true negative rate.

Predicting an individual patient's risk

Sensitivity (TPR) and specificity (TNR) describe to the scientist how well the test works, but they are not much use to the doctor who knows the test result (positive or negative) and wants to know how likely it is that the patient has the disease – or, in our example, that the baby will die. To estimate this we read Figure 5.1 horizontally rather than vertically.

First let us look at all the women with a positive result (Fig. 5.4). 18 of the 34 babies actually died, so the predictive value of a positive result is 18/34 or 53%. Note that the positive predictive value is *not* the same as the sensitivity (TPR), which we have already noted was 90%.

Of those who had a negative test (Fig. 5.5), 64 out of 66 babies eventually survived. The predictive value of a negative result is thus 64/66 or 97%. Again this is *not* the same as the specificity (TNR). We will see later that the predictive value of a test varies with the prevalence of the disease.

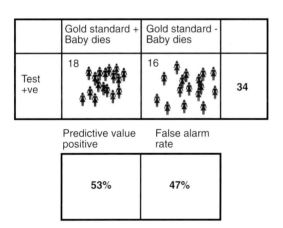

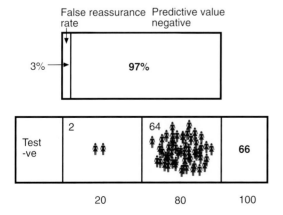

Fig. 5.4 **Positive predictive value.**

Fig. 5.5 **Negative predictive value.**

The effect of varying the test cut-off point

So far we have been discussing 'dichotomous' tests, i.e. tests that are simply either positive or negative. Most tests, however, give a range of results from strongly positive to strongly negative. Examples would include simple measures like haemoglobin concentration, or complicated measures like the fetal umbilical artery blood velocity.

Let us imagine that our test gives a result between 0 and 100. Figure 5.6 shows the distribution of results for patients with and without disease, i.e. gold standard positive and negative. If we take a cut-off value of 40, and call higher values 'positive' and lower 'negative', we get the same test characteristics as before.

Imagine what would happen if we varied the cut-off. The performance rates would change (Fig. 5.7). We could, for example, move the cut-off value right up to 75 so that all the results were negative. The false negative and true negative rates would then both be 100%. If we moved the cut-off down to a value of 5 so that all the results were called positive, the true and false positives would both be 100%.

To see what is happening we can plot how the true and false positive rates vary with the cut-off level (Fig. 5.8). We call the result a receiver operator characteristic or ROC curve (Box 5.1).

A perfect test and a useless test

It is instructive to compare the ROC curves for perfect and useless tests since both can achieve either high sensitivity or high specificity but only the 'perfect' test can do both at the same time. Typical results and the ROC curve for a perfect test are shown in Figure 5.9 and for a useless test in Figure 5.10.

It is meaningless to say that a test has a particular sensitivity without also giving the specificity. Ideally both sensitivity and specificity should be given for a range of cut-offs so that the test can be used in different ways for different indications.

Box 5.1

RECEIVER OPERATOR CHARACTERISTIC

This term comes from the early radar operators in England in the Second World War. These operators realized that if they made their receiving sets very sensitive they picked up all the incoming enemy aeroplanes, but also had a high false-positive rate from flocks of birds. If they turned the sensitivity down they got rid of the false positives due to birds, but also missed some incoming planes.

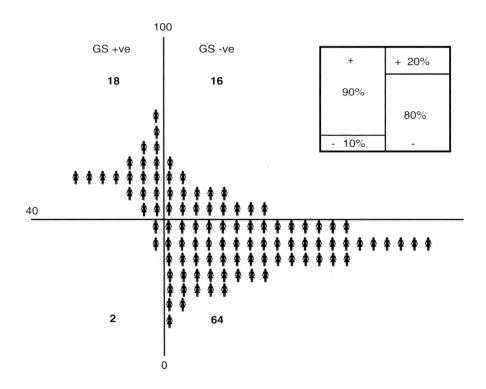

Fig. 5.6 **'Gold standard' (GS) positive and negative.**

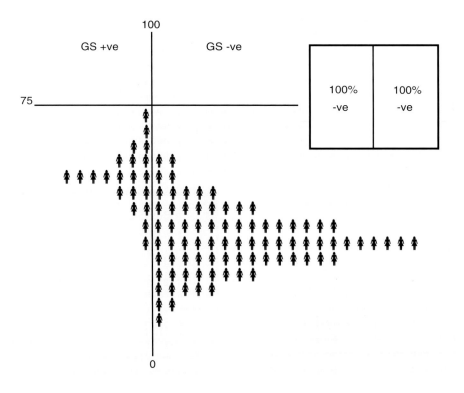

Fig. 5.7 **Varying the cut-off.** GS, gold standard.

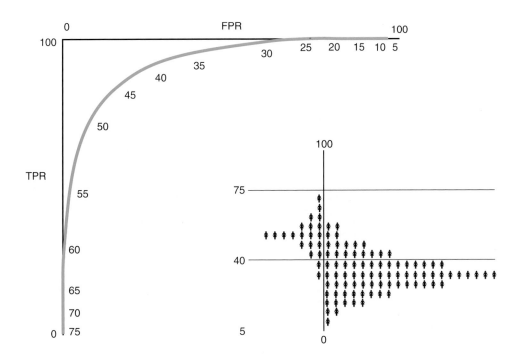

Fig. 5.8 **Receiver operator characteristic (or ROC) curve.** FPR, false positive rate; TPR true positive rate.

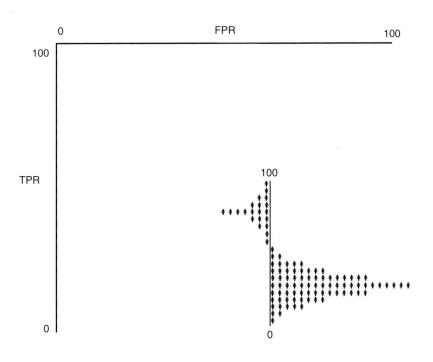

Fig. 5.9 **A perfect test.** FPR, false positive rate; TPR true positive rate.

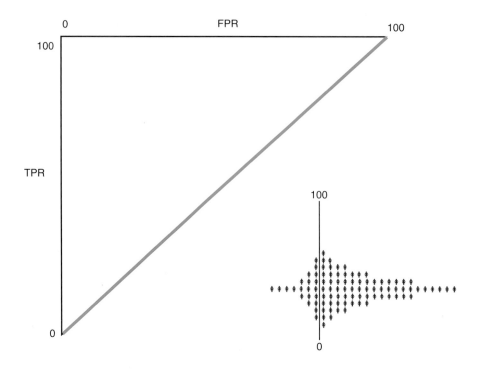

Fig. 5.10   **A useless test.** FPR, false positive rate; TPR true positive rate.

The influence of disease prevalence

We can see what happens if the disease prevalence is halved, simply by adding another 100 gold standard negatives to our original two-by-two table. The result is shown in Figure 5.11. All the new cases survived so they have been added to the right-hand column. Since the specificity of the test is 80%, 20 will show up as false positives and 80 will be true negatives.

The prevalence is now halved from 20 in 100, to 20 in 200. The sensitivity (TPR) is still 90% and the specificity (TNR) is unchanged at 80%. However, the predictive value of a positive result (PVP) has dropped from 18/34 (53%) to 18/54 (33%). The predictive value of a negative test has risen from 64/66 (97%) to 144/146 (98.5%). This is important. The predictive value of a test result varies with the disease prevalence. As clinicians often say, 'Common things are common.'

Bayes' theorem and likelihood ratios

Calculating the predictive value of a test result from the two-by-two table, as we did above, is only possible if the patient in front of you comes from a population with the same disease prevalence as that of the patients on whom the test was originally developed. This is often not the case. Tests are frequently developed on high-risk patients in teaching hospitals, and then applied to patients in a low-risk practice. Occasionally the reverse may happen, if we apply a test to someone we already know to be at particularly high risk.

Doctors need a way of calculating the predictive value of a test from the information that they are likely to have available, namely the prevalence of the disease and the test characteristics. It can be done. We will change all our rates to odds for the following section since this makes the mathematics easier. Remember a risk of 1 in 4 is the same as odds of 1 : 3. A risk of 90% is the same as odds of 90 : 10 or 9 : 1.

Let us return now to our original 2 × 2 table redrawn to show the crucial information (Fig. 5.12). The top row gives us the information we need – the predictive value positive. With a positive test the odds of having the disease are 18 : 16 or 9 : 8 (or slightly better than evens). The disease prevalence gives us the odds before the test result, i.e. 20 : 80 or 1 : 4. We call these the prior odds. What we need from the test is a single measure, the diagnostic value, that changes the prior odds of 1 : 4 to posterior odds of 9 : 8.

The answer is the ratio between the true-positive rate (90%) and the false-positive rate (20%). This is called the likelihood ratio of a positive result (LR +ve) because it is the ratio between the likelihood of having a positive result if the disease is present, and the likelihood of having a positive result if the disease is absent. The LR +ve for this test is thus 9 : 2. The relationship between these three figures is:

Prior odds	×	Likelihood ratio	=	Posterior odds
1 : 4	×	9 : 2	=	9 : 8

	Gold standard + Baby dies	Gold standard - Baby lives	
Test +ve	18	16	**34**
Test -ve	2	64	**66**
	20	**80**	**100**

PVP
53%

Prevalence 20/100
20%

	Gold standard + Baby dies	Gold standard - Baby lives	
Test +ve	18	36	**54**
Test -ve	2	144	**146**
	20	**180**	**200**

PVP
33%

Prevalence 20/200
10%

Fig. 5.11 **The positive predictive value falls with lower disease prevalence.** PVP, predictive value of a positive result.

	Gold standard + Baby dies	Gold standard - Baby lives	
Test +ve	18	16	**34**
Test -ve	2	64	**66**
	20	**80**	**100**

TPR 90%   FPR 20%

	Gold standard + Baby dies	Gold standard - Baby lives	
Test +ve	9	8	
Test -ve			
	1	4	

9   2

Prior odds X LR = Posterior odds
1/4 X 9/2 = 9/8

1:4 Prior odds
9:8 Posterior odds
9:2 Likelihood ratio

Fig. 5.12 **Prior odds × Likelihood ratio = Posterior odds.** FPR, false positive rate; TPR true positive rate.

Box 5.2

BAYES AND PREGNANCY TESTS: THE BAYESIAN'S WIFE

My wife felt pregnant but had a negative pregnancy test. Her doctor told her that 10% of pregnant women had a negative result on first testing but she was still disappointed. I calculated the probabilities as follows. I asked her how sure she had been that she was pregnant before the test and she said 95% certain. This gave prior odds of pregnancy of 19 : 1 which I rounded to 20 : 1. I assumed that the false positive rate was virtually nil so I got a LR for a negative test of 1 : 10 (likelihood of a negative result given pregnancy = 10% : likelihood of negative result given no pregnancy = 100%). This gave posterior odds that she was in fact pregnant of 20 : 1 × 1 : 10 = 2 : 1 and I converted this for her benefit into a probability of two in three. This estimate cheered her up and a couple of weeks later the pregnancy was confirmed.

This is one of the most famous theorems in statistics, named the Bayes theorem after its author, the Reverend Thomas Bayes. It comes in a number of different versions but this one, the odds-likelihood ratio form, is the most useful for doctors.

A dichotomous test (one that is either positive or negative) will have two likelihood ratios, one for a positive result and one for a negative result. If the test has a range of results the LR will vary also with the cut-off point chosen. It is possible to plot ROC curves as likelihood ratios. If the doctor knows the LR for the test result and the prior odds, calculation of the individual patient's risk is easy (Box 5.2).

A real example: Doppler ultrasound for the prediction of perinatal death

Fetal umbilical artery flow velocity waveforms can be measured by continuous wave Doppler (see p. 318). The test is negative if there is forward blood flow at the end of diastole and positive if the flow is absent or reversed (absent or reversed end-diastolic flow – ARED). The aim of the test is to predict babies who will die in utero or soon after birth, so that death can be avoided by delivering the baby early. The gold standard is thus baby survival or death.

Some figures from a series of studies are shown in Table 5.1. The sensitivity is 20/30 (66.6%), and the specificity 2876/2948 (98%). The prevalence of perinatal death in these series is 30/2978, i.e. approximately 1%. If we had applied the test to a patient whose prior risk of perinatal death was also 1% we could read off the positive predictive value directly as 20/92 (22%). However, we usually know that our patient has a much higher or lower risk than this, even before we do any test. Table 5.2 shows how the positive predictive value varies with disease prevalence. In the three parts of this table, the sensitivity (60%) and specificity (98%) do not change.

The chance of the baby dying is much greater if a positive result is found in a very high-risk patient than in a low-risk patient who is simply being screened for disease. Again remember predictive value varies with prevalence – common things are common.

Up till now we have used the Doppler result as if it was either positive or negative. In practice there are a range of results. The worst is reversed end-diastolic flow (EDF), followed by absent EDF and reduced EDF. The best result is normal EDF. Unfortunately few researchers have reported mortality for all these various cut-off points so we cannot plot an ROC curve for prediction of death. However, some workers have reported results for different cut-offs, for the surrogate endpoint of fetal hypoxaemia. We can use these LRs easily in practice.

Imagine a healthy woman undergoing a screening Doppler test. Her prior odds of hypoxaemia might be estimated at say 1 : 1000. The EDF is found to be reduced. The posterior odds become 1 : 1000 × 25 = 25 : 1000 or 1 in 40. Even with an abnormal result, therefore, the baby is still probably not hypoxaemic.

Conversely, imagine a high-risk woman (say, with high blood pressure and vaginal bleeding) whose baby has the same Doppler ratio. If we estimate her prior odds of hypoxaemia as evens (1 : 1) the posterior odds become 1 : 1 × 25 = 25 : 1. The baby is almost certainly hypoxaemic and her obstetrician may advise immediate delivery.

Table 5.1
Doppler ultrasound for the prediction of perinatal death

Gold standard Outcome following test	Positive Baby dies	Negative Baby lives	Total
Positive (ARED)	20	72	92
Negative (EDF present)	10	2876	2886
Total	30	2948	2978

Table 5.2
Effect of prevalence on predictive value

Gold standard Outcome following test	Positive Baby dies	Negative Baby lives	Total
A: Prevalence 5000/10 000 = 50%, i.e. very high risk			
Positive (ARED)	3000 (true +ve)	100 (false +ve)	3100
Negative (EDF present)	2000 (false −ve)	4900 (true −ve)	6900
Total	5000	5000	10 000
Positive predictive value 3000/3100 = 97%			
B: Prevalence 500/10 000 = 5%, i.e. moderately high risk			
Positive (ARED)	300 (true +ve)	190 (false +ve	490
Negative (EDF present)	200 (false −ve)	9310 (true −ve)	9510
Total	500	9500	10 000
Positive predictive value 300/490 = 61%			
C: Prevalence 10/10 000 = 0.1%, i.e. very low risk			
Positive (ARED)	6 (true +ve)	199 (false +ve)	205
Negative (EDF present)	4 (false −ve)	9791 (true −ve)	9795
Total	10	9990	10 000
Positive predictive value 6/205 = 2.9%			

Effective treatments: how to identify them

Some treatments of well-defined diseases are so much more effective than any alternative, that no one doubted early reports of their effectiveness. Examples are insulin for diabetes, salpingectomy for ruptured tubal pregnancy, or in vitro fertilization for bilateral tubal blockage.

Few treatments, however, are so clear-cut. More commonly, disease definitions are hazy, the prognosis is variable no matter what is done, and treatment is only partially effective. Frequently research studies appear to conflict, and clinical practice varies even between experts. How is the practising doctor to choose? One method of choosing the best treatment has recently achieved prominence – meta-analysis. This is a way of combining the results of all the randomized clinical trials of similar treatments for similar diseases.

Why are clinical trials necessary?

The best way to measure the effectiveness of a treatment is to compare a group of patients given the treatment (the intervention or treatment group), with another group not given it (the control group). If there is already an established treatment for the disease the control group will usually be given this treatment and the experimental group the new treatment. If the two groups are otherwise similar, and the treated patients have better outcomes, we conclude that the treatment was effective.

Bias

Difficulties arise if the two groups were not really comparable, or the play of chance misled us. Incomparable groups usually result from a poorly designed experiment, in which the results for one or other group are susceptible to bias.

Bias results from a systematic error as opposed to random variation. It cannot be eliminated simply by increasing the sample size. We can never be certain that there is no systematic error, but in a trial there is no problem so long as any bias affects treatment and control groups equally, and cancels itself out. Sometimes, however, some systematic error affects the measurements of one group and not the other. This can happen in many ways and is often extremely difficult to eradicate.

The simplest type of clinical study (apart from individual case reports) is to study a series of cases. This is of little use for evaluating treatment effectiveness unless the advance is dramatic.

All too often cases in a series are selected, e.g. by admission to a certain hospital, treatment by a certain doctor, or membership of a certain age, sex or racial group. If so, any conclusions cannot automatically be transferred to other patients.

Historical bias The results may be compared with treatments used in the past, but such historical comparisons will be subject to bias if other aspects of patient care are improving (see Box 5.3).

Bias of expertise Comparisons between patients treated by different doctors or in different hospitals are often

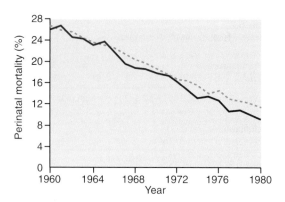

Fig. 5.13   **The perinatal mortality rates from Denmark (solid line) and Holland (dotted line) between 1960 and 1980.**

biased. The doctor evaluating the treatment is often an expert whose patients will do better than those treated by other doctors. Conversely an expert may be referred the more difficult cases, biasing the results against the new treatment. Yet again, an expert with special diagnostic skills may make the diagnosis in milder cases, thus biasing results in favour of the new treatment.

Selection bias   Even if the same doctor administers the treatment, a non-randomized comparison of treatments may be misleading. For example, comparisons of breech babies delivered vaginally with those delivered by caesarean section usually conclude that the latter are more likely to survive. However, babies delivered after a rapid labour, or who were thought unlikely to survive because they were very premature or abnormal, are all more likely to be delivered vaginally, thus biasing the results against vaginal delivery.

Association and causation

If two things appear to be changing together we can say that they are associated. However *association* does not necessarily imply *causation*. For example, perinatal mortality has fallen steadily over the last 30 years, during which time the proportion of deliveries in hospital has steadily increased. Some people have therefore concluded that hospital delivery prevents perinatal death. This conclusion, however, cannot be drawn. In Figure 5.13 the perinatal mortality rates from Denmark and Holland are shown. They fell dramatically in both countries. Home births, however, decreased from 50% to <1% in Denmark but fell much more slowly in Holland (from 70% to 40%). The years with the biggest change from home to hospital were those with the smallest drop in perinatal mortality (Fig. 5.14). Another factor or factors must therefore be responsible for most of the observed improvement.

Matching

If we know what factors influence the outcome of treatment, the cases and controls can be matched for these factors to make the two groups similar. For example cases of cancer can be matched for the stage of the disease. A staging procedure, however, may not cover all the variation in, say, spread of cancer. Two cancers may both be at the same stage but one may be a lot larger than the other. If the larger ones within each stage were more likely to be in the control group, the trial would be biased in favour of the treatment.

Another weakness of studies using matched patients is that we rarely know about all the possible factors that might affect outcome. An unknown factor can still bias results if it was unequally distributed between groups (see Box 5.4).

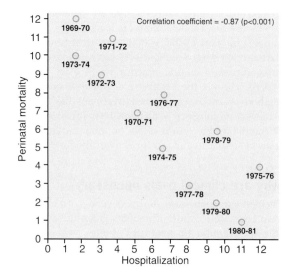

Fig. 5.14   **Scattergram of ranks of proportional changes in rates of hospitalization and perinatal mortality.** Rank 1 denotes the greatest increase in hospitalization and the greatest decrease in perinatal mortality. Rank 12 denotes the smallest increase in hospitalization and the only increase in perinatal mortality.

Box 5.4

CLOFIBRATE TRIAL

Men who had had a heart attack were allocated at random to receive the cholesterol-lowering drug clofibrate or placebo. There was no difference in 5-year mortality (20.0% clofibrate versus 20.9% placebo) and the investigators concluded correctly that the drug was ineffective. However, they noted that 20% of subjects had failed to take the drugs as prescribed, and that their mortality was higher (compliers 15.0%, vs non-compliers 24.6%). Strangely this difference was present to the same extent among those allocated to placebo (compliers 15.1%, vs non-compliers 28.2%). If the investigators had simply been comparing people who had taken the drug with those who did not, they might have concluded mistakenly that the treatment was highly effective. Compliers started off with fewer risk factors than non-compliers but the differences were far too small to explain the observed difference in mortality. Non-compliance was the strongest risk factor. Since this had not been known to be a risk factor, it could not have been matched for in a non-randomized study.

Box 5.5

ENTRY BIAS

A trial compared oxytocin infusion with prostaglandin pessary, as treatment for pregnant women whose membranes ruptured before labour began. Allocation was by the final digit of the hospital number. Most staff believed, rightly or wrongly, that prostaglandin was the better treatment if the cervix was tightly closed. If a woman with a soft open cervix was admitted, she was entered in the trial without problems. However, when a woman with a tight cervix came in, she was entered in the trial only if the digit was even (allocation was to prostaglandin); if it was odd some staff did not enter her, and instead gave prostaglandin anyway outside the trial. Thus among women in the trial those who got prostaglandin tended to be the ones with the more tightly closed cervices. Not surprisingly prostaglandin appeared to give worse results than oxytocin.

Randomization

The best way to ensure that two groups of patients are matched for unknown, as well as known, risk factors is to select them at random. This means using the toss of a coin, random number tables, or other forms of computer-generated random numbers, to select which patients get the new treatment and which are given placebo or control therapy.

Frequently patients are allocated to treatment or placebo groups alternately, by day of the week, or last digit of hospital number. At first sight this may seem satisfactory but since the doctors know the group allocation when they enter the trial there is scope for entry bias (see Box 5.5).

Exclusions

Bias can also occur if patients are more likely to be excluded from the trial in one group than the other. For example, we might wish to compare two policies for dealing with the membranes in labour: leave them intact or rupture them. Women are allocated at random in early labour – half to have the membranes ruptured, and half left intact. Some women allocated to the membrane rupture group are likely to make slow progress and eventually get the membranes ruptured anyway. If we remove them from analysis we will be biasing results against the membrane rupture policy, because

we will be removing women with difficult labours from the 'leave intact' group. The situation will be even worse if some women in the 'rupture' group labour so quickly that there is no time to artificially rupture the membranes. If we exclude them from the 'rupture' group we will again be biasing results against rupture by excluding the most favourable cases from that group. We avoid the problem by analysing the trial by 'intention to treat'.

Intention to treat

If we analyse the trial by comparing the two groups as chance allocated them, we can be sure that no bias has crept in. It may seem strange to include the results for some women who had the membranes left intact in the 'rupture' group and some women who had them ruptured in the 'leave intact' group, but there is no other way to avoid bias. Of course we must ensure that compliance is high, if we really want to find out if a drug or procedure can work.

Biased assessment of outcome

Even if the two groups of patients in a trial are exactly comparable, bias may be introduced if the investigators recording the outcomes know which form of care has been received. For example, it is widely believed that amniotomy causes neonatal infection. If the doctors caring for the babies know that the membranes were ruptured early in labour they might do more tests for infection, and make the belief a self-fulfilling prophecy.

If the doctors are not told which group the patient is in, they are said to be blinded, and their assessment of outcome cannot be influenced. This is a particular problem with 'soft' outcomes, i.e. those whose measurement is not totally objective.

The placebo effect

If the patient believes that the treatment she has received works, that may also result in a self-fulfilling prophecy. This is called the placebo effect. Trials of many treatments for premenstrual tension (see p. 229) have shown high cure rates among patients given inactive medicine. Usually the active treatment has been no better, and investigators have concluded that the treatment was ineffective. If no placebo had been used, the treatment might have been wrongly given the credit for the improvement. Patients are also said to be 'blinded' when they do not know which treatment they are receiving. A trial is said to be 'double blind' when neither the patient nor the investigator knows which treatment is being given.

Blinding is not always necessary. If the endpoint is unambiguous – like death, or caesarean section – blinding at the stage of outcome assessment is unnecessary, although it may still be necessary during the treatment period. If blinding is not possible, but the outcome is susceptible to observer bias, it may be possible to eliminate it by having independent observers make the assessment.

Some of the problems which may occur in clinical research and their solutions are summarized in Table 5.3.

Statistical problems

These occur because of random variation – the play of chance. Random variation differs from bias in that increasing the sample size will reduce it. There are two ways that the play of chance can mislead.

1. We may think there is a difference, when all we saw was chance variation. This is called a type 1, or alpha, error.
2. We may fail to realize that there is a real difference. This is called a type 2, or beta, error.

A number of statistical tests have been used to avoid making these errors.

Type 1 and type 2 errors
Tests to avoid type 1 error

The results of an experiment usually take the form of a series of observations on a treatment and control group. These may be continuous measures such as birth weights or dichotomous variables such as death rates. We will concentrate on dichotomous outcomes.

If the mortality rates are identical between treatment and control groups we will not be misled into a false belief that the treatment was effective. The difficulty arises when there is a difference and we want to know whether it occurred by chance or was caused by the treatment. Most statistical tests tell us how likely it was to occur by chance. This is the familiar 'p' value. By convention we call $p < 0.05$ 'statistically significant'. This means that there was a less than 5% chance that

Table 5.3
Research problems and their solutions

Problem	Solution
Imbalance in known and measurable risk factors	Matched controls
Imbalance in subtle and difficult to measure risk factors	Randomized controls
Imbalance in unknown risk factors	Randomized controls
Biased entry	'Blind' the researchers
Biased entry but impossible to blind researchers	Enter patients irreversibly before randomization, e.g. telephone randomization, or monitor randomization closely
Biased assessment of outcomes	'Blind' researchers
Placebo effect	Use placebo, and 'blind' patients
Biased exclusions after randomization	Analysis by 'intention to treat'
Type 1 error (see text)	Increase sample size. Search for unpublished trials and perform meta-analysis
Type 2 error (see text)	Increase sample size. Search for unpublished trials and perform meta-analysis

the difference we observed would occur by chance if the treatments were equally effective.

Although hallowed by tradition, this method of presenting results simply tells us that we have not made a type 1 error. If 'p' is greater than 0.05 we do not know whether there really is no important difference, or whether our trial was too small. Nor does the 'p' value tell us the likely size of any difference. A very small and clinically unimportant difference, may be statistically highly significant if a large study has been performed.

Type 2 error

Here we are concerned with the probability that a trial has failed to show a real effect, i.e. a false negative result (Box 5.6). The probability of a negative result depends on the size of the treatment effect we wish to detect.

It is possible to quantify the probability of failing to detect a particular size of effect. The size of effect that is really important is a clinically meaningful effect – one that would cause doctors to change treatment. A particular trial can exclude a large effect more reliably than a small effect. We call this the power of the trial (Box 5.7).

Odds ratios and their confidence intervals

A good way to look at treatment effects is to consider the risks or 'odds' of the bad outcome after treatment versus

---

Box 5.7

THE POWER OF RANDOMIZED TRIALS

The importance of evidence from randomized controlled trials (RCTs) is well recognized. A well-conducted randomized trial is usually more influential than almost any other form of clinical research. In 1954, seven key observational studies were published linking smoking and lung cancer. All of them were susceptible to one form of bias or another, and only after many years, many further observational studies and much argument, was it generally accepted that smoking did cause lung cancer, with a relative risk of about 10. In contrast, the same year, 1954, the polio vaccine trial, a randomized double-blind placebo-controlled trial, demonstrated that vaccination cut the polio rate by a factor of about 2.5. This much smaller effect was established once and for all, by this single experiment.

---

control therapy. The effect of the treatment is given in the form of a relative risk (RR) or more commonly an odds ratio (OR).

An OR of 1 indicates that the treatment does not alter the adverse outcome. An OR below 1 indicates that the chances of adverse outcome are reduced by treatment. An OR above 1 indicates that treatment increases these odds. An OR of 0.5 indicates a halving of the odds, and an OR of 2 a doubling.

The 95% confidence intervals (CI) can be calculated. An OR of 0.5 with 95% CI 0.25–1, indicates that we have found a halving in the odds of the outcome and can be 95% confident that the true effect lies between an OR of 0.25 and 1.

This corresponds to a p value of 0.05 since the confidence interval just includes 1. If the 95% CI fails to reach 1, the p value is less than 0.05, i.e. it is significant. If the 95% CI includes 1 the p value is greater than 0.05, i.e. the result is not statistically significant.

Graphs such as that in Figure 5.15 occur frequently in the scientific literature. By convention, in their titles the 'treatment' is named first and odds ratios are almost always given for 'adverse' outcomes.

A point estimate to the left of the line indicates a beneficial effect of treatment and to the right an adverse effect. If the 95% confidence interval includes 1 (no effect of treatment), there is a greater than 5% probability that the observed difference occurred by chance, and the result is not statistically significant at the conventionally accepted level. Note also that the scale for odds ratios is logarithmic.

Box 5.6

POSTURAL TREATMENT FOR BREECH

Some experts had the idea that if a pregnant woman gets into the knee–chest position this might encourage breech babies to turn spontaneously to cephalic. They did a trial on 55 women with breech babies, randomly allocated to assume the knee–chest position. 26/30 in the treatment group were still breech at delivery and 20/25 in the control group (relative risk 1.08). To measure the chance that this difference was due to a type 1 error they did a chi-square test. The result was $p = 0.76$ and they concluded that there was a high probability that this observed difference was simply a chance effect and they reported the result as not statistically significant.

However, this is not the same as saying that there is no effect. The 95% confidence interval for the relative risk ranges from 0.85–1.38. This means that, although the trend was towards a detrimental effect, the knee–chest position could easily reduce the rate of breech babies at delivery by, say, 10%.

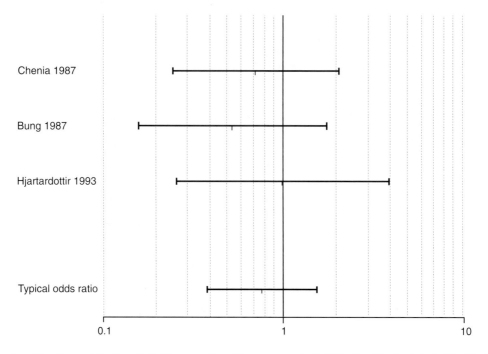

Fig. 5.15 **An odds ratio graph for the effect of knee–chest position on non-cephalic births.** A point estimate to the left of the line indicates a beneficial effect of treatment and to the right an adverse effect.

Meta-analysis

Type 2 errors are minimized by very large trials. Unfortunately these are difficult and expensive to perform. One solution is to combine the results of small and medium-sized trials. The statistics need not concern us here, but the results can be conveniently presented as odds ratios for each trial separately. Beneath them is plotted the typical odds ratio and CI for all the trials combined.

Here are four contrasting examples:

Example 1: Knee–chest position for breeches

Two other groups of researchers have performed randomized trials of postural treatment to encourage spontaneous version of breech babies (see Box 5.6). None of them showed a significant effect, but meta-analysis allows us to test whether there was a significant effect overall. We can see that all the trials show a small reduction in non-cephalic presentation at delivery but that since the typical odds ratio still includes 1, conventional levels of significance have not been reached. Since the lower limit for the 95% CI includes an odds ratio of 0.4 and such a reduction in non-cephalic presentation would clinically be very important, more trials are needed.

Conclusion   It is important to continue this research.

Example 2: Steroids to prevent respiratory distress syndrome

This meta-analysis graph is one of the classics of obstetrics (Fig. 5.16). The very first trial demonstrated that steroids were effective. Unfortunately that trial was followed by a series of small trials, many of which failed to reach conventional levels of significance and many readers mistakenly assumed that the effectiveness of steroid therapy was controversial. It was only when graphs like this one were published that it became clear that apparently conflicting results were simply an effect of small trials.

Conclusion   It is now universally recognized that steroids are effective in preventing respiratory distress syndrome among preterm babies.

Example 3: Transcutaneous electronic nerve stimulation

Transcutaneous electronic nerve stimulation (TENS) is a non-drug method for pain relief in labour. It involves strapping a flexible metal plate to the mother's lumbar region and passing pulses of electric current. There is likely to be a placebo effect, so the best trials have attached a dummy plate to the control group of women. Meta-analysis of such trials suggests that TENS increases the rate of severe pain (Fig. 5.17). However, it is clear from the graph that some trials have given conflicting results.

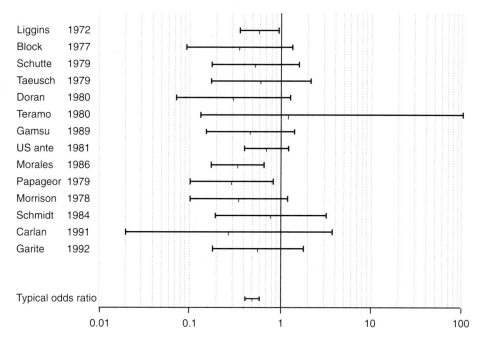

Fig. 5.16   **The effect of steroids prior to preterm delivery on respiratory distress syndrome in the baby.**

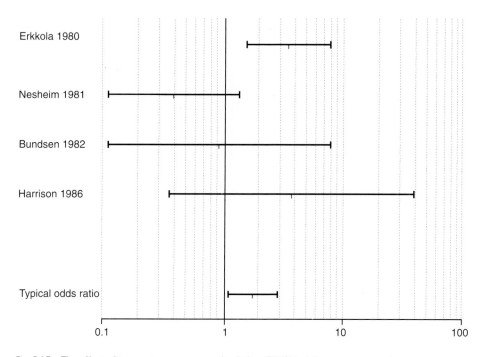

Fig. 5.17   **The effect of transcutaneous nerve stimulation (TENS) in labour on severe pain.**

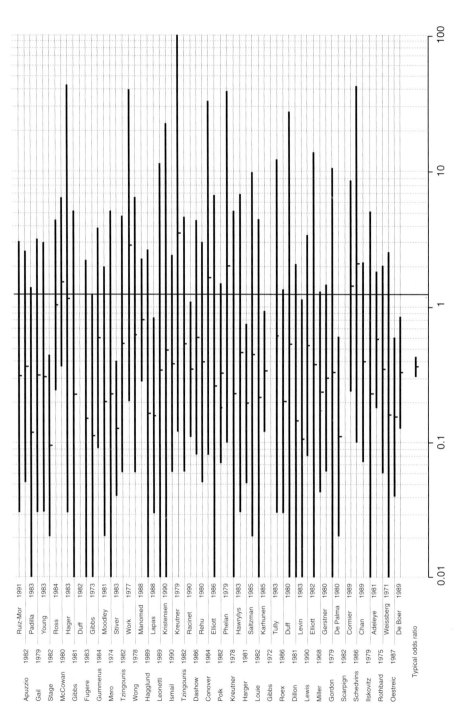

Fig. 5.18 **The effect of prophylactic antibiotics for caesarean section on maternal wound infection.**

Conclusion   Although some of the difference may be chance effects it is probably worthwhile doing more research. (Note that despite the apparent ineffectiveness of TENS it is popular with patients (see Ch. 46).)

Example 4: Prophylactic antibiotics for caesarean section

The message of the graph Figure 5.18 is firstly that prophylactic antibiotics are effective in reducing wound infection. It also shows us that too many trials have been performed already.

Conclusion   There is no need for any more research. Researchers should tackle other questions.

Key points

- Randomized comparisons are now regarded as the scientifically most rigorous way to compare interventions. The authors of this textbook believe that new treatment should not be introduced without first being evaluated by randomized controlled trials.

- An exception may be made for those interventions whose effect is so dramatic that the benefit is obvious, e.g. insulin for diabetes or anti-D prophylaxis to prevent rhesus immunization.

- What about treatments already in use? Every effort should be made to perform randomized controlled trials to evaluate them. If they are effective they should be used unless there is a good reason otherwise. If they are ineffective they should be abandoned.

- The specialty of obstetrics is particularly well placed to put treatment on such a rational footing since all the randomized controlled trials have been collected, and meta-analyses of many interventions have been published, and regularly updated by the National Perinatal Epidemiology Unit in Oxford.

6

Human embryogenesis

Introduction

In obstetric practice it is common to use 280 days (40 weeks) from the first day of the last menstrual period (LMP) to estimate the delivery date of a full-term pregnancy. This period has also become a convenient but inaccurate description of the number of weeks of 'pregnancy'. This is an obvious source of confusion since embryologists refer to the number of gestational days, i.e. days since fertilization, when discussing early human development. Since conception requires male and female gametes to be in the same place (the ampulla of the fallopian tube) at the same time (within a few hours of ovulation and within 6 days of intercourse), it can be approximated to:

- ~14 days after the first day of the LMP, i.e. roughly the day of ovulation in a woman with a regular 28-day cycle (p. 123)
- the day of ovulation as judged by a change in basal body temperature, serum luteinizing hormone (LH) and/or oestrogen to progesterone ratios
- 6 days prior to the rapid increase in chorionic gonadotrophin levels that is associated with implantation of the embryo.

In most pregnancies only the first of these options is available and thus 8 weeks of 'pregnancy' implies 42 gestational days (GD).

Nomenclature

Embryology has a long and distinguished history and is thus cursed with a dense classically-based nomenclature. Attempts at standardization have often led to the same structure having at least two different names (e.g. yolk sac and umbilical vesicle; branchial and pharyngeal arches) and/or the same structure changing its name at different stages of development (e.g. allantois → urachus → medial umbilical ligament). This complexity can be disheartening so only the most up-to-date terms will be used and these will be related to the mature tissues wherever possible. Some transient structures are important in understanding malformations and these will be highlighted.

To start with the most obvious piece of nomenclature, the boundary between embryonic and fetal life is ~ 56 GD (i.e. ~ 10 weeks post-LMP). This is an arbitrary but useful boundary that is based on the fact that 90%

of adult structures are recognizable at this stage. One of the most important concepts in embryogenesis is the establishment of the three main embryonic axes: (1) rostrocaudal; (2) dorsoventral; (3) left–right (Box 6.1, Fig. 6.1).

Fertilization to implantation (0–6 GD)

In vitro fertilization has greatly increased our understanding of the early cellular and molecular events in human embryogenesis (Fig. 6.2). Sadly for the male ego, the sperm has only three essential roles in embryogenesis:

1. to stimulate a change in the zona pellucida that prevents further sperm entering the cell
2. to deliver a paternally imprinted haploid genome (see Box 6.2) in order to reconstitute a diploid chromosome number
3. to stimulate the second meiotic division in the egg with subsequent production of the second polar body.

In contrast to the sperm, the egg is a complex cell with many subcompartments, each with a critical role. At the most basic level the egg carries a maternally imprinted haploid genome (Box 6.2). It also determines the orientation of at least one of the 'axes' in the early embryo (Box 6.1), and it provides all the RNA and protein synthesis requirements until the embryonic genome becomes transcriptionally active at 2–3 days post-fertilization.

The first mitotic division occurs 36 hours after fertilization. The next four mitoses are at intervals of ~ 17 hours and produce a ball of cells called a blastomere. After the fifth mitotic division the blastomere becomes polarized as a sphere with a single-cell-layered wall (trophoblast) and an inner cell mass. The inner cell mass of this blastocyst contains the cells that will form the embryo itself. The 128 cells that are present following the seventh mitotic division still occupy the same volume as the initial fertilized egg, i.e. there has been no physical growth. The embryo sheds the zona pellucida at about this time, a process termed fancifully as 'hatching'. Over these first 5 days the embryo is transported along the fallopian tube and becomes attached to the uterine wall around 6 GD.

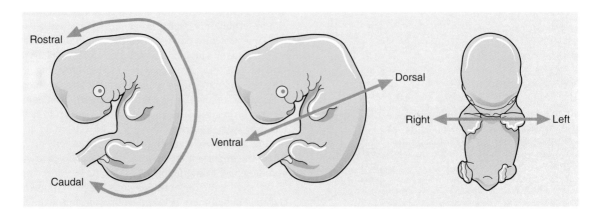

Fig. 6.1 **The rostral–caudal, dorsal–ventral and left–right embryonic axes.**

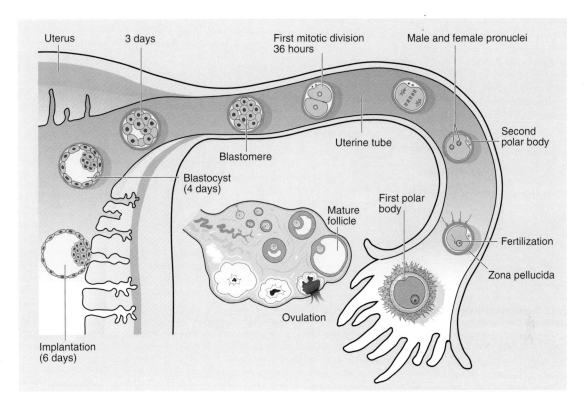

Fig. 6.2 **Fertilization occurs in the fallopian tube.** The embryo is then transported along the fallopian tube and implants in the uterine wall around 6 GD.

Box 6.2

IMPRINTING

The male and female gamete both contain 23 chromosomes, one copy of each autosomal chromosome (numbered 1–22 in decreasing order of size) and one sex chromosome (X in egg and X or Y in sperm). The DNA sequence of each pair of chromosomes is essentially identical, but the copy we have inherited from one parent can function very differently from the one inherited from the other parent. For example, the short arm of chromosome 11 contains the gene insulin-like growth factor type 2 (*IGF2*). Although there are two copies of *IGF2* in each cell, only one is ever active and this is always on the paternally inherited chromosome 11. *IGF2* produces a protein which promotes fetal growth (the 'male' drive) but is silenced on the maternal copy (the 'female' drive). This particular mechanism probably evolved to balance the conflict between the advantage to the male of having a large offspring at birth against the risk to the mother of delivering such a large offspring.

Differential gene activation is the result of the silencing of one copy of a gene via covalent modifications of both the DNA itself (methylation) and histone proteins (acetylation) which are intimately associated with the double-stranded DNA molecule. These parent-of-origin-specific modifications are known as 'genomic imprinting'. Beckwith–Wiedemann syndrome is caused by specific genetic mutations that result in a fetus having two active copies of *IGF2*. This result in an infant that is large for gestational age and who is prone to tumour formation, particularly Wilms' tumour. Several other examples of imprinting mutations are known.

Implantation and formation of the germ layers (7–18 GD)

At implantation the trophoblast buries itself in the endometrium. The embryo thus gains access to the maternal circulation and behaves as an efficient paracytic organism which enables a very rapid period of growth. The inner cell mass begins to differentiate and the embryo takes on the appearance of a disc consisting of two layers of morphologically distinct cells: the epiblast (the dorsal region) and the hypoblast (the

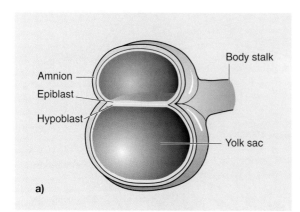
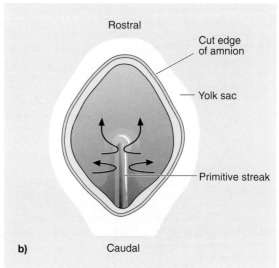

Fig. 6.3 **Formation of the germ layers. (a)** The inner cell mass takes on the appearance of a disc comprising two layers of morphologically distinct cells: the epiblast (the dorsal region) and the hypoblast (the ventral region). **(b)** 'Gastrulation' describes the process where epiblastic cells in the disc migrate towards a groove in the caudal end of the disc known as the primitive streak. These migrating cells pass through the primitive streak to form the embryonic endoderm.

ventral region, Fig. 6.3a). This is the first real evidence of embryonic polarity. The largest embryonic cavity at this stage is the umbilical vesicle which is lined with hypoblast cells. The amniotic cavity begins to form by 9 GD and is lined with epiblast cells.

By day 16 the embryonic disc takes on an oval shape and a second axis (rostrocaudal or head–tail axis) becomes apparent. This is accompanied by a process known as gastrulation where epiblastic cells migrate towards a groove in the caudal end of the disc known as the primitive streak (Fig. 6.3b). The migrating cells pass though the primitive streak and form a new embryonic compartment or 'germ layer' called the mesoderm. The dorsal epiblast now becomes known as embryonic ectoderm and the hypoblastic region as embryonic endoderm. The embryo now has three layers bounded by the umbilical vesicle ventrally and the amniotic cavity dorsally.

Organogenesis (20–56+ GD)

A full description of organogenesis would require many volumes, and the descriptions given here are necessarily brief. For simplicity, organogenesis is divided into five main areas:

1. neural tube and brain
2. gut tube and derivatives
3. heart and liver
4. face
5. limbs and skeletal muscle.

Neural tube and brain

Formation of the neural tube and primitive brain is the first evidence of organogenesis. It begins at 19 GD when a midline groove forms on the dorsal ectodermal surface, rostral to the primitive streak. This change in the surface ectoderm is induced by a strip of specialized midline mesodermal cells called the notochordal process (Fig. 6.4). Two important paired structures form on either side of this groove:

- the neural folds
- the somites.

The neural folds grow rapidly and begin to fuse across the midline in the cervical region to form the neural tube by 22 GD. At the same time paired, segmental condensations of the mesoderm (somites) are beginning to form blocks of tissue on either side of the midline (paraxial mesoderm). A new pair of somites appears every 6.6 hours in a rostrocaudal direction. The somites are critical for establishing the adult body plan and their formation has been studied in great depth as the paradigm for repeated segment (metameric) pattern formation in embryogenesis (Box 6.3).

Fusion of the neural tube proceeds rapidly in both rostral and caudal directions. This apparently simple tube will give rise to the entire central nervous system (CNS). At either end of the embryo the neural tube remains open for a short time, and these openings are referred to as the rostral and caudal neuropores. The rostral neuropore closes by 23 GD, and failure of this

6

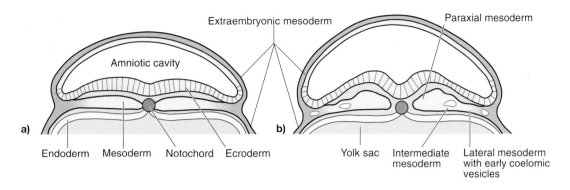

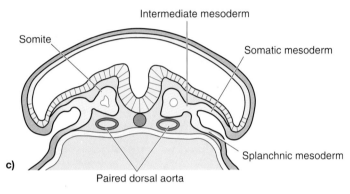

Fig. 6.4 **Formation of the neural tube.** This begins with the appearance of a midline groove on the dorsal ectodermal surface, induced by a strip of specialized midline mesodermal cells called the notochordal process. This fold fuses across the midline in the cervical region to form the neural tube. Failure of this tube to close cranially results in anencephaly, and failure caudally leads to spina bifida.

Box 6.3

PATTERN FORMATION

Pattern formation is a fascinating process in the embryo whereby the future fate of a group of cells is determined before any morphological change has occurred. This process is now known to be effected by the activation of specific sets of transcription factors which in turn is a response to a combination of gradients of signalling molecules within the embryo. The best-known example of this is the combination of *Hox* gene activation that predicts and determines the formation of individual somites along the rostrocaudal axis (Fig. 6.5). However, these same *Hox* genes also play a role in patterning the limb bud and are only one of a number of different classes of transcription factors that are vital for pattern formation.

Defects in these patterning processes are likely to underlie many types of malformation. For example, mutations in an important transcription factor *PAX6* result in failure of iris formation (aniridia; Fig. 6.6a), whereas mutations in the related gene *PAX9* cause the absence of particular teeth (hypodontia). As the same genes are involved in different parts of the fetus, a gene defect may produce abnormalities at different sites which may, in some cases, explain why certain syndromes have a particular combination of malformations. Other malformation combinations may be explained by the fact that certain genes lie close to each other on a given chromosome, and deletion of a particular segment means that both genes will be missing, e.g. the *PAX6* of aniridia mentioned above and the Wilms' tumour suppressor gene *Wt1*, both of which are usually near to each other on chromosome 11.

process results in one of the most severe of human malformations, anencephaly (p. 343). The caudal neuropore is the last part of the neural tube to close at 26 GD, and failure of this closure leads to spina bifida (p. 344).

The rostral half of the neural tube is more complex and forms the future brain. The caudal part forms the spinal cord. In common with many other embryological structures, the formation of the CNS is best viewed as a tube which is segmented along the long axis, each linear segment then undergoes complex subsegmental growth

59

Fundamentals

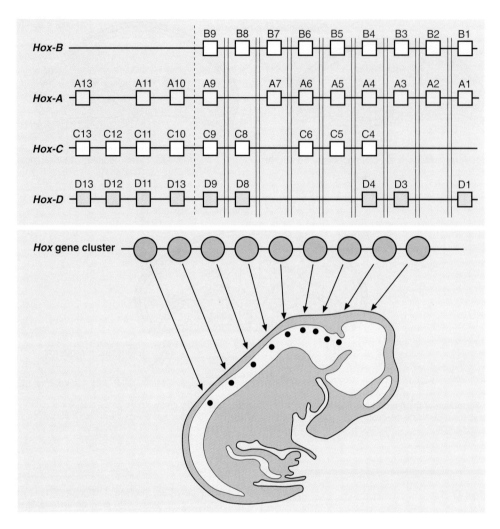

Fig. 6.5 **Formation of somites.** *Hox* gene activation determines the formation of individual somites along the rostrocaudal axis. The same genes also play a role in patterning the limb bud.

and differentiation to produce the final adult form. At day 26 the CNS is a tube with four main segments:

1. forebrain – prosencephalon
2. midbrain – mesencephalon
3. hindbrain – rhombencephalon
4. spinal cord.

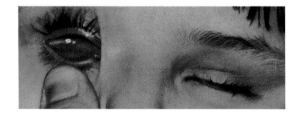

Fig. 6.6 **Aniridia.** The eye socket is empty.

The forebrain

The prosencephalon is initially subdivided into three segments. The most rostral is the telencephalon medium, then come the D1 and D2 compartments of the diencephalon. All three segments surround the future third ventricle (Fig. 6.7). D1 will give rise to the bilateral optic evaginations by day 28 (see Face, below) and D2 will form the thalamus, hypothalamus, pineal gland and part of the pituitary (neurohypophysis). The telencephalon medium forms as a rostral out-pouching of the third ventricle. By day 32 a midline crest separates the two future cerebral hemispheres. Failure of this process results in a malformation called holoprosencephaly (Fig. 6.8). Subsequent development of telencephalic structures is extremely complex and much of it occurs during fetal and postnatal life rather than during embryogenesis. In addition to the cerebral hemispheres

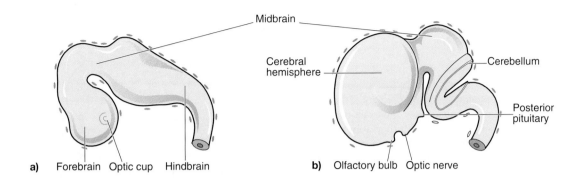

a) Forebrain Optic cup Hindbrain

b) Olfactory bulb Optic nerve

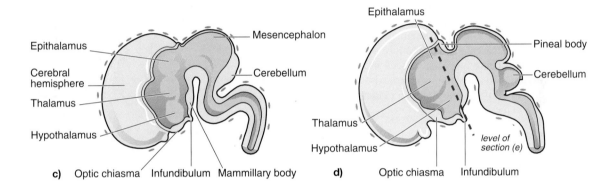

c) Optic chiasma Infundibulum Mammillary body

d) Optic chiasma Infundibulum

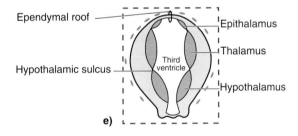

e)

Fig. 6.7 **Development of the CNS. (a)** At day 26 the CNS is a tube with four main segments: forebrain (prosencephalon), midbrain (mesencephalon), hindbrain (rhombencephalon) and spinal cord. **(b–e)** Morphological changes in **(b,c)** the 7th week, and **(d,e)** the 8th week.

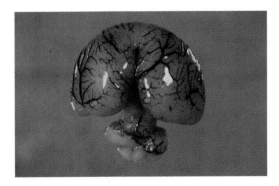

Fig. 6.8 **Holoprosencephaly occurs when there is failure of division between the two future cerebral hemispheres.** The condition is associated with profound cerebral impairment.

the telencephalon gives rise to the caudate and lentiform nuclei (derivatives of the corpus striatum) and the connections between the hemispheres derived from the lamina terminalis (anterior commissure, hippocampal commissure and corpus callosum).

The midbrain

The mesencephalon is less complicated than the forebrain. It segments dorsally to form the superior and inferior colliculi (roles in integrating visual and auditory signals respectively) and ventrally to form the tegmentum (oculomotor nuclei of cranial nerves III and IV). This typifies a general pattern within the neural tube where dorsal grey matter has a sensory function and ventral grey matter has a motor function. Later in development the cerebral peduncles occupy a significant proportion of the midbrain.

The hindbrain

The rhombencephalon is highly segmented into eight regions known as rhombomeres. The exact function of each rhombomere is not clear but they appear to have a role in forming the motor components of cranial nerves V, VII, IX and X. More rostrally the rhombencephalon forms the pons and the cerebellum. Like the cerebral hemispheres, the cerebellum continues to develop throughout intrauterine life.

The spinal cord

The spinal cord itself is unsegmented along the rostrocaudal axis. The adjacent somites produce the repeated pattern of spinal nerve roots that is seen in adult life. The cord is patterned in the dorsoventral axis and maintains the dorsal/sensory, ventral/motor pattern for grey matter function mentioned above.

Gut tube and its derivatives

Initially the primitive gut is simply a concavity within the embryo that is lined with embryonic endoderm and it has a large direct connection to the umbilical vesical (Fig. 6.9). As development progresses the gut becomes a tube with a fundamental role in the development of many organs. The most important of these in rostrocaudal order are:

- the thyroid and pituitary glands
- the lungs
- the pancreas
- the bile ducts and gall bladder (covered in the section on Heart and liver, below)
- the urogenital system.

Excepting the urogenital system, these structures all arise as midline invaginations of the gut tube endoderm into the underlying mesoderm. The gut tube, like the neural tube, is strictly patterned along the long axis with complex subsegmental development. Also like the neural tube, morphogenesis broadly proceeds in rostrocaudal temporal sequence.

Thyroid and pituitary glands

The tongue develops from a bud of tissue on the ventral wall of the gut tube. Just caudal to this, the thyroid primordium is evident from day 20 as a midline ventral invagination of endoderm. The base of the invagination hypertrophies and differentiates to form the thyroid gland itself. By 40 GD, the thyroid gland has 'descended'

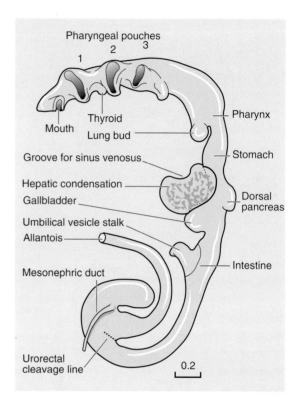

Fig. 6.9 **Formation of the gut.** Initially the primitive gut is simply a concavity within the embryo lined with embryonic endoderm, with a large direct connection to the umbilical vesical. As development progresses the gut becomes a tube with a fundamental role in the development of the gastrointestinal tract, the thyroid and pituitary glands, the lungs, the pancreas, the bile ducts and gall bladder and the urogenital system.

and is lying at the level of the second and third tracheal cartilage. Terms such as 'descended' are often used in descriptions of morphogenesis but refer to differential growth of surrounding tissue rather than active burrowing of the structure. The stalk of the invagination (thyroglossal duct) usually regresses, apart from a small pit at the base of the tongue called the foramen caecum. Remnants of the thyroglossal ducts can persist in the form of ectopic thyroid tissue and thyroglossal cysts.

The pituitary is formed by the meeting of two different invaginations, one from the dorsal wall of the rostral gut tube (Rathke's pouch) and the other from the floor of the diencephalon. Neoplastic change in the stalk of the former results in the rare hormone-secreting tumour craniopharyngioma.

The lungs

The respiratory diverticulum is first seen as an invagination of the ventral wall of the gut tube at 26 GD. This diverticulum elongates so that the trachea lies immediately ventral to the oesophagus. The development of both of these structures is intimately related and developmental problems may result in tracheo-oesophageal fistulae and/or oesophageal atresia. The development of the airways proceeds by a process known as branching morphogenesis, in which there is bifurcation of the invaginating tube-like structures at regular intervals. The earliest branching events show evidence of the left–right asymmetry apparent in adult life (Fig. 6.10).

The pancreas

The pancreas develops as separate dorsal and ventral invaginations in the gut tube, caudal to the developing stomach. The ventral pancreas develops in the same region as the hepatic ducts and gall bladder (see below) and their ductal systems are connected. The dorsal pancreas is larger and its duct drains directly into the duodenum. At some point after 42 GD the dorsal and ventral pancreas fuse and the ducts of both structures anastomose.

The urogenital system

The development of the renal, genital and anorectal systems are closely related. The paired primitive kidney (mesonephros) develops from intermediate mesoderm

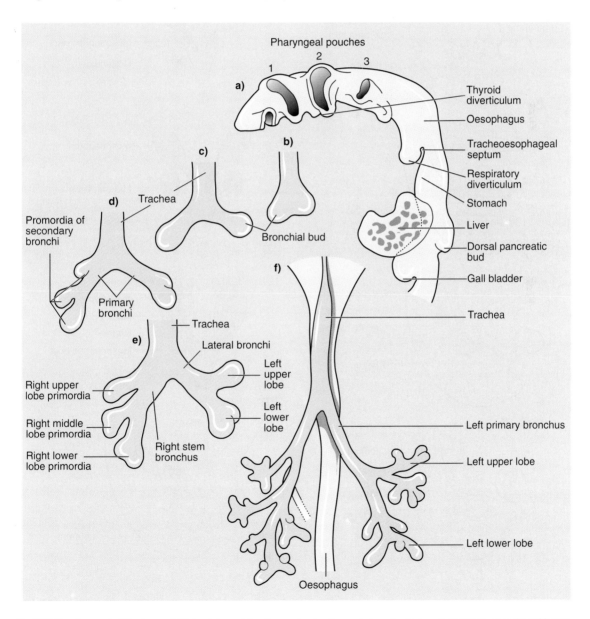

Fig. 6.10 **Development of the lungs. (a)** Lateral views of the pharynx showing the respiratory diverticulum. **(b–f)** Anterior view: **(b)** at 28 days; **(c)** at 32 days; **(d)** at 33 days; **(e)** at the end of the 5th week; **(f)** early in the 7th week.

Fundamentals

on either side of the gut tube. The mesonephros is connected to a specialized midline region of the caudal gut (the cloaca) via the metamerically patterned mesonephric (Wolffian) ducts. The caudal end of the mesonephric duct, called the ureteric bud, induces the surrounding mesenchyme to form the mature kidney (metanephros) (Fig. 6.11). Failure of this process results in renal agenesis. The primitive gonad develops at the rostral end of the mesonephric duct at the level of the stomach. At 46 GD a second paired-duct system, the

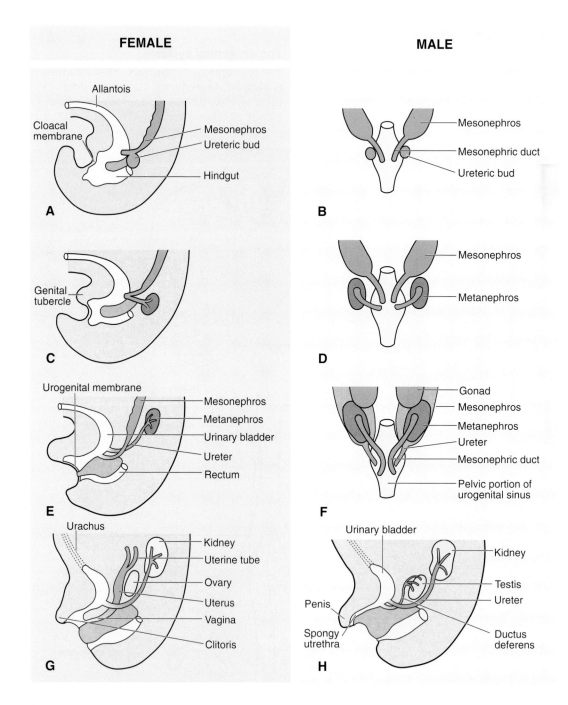

Fig. 6.11 **Development of the urogenital system.** At 46 GD a paired duct system, the paramesonephric (Müllerian) duct, forms parallel to the mesonephric duct. In male embryos a cascade of gene activation initiated by SRY protein causes the primitive gonad to become a testis and the mesonephric duct to form the vas deferens; the paramesonephric duct regresses. In female embryos, the primitive gonad becomes the ovary, the mesonephric duct regresses and the paramesonephric ducts form the fallopian tubes, uterus and upper vagina.

paramesonephric (Müllerian) duct, forms parallel to the mesonephric duct. In male embryos a cascade of gene activation initiated by SRY protein causes the primitive gonad to become a testis and the mesonephric duct forms the vas deferens; the paramesonephric duct regresses. In female embryos, the primitive gonad becomes the ovary, the mesonephric duct regresses and the paramesonephric ducts form the fallopian tubes, uterus and upper vagina. This sexually dimorphic development occurs during late embryogenesis and early fetal life, and molecular analysis of this system has been very useful in understanding intersex states (Ch. 10). The mesonephros regresses in both sexes.

The cloaca separates dorsally to form the rectum and ventrally to form the bladder, urethra and the lower part of the vagina. The external genitalia develop from swellings on the ectodermal surface of the embryo: the midline genital tubercle which forms the penis and clitoris; the paramedial genital fold which forms part of the penile urethra and the labia minora; and the paired lateral genital swellings which form the scrotum and labia majora. Development of the external genitalia is a late event and it is often difficult for a non-expert to correctly assign the sex of a mid-gestation fetus by external morphology.

Heart and liver

The heart and liver are derived from a condensation of mesenchyme that forms by day 20 in the very rostral part of the embryo, between the forebrain and the endoderm. This mesenchyme forms the heart tube, which then shows highly programmed regional growth over the next 2 days to become asymmetrically looped. This 'cardiac looping' is the first evidence of a left–right axis in the embryo. The heart tube (like the neural tube and gut tube) is highly organized along its long axis to form, in a caudorostral direction, the atria, the left ventricle, the right ventricle and the conotruncal region. The subsegmental growth of the heart tube continues until four chambers are recognizable but retain a common connection (Fig. 6.12). Separation of the chambers and the formation of AV valves is dependent on the fusion of ridges of tissue within the heart (the endocardial cushions). Failure of this process results in a heart malformation not infrequently found in Down's syndrome, an AV canal defect. The aorta at this stage consists of a ventral root that feeds four paired vessels (aortic arches) which supply the rapidly growing pharyngeal arches (see below). A combination of regression and differential growth of these arches eventually shapes the mature thoracic aorta. The right side of the fourth arch, for example, becomes the right subclavian artery whereas the left side of the fourth arch becomes part of the aortic arch.

The first evidence of liver formation is on day 22 as a condensation of mesenchyme in the cardiac region

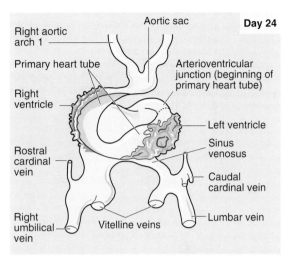

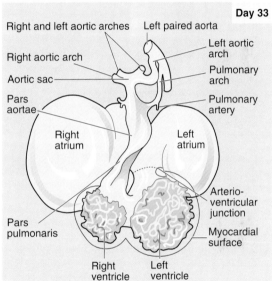

Fig. 6.12 **Development of the heart.** The primary cardiac loop which forms, in a caudorostral direction, the atria, the left ventricle, the right ventricle and the conotruncal region. Growth of the heart tube continues until four chambers are recognizable.

overlying a thickened region of gut endoderm (hepatic plate). The ductal system of the liver and the gall bladder is derived from an invagination of the hepatic plate, whereas the hepatocytes are mesenchymal in origin.

Face

The face develops around the primitive oral cavity at the rostral end of the gut tube. The major early morphogenic events involve:

- the paired sensory placodes
- the facial processes.

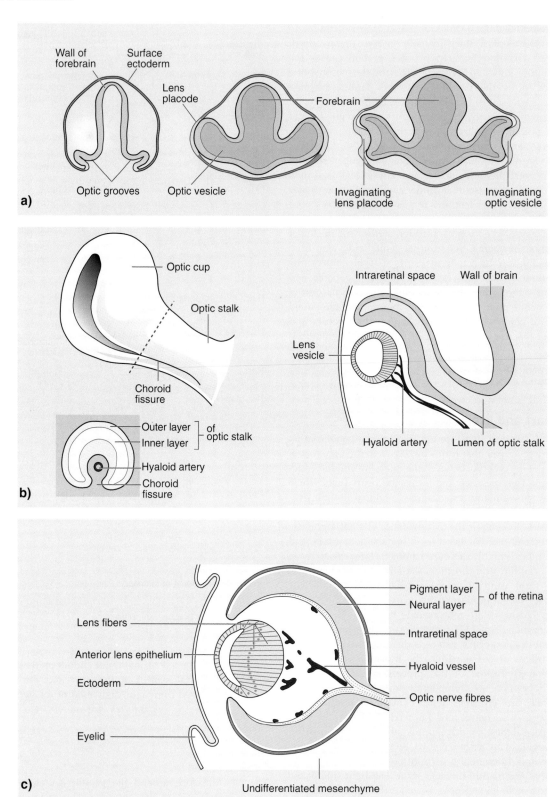

Fig. 6.13 **Development of the eye. (a)** The invaginating lens placode becomes separated from the surface ectoderm. **(b,c)** The retina is formed from an outpouching of the forebrain (the optic cup).

The paired sensory placodes

The otic, nasal and optic placodes are defined thickenings on the surface ectoderm. The otic placode is the first to appear at 20 GD on the lateral wall of the hindbrain. This placode gradually invaginates to become the otic cyst and then undergoes complex morphogenesis to form the semicircular canals and cochlea. The external ear develops from mounds of tissue (auricular hillocks) on the first and second pharyngeal arches (see below). The middle ear develops from the tissue between these arches. The nasal placode is first evident on the frontonasal process by 30 GD and invaginates to form the nasal air passages. The optic placode is induced at ~ 28 GD by signals emanating from the bilateral optic evagination (optic stalks) arising from the diencephalon. The optic placode invaginates to form the optic vesicle that will ultimately become the lens of the eye (Figs 6.13 and 6.14). The cupped end of the optic stalk becomes the neural retina and the stalk itself the optic nerve. Failure of any part of this process will result in anophthalmia.

The facial processes

By 22 GD paired tubes of tissue form ventral to the hindbrain. These 'pharyngeal arches' have a fundamental role in the morphogenesis of the head and neck. There are usually only three pharyngeal arches visible in the embryo, and the cells that form the arches contain a significant number of migratory neural crest cells (Box 6.4). The first pharyngeal arch is the most important in face development and through differential growth this tube of tissue becomes c-shaped; the top arm forms the maxillary process and the bottom arm the mandibular process (Fig. 6.14). The upper lip is formed at ~ 40 GD by fusion of the maxillary process with the midline unpaired frontonasal process. Failure to fuse results in unilateral or bilateral cleft lip (Fig. 6.15a). The lower jaw is formed by fusion of the mandibular processes in the midline. The secondary palate forms from outgrowths of palatal shelves from the maxillary process within the oral cavity. These initially grow down beside the tongue and then elevate to fuse in the midline. Failure to do so results in cleft palate (Fig. 6.15b).

Limbs and skeletal muscle

The upper limbs develop first, but the sequence of events is similar in both the upper and lower limbs. Limb formation begins as a ridge of cells on the lateral aspect of the embryo opposite somites 8–10 at ~ 26 GD.

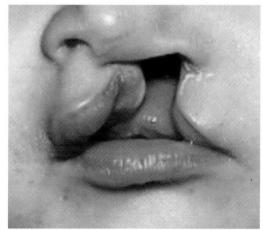
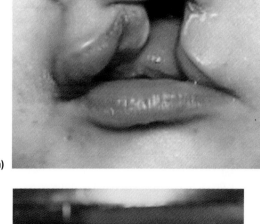

(a)

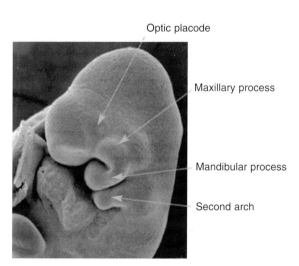

Optic placode

Maxillary process

Mandibular process

Second arch

Fig. 6.14 **Face development.** By 22 GD paired tubes of tissue form ventral to the hindbrain – the 'pharyngeal arches'. The first pharyngeal arch becomes c-shaped. The top arm of the 'c' forms the maxillary process and the bottom arm the mandibular process.

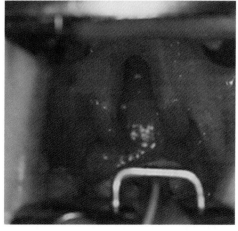

(b)

Fig. 6.15 **Formation of the lips and palate. (a)** The upper lip is formed by fusion of the maxillary process with the midline unpaired frontonasal process. Failure of this process results in unilateral or bilateral cleft lip. **(b)** The lower jaw is formed by fusion of the mandibular processes in the midline. Failure of this process results in cleft palate.

Box 6.4

NEURAL CREST CELLS

Neural crest cells are migratory cells that originate in the dorsal region neural fold throughout the length of the embryo. They have many important functions including the formation of pigment cells, enteric glial cells and the adrenal medulla. Cranial neural crest cells make major contributions to the facial skeleton, the musculature and the outflow tract of the heart. Much of the mesenchyme of the pharyngeal arches is of neural crest origin. Several human conditions are the result of failure of normal migration of neural crest cells. One of the best studied of these is Waardenburg syndrome which is characterized by sensorineural deafness, heterochromasia (different-coloured eyes), Hirschsprung's disease and patchy depigmentation of the skin (Fig. 6.16). The same condition can be caused by mutations in two different transcription factors *PAX3* and *MITF*, which appear to be critical to neural crest cell survival in the embryo.

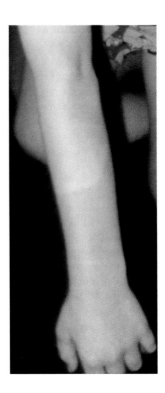

Fig. 6.16 **Neural crest cell migration.** Neural crest cells have many important functions including the formation of pigment cells, enteric glial cells and the adrenal medulla. Failure of normal migration of these cells is associated with patchy depigmentation of the skin.

Rapid division of cells under this apical ectodermal ridge results in paired limb buds (the lower limb bud is visible by 28 GD). These limb buds elongate and a terminal hand plate becomes apparent by 33 GD. By 41 GD finger rays can be seen. The fingers are then formed by a remarkable process of apoptosis, or programmed cell death, in the interdigital spaces (Fig. 6.17). Failure of this process results in syndactyly. The molecular signals that pattern the hand plate are reminiscent of those that pattern the neural tube, as well as other structures in the embryo (Box 6.3). Failure of this patterning can lead to polydactyly (Fig. 6.18).

The cells that form the muscle of the trunk and the limbs are also patterned and migrate from the paraxial mesoderm of the somites. Their fate is determined by their somite of origin. Other tissue derived from the paraxial mesoderm include the vertebrae and the dermis.

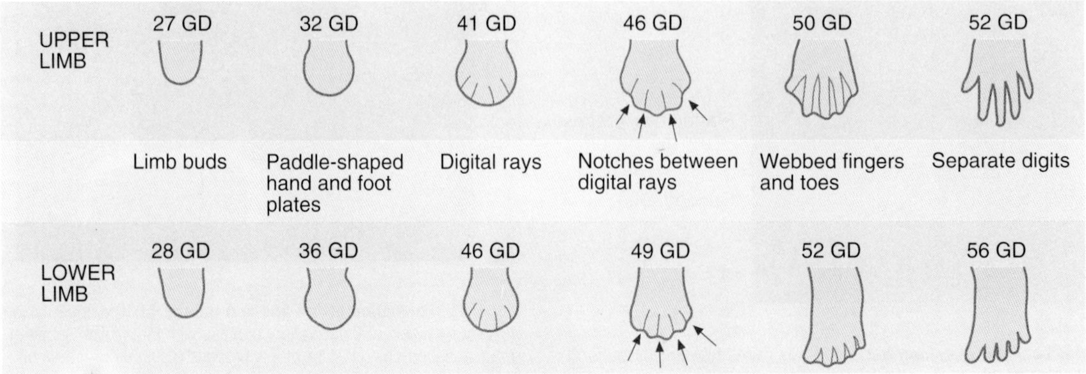

UPPER LIMB
27 GD
32 GD
41 GD
46 GD
50 GD
52 GD
Limb buds
Paddle-shaped hand and foot plates
Digital rays
Notches between digital rays
Webbed fingers and toes
Separate digits
LOWER LIMB
28 GD
36 GD
46 GD
49 GD
52 GD
56 GD

Fig. 6.17 **The development of the hands and feet between the fourth and eighth week.**

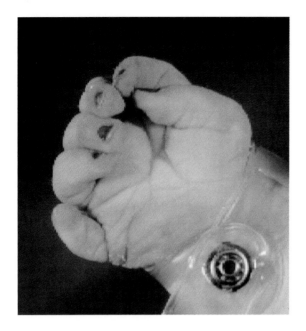

Key point

● Embryology is a fascinating subject and it can be very helpful when learning normal human anatomy. It becomes vital when trying to understand, prevent or treat birth defects.

Fig. 6.18 **Extra digit (polydactyly).** This results from the failure of normal pattern formation in the hand plate.

Introduction

A thorough understanding of pelvic anatomy is essential for clinical practice. Not only does it facilitate an understanding of the process of labour, it also allows an appreciation of the mechanisms of sexual function and reproduction, and establishes a background to the understanding of gynaecological pathology. Congenital abnormalities are discussed in Chapter 9.

Obstetric anatomy

The bony pelvis

The girdle of bones formed by the sacrum and the two innominate bones has several important functions (Fig. 7.1). It supports the weight of the upper body, and transmits the stresses of weight bearing to the lower limbs via the acetabula. It provides firm attachments for the supporting tissues of the pelvic floor, including the sphincters of the lower bowel and bladder, and it forms the bony margins of the birth canal, accommodating the passage of the fetus during labour.

The birth canal is bounded by the true pelvis, i.e. that part of the bony girdle which lies below the pelvic brim – the lower parts of the two innominate bones and the sacrum. These bones are bound together at the sacro-iliac joints, and at the symphysis pubis anteriorly. The brim is outlined by the promontory of the sacrum, the sacral alae, the iliopectineal lines, and the symphysis.

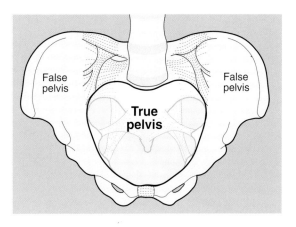

Fig. 7.1 **The 'true' and 'false' pelvis.**

The pelvic outlet is bounded by bone and ligament including the tip of the sacrum, the sacrotuberous ligaments, the ischial tuberosities, and the subpubic arch (of rounded 'Norman' shape) formed by the fused rami of the ischial and pubic bones. In the erect posture the pelvic brim is inclined at an angle of 65–70° to the horizontal. Because of the curvature of the sacrum, the axis of the pelvis (the pathway of descent of the fetal head in labour) is a J-shaped curve (Fig. 43.4).

The change in the cross-sectional shape of the birth canal at different levels is fundamentally important in understanding the mechanics of labour. The canal can be envisaged initially as a sector of a curved cylinder of about 12 cm diameter (Fig. 7.2). The stresses of weight bearing at the brim level in the average woman tend to flatten the inlet a little, reducing the anteroposterior diameter, but increasing the transverse diameter. In the lower pelvis, the counterpressure through the necks of the femora tends to compress the pelvis from the sides, reducing the transverse diameters of this part of the pelvis (Figs 43.2 and 43.3). At an intermediate level, opposite the third segment of the sacrum, the canal retains a circular cross-section. With this picture in mind, the 'average' diameters of the pelvis at brim, cavity, and outlet levels can be readily understood (Table 7.1).

The distortions from a circular cross-section, however, are very modest. If, in circumstances of malnutrition or metabolic bone disease, the consolidation of bone is impaired, more gross distortion of pelvic shape is liable to occur, and labour is likely to involve mechanical difficulty (see p. 428). This is termed cephalopelvic disproportion. The changing cross-sectional shape of the true pelvis at different levels – transverse oval at the brim

Table 7.1
Average pelvic diameters

Level	Diameter	
	Direction	Size
Inlet	Anteroposterior	11.5 cm
	Transverse	13 cm
Cavity	All diameters	12 cm
Outlet	Anteroposterior	12.5 cm
	Transverse intertuberous	11 cm
	Interspinous	10.5 cm

and anteroposterior oval at the outlet – usually determines a fundamental feature of labour, i.e. that the ovoid fetal head enters the brim with its longer (anteroposterior) diameter in a transverse or oblique position, but rotates during descent to bring the longer head diameter into the longer anteroposterior diameter of the outlet before the time of birth. This rotation is necessary because of the relatively large size of the human fetal head at term, which reflects the unique size and development of the fetal brain (Fig. 48.1).

In most affluent countries, marked pelvic deformation is rare. Pelvimetry using X-rays, CT, or MRI scans can be used to measure the pelvic diameters but is of limited clinical value in predicting the likelihood of a successful vaginal delivery. Mechanical difficulty in labour is assessed by close observation of the progress of dilatation of the cervix, and of descent, assessed by both abdominal and vaginal examination.

The pelvic organs during pregnancy

The uterus

The uterus is a remarkable organ, composed largely of smooth muscle, the myometrium, which increases in weight during pregnancy from about 40 g to around 1000 g as the myometrial muscle fibres undergo both hyperplasia and hypertrophy (Fig. 7.3). It provides a 'protected' implantation site for the genetically 'foreign' fertilized ovum, accommodates the developing fetus as it grows, and finally expels it into the outside world during labour.

Whereas the body of the uterus is formed from a thick layer of plain muscle, the cervix, which communicates with the upper vagina, is largely composed of denser collagenous tissue. This forms a rigid collar, retaining the fetus in utero as the myometrium hypertrophies and stretches. The junctional area between the body and cervix is known as the isthmus which, in late pregnancy and labour, undergoes dilatation and thinning, forming the lower segment of the uterus. It is through this thinned area that the uterine wall is incised during caesarean section.

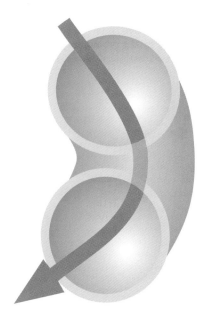

Fig. 7.2 **The birth canal resembles a curved cylinder.**

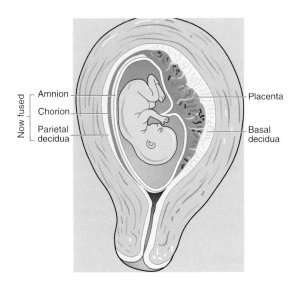

Now fused

Amnion
Chorion
Parietal decidua

Placenta

Basal decidua

Fig. 7.3 **The uterus and developing fetus at 12 weeks' gestation.**

The uterine arteries, branches of the anterior division of the internal iliac arteries, become tortuous and coiled within the uterine wall (Fig. 7.4). Innervation of the uterus is derived from both sympathetic and parasympathetic systems, and the functional significance of the motor pathways is incompletely understood. Drugs which stimulate alpha-adrenergic receptors activate the myometrium, whereas beta-adrenergic drugs have an inhibitory effect, and both beta-agonists and alpha-antagonists have been used in attempts to inhibit premature labour (see p. 378). Afferent fibres from the cervix enter the cord via the pelvic splanchnic (para-sympathetic) nerves (S2,3,4). Pain stimuli during labour from the fundus and body of the uterus travel via the hypogastric (sympathetic) plexus, and enter the cord at the level of the lower thoracic segments.

The cervix

This becomes more vascular and softens in early pregnancy. The mucous secretion from the endocervical glands becomes thick and tenacious, forming a mechanical barrier to ascending infection. In late pregnancy the cervix 'ripens' – the dense mesh of collagen fibres loosens, as fluid is taken up by the hydrophilic mucopolysaccharides which occupy the interstices between the collagen bundles. This allows the cervix to become shorter as its upper part expands.

Additional changes

The ligaments of the sacroiliac and symphyseal joints become more extensible under the influence of pregnancy hormones. As a result the pelvic girdle has more 'give' during labour. The increased mobility of the joints may result in backache or symphyseal pain.

The urinary tract in pregnancy

Frequency of micturition is often noticed in early pregnancy. As pregnancy advances the ureters become dilated, probably due to the relaxing effect of progesterone on the smooth muscle wall, but also in part to the mechanical effects of the gravid uterus. The urinary tract is therefore more vulnerable to ascending infection (acute pyelonephritis) in comparison to non-pregnancy.

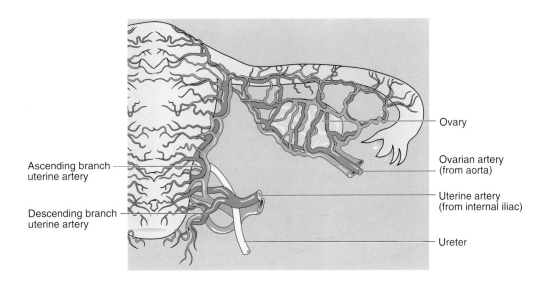

Ascending branch uterine artery

Descending branch uterine artery

Ovary

Ovarian artery (from aorta)

Uterine artery (from internal iliac)

Ureter

Fig. 7.4 **The blood supply of the uterus, fallopian tube and ovary (posterior view).**

The perineum

This term usually refers to the area of skin between the vaginal orifice and the anus. The underlying musculature at the outlet of the pelvis, surrounding the lower vagina and the anal canal, is important in the maintenance of bowel and urinary continence, and in sexual response. The muscles intermesh to form a firm pyramidal support, the perineal body, between the lower third of the posterior vaginal wall and the anal canal (Fig. 7.5). The tissues of the perineal body are often markedly stretched during the expulsive second stage of labour and may be torn as the head is delivered. Injury to the anal sphincters may lead to impaired anal continence of faeces and/or flatus. Poor healing of an episiotomy or tear is liable to result in scarring, which may cause dyspareunia (pain during intercourse).

Anatomical points for obstetric analgesia

Pudendal nerve block

Knowledge of the pudendal nerves is important in obstetrics because they may be blocked to minimize pain during instrumental delivery, and because their integrity is vital for visceral muscular support and for sphincter function. These nerves, which innervate the vulva and perineum, are derived from the 2nd, 3rd and 4th sacral roots (Fig. 46.2). On each side the nerve passes behind the sacrospinous ligament close to the tip of the ischial spine, and re-enters the pelvis along with the pudendal blood vessels in the pudendal canal. After giving off an inferior rectal branch, they divide into the perineal nerves and the dorsal nerves of the clitoris. Motor fibres of the pudendal nerve supply the levator ani, the superficial and deep perineal muscles, and the voluntary urethral sphincter. Sensory fibres innervate the central areas of the vulva and perineum. The peripheral skin areas are supplied by branches of the ilioinguinal nerve, the genitofemoral nerve, and the posterior femoral cutaneous nerve (Fig. 7.6). The pudendal nerve can be blocked by an injection of local anaesthetic injected just below the tip of the ischial spine as described on page 421.

Spinal block

The spinal cord ends at the level of L1–2. A spinal injection at the level of the L3–4 space will produce excellent analgesia up to around the level of the T10 nerve root or above depending on the position of the patient and the volume of local anaesthetic used.

Epidural block

The epidural space, between the dura and the periosteum and ligaments of the spinal canal, is about 4 mm deep. Epidural injection of local anaesthetic blocks the spinal nerve roots as they traverse the space.

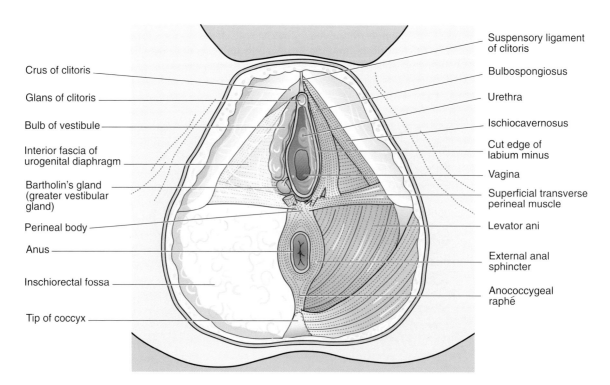

Crus of clitoris
Glans of clitoris
Bulb of vestibule
Interior fascia of urogenital diaphragm
Bartholin's gland (greater vestibular gland)
Perineal body
Anus
Inschiorectal fossa
Tip of coccyx

Suspensory ligament of clitoris
Bulbospongiosus
Urethra
Ischiocavernosus
Cut edge of labium minus
Vagina
Superficial transverse perineal muscle
Levator ani
External anal sphincter
Anococcygeal raphé

Fig. 7.5 **The perineum.** A view from below the pelvic outlet showing the intermeshing muscles.

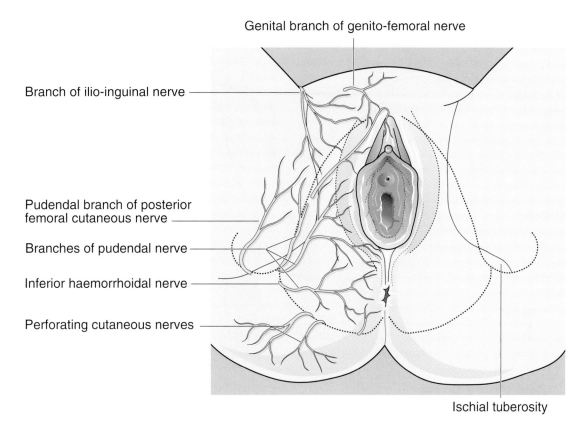

Genital branch of genito-femoral nerve

Branch of ilio-inguinal nerve

Pudendal branch of posterior femoral cutaneous nerve

Branches of pudendal nerve

Inferior haemorrhoidal nerve

Perforating cutaneous nerves

Ischial tuberosity

Fig. 7.6 **Innervation of the vulva.**

Gynaecological anatomy

The uterus

The uterus has the shape of a slightly flattened pear, and measures $7.5 \times 5.0 \times 2.5$ cm. Its principal named parts are the fundus, the cornua, the body, and the cervix (Fig. 7.7).

It forms part of the genital tract, lying in close proximity to the urinary tract anteriorly, and the lower bowel behind. All three tracts traverse the pelvic floor in the hiatus between the two bellies of the levator ani muscle. Clinically this means that a problem in one tract can readily affect another (Fig. 7.8).

The uterine cavity is around 6 or 7 cm in length, and forms a flattened slit, with the anterior and posterior walls in virtual contact. The wall has three layers: the endometrium (innermost); the myometrium; and the peritoneum (outermost).

Endometrium

The endometrium is the epithelial lining of the cavity. The surface consists of a single layer of columnar ciliated cells, with invaginations forming uterine mucus-secreting glands within a cellular stroma. It undergoes

cyclical changes in both the glands and stroma, leading to shedding and renewal about every 28 days.

There are two layers – a superficial functional layer which is shed monthly, and a basal layer which is not shed, and from which the new functional layer is regenerated. The epithelium of the functional layer shows active proliferative changes after a menstrual period until ovulation occurs, when the endometrial glands undergo secretory changes. Permanent destruction of the basal layer will result in amenorrhoea. This fact forms the basis for ablative techniques for the treatment of menorrhagia.

The normal changes in endometrial histology during the menstrual cycle, described on page 121, are determined by changing secretion of ovarian steroid hormones. If the endometrium is exposed to sustained oestrogenic stimulation, whether endogenous or exogenous, it may become hyperplastic. Benign hyperplasia may precede malignant change.

Myometrium

The smooth muscle fibres of the uterine wall do not form distinct layers. While the outermost fibres are predominantly longitudinal, continuous with the musculature of

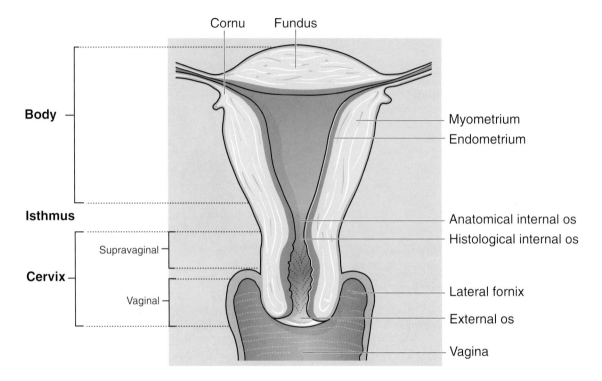

Fig. 7.7 **Coronal section of the uterus.**

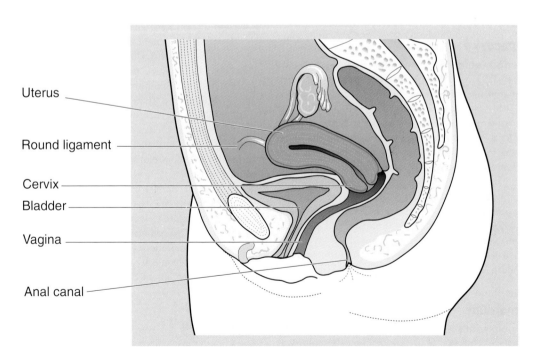

Fig. 7.8 **Female pelvic organs: sagittal view.**

the uterine tubes above and the vaginal wall below, the main thickness of the uterine wall is formed from a mesh of criss-crossing spiral strands, The individual muscle cells contain filaments of actin and myosin, which interact to generate contractions. During labour the propagation of contractile excitation throughout the uterine wall is facilitated by the formation of 'gap-junctions' between adjacent muscle cells. As a result, the spread of excitation resembles that in a syncytium.

Peritoneum

The posterior surface of the uterus is completely covered by peritoneum, which passes down over the posterior fornix of the vagina into the pouch of Douglas. Anteriorly the peritoneum is reflected off the uterus at a much higher level onto the superior surface of the bladder.

The cervix

The cervix connects the uterus and vagina, and projects into the upper vagina. The 'gutter' surrounding this projection comprises the vaginal fornices – lateral, anterior and posterior. The cervix is about 2.5 cm long; the shorter part of it, which lies above the fornices, is termed the supravaginal part. The endocervical canal is fusiform in shape between the external and internal os. After childbirth the external os loses its circular shape and resembles a transverse slit. The epithelial lining of the canal is a columnar mucous membrane with an anterior and posterior longitudinal ridge, from which shallow palmate folds extend; hence the name arbor vitae.

There are numerous glands secreting mucus, which becomes more abundant and less viscous at the time of ovulation in mid-cycle. The vaginal surface of the cervix is covered with stratified squamous epithelium, similar to that lining the vagina. The squamocolumnar junction (histological external os) commonly does not correspond to the anatomical os, but may lie either above or external to the anatomical os. This 'tidal zone', within which the epithelial junction migrates at different stages of life, is termed the transformation zone. The ebb and flow of the squamocolumnar junction is influenced by oestrogenic stimulation. In the newborn female, and in pregnancy particularly, outgrowth of the columnar epithelium is very common, forming a bright pink 'rosette' around the external os. This appearance has been misnamed an 'erosion', but the epithelial covering, though delicate, is intact. In cases where the cervix has undergone deep bilateral laceration during childbirth, the resulting anterior and posterior lips tend to evert, exposing the glandular epithelium of the canal widely. This appearance is termed ectropion.

Clinical aspects

The transformation zone is typically the area where precancerous change occurs. This can be detected by microscopic assessment of a cervical cytological smear. If the duct of a cervical gland becomes occluded, the gland distends with mucus to form a retention cyst (or Nabothian follicle). Multiple follicles are not uncommon, giving the cervix an irregular nodular feel and appearance. The body of the uterus is usually angled forward in relation to the cervix (anteflexion), while the uterus and cervix as a whole lean forward from the upper vagina (anteversion). In about 15% of women the uterus leans backwards towards the sacrum, and is described as retroverted. The cervical os then faces down the long axis of the vagina, rather than at right angles to it. In most instances retroversion is an asymptomatic variant of normality.

It is especially important to distinguish retroversion from anteversion before introducing a sound or similar instrument into the uterine cavity, to avoid perforation of the uterine wall. After the menopause the uterus and cervix gradually become atrophic, and cervical mucus is scanty. The amount of cervix projecting into the vagina also diminishes.

Because the uterus lies immediately behind the bladder, and between the lower parts of the ureters, particular care must be taken not to damage these structures during hysterectomy (Fig. 7.9). The endometrium and uterine cavity can be examined by hysteroscopy. The tubal ostia can be seen (Fig. 7.10). Because the anterior and posterior walls are normally in contact, the cavity must be inflated with gas or fluid to obtain an adequate view of the surfaces.

The uterine attachments and supports

Structures attached to the uterus include (Fig. 7.11a,b):

- round ligament
- ovarian ligament
- uterosacral ligament or fold
- cardinal ligament/transverse cervical ligament (of Mackenrodt).

The broad ligament is merely a double fold of peritoneum extending laterally from the uterus towards the pelvic sidewall. The hilum of the ovary arises from its posterior surface. The portion of the fold lateral to the ovary and tube is termed the infundibulopelvic ligament. Between the leaves of this fold, the uterine and ovarian blood vessels form an anastomotic loop. The ovarian ligament forms a ridge on the posterior leaf of the broad ligament, from the cornu of the uterus to the medial pole of the ovary. Developmentally it is part of the gubernaculum of the ovary, in continuity with the round ligament, which curves round anteriorly from the cornu towards the inguinal canal, through which

Fundus of anteverted uterus

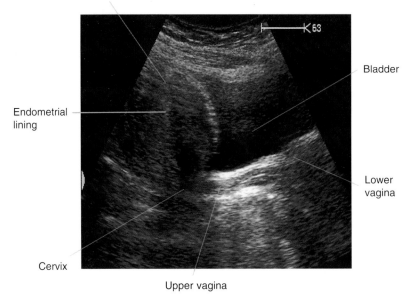

Endometrial
lining

Bladder

Lower
vagina

Cervix

Upper vagina

Fig. 7.9 **Transabdominal scan of the bladder, uterus and vagina.**

it passes. The uterosacral ligaments pass upwards and backwards from the posterior aspect of the cervix towards the lateral part of the second piece of the sacrum. In their lower part they contain plain muscle along with fibrous tissue and autonomic nerve fibres. In their upper part they dwindle to shallow peritoneal folds. The ligaments divide the pouch of Douglas from the pararectal fossa on each side.

The main ligaments providing support to the internal genital organs are the cardinal ligaments. The traditional name 'transverse cervical ligaments' is a misnomer. The cardinal ligaments are essentially dense condensations of connective tissue around the venous

and nerve plexuses and arterial vessels which extend from the pelvic sidewall towards the genital tract. Medially they are firmly fused with the fascia surrounding the cervix and upper part of the vagina. They pass upwards and backwards towards the root of the internal iliac vessels. These condensations of fibrous and elastic tissue, together with plain muscle fibres, are sometimes referred to as the parametrium. They support the upper vagina and cervix, helping to maintain the angle between the axis of the vagina and that of the anteverted uterus. Inferiorly they are continuous with the fascia on the upper surface of the levator muscles.

The pelvic diaphragm

Below the level of the cardinal ligaments, the pelvic organs are supported by a sloping shelf of muscle on each side, formed by the levator ani muscle (Fig. 7.12). The disposition of the muscle bundles is comparable to that of the abdominal musculature. Near to the midline there is a longitudinal muscle bundle, the puborectalis (cf. the rectus abdominis). Laterally the muscle sheets (iliococcygeus and ischiococcygeus) are oblique/transverse. The most medial fibres of puborectalis are inserted into the upper part of the perineal body. The succeeding fibres turn medially behind the anorectal flexure, and are inserted into the anococcygeal raphe and the tip of the coccyx, along with the fibres of ilio- and ischiococcygeus. Thus all three visceral tubes reach the body surface via a hiatus between the medial margins of puborectalis, and all are supported from behind by the sling action of the muscle when it con-

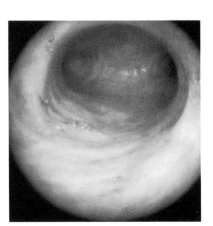

Fig. 7.10 **Normal hysteroscopic view of the endometrial cavity, showing both tubal osteae.**

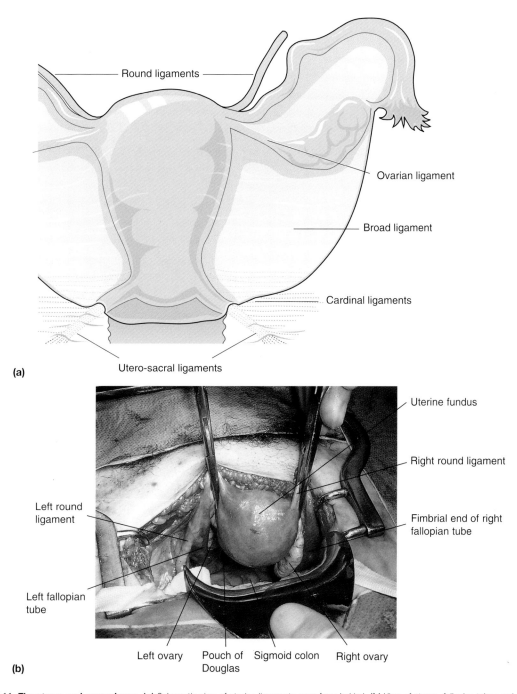

(a)

(b)

Fig. 7.11 **The uterus and appendages. (a)** Schematic view of uterine ligaments seen from behind. **(b)** View of uterus, fallopian tubes and ovaries at abdominal hysterectomy.

tracts. Innervation is from the pudendal nerve (S2,3,4). The fascia on the upper surface of the pelvic diaphragm blends with the lower part of the cardinal ligaments. The fascia on the inferior surface of levator ani forms the roof of the ischiorectal fossa.

The main blood supply of the uterus is from the uterine arteries, which are branches of the internal iliac vessels (Fig. 7.13). Each passes medially in the base of the broad ligament above the ureter, and ascends along the lateral aspect of the uterus, forming an anastomotic

Fundamentals

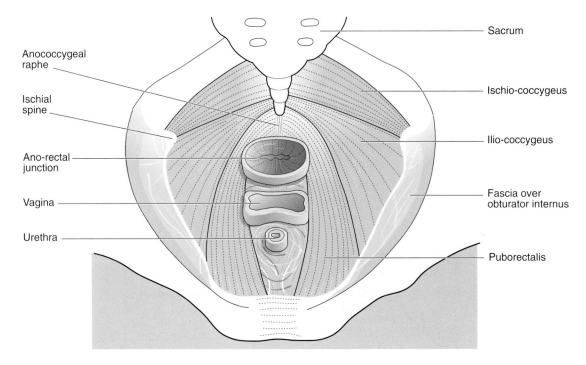

Fig. 7.12 **The urogenital diaphragm from above.**

Sacrum

Anococcygeal raphe

Ischial spine

Ano-rectal junction

Vagina

Urethra

Ischio-coccygeus

Ilio-coccygeus

Fascia over obturator internus

Puborectalis

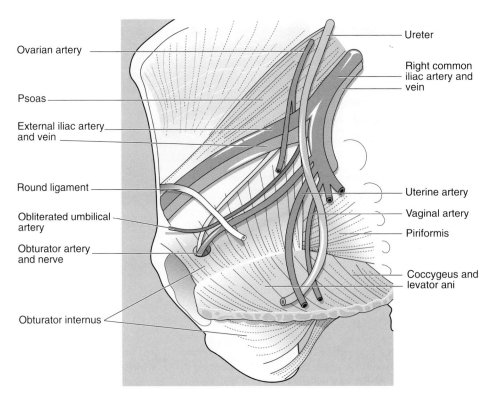

Ovarian artery

Psoas

External iliac artery and vein

Round ligament

Obliterated umbilical artery

Obturator artery and nerve

Obturator internus

Ureter

Right common iliac artery and vein

Uterine artery

Vaginal artery

Piriformis

Coccygeus and levator ani

Fig. 7.13 **The lateral pelvic sidewall.**

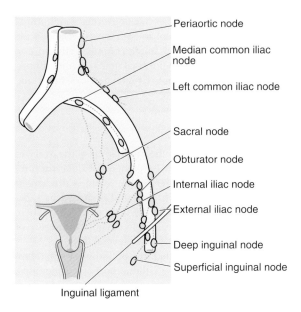

Periaortic node

Median common iliac node

Left common iliac node

Sacral node

Obturator node

Internal iliac node

External iliac node

Deep inguinal node

Superficial inguinal node

Inguinal ligament

Fig. 7.14 **Lymphatic drainage of the uterus.** The lymph channels follow the blood supply.

loop in the broad ligament with the ovarian artery, below the uterine tube (see Fig. 7.4). The uterine veins form a plexus in the parametrium below the uterine arteries, draining into the internal iliac veins. The principal lymph drainage is to iliac and obturator glands on the pelvic sidewall. From the fundus and cornua lymph drains via the ovarian pathway to aortic nodes, while a few lymphatics in the round ligaments drain into the inguinal nodes (Fig. 7.14). The uterus is supplied by sympathetic and parasympathetic nerves, the exact functional significance of which is uncertain.

Congenital abnormalities of the uterus

Most of the female genital tract develops from the two paramesonephric (Müllerian) ducts, the caudal portions of which approximate in the midline and fuse to form the uterus, cervix, and upper part of the vagina. The upper divergent portions of the ducts form the uterine tubes.

Congenital abnormality can result from:

● failure of or incomplete fusion
● failure of canalization
● asymmetrical maldevelopment.

The diagrams in Figure 9.4 (p. 111) illustrate some of abnormalities which may be encountered. Failures of canalization are likely to present at puberty as menstrual blood has no way to escape (p. 128). Incomplete fusion is associated with late miscarriage, preterm labour, and malpresentation. Because of the intimate association during development, congenital abnormality of the

female genital tract is commonly associated with abnormality of the urinary tract.

The vulva

The term vulva generally encompasses all the external female genitalia, i.e. the mons pubis, the labia majora and minora, the clitoris, and the structures within the vestibule – the external urinary meatus and the hymen. The mons pubis is a thickened pad of fat, cushioning the pubic bones anteriorly. The labia majora contain fatty tissue overlying the vascular bulbs of the vestibule and the bulbospongiosus muscles. The skin of the labia majora bears secondary sexual hair on the lateral surfaces only. There are abundant sebaceous, sweat, and apocrine glands. The folds of the labia minora vary considerably in size, and may be concealed by the labia majora or may project between them. They contain no fat, but are vascular and erectile during sexual arousal; the skin contains many sebaceous glands. Anteriorly the folds bifurcate before uniting to form a hood above the clitoris and a frenulum along its dorsal surface. Posteriorly the labia minora are linked by a fine ridge of skin, the fourchette.

The labia minora and the fourchette form the boundaries of the vestibule. Between the fourchette and the posterior part of the hymen there is a crescentic furrow termed the navicular fossa. The urethral meatus lies within the vestibule, close to the anterior margin of the vaginal orifice. There are pairs of small mucus-secreting paraurethral glands in the lower part of the posterior wall of the urethra. These rudimentary tubules are homologous with the glands in the male prostate. If they become infected and blocked, they may form a paraurethral abscess, cyst, or urethral diverticulum. Two mucus-secreting glands, known as Bartholin's glands (or greater vestibular glands), lie posterolateral to the vaginal orifice on each side, embedded in the posterior pole of the vascular vestibular bulb (see Fig. 7.5). Their ducts open near the lateral limits of the navicular fossa. The glands only become palpable, and the duct orifices become visible, if infection is present.

Blood supply

The main sources of the vascularity of the vulva are branches of the internal pudendal arteries. There are also branches from the superficial and deep external pudendal arteries.

Nerve supply

The main sensory supply to the vulva is via the pudendal nerves. Peripheral parts of the vulvar skin are supplied by filaments from the iliohypogastric and ilioinguinal nerves, and from the perineal branches of the posterior cutaneous nerves of the thigh (see Fig. 7.6).

Fundamentals

The pudendal nerve provides motor fibres to all the muscles of the perineum, including the voluntary urinary and bowel sphincters, as well as the levator ani.

Lymph drainage

The main pathway of drainage is to the superficial inguinal glands, and on through the deep inguinal to the external iliac glands. Some lymphatics from the deeper structures of the vulva pass with vaginal lymphatics to the internal iliac nodes.

The fallopian tubes

The tube extends on each side from the cornu of the uterus within the upper border of the broad ligament for about 10 cm. The tubes and ovaries together are commonly described as the uterine appendages, or adnexa (Fig. 7.15).

The tube can be divided into four parts (Fig. 7.16). The interstitial (intramural) part forms a narrow passage through the thickness of the myometrium. The isthmus, extending out from the cornu for about 3 cm, is also narrow. The ampulla is thin-walled, 'baggy', and tortuous; its lateral portion is free from the broad ligament, and droops down behind it towards the ovary. Near its lateral limit the abdominal ostium is constricted, but opens out again to form the infundibulum. This trumpet-shaped expansion is fringed by a ring of delicate fronds (or fimbriae), one of which is attached to the surface of the ovary.

The walls of the tubes include outer longitudinal and inner circular layers of smooth muscle. The delicate lining (endosalpinx), containing columnar ciliated and secretory cells, has longitudinal folds in the isthmic segment, which change into a highly intricate branching pattern in the ampulla.

Tubal function

At the time of ovulation the fimbriae clasp the ovary in the area where the stigma (or point of follicular rupture) is forming. Usually, therefore, the ovum is discharged into the infundibulum (funnel) and is carried by tubal peristalsis into the ampulla of the tube, which is where fertilization occurs. Transit of the zygote to the site of implantation in the uterus takes several days.

Sterilization is effected by occluding both tubes, preferably in the narrow isthmic portion, using clips, sutures, rings, or diathermy.

Patency of the tubes can be tested by injecting a watery dye (methylthioninium chloride (methylene blue)) through the cervix, and observing spill from the abdominal ostia by laparoscopy. The contours of the uterine cavity and tubal lumen may be demonstrated with radio-opaque fluid during a hysterosalpingogram.

The vagina

The vagina, which links the external and internal parts of the female genital tract, has a dual function: it forms the coital canal, affording access for spermatozoa

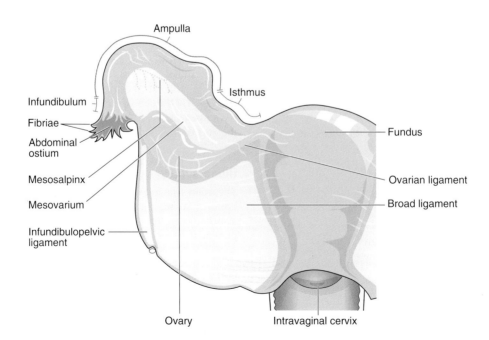

Fig. 7.15 **Posterior view of the uterus and broad ligament.**

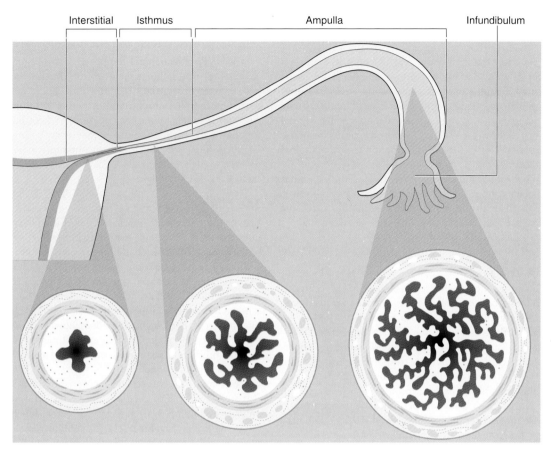

Fig. 7.16 **The oviduct, showing the structure of the mucosal layer.**

to reach the cervix and, with the cervix, it forms the soft-tissue birth canal. It lies in close proximity to the urethra and bladder anteriorly, and to the anal canal and rectum posteriorly. All three canals traverse the pelvic floor, passing between the medial (puborectalis) portions of the levator ani muscles. The insertion of these muscle fibres into the anococcygeal raphe creates a sling behind the bowel so that, at the junction of the lower rectum and the anal canal, a sharp angle is created which is opened when the muscle relaxes. Other muscle fibres are inserted into the perineal body near its apex, creating a similar sling which angulates the axis of the vagina at that level. In turn, the anterior vaginal wall in the area of the bladder neck receives support.

There are differences in the anatomy of the vagina above and below this level. The lower third of the vagina is closely invested by the superficial and deep muscles of the perineum. It:

- incorporates the urethra in its anterior wall
- is separated from the bowel by the perineal body
- has a rich arterial blood supply from branches of the vaginal arteries, and from both external and internal pudendal vessels.

The upper two-thirds of the vagina, above the levator shelf:

- is not invested by muscles, but is wide and capacious
- is in apposition with the bladder base anteriorly, and with the rectum (and, above that, the pouch of Douglas) posteriorly
- is supported laterally and at the vault by the parametrium (cardinal and uterosacral ligaments). During sexual arousal the smooth muscle fibres within the parametrium elevate the vaginal vault and cervix, thereby elongating the vagina, and straightening its long axis.

Vaginal structure

The vaginal walls form an elastic fibromuscular tube with a multilayered structure. The lining of stratified squamous epithelium is corrugated into transverse folds (or rugae), which facilitates stretching during child birth. The epithelium contains no glands, but during the reproductive years the more superficial cells contain abundant glycogen. This polysaccharide is broken down by lactobacilli which form the normal flora of the vagina, producing lactic acid. This accounts for the low pH in the vaginal lumen (average pH 4.5).

Between the epithelium and the muscle there is a layer of areolar tissue containing an extensive venous plexus. Vascular engorgement during sexual arousal, analogous to erection in the male, is most marked in the lower part of the vagina, encroaching on the vaginal lumen as the rugae distend. The vasocongestive response also results in increased transudation into the vaginal lumen.

The smooth muscle layers (outer longitudinal, inner circular) are not distinct, and an interlacing pattern is usual. Deep to the muscle there is another extensive plexus of veins, within the outer vaginal fascia.

The ovary

The ovaries are attached on each side to the posterior surface of the broad ligaments through a narrowed base termed the hilum. The ovaries are also attached to the cornua of the uterus by the ovarian ligaments. Developmentally these are the upper portions of the gubernacula ovarii, and they are responsible for drawing the ovaries down into the pelvis from the posterior wall of the abdominal cavity. Typically, each ovary lies in an ovarian fossa, a shallow peritoneal depression lateral to the ureter, near the pelvic sidewall. The position may vary, however, and when the uterus is retroverted, one or both ovaries may lie in the pouch of Douglas.

The ovaries are ovoid in shape, with an irregular surface and a firm, largely solid, stroma which can be divided indistinctly into an outer cortex and an inner medulla. The surface epithelium of cuboidal coelomic cells forms an incomplete layer, beneath which is a fibrous investment – the tunica albuginea. The germ cells from which the ova are derived are embedded in the substance of the ovaries.

The ovarian blood vessels and nerves enter through the hilum from the broad ligament. The ovarian arteries are direct branches of the aorta. Within the broad ligaments they form an anastomotic loop with branches of the uterine arteries.

Anatomy of the lower urinary tract

The descending ureters are narrow thick-walled muscular tubes which cross into the pelvis close to the bifurcation of the common iliac arteries. They lie immediately under the peritoneum of the pelvic sidewall, behind the lateral attachment of the broad ligaments. Curving medially and forwards, they pass through the base of the broad ligaments below the uterine arteries, about 2 cm lateral to the supravaginal part of the cervix, a short distance above the lateral fornices of the vagina.

Approaching the bladder, the ureters pass medially in front of the upper vagina, and enter the bladder base obliquely at the upper angles of the trigone.

The wall of the ureter is composed of three elements: an external fibrous sheath, layers of smooth muscle, and a lining of transitional epithelium. There may be partial or complete duplication of one or both ureters. An ectopic ureter is one that opens anywhere but the trigone of the bladder, and this may even be into the vagina or the vestibule. Urinary incontinence inevitably results.

The bladder

The urinary reservoir, lined with transitional epithelium, has the shape of a tetrahedron when empty, but the mesh of smooth muscle in the bladder wall can readily distend to contain a volume of half a litre or more. This muscle coat (the detrusor muscle) is thus normally relaxed and capable of considerable stretching without a contractile response. If urinary outflow during micturition is chronically impeded, however, the detrusor muscle becomes irritable and ultimately hypertrophic, producing prominent trabecular bands visible at cystoscopy.

The bladder is covered with peritoneum on its superior surface only. The peritoneum is reflected onto the anterior abdominal wall at a varying level, dependent on the degree of bladder filling. The oblique passage of the terminal part of each ureter through the bladder wall creates a one-way valve, which normally prevents urinary backflow from the bladder. This protects the kidneys from ascending infection. The triangular area within the bladder base defined by the two ureteric orifices and the internal urethral orifice is termed the trigone. Over this area the epithelium remains smooth, even when the bladder is empty.

The urethra

The female urethra is about 4 cm long. Below the bladder neck it is embedded in the anterior vaginal wall, and the smooth muscle layers of the two structures intermingle. The urethral tissues also reflect the vascularity and turgidity of the vagina itself. Many of the urethral muscle fibres near the bladder neck are longitudinal and continuous with those of the bladder above, forming a funnel which opens out when these fibres contract, flattening the angle between the bladder base and the upper urethra. There are also abundant elastic fibres at this level, whose action helps to restore urethral closure after micturition. Around the lower part of the urethra there is a fusiform collar of voluntary muscle – the external urethral sphincter. This segment of the urethra passes through the perineal membrane, which keeps it in a stable position. The upper urethra, on the other hand, shares the mobility of the bladder neck. The urethra is lined by transitional epithelium in its upper part, and by squamous epithelium below.

Nerve supply

Apart from the external sphincter, the efferent nerve supply controlling bladder function is from the pelvic parasympathetic system (S2,3,4) which provides the main motor fibres to the detrusor muscle. Afferent fibres conveying the normal sensations of bladder filling also return through the parasympathetic pathway, though some sympathetic sensory fibres convey the feelings of bladder overdistension via the hypogastric plexus. At the level of the 2nd, 3rd and 4th sacral segments of the spinal cord, the sensory and motor parasympathetic nerves form spinal reflex arcs, which are moderated by interaction with higher centres in the brain. Urinary continence depends upon a variety of factors. These include the elastic fibres surrounding the bladder neck which normally maintain urethral closure; and the tone or reflex contraction of the levator ani muscles which, through their insertion into the perineal body, elevate the urethrovesical junction, creating an angulation at the junction of the mobile (upper) and fixed (lower)

portions of the urethra. The turgidity of spongy tissue underlying the urethral epithelium also assists in occluding the urethra, as does the action of the voluntary sphincter.

Key points

- Without understanding the anatomy of the pelvis it is impossible to understand the mechanisms of labour.

- The cross-sectional shape of the birth canal is different at different levels. At the pelvic brim it is oval in shape, and the widest part of this oval is in the lateral plane from one side to the other. The outlet is also oval, with the widest part in the anteroposterior plane. The head enters the pelvic brim in the transverse position, as the inlet is widest in this plane, but rotates 90° at the pelvic floor to the anteroposterior plane before delivery. The shoulders also follow the same rotation.

History and examination

In general, history and examination cannot be divided neatly into different specialties, and questions relating to obstetrics and gynaecology should form part of the assessment of any woman presenting to any specialty. There may be embarrassment and recrimination, for example, when a suspected appendicitis turns out to be a pelvic infection secondary to an unsuspected intra-uterine contraceptive device. Similarly, not all problems presenting to obstetricians and gynaecologists are obstetrical or gynaecological in nature. It is therefore important to take a full history and perform an appropriate examination in all cases. The key points of gynaecological and obstetrical history and examination are emphasized below.

Gynaecological history

A gynaecological history should follow the usual model for history-taking with questions about the presenting complaint, its history and associated problems. It should include a past medical history and information about prescription and non-prescription drugs used and known allergies. After questions about social circumstances and activities, and family history, the history is completed with a general systemic enquiry. However, during a gynaecological history there are specific key areas to be expanded upon. These include menstrual, fertility, pelvic pain, urogynaecological and obstetric histories.

Menstrual history
The pattern of bleeding

The simple phrase *'tell me about your periods'* often elicits all the information required. The bleeding pattern of the menstrual cycle is expressed as a fraction, such that a cycle of 4/28 means the woman bleeds for 4 days every 28 days. A cycle of 4–10/21–42 means the woman bleeds for between 4 and 10 days every 21 to 42 days. Asking the shortest time between the start of successive periods, the longest time between periods and the average time between periods helps determine the cycle characteristics.

Fundamentals

Bleeding too little

Amenorrhoea is the absence of periods. Primary amenorrhoea is when someone has not started menstruating by the age of 16. Secondary amenorrhoea means that periods have been absent for longer than 6 months. Oligomenorrhoea means the periods are infrequent, with a cycle of 42 days or more.

The climacteric is the perimenopausal time when periods become less regular and are accompanied by increasing menopausal symptoms. The menopause is the time after the last ever period, and can only therefore be assessed retrospectively.

Irregular periods, oligomenorrhoea or amenorrhoea, suggest anovulation or irregular ovulation. Specific questions about weight, weight change, acne, greasy skin, hirsutism, flushes or galactorrhoea may help identify the nature of the ovarian dysfunction.

Bleeding too much

It is very difficult to find out how heavy someone's periods are. If menstrual blood loss is accurately measured, an average of 35 ml of blood is lost each period. Menorrhagia is defined as loss of more than 80 ml during regular menstruation. Some women will complain of very heavy periods with a normal blood loss while others will not complain in the presence of menorrhagia. Asking how often pads or tampons have to be changed and using pictorial charts can provide more objective information. Whether menstrual loss is excessive, however, is a largely subjective assessment.

Specific symptoms can indicate abnormally heavy menstruation. Although small pieces of tissue are normal, blood clots are not. 'Flooding' is when menstrual blood soaks through all protection. It is both abnormal and distressing. Symptoms of anaemia may also be present. A history of the menstrual cycle since menarche (the first period) can reveal changes in the bleeding pattern. However, an emphasis on the effect on lifestyle and treatments tried previously is particularly important.

Bleeding at the wrong time

It is important to ask specifically about bleeding or brown, or bloody, discharge between periods (intermenstrual bleeding (IMB)), or after intercourse (postcoital bleeding (PCB)). These symptoms can point to significant abnormalities of the cervix or uterine cavity. Postmenopausal bleeding (PMB) is defined as bleeding more than 1 year after the last period. Undiagnosed abnormal bleeding requires further investigation.

Fertility history

Last menstrual period (LMP)

This question is vital and should be followed with whether that period came at the expected time and was of normal character. As well as alerting to the possibility of pregnancy, the information is important because some investigations need to be performed at specific times of the menstrual cycle.

Contraception

It is useful to establish whether the woman is sexually active, perhaps with something like 'Are you currently in a physical sexual relationship?' and then 'Are you using any contraception at present?' A further discussion about fertility issues, unprotected intercourse and risk factors for certain diseases may be appropriate. A contraceptive history should include any problems with chosen contraceptives and why they were stopped. Questions may be followed up with 'Are you hoping for a pregnancy?' if the situation is not clear.

If there are any infertility issues, their duration and the results of any investigation or treatment may be of interest. If the woman is postmenopausal, enquiry should be made about past or current use of hormone replacement therapy and whether she has any symptoms attributable to the menopause.

Cervical smears

The date of the woman's last smear should be noted, and when it was recommended that she had her next smear. Any previous abnormalities should also be noted, and whether she has had any colposcopic investigation or treatment. If she is over 50 it may be relevant to discuss breast screening.

Pelvic pain history
Painful periods

Dysmenorrhoea is a common problem and its effects on lifestyle are important. The cramping pain of primary dysmenorrhoea is at its most intense just before and during the early stages of a period. Young women are particularly affected and the pain has usually been present from the time of the first period. It is not usually associated with structural abnormalities and may improve with age or pregnancy. Secondary dysmenorrhoea is when menstruation has not tended to be painful in the past and is slightly more likely to indicate pelvic pathology. In particular, progressive dysmenorrhoea, where the intensity of the pain increases throughout menstruation, can suggest endometriosis.

Pelvic pain

The relationship of pelvic pain to the menstrual cycle is important. Mittelschmertz is a cramping pelvic pain that can be midline or unilateral. It occurs 2 weeks before a period and is caused by ovulation. Intermittent discomfort may suggest some scarring or ovarian pathology but it is more commonly non-gynaecological. It is vital to take a urinary and lower gastrointestinal history as urinary tract infection or irritable bowel syndrome may present with pelvic pain. Any pain is likely to be worse if the person is anxious, stressed or depressed. Chronic pelvic pain is particularly affected by psychosomatic factors, and recognizing this during history-taking is important.

Pain on intercourse

There are two main types of dyspareunia, superficial and deep. They can be differentiated by asking 'Is it painful just as he begins to enter, or when he is deep inside?' Deep dyspareunia is associated with pelvic pathology such as scarring, adhesions, endometriosis or masses that restrict uterine mobility. Superficial dyspareunia can arise from local abnormalities at the introitus or from a lack of lubrication. It can also be due to a voluntary or involuntary contraction of the muscles of the pelvic floor referred to as vaginismus (see also p. 187).

Vaginal discharge

Discharge can be normal or be associated with cervical ectopy and, particularly if offensive or irritant, can indicate infection. It can also suggest neoplasia of the cervix or endometrium. Enquire about the duration, amount, colour, smell and relationship to cycle.

Urogynaecological history
Urinary incontinence

A good initial question to ask is 'Do you ever leak urine when you don't intend to?'. If so, find out what provokes it, how it affects her lifestyle and what steps she takes to avoid it. 'Do you ever not make it to the toilet in time?' can help identify urge incontinence as can a history of frequency and small volumes passed after desperation. Incontinence after exercise, coughing, laughing or straining can suggest stress incontinence. It can be difficult to differentiate stress incontinence and urge incontinence, however, as there is often a mixed picture.

Other urinary symptoms

Enquiry should be made about frequency and nocturia. If present, small volumes and an inability to interrupt the flow may suggest detrusor instability. If large volumes are passed, ask about thirst and fluid intake. A history of dysuria or haematuria may suggest bladder

infection or pathology. 'Strangury' is constant desire to pass urine and suggests urinary tract inflammation.

Prolapse

Prolapse may be associated with vaginal discomfort, a dragging sensation, the feeling of something 'coming down' and possibly backache. Although the uterus, anterior vaginal wall and posterior vaginal wall can prolapse, it is difficult to separate these by history. Bladder and bowel function should be explored, including a question about the need to digitally manipulate the vagina in order to be able to void.

Gynaecological examination

Signs of gynaecological disease are not limited to the pelvis. A full examination may reveal anaemia, pleural effusions, visual field defects or lymphadenopathy in gynaecological conditions. However, passing a speculum, taking a cervical smear and performing a bimanual pelvic examination are the key skills to master. A great deal of sensitivity is required in their use.

Passing a speculum
Preparation

The patient should empty her bladder and remove sanitary protection. The examination room should be quiet and have a private area for the patient to undress. It should contain an examination couch with a modesty sheet and good adjustable lighting. A female chaperone should always be present. The examination requires full explanation and verbal consent.

Stand on the right of the patient with gloves, speculum and lubricating gel immediately to hand. The patient should lie back, bend her knees, put her heels together and let her knees fall apart. The light should be adjusted to give a good view of the vulva and perineum and the modesty sheet should cover the patient's abdomen and thighs.

Inspection

Inspect the hair distribution and vulval skin. Hair extending towards the umbilicus and onto the inner thighs can be associated with disorders of androgen excess, as can clitoromegaly. The vulva can be a site of chronic skin conditions such as eczema and psoriasis, specific conditions such as lichen sclerosis and warts, cysts of the Bartholin's glands and cancers. Ulceration may imply herpes, syphilis, trauma or malignancy.

Look at the perineum (Fig. 8.1) and gently part the labia to inspect the introitus. Perineal scars are usually secondary to tears or episiotomy during childbirth. A

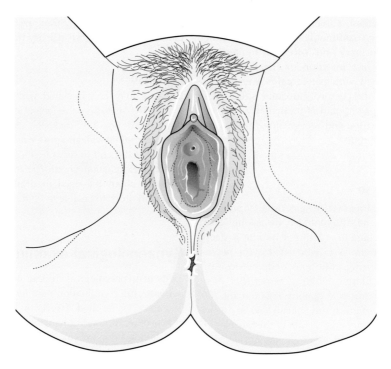

Fig. 8.1 **Inspection of the perineum.**

red papule around the urethral opening is usually a prolapsed area of urethral mucosa. A white, plaque-like discharge may suggest thrush, and pale skin with punctate red areas implies atrophic vaginitis. Asking the woman to cough may reveal demonstrable stress incontinence or the bulge of a prolapse.

Speculum examination

Disposable speculums are all one size but smaller and larger metal speculums are available if required. Ensure the speculum is warmed, working normally and lubricated with gel. Hold the speculum so that its blades are oriented in the same direction as the vaginal opening. Part the labia and slowly insert the speculum, rotating it gently until the blades are horizontal (Fig. 8.2a,b,c).

If the patient is in the lithotomy position at the edge of the couch, the speculum can be turned downwards to avoid pressure on the clitoris. If the patient is lying on the couch itself, it is usually easier to rotate the speculum upwards. It should be inserted fully in a slightly posterior direction, before firmly, but gently, opening to visualize the cervix (Fig. 8.3). The speculum can be closed a little when the cervix pops into view.

If the cervix is not visible it is often because the speculum has not been inserted far enough before opening. If this is not the case, the cervix is either above or below the blades. As most uteri are anteverted, it is usually below the blades and the speculum should be angled more posteriorly before re-opening. Otherwise, gently insert a finger to determine its position.

Inspect the vagina for atrophic vaginitis and discharge. A creamy or mucousy discharge is normal. A yellow-greenish frothy discharge is seen with *Trichomonas vaginalis* and a grey-green fishy discharge suggests bacterial vaginosis. There may be a purulent cervical discharge with gonorrhoea, and an increased mucousy discharge may occur with chlamydial cervicitis. Swabs, if required, should be taken from the vaginal fornices (high vaginal) or the cervical canal (endocervical).

The cervical os is small and round in the nulliparous and bigger and more slit-like in parous women. Threads from an IUCD may be present. Translucent lumps or cysts around the os are Nabothian follicles but warts and tumours can sometimes be seen. An ectopy is red, mucousy, epithelium of the cervical canal on the surface of the cervix. It varies across the cycle and should be looked on as normal, although it may be associated with contact bleeding or increased discharge.

The speculum should be opened further and withdrawn beyond the cervix before rotation back again and removal.

Taking a cervical smear

Smears should ideally be performed in the mid to late follicular phase and not during menstruation. Confirm the woman's details and clearly print her name and date

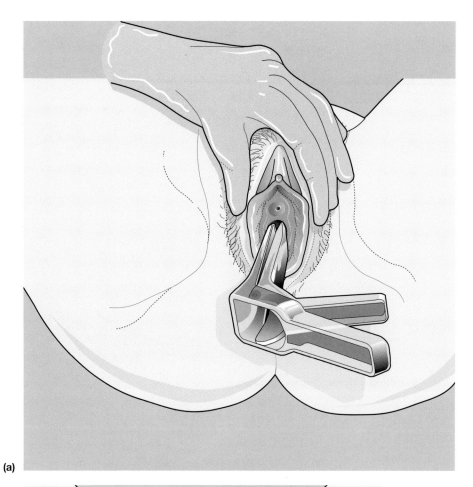

(a)

(b)

Fig. 8.2a,b **Insertion of a bivalve (Cuscoe's) speculum (Fig. 8.2c continues on next page.)**

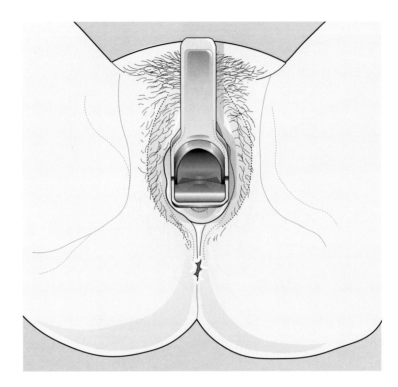

(c)

Fig. 8.2c **Insertion of a bivalve (Cuscoe's) speculum.**

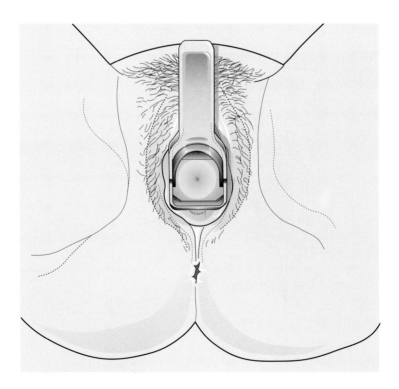

Fig. 8.3 **Visualization of the cervix.**

of birth on the frosted end of the slide with a pencil. Run the speculum under warm water to provide appropriate lubrication and visualize the cervix.

An Aylesbury spatula should be used to obtain the sample from the transformation zone in non-pregnant women. Rest the pointed tip of the spatula within the os and rotate it 360 degrees in a clockwise direction and then 360 degrees in an anticlockwise direction exerting pencil pressure and ensuring the spatula has contact with the cervix at all times (Fig. 8.4).

Quickly spread both sides of the spatula onto the slide using clean straight sweeps and place the slide immediately in the fixative (industrial methylated spirits) for between 10 and 90 minutes. High-risk specimens should be placed in a separate jar and be left in the fixative for at least 1 hour.

Complete and check the cytology request form, ensuring that all the information required is provided, and marry this to the smear for transport to the laboratory. Inform the woman how long the result will take and how it will be delivered.

A bivalve speculum holds open the vaginal walls and obscures any cystocele or rectocele. A univalve speculum can demonstrate these. The patient lies in the left-lateral position with her knees drawn up. The lubricated blade of the speculum is used to hold back the anterior vaginal wall. Coughing will show a bulge of the poste-rior wall if a rectocele is present. When the posterior wall is held back, coughing will demonstrate the bulge of a cystocele and uterine descent (Figs 8.5 and 8.6).

Pelvic examination (Fig. 8.7)

Apply lubricating gel to the gloved fingers of the right hand. Part the labia with the index and middle fingers of the left hand. Gently slip the right index finger into the vagina. If comfortable, slip the middle finger in below the index finger making room posteriorly to avoid the sensitive urethra. The cervix feels like the tip of a nose and protrudes into the top of the vagina.

Feel the cervix and record irregularities or discomfort. 'Cervical excitation' is when touching the cervix causes intense pain and it implies active pelvic inflammation. The dimple of the os can be felt and the firmness of the uterine body lies above or below the cervix. A vaginal cyst may be an embryological duct remnant, and vaginal nodules may represent endometriosis.

Assess the position of the uterus. It is usually ante-verted with the cervix posterior and the uterine body anterior. If the uterus is retroverted, the cervix is anterior and the uterine body lies posteriorly. The fingers should be manipulated behind the cervix to lift the uterus. With the left hand above the umbilicus, feel through the

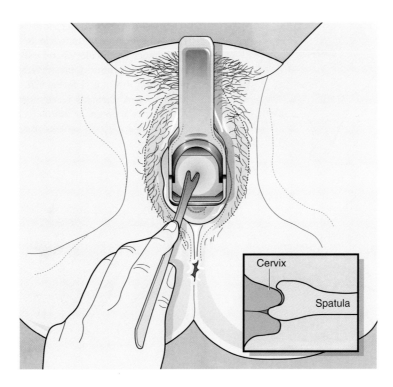

Cervix

Spatula

Fig. 8.4 **Taking a cervical smear.**

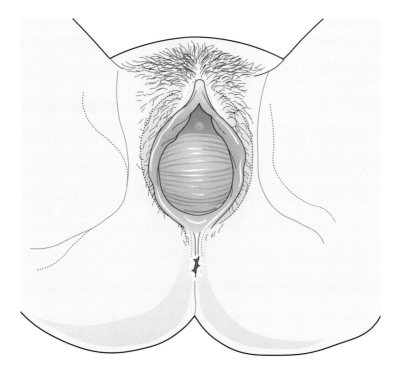

Fig. 8.5 **The bulge of a prolapse.**

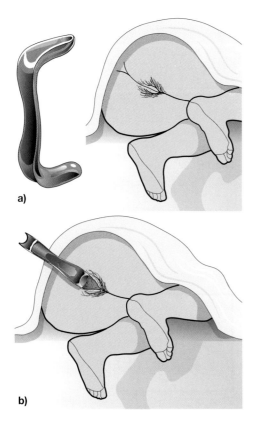

a)

b)

Fig. 8.6 **Examination with a univalve (Sims') speculum.**

abdomen for the moving uterus (Fig. 8.8). If the uterus cannot be palpated, the hand should be moved gradually down until the uterus is between the fingers.

Assess the mobility, regularity and size of the uterus. The adhesions of endometriosis, infection, surgery or malignancy fix the uterus and make bimanual examination more uncomfortable. Asymmetry of the uterus may imply fibroids. Uterine size is related to stage of pregnancy. A normally sized uterus feels like a plum. At 6 weeks a pregnant uterus feels like a tangerine, at 8 weeks an apple, at 10 weeks an orange and at 12 weeks

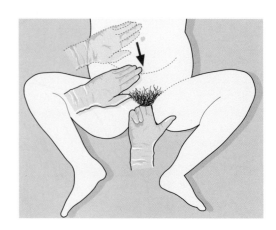

Fig. 8.7 **Digital pelvic examination.**

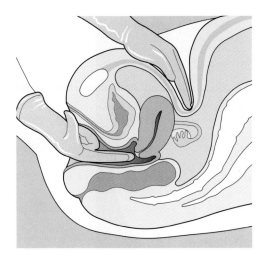

Fig. 8.8 **Bimanual examination.**

a grapefruit. At 14 weeks the uterus can be felt on abdominal palpation alone.

Feel for adnexal masses in the vaginal fornices lateral to the cervix on each side. Push up the tissues in the

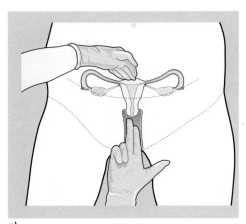

a)

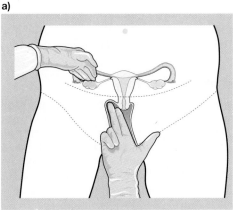

b)

Fig. 8.9 **Examination of the uterus and adnexa.**

adnexa and, starting with a hand above the umbilicus, bring it down to the appropriate iliac fossa trying to feel a mass bimanually (Fig. 8.9). In thin women the ovaries can just be felt, but a definite adnexal mass is abnormal and should be investigated further. As large adnexal masses tend to move to the midline it can be difficult to differentiate a large ovarian cyst from a large uterus.

Obstetrical history

An obstetrical history follows the usual model for history-taking. However, as with gynaecological histories, there are several unique things to be covered. A history from a pregnant woman starts with calculating the gestation and putting this pregnancy in the context of previous pregnancies. The presenting complaint is next and this encompasses a record of what is happening now, risk factors and symptom progression. It is followed by a complete history of this pregnancy and previous pregnancies. After this, medical, gynaecological, drug, social and family histories are expanded. However, these are often straightforward as pregnant women are usually young and generally healthy.

Establishment of the estimated day of delivery (EDD)

Term is between 37 and 42 weeks' gestation but the actual EDD is 40 weeks after day 1 of the last menstrual period (LMP). This can cause confusion as gestation is calculated from the LMP not conception. When someone is 12 weeks' pregnant she conceived 10 weeks ago. Gestational wheel calculators allow the easy calculation of EDD and current gestation from the LMP (Fig. 8.10). In the absence of a calculator, Naegele's rule can be used. To calculate the EDD, subtract 3 months from the LMP and add 10 days.

These methods assume a regular 4-week cycle. If this is not the case, the EDD may require adjustment. With a regular 5-week cycle, the true EDD will be 1 week later than calculated. An ultrasound scan (USS) is used to confirm the final EDD. However, scans have an associated error that increases with gestation, and in the early second trimester this is approximately plus or minus 1 week. In general, the EDD from the LMP is used, unless the USS date differs by more than a week.

Obstetrical summary

Parity is a summary of a woman's obstetrical history and two numbers are used to document this. Added together the numbers give the number of previous pregnancies. Someone who is para 0+0 has never been pregnant before. The first number is the total number of live births, plus the number of stillbirths after 24 weeks'

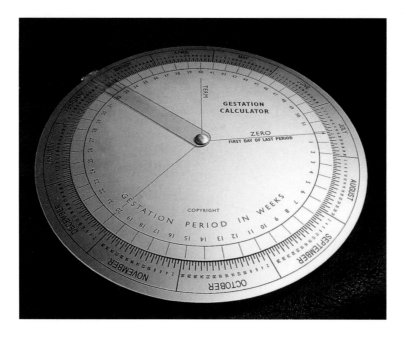

Fig. 8.10 **Gestational wheel.**

gestation. The second number is the number of pregnancies before 24 weeks in which the baby was not born alive.

A woman who is para 3+3 has been pregnant six times. The first '3' might represent a normal term delivery, a live birth at 23 weeks after which the baby died, and a stillbirth at 25 weeks' gestation. The other three pregnancies may have been a spontaneous miscarriage at 23 weeks, an early ectopic pregnancy and a first trimester pregnancy termination. The numbers relate to pregnancies rather than babies so that the mother of twins would be para 1+0. A woman who is primiparous is pregnant and para 0. A parous woman is pregnant and para 1 or more.

What is happening now?

The next stage is the presenting complaint and its history. Assuming there is a specific problem, the history should include when it was first noticed, its progress, management and associated symptoms. It may also be useful to ask about important risk factors, for example a past history of placental abruption, chronic hypertension, smoking or pre-eclampsia.

Remember that there are two patients. The fetus should be assessed by asking about movements, abdominal growth, any recent tests of fetal well-being. Fetal movements are first felt around 20 weeks, a time referred to as the 'quickening', but it can be as early as 16 weeks. Normally, there are several movements each hour but they are more frequently noticed when concentrated on. Kick charts usually involve noting the time when 10 movements have occurred and seeking help if this has not happened by mid-afternoon.

History of this pregnancy

This pregnancy should now be covered in detail. The first thing to ask about is pre-conceptual folic acid followed by the diagnosis of pregnancy and problems such as bleeding, excessive vomiting or pain in the first trimester. The next thing to ask about is the booking appointment, results of investigations, including USS and prenatal screening tests, and any specific plans. Then cover subsequent antenatal care, including clinics, parentcraft and day unit assessment. The reason for and outcome of any additional USS should be reported. Any concerns, problems identified or emergency attendance at hospital should be documented along with plans for the rest of the pregnancy and delivery.

Past obstetric history

Each of the woman's previous pregnancies should be discussed chronologically. Information required includes the date, the gestation and outcome. If the pregnancy ended in the first or second trimester, the diagnosis and management, including any operative procedures, should be recorded. For other pregnancies, information about the method of delivery, the reason for an operative delivery, the sex, weight, health and method of feeding of the baby should be obtained. In particular, any pregnancy and postnatal complication should be highlighted.

Medical history

The medical history should include previous operations, hospitalizations and medical problems. Continuing medical problems are of great importance because they may have an effect on the pregnancy and make complications more likely or complex. In addition, pregnancy may have an effect on medical problems, resulting in their deterioration, improvement or an alteration in management.

Gynaecological history

All or some of the gynaecological topics may be important in the history. Infertility treatment, particularly the use of assisted reproductive technologies such as intracytoplasmic sperm injection (ICSI), may suggest the need for additional counselling and tests. The date of the last cervical smear is important.

Drug history

It is important to record drugs taken, both over-the-counter and prescribed, and the reasons for their use. The need to continue the drug, or change its dose, as well as any possible teratogenic effects should be considered.

Family history

In a pregnant woman, it is a family history of fetal abnormalities, genetic conditions or consanguinity that is particularly important. In addition, some obstetrical conditions such as twins, pre-eclampsia, gestational diabetes and obstetric cholestasis may have a familial element.

Social history

It is important to assess the facilities for the forthcoming baby and determine whether further support is required. The woman's occupation and her plans for working during the pregnancy should be noted. It is also important to ask about smoking, drinking and other drugs of misuse.

Systemic enquiry

Often the systemic enquiry will be covered in the history of the presenting complaint. Remember, however, that many symptoms are more common in pregnancy including urinary frequency, shortness of breath, tiredness, headache, nausea and breast tenderness.

Low-risk versus high-risk pregnancy

The key to good antenatal care is to recognize which women are more likely to develop problems in pregnancy before they happen. Clearly all women can develop problems but women at extremes of age and weight, those with pre-existing medical conditions like diabetes, hypertension and epilepsy, those with significant past or family histories of obstetric problems, and those who smoke heavily, misuse drugs or have poor social circumstances, are all more likely to develop problems. In these high-risk pregnancies, antenatal care should be tailored to meet the increased needs of the woman and fetus.

Obstetrical examination

In an obstetrical examination the areas to focus on should be guided by the clinical history. It is only by becoming familiar with examination findings in normal pregnancy that deviations from normal can be fully appreciated. In the hyperdynamic circulation of pregnancy, for example, cardiac murmurs are common. The vast majority of these are flow murmurs but unrecognized pathological murmurs occasionally become apparent. Likewise in normal pregnancy skin changes and increasing oedema are common.

A systematic approach is preferable. Starting with the hands and working up to the head and down to the abdomen and legs will avoid missing important signs. Examination of the skin, sclera, conjunctiva, retina, thyroid, liver, and tendon reflexes may reveal important abnormalities that may otherwise be missed. There are three elements of obstetrical examination, however, that are particularly important: blood pressure assessment, abdominal palpation and vaginal examination.

Blood pressure assessment

The pregnant woman should lie in a semirecumbent position at an approximately 30° angle and time should be taken to ensure that she is relaxed. The room should be quiet, and any tight clothing on her arm removed. The blood pressure should be taken from her right arm, supported at the level of the heart (Fig. 8.11).

An appropriately sized cuff should be used, as too small a cuff will overestimate the blood pressure. The best cuffs have an indication of acceptable arm circumference on them. Ideally the cuff bladder should cover 80% of the arm circumference and the width of the bladder should be 40% of the arm circumference. Problems occur if the bladder length is less than 67% (this usually means the arm circumference is more than 34 cm). In such cases a large or thigh cuff should be used.

Place the centre of the cuff bladder directly over the brachial artery on the inner side of the right upper arm, at the same level as the sternum at the fourth intercostal space. Apply the cuff all round, evenly and firmly but not tightly, with the connecting tubes pointing upwards and the antecubital fossa free. Palpate the brachial

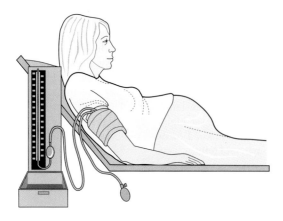

Fig. 8.11 **Blood pressure measurement.**

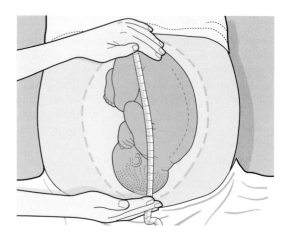

Fig. 8.12 **Measurement of symphysiofundal height.**

artery in the antecubital fossa and place the bell end of the stethoscope over it without undue pressure.

Rapidly pump the pressure in the sphygmomanometer cuff to 20–30 mmHg above the point where brachial artery pulsation ceases. Let the air out at 2–3 mmHg per second. The systolic blood pressure is the point where the first clear tapping sound is heard. Read the top of the meniscus or needle to the nearest 2 mmHg. The diastolic blood pressure is the point where the Korotkoff sounds first become muffled (phase IV) rather than where they disappear (Korotkoff V). Ideally, the record should detail which phase was used, and if there is uncertainty, the measurement can be repeated.

Abdominal palpation

Ensure the patient has privacy, is comfortable and relaxed. Although pregnant women should avoid lying flat on their back for any period of time as this can compress major vessels, the woman should be examined in the recumbent position.

Initially the abdomen is inspected. During inspection look for the distended abdomen of pregnancy and note asymmetry, fetal movements and tense stretching. The skin may reveal old or fresh striae gravidarum, a midline pigmented linea nigra and any scars from previous surgery. The most common scars to see are the Pfannenstiel scar of previous pelvic surgery, the small subumbilical and suprapubic scars of laparoscopy and the gridiron incision of a previous appendicectomy.

The next stage is palpation. This begins with the symphysiofundal height (SFH) (Fig. 8.12). The uterus is palpated with the palm of the left hand, moving it upwards and pressing with the lateral border. There is a 'give' at the fundus. Hold the end of a tape measure, measuring (i.e. cm) side down, at the fundus and mark the tape at the upper border of the pubic symphysis.

At 20 weeks' gestation, the uterus comes up to around the umbilicus and the SFH is ≈ 20 cm. Each week the uterus grows 1 cm, so that at 28 weeks it is ≈ 28 ± 2 cm and at 32 weeks it is ≈ 32 ± 2 cm. Metric measurement is therefore a reasonable guide to the size for gestation, and is useful in identifying those that are large or small for dates.

The next stage is to feel the uterus using gentle pressure of both hands and noting any irregularities, any tender areas and the two fetal 'poles', head and bottom. The 'lie' of the fetus refers to the axis of the poles in relation to the mother. It is usually longitudinal but can be transverse or oblique. The presentation refers to the part of the baby that is entering the pelvis. Generally it is a head (cephalic) or a bottom (breech) but it can be the back or limbs (Figs 8.13–8.16). In twins, it should be possible to feel at least three fetal poles.

The 'engagement' of the head refers to how far into the pelvis it has moved (Figs 8.17–8.21). This may be palpated by turning to face the woman's feet and

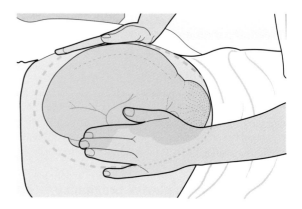

Fig. 8.13 **Palpation of the lie and liquor volume.**

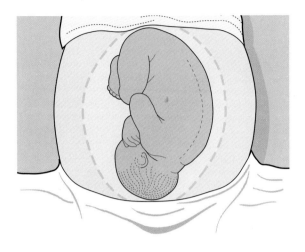

Fig. 8.14 **Longitudinal cephalic.**

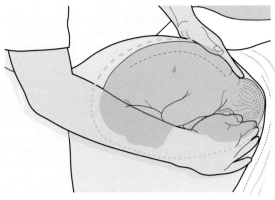

Fig. 8.17 **Palpation of the descent of the fetal head.**

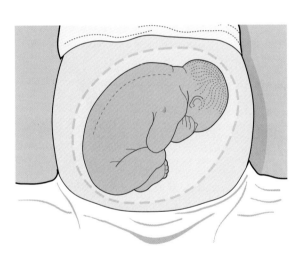

Fig. 8.15 **Oblique breech.**

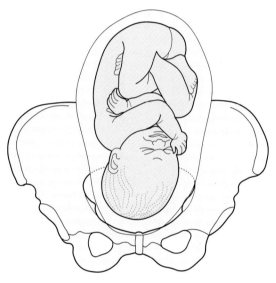

Fig. 8.18 **Head 5/5 palpable (free).**

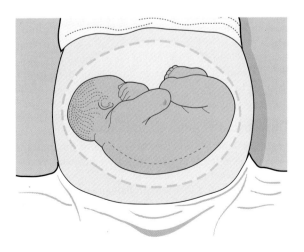

Fig. 8.16 **Transverse (back presenting).**

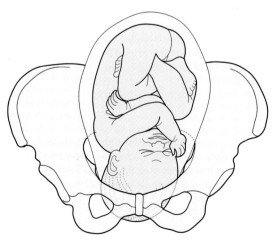

Fig. 8.19 **Head 4/5 palpable.**

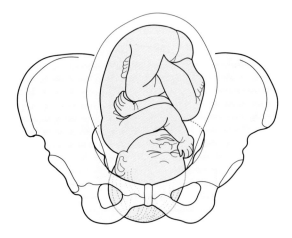

Fig. 8.20 **Head 2/5 palpable (engaged).**

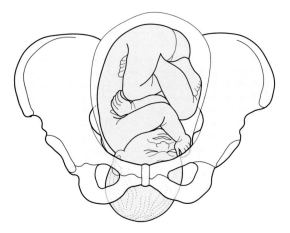

Fig. 8.21 **Head 0/5 palpable (fully engaged).**

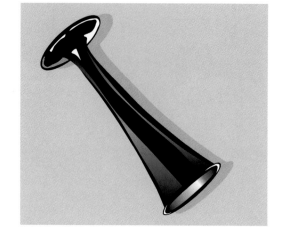

Fig. 8.22 **A Pinard stethoscope.**

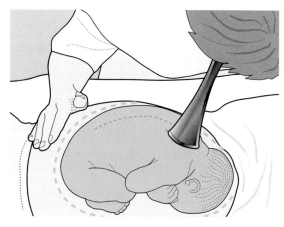

Fig. 8.23 **Using the Pinard stethoscope.**

pushing suprapubically, trying to ballot the head between the fingers. The descent can be likened to a setting sun and is recorded as fifths palpable. It is 'engaged' when the maximum diameter of the fetal head has passed through the pelvic brim. Therefore at three-fifths (3/5) palpable it is not engaged but at two-fifths (2/5) palpable it is.

An attempt should be made to get an idea of the liquor volume, particularly if the SFH is abnormal. In oligohydramnios, fetal parts can often be felt easily while in polyhydramnios the uterus is usually tense and fetal parts are difficult to feel. Also feel for the back of the fetus. It is firmer than the limbs (the side of most movements) and lies to one side. This helps work out the position of the fetus and where to pick up the fetal heart. It runs at a rate of 110–150 b.p.m. and is heard over the shoulder.

The fetal heart is heard using a Doppler USS transducer or a Pinard stethoscope (Figs 8.22 and 8.23).

To use a Pinard stethoscope, place the funnel over the anterior shoulder of the fetus and an ear at the other end, and listen carefully without holding on. It can be tricky, and is rather like listening to a clock ticking behind a waterfall. At the end of the examination ensure that the woman is comfortable, cover her abdomen, and help her to sit up.

Obstetrical vaginal examination

Vaginal examination is the cornerstone of intrapartum management, but is also a key skill in antenatal assessment. It is used in the diagnosis of pre-labour rupture of membranes and to assess pre-labour cervical change.

Although the diagnosis of membrane rupture is often made from the clinical history, a speculum examination is important for three reasons. The first is to look for evidence of liquor in the vagina. The technique is similar to gynaecological speculum examination with careful aseptic technique. A pool of fluid, sometimes containing white flecks of vernix, can usually be seen in the posterior vagina or coming from the cervix on coughing. The second is to allow a high vaginal swab to be taken, looking particularly for pathogenic bacteria, notably group B β-haemolytic streptococci. The third is to allow a visual inspection of the cervix to avoid digital examination.

Digital examination assesses pre-labour cervical change in preterm and post-term pregnancies. This helps determine those at risk of preterm delivery and is useful in the management of labour induction. After abdominal palpation, the vaginal examination is performed in the same way as a gynaecological examination. In addition, however, it is important to note the ischial spines posterolaterally, as the 'station', or degree of descent, is with reference to this point.

Feel for the cervix and note its position. Is it anterior or posterior and difficult to reach? Note its length. The cervix shortens from 3–4 cm until it is flush with the fetal head and does not protrude into the vagina. This is called effacement. What is its consistency, is it soft like a cheek or hard like a nose? Feel for the os and how much it is dilated. Note if it is closed or whether one or two fingers can be inserted. The station of the presenting part is determined as above.

The cervix is assessed by the modified Bishop's score (Table 45.2, p. 416). As the cervix ripens, it becomes softer, shorter, more anterior, more dilated and the fetal head descends. As labour approaches, the Bishop's score increases.

Key points

- Taking a history is never the same for any two patients, and many questions will follow from previous answers.
- Never miss out on a chance to practise these skills.

Gynaecology

9 Paediatric gynaecology

Puberty should transform a girl into a fertile woman, and its social importance is so great that any deviation from normality may be the cause of considerable embarrassment and anxiety. This chapter describes normal puberty and outlines the management of both delayed puberty and precocious puberty. There is also a short discussion about sexual abuse.

Normal puberty

Puberty encompasses:

- adolescent growth spurt
- acquisition of secondary sexual characteristics
- onset of menstruation or menarche
- establishment of ovulatory function.

Endocrine changes

Puberty begins with the reactivation of the hypothalamo-pituitary–ovarian axis, which has lain in abeyance from the third or fourth month of postnatal life. During childhood the hypothalamus and pituitary are highly sensitive to suppression by low levels of gonadal steroids. With the onset of puberty this extreme sensitivity is lost.

The first recognized endocrine event is the appearance of sleep-related, pulsatile release of gonadotrophins. As puberty progresses these extend throughout the 24 hours of the day. These gonadotrophins lead to production of ovarian oestrogen, which initiates the physical changes of puberty. Changes in the ovaries are evident at an early stage. In normal girls, before any physical signs of puberty are apparent, ultrasonography demonstrates a progressive increase in the size of ovarian follicles, such that after the age of $8^{1}/_{2}$ years a multicystic appearance of the ovaries (defined as more than six follicles greater than 4 mm in diameter, in each ovary) can often be demonstrated.

Signs of puberty

The external signs of puberty usually (but not always) occur in a specific order (Fig. 9.1).

The onset of the adolescent growth spurt is an early feature of puberty in girls and this may enable a girl to temporarily outstrip an older brother in height. This acceleration in growth is dependent on growth hormone as well as gonadal steroids.

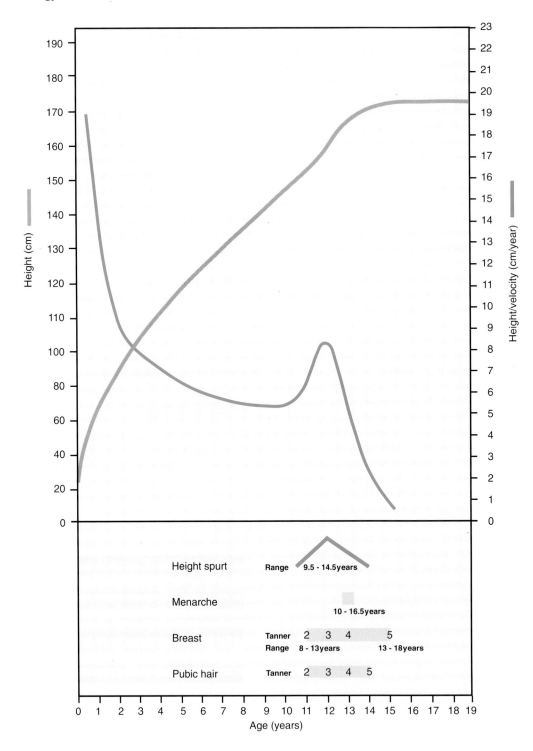

Fig. 9.1 **Schematic representation of puberty.**

Almost at the same time, the subareolar breast bud appears (thelarche). Breast development, which is primarily under the control of ovarian oestrogens, is described in five stages (Fig. 9.2). The appearance of the breast bud is followed shortly afterwards by pubic and axillary hair (pubarche), mainly under the influence of ovarian and adrenal androgens (Fig. 9.3). Menarche is a late feature in the course of puberty.

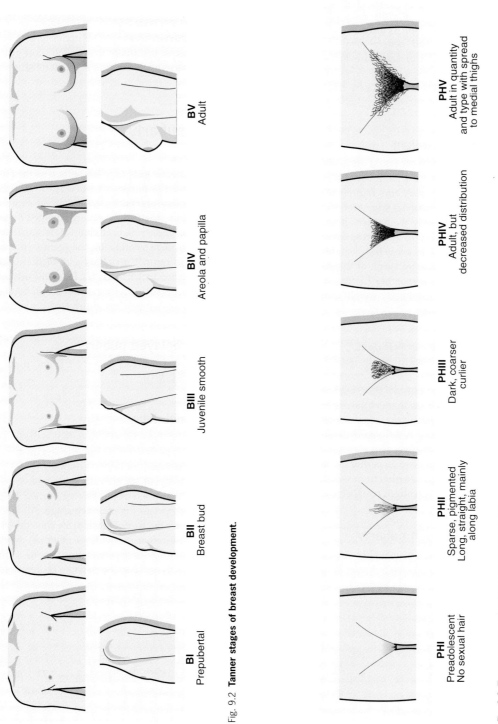

BI
Prepubertal

BII
Breast bud

BIII
Juvenile smooth

BIV
Areola and papilla

BV
Adult

Fig. 9.2 **Tanner stages of breast development.**

PHI
Preadolescent
No sexual hair

PHII
Sparse, pigmented
Long, straight, mainly
along labia

PHIII
Dark, coarser
curlier

PHIV
Adult, but
decreased distribution

PHV
Adult in quantity
and type with spread
to medial thighs

Fig. 9.3 **Tanner stages of pubic hair development.**

Age of menarche

Since the turn of the 20th century the average age for the onset of puberty has become progressively younger. In 1900 the average age of the menarche was approximately 15.5 years, while currently it is 12.8 years. This has been attributed to improvement in socio-economic conditions, nutrition and general health. This trend appears to have slowed or ceased in Western Europe and the USA during the past 30 years, as might be expected once nutrition and child care had reached an optimum level.

Influence of body weight

It had previously been proposed that the menarche was closely related to the attainment of a critical body weight, which in the USA and Europe was approximately 48 kg. Further analysis suggested that the significant component of body weight was body fat, which during the adolescent growth spurt increases to about 22% of body weight. This converts a lean body weight-to-fat ratio of 5 : 1 at the initiation of the growth spurt to one of 3 : 1 at the menarche. Factors which delay the attainment of a critical body weight may delay the menarche. These include:

- Malnutrition.
- Slow growth before and after birth.
- Twins, who have a later menarche than singletons of the same population.
- Athletic training, as it results in an increased proportion of lean body mass at the expense of adipose tissue. For each year of premenarcheal training, the menarche is delayed by 5 months.
- Environmental factors may also play a role. Urban communities tend to have an earlier menarche than rural communities, as do girls from social class I when compared to girls from social classes II and III.

Progression through puberty

95% of normal girls attain stage 2 breast development (the appearance of the subareolar breast bud) by the age of 13.2 years. 50% will complete all stages of puberty in 2–3 years while 97% will do so in 5 years.

The bone age, which is an index of physiological maturation, correlates closely with the menarche. It can be measured by an X-ray of the hand. 80% of girls begin to menstruate at a bone age of 13–14 years.

After the menarche, menstrual cycles tend to be irregular as ovulation is initially infrequent. Most girls take several months or even a year or so to establish a regular cycle.

Delayed puberty

Definition

Delayed puberty in girls may be defined as the absence of physical manifestations of puberty by the age of 13 years. Primary amenorrhoea is defined as no menstruation by the age of 14 years accompanied by failure to develop secondary sexual characteristics. It is also defined as no menstruation by the age of 16 years in the presence of normal sexual development and this is discussed further in Chapter 12. In some instances a girl may enter puberty but the normal progression is not maintained. This is described as arrested puberty.

Causes of delayed puberty

These features of delayed puberty fall into three main categories (Table 9.1).

Constitutional delay

Constitutional delay – in other words the girl is normal but inherently late in entering puberty – is the commonest cause of delayed puberty. Although these individuals are usually of short stature, and have usually been shorter than their peers for years, their height is generally appropriate for their bone age. All stages of development are delayed. They may be considered to be physiologically immature, with a functional deficiency of gonadotrophin-releasing hormone for their chronological age, but not for their stage of physiological

Table 9.1
Differential features of delayed puberty

	Stature	Gonadotrophins	Gonadal steroids	Karyotype
Constitutional delay	Short	Prepubertal	Low	Normal
Hypogonadotrophic hypogonadism	Normal	Low	Low	Normal
Primary gonadal failure:				
Turner's syndrome and variants	Short	High	Low	XO and variants
Gonadal dysgenesis	Normal	High	Low	XX or XY

development. There is frequently a history of delayed menarche in their mothers.

In these patients bone age shows a better correlation with the onset and progression of puberty than chronological age. On attaining a bone age of 11–13 years they can be expected to enter puberty.

Hypogonadotrophic hypogonadism

This arises from a defect of gonadotrophin-releasing hormone (GnRH) secretion, and consequently of follicle-stimulating hormone (FSH) and luteinizing hormone (LH). It may be associated with:

- Conditions affecting body weight, such as chronic systemic disease, malnutrition or anorexia nervosa.
- Central nervous system tumours, which may lead to interference with GnRH synthesis or secretion, or with its stimulation of the pituitary gonadotrophs. The most common of these rare conditions is craniopharyngioma.
- Isolated gonadotrophin deficiency is very rare. Such patients are generally of appropriate height for chronological age, in contrast to patients with central nervous system tumours who usually have associated growth hormone deficiency, and to those with constitutional delay, who are short for chronological age. The commonest form is Kallmann's syndrome, in which anosmia arising from agenesis or hypoplasia of the olfactory bulbs is associated with GnRH deficiency.

Primary gonadal failure (hypergonadotrophic hypogonadism)

Although gonadal dysgenesis may occur in isolation, it is most commonly associated with chromosomal anomalies, particularly Turner's syndrome (p. 115). Gonadal failure may also occur following chemotherapy or radiotherapy, as the result of germ cell damage.

Other causes

These include hyperprolactinaemia and hypothyroidism.

Investigation and management of delayed or arrested puberty

The scheme of investigation follows logically from the differential diagnosis discussed above:

1. Plasma FSH, LH, oestradiol, prolactin and thyroid function tests
2. Karyotype
3. X-ray for bone age
4. Cranial CT or MRI scan.

Constitutional delay

Often reassurance and continued observation are sufficient. It is important to reassure the parents as well as the girl herself. Where psychological problems arise as a result of comparison with her peers, treatment may be indicated. This may take the form of 3 months' therapy with low-dose estradiol, 2 µg daily. If necessary this can be repeated.

Hypogonadotrophic hypogonadism

In those with low weight, restoration of weight usually results in spontaneous onset of puberty. Those with central nervous system tumours require appropriate neurosurgical treatment.

Where the defect lies at hypothalamic level, for example with Kallmann's syndrome, pulsatile administration of GnRH via an infusion pump results in progress through all stages of puberty in the course of 12 months. It is, however, a very demanding form of treatment and in most cases replacement therapy with estradiol is usually employed for physical maturation. Pulsatile GnRH treatment, however, is necessary if ovulation induction is required.

Primary gonadal failure

Girls with pure Turner's syndrome or complete ovarian dysgenesis will usually be infertile and will require hormone replacement therapy throughout their lives until the age of 50. The first stage in treatment is to achieve apparently normal progress through puberty, and this is achieved by estradiol replacement therapy. As above, it is commenced at a low dose (2 µg daily) until breast development is adequate. It is important not to begin with higher doses as this may result in poor breast development. Subsequently, higher doses of 10–20 µg daily may be introduced and a progestagen added to avoid unopposed oestrogen stimulation of the endometrium.

Precocious puberty

The appearance of signs of sexual maturation prior to the age of 8 years constitutes precocious puberty.

Causes of precocious puberty
Constitutional

80% of cases are constitutional, with the normal sequence of pubertal development occurring at an early age. The growth spurt is a striking feature, but frequently it is the occurrence of menstruation which brings the girl to medical attention. Caution should be exercised in accepting blood loss as menstrual in origin before excluding a local lesion, such as a foreign body or even neoplasia of the vagina or cervix.

Intracranial lesions

This is the next most likely cause, particularly in younger girls. An intracranial lesion resulting from encephalitis, meningitis or hydrocephaly, or a small space-occupying lesion, may trigger premature reactivation of the hypothalamo-pituitary–ovarian axis.

Feminizing tumours

Feminizing tumours of the ovary or adrenal may give rise to vaginal bleeding without signs of pubertal development.

Other causes

Other possible causes are hypothyroidism, and the very rare McCune–Albright syndrome in which cystic cavities develop in the long bones (polyostotic fibrous dysplasia) and *café au lait* skin pigmentation is evident.

Investigation and management of precocious puberty

1. Plasma FSH, LH, oestradiol and thyroid function tests.
2. X-ray of the hand to determine bone age, which is advanced in the constitutional and cerebral forms.
3. Ultrasound scan of the abdomen and pelvis.
4. Radiological skeletal survey of the long bones. Changes in the McCune–Albright syndrome may be restricted to one side of the body.
5. Cranial CT or MRI scan.

Ultrasound examination by an experienced sonographer has become the mainstay of diagnosis. In the constitutional and cerebral forms, the ovaries will show the multicystic appearance previously described in normal puberty. It will also distinguish between a follicular cyst, which may be expected to subside spontaneously, and a predominantly solid oestrogen-secreting granulosa/theca cell tumour of the ovary, which will require surgical removal.

With precocious puberty the aims of treatment are:

1. to arrest or induce regression of the physical signs of puberty, and in particular menstruation, for obvious social reasons
2. to avert the rapid advance in bone age, as premature fusion of the epiphyses would compromise the final height of the child.

The introduction of GnRH agonists, which suppress gonadotrophin secretion, has revolutionized the treatment of constitutional and cerebral precocious puberty.

Preparations are available which may be used intra-nasally or as a depot injection, and treatment can be continued for 2–3 years without significant side-effects.

Abnormal genital tract development

Vagina

There may be horizontal septae, vertical septae or the vagina may be absent.

Horizontal septae

There may be cryptomenorrhoea with cyclical pain and a haematocolpos. If obstruction is caused simply by the hymen (blood looks blue behind it) then a cruciate incision, usually under anaesthesia, is all that is required. If the septum looks pink rather than blue the situation is potentially more serious and should be referred to a specialist surgeon. If the septum is in the low or mid-portion of the vagina, *total* excision and re-suturing is necessary. If the septum is high, a combined abdominal and vaginal approach may be required. Pregnancy rates are excellent with low septae but only around 25% for those higher in the vagina.

Vertical septae

These may be associated with abnormal uterine development. Although presentation may be with dyspareunia, infertility or occasionally in advanced labour, the septum is often asymptomatic. It can be surgically removed.

Vaginal atresia

This is associated with an absent, or only a rudimentary, uterus and is known as the Rokitansky syndrome. Presentation is at puberty with amenorrhoea (or cryptomenorrhoea) in the presence of normal secondary sexual characteristics. If the uterus is non-functioning it is possible to create a vagina with regular use of vaginal dilators, or by one of a variety of surgical techniques. Surrogacy is an option for childbearing.

Uterus

Abnormal uterine shapes (Fig. 9.4) are usually asymptomatic but may present with primary infertility, recurrent pregnancy loss or menstrual dysfunction (oligomenorrhoea, dysmenorrhoea or menorrhagia). In pregnancy, there may be miscarriage, pre-term labour or abnormal fetal lie.

Unicornuate uterus   With this there is a higher miscarriage rate and risk of preterm labour.

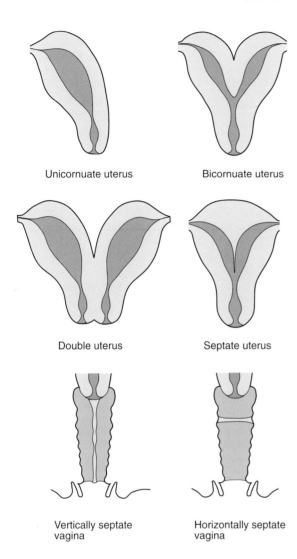

Unicornuate uterus   Bicornuate uterus

Double uterus   Septate uterus

Vertically septate vagina   Horizontally septate vagina

Fig. 9.4 **Common genital tract malformations.**

Bicornuate uterus This may carry a pregnancy to an adequately advanced gestation, and the chance of this probably increases with successive pregnancies. A 'Strassman' procedure will correct the defect, but the benefits for pregnancy are unproven. A bicornuate uterus may be asymmetrical with one side hypoplastic (Fig. 9.4). Pregnancy in the hypoplastic horn carries a risk of rupture.

Septate uterus If it is appropriate to remove the septum, a hysteroscopic approach is probably the most appropriate.

Sexual abuse

This is the involvement of dependent sexually immature children and adolescents in sexual activity they do not truly comprehend, to which they are unable to give informed consent and which violates social taboos or family roles. The abuser is usually male and well known to the child and family. It may present to the medical services acutely, following injury or allegation, or may be suggested by precociousness and other behavioural disorders.

There are numerous pitfalls to the clinical examination, and a depth of experience is required if the results of an examination are to stand up in court. Early senior multidisciplinary help is essential in this highly emotive area where incorrect interpretation of the signs may have major consequences. The use of a colposcope is important and photographic records are extremely useful.

The history should be carefully taken and documented, and the social work team involved if appropriate. Swabs (which may include swabs for DNA analysis) should be taken with a 'secure chain of evidence'

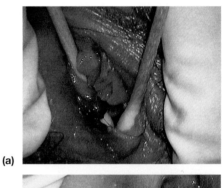

(a)

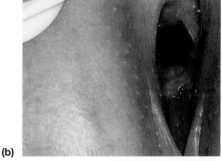

(b)

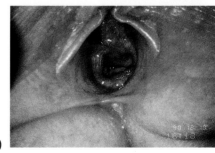

(c)

Fig. 9.5 **It is essential to differentiate normal hymenal views from those that are pathological. (a)** Acute tearing. **(b)** Partial thickness tear at the posterior margin. **(c)** Concavities in the hymen.

in case required for a later legal action. Particular attention should be paid to bleeding, bruising or any other area of injury, particularly lacerations at the posterior fourchette and perineal abrasions.

A normal hymen has a number of different shapes (annular, crescentic, fimbriated, septate, sleeve or funnel shaped) and these should not be confused with tears (Fig. 9.5a,b). Notches and clefts can be highly suggestive of penetrating injury, but may be normal if associated with an intravaginal ridge above them (Fig. 9.5c); they are very rare in the posterior segment in non-abused girls. 'Straddle injuries', caused by falling astride an object such as a fence, very rarely affect the hymen and there is much more likely to be bruising anterior to the vagina or laterally (e.g. labia majora). It is also rare for tampon use to cause hymenal injury (although it may increase the diameter slightly), and there are no reported cases of congenital absence of the hymen. Conversely a normal prepubertal hymen does not exclude abuse.

Paediatric vaginal discharge

Such a symptom raises the possibility of, but does not necessarily imply, sexual abuse.

Non-microbial causes

Threadworms are possible. Foreign body insertion is rare.

Microbial causes

Investigation is difficult to interpret as there are few data on the commensal profile of children. In those with discharge, the Group A streptococcus is commonly found, followed by *Haemophilus influenzae* and *Candida* species. Bowel flora are also common. *Gardnerella* and *Trichomonas vaginalis* are probably not commensals. Swabs should also be checked for *Chlamydia* and *Neisseria gonorrhoeae*.

Key points

- Delayed puberty, the absence of physical manifestations of puberty by the age of 13 years, is most commonly a variant of normality referred to as 'constitutional delay'. It may, however, be caused by hypogonadotrophic hypogonadism, Turner's syndrome, or gonadal dysgenesis. It may be worth checking gonadotrophin levels and a karyotype.

- Precocious puberty, the appearance of signs of sexual maturation prior to the age of 8 years, may also be constitutional but is also associated with intracranial lesions, feminizing tumours and the very rare McCune–Albright syndrome.

10

Intersex

Introduction

Sex is not, as society regards it, a simple binary phenomenon. Biologically, sex is a spectrum involving a set of characteristics with bimodal distribution (Fig. 10.1). There are some individuals in mid-spectrum to whom it is not scientifically possible to allocate a sex, e.g. XXY, XX/XY chromosomal states, and ovotesticular states. Social and legal convention forces a choice but this is administrative simplification of biological reality.

Definitions

A prosaic but useful definition of 'sex' is: 'a species dimorphism, represented at different planes by chromosomes and the genes they carry, gonads, sex ducts, external genitalia, bodily habitus, secondary sex characters and behaviour or psychological attitudes'.

'Phenotypic sex' is the apparent sex, judged by external characteristics. The term 'intersex' is used when there is contradiction between, or poor development of, sex characteristics. It is convenient for medical use but is likely to cause distress to patient or relative.

Cases with purely mental rather than physical sex contradictions – transsexuals, homosexuals, etc. – rarely present to gynaecologists and are not discussed here.

Some fundamental principles

1. The chromosomal complement of the zygote normally determines the sex of the gonads. The gonads normally determine the phenotypic sex.
2. Female corresponds closely to 'neutral' in humans. Thus in XO (Turner's syndrome) with no second – or 'differentiating' – sex chromosome (X or Y) and no gonadal development, the phenotype is female.
3. Male development requires some positive influence. If a Y chromosome is present, it will tend to dominate.
4. 'Sex change' does not happen in humans, despite all the prurient press may say. Sex of registration may be altered if it is shown that the birth assignation was erroneous. Endocrine factors and plastic surgery can alter secondary characteristics but this does not affect the basic sexual composition.

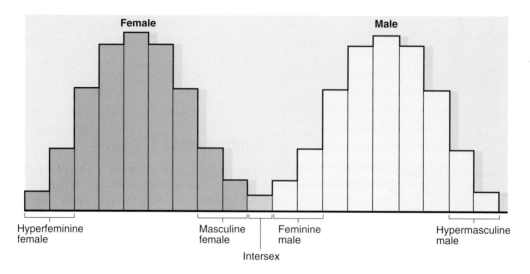

Fig. 10.1 **Bimodal distribution of sex characteristics.** Sex involves a spectral distribution of characters of bimodal type. In the centre it may be possible to allocate a sex on a strictly scientific basis.

Normal sex differentiation

The chromosomes

Chromosomal complement is the only sex characteristic of the early conceptus. Central to the accumulation of knowledge of sex chromosome anomalies was the discovery of the nuclear chromatin body, a microscopic blob found under the nuclear membrane of all female cells. It is now clear that one X chromosome is necessary for cell viability but once ovarian differentiation has been initiated the second X has no function and condenses to form the Barr body (Fig. 10.2). More than two X chromosomes will mean that there are additional bodies – the formula being 'X chromosomes – 1 = number of Barr bodies' (see Fig. 10.3). Early studies were on cases with evident abnormality; only when total population studies were carried out did the picture become clear.

The Y chromosome

It has long been known that the short arm of the Y chromosome controlled testicular development, but

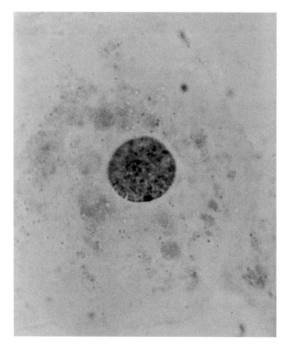

Fig. 10.2 **Nuclear chromatin (Barr) body seen beneath nuclear membrane close to 6 o'clock.**

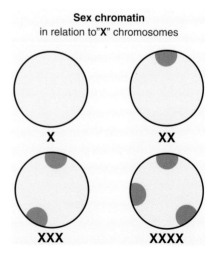

Fig. 10.3 **Sex chromatin in relation to X chromosomes.** Barr bodies are peripheral blobs consisting of nuclear chromatin. There is always one less Barr body than the number of X chromosomes.

identification of the gene has proved a long task. Studies were based on intersex cases in which the gonads and other sex features were contrary to the chromosomes, so-called 'sex reversal'.

After several false proposals (e.g. *H-Y* and *ZFY*), it has recently become accepted that a gene called *SRY* (sex-determining region of Y) is responsible. It encodes a DNA-binding protein which probably influences other genes to produce differentiation of the primitive gonadal streak into testis. The detail of *SRY*'s mode of action is now the focus of attention. A very few XX males do not have *SRY*, so some other genetic material must, in certain circumstances, be able to induce testicular differentiation.

Mixed chromosomes

It is not uncommon for lymphocytes to have mixed sex chromosome complements. This can be due to mosaicism arising from post-fertilization mitotic errors or very rarely to chimaerism, when the cell-mix derives from two separate acts of syngamy (union of gametes). Surrogacy may result from dispermic conceptions – one sperm fertilizing the ovum nucleus and another uniting with an unextruded second polar body (see Fig. 10.4) – or from dizygous twins with transfer of tissue soon after conception.

Genital differentiation

So-called 'inductors' cause the primitive gonad to develop, with medullary growth predominating in the male to form testes and cortical growth in females forming ovaries.

In males, testosterone leads to Wolffian (mesonephric) duct development (Fig. 6.11). Atrophy of the Müllerian (paramesonephric) ducts occurs because of the presence of Müllerian inhibiting factor (MIF) from the Sertoli cells of the testis. Testosterone also induces the positive development of the external genitalia, the enzyme

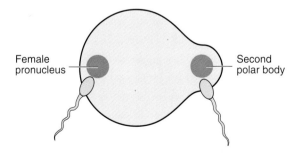

Fig. 10.4 **Dispermic conception.** Very rarely an extruded second polar body may be fertilized in addition to the haploid ovum nucleus; if the sperms involved are of different sexes an XX/XY chimaera will result.

5-alpha-reductase being required to produce the active form, dihydrotestosterone. Male sex hormones also influence cerebral sex centres.

In females, absence of MIF allows the Müllerian ducts to form the uterus, fallopian tubes and upper vagina. In the absence of testosterone the external genitalia develop in the female form.

Incidence of intersex

The incidence of intersex conceptions is impossible to define precisely as many end in miscarriage – most XO conceptuses are not born alive, though others survive without problems. Minimal rates of conditions, however, can be calculated and summation makes it clear that intersex is far from being the rarity imagined.

For practical purposes it is enough to realize that one GP can expect to have a dozen or so cases on his or her list, perhaps not all identified; most will be chromosomal. The problems of intersex are of such complexity and sensitivity that they assume a clinical importance quite disproportionate to incidence or mortality rates.

Classification of intersex states

Cases can be grouped according to the level at which the basic anomaly operates:

- Chromosomal
- Gonadal
- Secondary sex characteristics:
  - partial masculinization of females
  - incomplete masculinization of males.

Chromosomal anomalies

Turner's syndrome (XO) occurs in 1 out of 2500 phenotypic female births. It is the best known of these conditions but is a syndrome with many atypical forms. Nevertheless, most XO cases have the major features (Fig. 10.5). These are:

- dwarfism
- sexual infantilism
- neck webbing
- streak gonads.

Other features ('Turners stigmata') may be present more frequently than in normals, for example:

- shield chest
- high arched palate
- low-set ears
- lymphoedema
- deafness
- coarctation of the aorta
- pigmented moles.

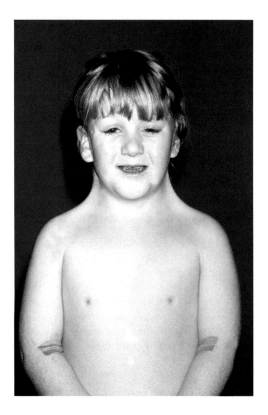

Fig. 10.5 **Classic Turner's syndrome.** This picture illustrates neck webbing. There was also short stature and subsequent primary amenorrhoea.

XX/XO mosaicism) a few primordial follicles may mature in early reproductive life.

Klinefelter's syndrome (XXY) occurs in 1 in 500 phenotypic males. The leading feature are:

- azoospermia
- gynaecomastia
- atrophic testes.

As there is no pubertal surge of steroids, epiphyseal closure is delayed so the patients are tall and lanky. Facial hair is scant, prostates small and gonadotrophin levels high. Infertility leading to discovery of azoospermia is the usual presentation. The testicular histology is 'seminiferous tubule dysgenesis' (Fig. 10.6) and the term has much to commend it as a diagnostic label.

XX/XY chimaerism is an extreme rarity usually due to dispermic conception. There are similarities to mixed gonadal dysgenesis.

Mixed gonadal dysgenesis describes cases with a gonad on one side and an atrophic streak on the other. Usually there is 45XO/46XY mosaicism. The 'streak' may be replaced by a malignant tumour – seminoma or dysgerminoma.

Other sex chromosome abnormalities include females with an extra X (XXX) and males with an extra Y (XYY) as well as an infinite range of mosaics.

The usual chromosome complement is 45XO but some are reported '46XXp-' (deletion of the short arm of one X). Mosaicism is common and the clinical features merge at one extreme with normal male and at the other with normal female.

```
   Normal              Typical              Normal
   male               Turner's             female
XY ◄──────► XO/XY ◄── XO ──► XO/XX ◄──────► XX
             or    or XXqi or XXr   or
            XY-                     XX-
```

XY- and XX- = deletion of part of X or Y
XXqi = isochromosome of the long arm of X
XXr = ring chromosome of an X

Thus the situation with Turner's syndrome is similar to male/female differentiation – there are no sharp borders, only regions of a spectrum. While primary amenorrhoea and sterility are to be expected, there are recorded exceptions. Commonly there is only a fibrous streak at the gonadal site, but occasionally (usually with

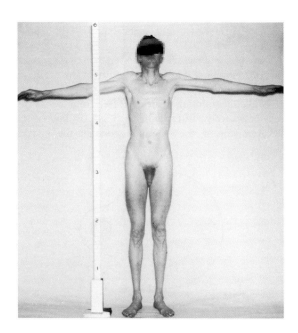

Fig. 10.6 **Seminiferous tubule dysgenesis (Klinefelter's syndrome)** showing tall stature, scant pubic hair and small testes but, in this case, little gynaecomastia.

Gonadal intersex

Three types of gonadal intersex exist:

Ovotesticular states (hermaphroditism) involve the presence of ovarian and testicular tissue in the same individual, either as separate gonads or as 'ovotestes'. Such cases are true hermaphrodites, but the word 'hermaphrodite' has lost its medical value through loose usage for any form of intersex. Though it is extremely rare in humans, in other species it is the norm, e.g. marine invertebrates, the more exotic of which are male or female in alternate seasons.

Most cases are 46XX. Occasionally an abnormal karyotype is found but only rarely is this XX/XY – the karyotype which might be expected (Fig. 10.7). It is commoner amongst the Bantu of South Africa.

As the proportion of ovarian and testicular tissue varies, there is no classical clinical picture. Other forms of intersex have fairly standard clinical patterns and can be confirmed by specific tests: ovotesticular states are suspected by excluding these other diagnoses and are confirmed by histological evidence of both types of gonadal tissue – usually a rather major undertaking.

'Pure' gonadal dysgenesis (or 'agenesis') cases have only a primitive streak, undeveloped gonads (like Turner's

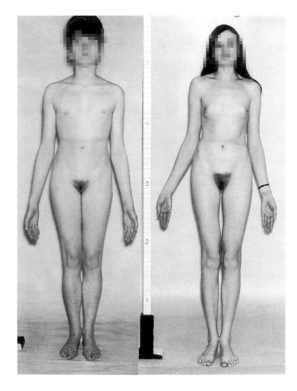

Fig. 10.8 **Two examples of pure gonadal dysgenesis.** Each had normal chromosomes but one was XX (left) and the other XY (right).

syndrome) but normal chromosomes – either XX or XY. Regardless of chromosomes, all are phenotypic females (Fig. 10.8). They have none of the 'Turner's stigmata' but they lack the secondary features which are dependent on gonadal activity. XY cases have an increased risk of cancer (see later).

Contrary gonadal development (sex inversion or reversal) leads to XY females and XX males. These cases have gonads contrary to the chromosomes, because of deletion or mutation of the *SRY* gene.

Secondary sex characteristics

Partial masculinization of females

Steroid synthesis errors due to enzyme deficiencies account for most cases. The disorder depends on the site of action and the existence of alternative pathways in the steroid metabolic pathways. Other names for this group of disorders are congenital adrenal hyperplasia and the adrenogenital syndrome.

The commonest of the errors (incidence about 1 in 12 000) is 21-hydroxylase deficiency, which has an autosomal recessive inheritance. It is unique in that specific treatment is available and can make childbearing possible. The enzyme 21-hydroxylase metabolizes 17-alpha-hydroxyprogesterone en route to cortisol (Fig. 10.9).

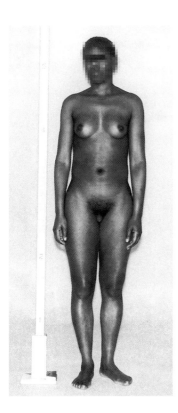

Fig. 10.7 **Hermaphrodite.** Male from South Africa who presented because of embarrassment when playing football on account of the size of his breasts. Histology of bisected intra-abdominal gonads revealed ovarian and testicular tissue.

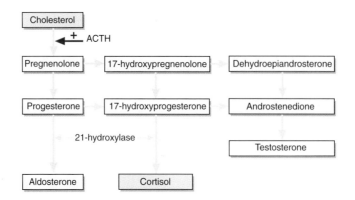

Fig. 10.9 **Synthesis of steroid hormones.** Deficiency of 21-hydroxylase enzyme leads to a build-up of precursors, particularly the weak androgens dehydroepiandrosterone and androsterone.

Deficiency of this enzyme means there is less cortisol to feed back on the pituitary. Adrenocorticotrophic hormone (ACTH) therefore increases, leading to adrenal hyperactivity – hence the term 'congenital adrenal hyperplasia'.

17-alpha-hydroxyprogesterone is also a precursor for testosterone, via a pathway which is not dependent on the 21-hydroxylase enzyme. There is therefore a build-up of androgenic steroids and, as a result, affected females show variable masculinization – clitoral hypertrophy, labial fusion, etc. – hence the term 'adrenogenital syndrome'.

The condition can also occur with associated aldosterone deficiency when the zona fasciculata of the adrenal gland is also involved. In this 'salt-losing' type, the consequent electrolyte disturbance can be rapidly fatal. Diagnosis is by steroid metabolite measurement. Treatment is with hydrocortisone (along with fludrocortisone for salt losers) and plastic surgery as necessary.

Molecular genetics now allows prenatal diagnosis. Prenatal therapy is possible with dexamethasone, which crosses the placenta. Other steroid synthesis errors also involve enzyme deficiencies but these are much rarer than 21-hydroxylase deficiency.

Steroid administration in pregnancy can cause masculinization of a female fetus. For example, some progestogens – the 19-nortestosterone derivatives (e.g. norethisterone) – have androgenic properties, as does danazol. The risk of pharmacological doses causing masculinization is small.

Incomplete masculinization of males

Four types of intersex occur in chromosomal males with testes.

Androgen insensitivity syndrome ('testicular feminization syndrome') is the commonest and most remarkable. The condition is inherited on an X-linked recessive basis, the defect being an absence of androgen receptors. There is as a consequence a normal female phenotype despite testes (Fig. 10.10). These are usually sited in groins or abdomen. There is a short, blind vagina. The

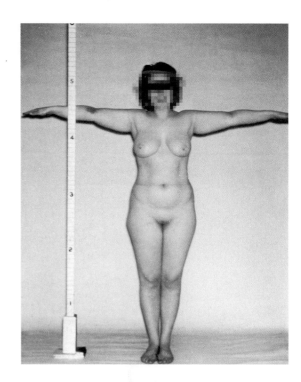

Fig. 10.10 **Androgen insensitivity syndrome.** 46/XY patient with extremely feminine physique.

feminizing component relates to peripheral conversion of thwarted androgens to oestrogens. Female pubertal development therefore occurs, and the patient often has an attractive feminine appearance.

Cases usually present with primary amenorrhoea: such individuals rarely have any worry about sexual identity and genial self-confidence is a feature. Diagnosis is easily confirmed by chromosome analysis, elevated plasma luteinizing hormone (LH) levels and testosterone at or above the male range. Treatment is not usually necessary except that post-pubertal gonadectomy is usually performed because of the neoplastic risk, common to undescended testes. However, unlike dysgenetic gonads in XY cases, these tumours are rarely malignant. Incomplete forms occur, and in some the feminizing component is absent. Again the condition is a spectrum with no clear demarcations; different members of the same family may even show different forms.

Failure of peripheral conversion of testosterone to dihydrotestosterone because of 5-alpha-reductase deficiency has been regarded as a variant of the testicular feminization syndrome but the mechanism is distinct and inheritance is autosomal recessive. Activity of testosterone is dependent on this conversion. The deficiency is not complete, so the increase in circulating testosterone at puberty leads to virilization of phenotypic females, often wrongly described as 'sex change'. In the Dominican Republic, where it is common, this is accepted with equanimity.

Failure of androgen production occurs very rarely. It is due to a range of steroid enzyme deficiencies.

Failure of Müllerian inhibitory factor production is held responsible for states in which there is inappropriate Müllerian tissue in males.

Presentation

Intersex states can present at a number of different times. At birth, the child's sex may be unclear. In deciding the sex, it is important not to simply take a guess as, if you are wrong, the social consequences can be disastrous. A few simple and quick investigations and the advice of a plastic surgeon will allow confident sex allocation. Starting school can also be a significant time to present, not least because an essential anatomical feature of masculinity is the ability to pass urine in the erect posture.

Puberty may fail to materialize, or may do so with the development of contrary features. After puberty,

disqualification from athletic competition may bring the first, traumatic realization of a problem. XY females and 21-hydroxylase-deficient XX girls, whose high androgens make good muscles, are often top performers and may be subjected to tests. In adult life, primary infertility investigations may reveal seminiferous tubule dysgenesis (XXY) or, rarely, other intersex states.

Management and prospects

Most of the action is in communication because specific treatment is rarely possible. Doctors can give the explanations and support, and how they do so is critical. Appropriate management advice may be quite opposite to what seems logical from the scientific findings but these decisions have to be based on what is practicable surgically, medically and socially. Only very rarely is it appropriate to consider re-registration from the original sex decision, but it remains an option if developments are making life in the original impossible.

The consultant chosen should have a special interest in the problem and work in cooperation with other experts. This is best managed through case conferences to avoid drifting round the clinics. Most outpatient clinics are ill-suited to these patients and the privacy of a side-room or office is desirable.

A comprehensive range of investigations should be planned. A plastic surgeon's help will often be needed.

At the major post-investigation consultation a frank and simple description of the situation and its implications is appropriate. Any treatment options should be discussed directly with the individual. Even relatively young children have a remarkable capacity for grasping the essentials and reacting logically, bravely and unemotionally.

Many patients who have been aware of their sexual ambiguity are tremendously grateful when they realize that its nature has been understood – the investigation provides the therapy. They often form a bond with the doctor concerned that should be maintained as far as possible either until matrimony (many do marry) or a close personal relationship, or adaptation to the state and prospect of a single existence seems complete.

When there has been no suspicion of sex anomaly, e.g. in seminiferous tubule dysgenesis or androgen insensitivity, it may be prudent, rather than telling an unworried man that he is chromosomally neuter or a blossoming young woman that she is chromosomally a male and has got testes, to explain the situation truthfully in terms of the testicular pathology or the receptor defect respectively. ('Gonad' is a very useful word in these conversations.)

Quite a number of types of intersex are regularly associated with a remarkably fulfilled and contented life, particularly cases of androgen insensitivity and pure gonadal dysgenesis. Many become high fliers in business or academia, which provide an outlet for positive drive that compensates for childlessness. Coitus is not usually a problem and successful sexual relationships frequently occur.

At the other end of the scale, patients with Turner's syndrome and 21-hydroxylase deficiency tend to fare less successfully. In part this is due to their small stature and often 'odd' appearance. There may be difficulty in securing employment and sexual relationships are less easy. A rewarding career may therefore be important. Help towards preferential treatment in the job market can be important.

The malignancy risk with XY chromosomes and dysgenetic intra-abdominal gonads is so high (50%) that it is usually wise to recommend excision.

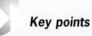

Key points

- Gender can be defined according to the chromosomes, gonads, genital sex or psychological status of an individual.

- The female state is neutral: development of the male requires a Y chromosome, testosterone production and functioning androgen receptors.

- Intersex states can be classified as chromosomal (e.g. Turner's syndrome or Klinefelter's syndrome), gonadal (true hermaphroditism, which is rare, or pure gonadal dysgenesis), endocrine abnormalities (e.g. steroid synthesis errors or androgen insensitivity syndrome), or Müllerian duct abnormalities.

- Management of intersex requires tact from everyone and expertise from a consultant with special interest in the topic.

11

The normal menstrual cycle

Introduction

Evolutionary aspects

Humans are one of the few species which have a monthly reproductive cycle. Most mammals ovulate less frequently than once a month – for example, sheep ovulate once a year and rabbits ovulate in response to coitus. In these species insemination usually leads to pregnancy, but in normal humans there is only a 30% chance of conception at each ovulation. The high frequency of ovulation in our species compensates for our relatively low fertility.

At some point in evolution, the human reproductive cycle became the same length as the lunar cycle – 28 days. The reason for this is unknown. From a biological point of view the length of the cycle is quite arbitrary. Regular periods in themselves are not necessary to health. Indeed, heavy periods may cause problems such as anaemia and it can be argued that in general women would be healthier if they did not have monthly periods.

Overview of the cycle

The menstrual cycle can be described by referring to either the uterus or the ovary. The uterine cycle results from the growth and shedding of the uterine lining – the endometrium. At the end of the menstrual phase the endometrium thickens again – the proliferative phase. After ovulation endometrial growth stops and the glands become more active – the secretory phase.

These endometrial changes are controlled by the ovarian cycle. The average duration of the cycle is 28 days and it is composed of:

- a follicular phase
- ovulation
- a postovulatory or luteal phase.

If the cycle is prolonged, the follicular phase lengthens but the luteal phase remains constant at 14 days. Fundamental to the normal menstrual cycle are:

- an intact hypothalamo–pituitary–ovarian endocrine axis
- the presence of responsive follicles in the ovaries
- a functional uterus.

Endocrine control of the menstrual cycle

Control of follicular maturation and ovulation is exercised by the hypothalamo–pituitary–ovarian axis (Fig. 11.1). The hypothalamus controls the cycle, but it can itself be influenced by higher centres in the brain, allowing factors such as anxiety or stress to affect the cycle. It acts on the pituitary gland by secreting gonadotrophin-releasing hormone (GnRH), a deca-peptide which is secreted in a pulsatile manner by the hypothalamus. The pulses are secreted approximately every 90 minutes. GnRH travels through the small blood vessels of the pituitary portal system to the anterior pituitary, where it acts on the pituitary gonadotrophs to stimulate the synthesis and release of follicle-stimulating hormone (FSH) and luteinizing-hormone (LH). Although there are two gonadotrophins, it appears that there is a single releasing hormone for both.

Follicle-stimulating hormone is a glycoprotein which stimulates follicular maturation during the follicular phase of the cycle. It also shares with LH the role of stimulating steroid hormone secretion, predominantly of oestrogen, by the granulosa cells of the mature ovarian follicle.

Luteinizing hormone is also a glycoprotein. In addition to its contribution to steroidogenesis in the follicle, it plays an essential role in ovulation, as this is dependent upon the mid-cycle surge of LH. Production of progesterone by the corpus luteum is also under the influence of LH.

Both FSH and LH and the other two glycoprotein hormones – thyroid-stimulating hormone (TSH) and human chorionic gonadotrophin (hCG) – are composed of two protein subunits, the alpha chain and the beta chain. The amino acid sequence of the alpha subunit is common to all four glycoproteins, but the beta chains are distinctive to each hormone. Sensitive assays for these hormones therefore have to be specific for the beta chain.

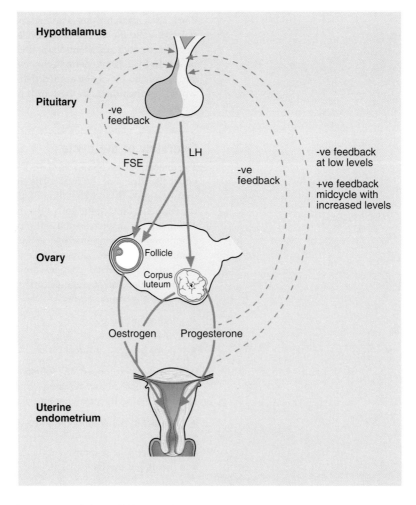

Fig. 11.1 **Hypothalamo–pituitary–ovarian–uterine axis.**

The cyclical activity within the ovary which constitutes the ovarian cycle is maintained by the feedback mechanisms which operate between the ovary, the hypothalamus, and the pituitary. These are described in the next section.

The ovarian cycle

Follicular phase

Days 1–8

At the start of the cycle, levels of FSH and LH are relatively high and these stimulate development of 10–20 follicles, resulting in full maturation of – almost invariably – a single 'dominant' follicle. This dominant follicle appears during the mid-follicular phase, whilst the remainder undergo atresia. The relatively high levels of FSH and LH have been triggered by the fall of oestrogen and progesterone at the end of the preceding cycle. During and immediately after the menses oestrogen levels are relatively low but they begin to increase as follicular development occurs.

Days 9–14

As the follicle increases in size, localized accumulations of fluid appear among the granulosa cells and become confluent, giving rise to a fluid-filled central cavity called the antrum (Fig. 11.2), which transforms the primary follicle into a Graafian follicle in which the oocyte occupies an excentric position, surrounded by two to three layers of granulosa cells termed the cumulus oophorus.

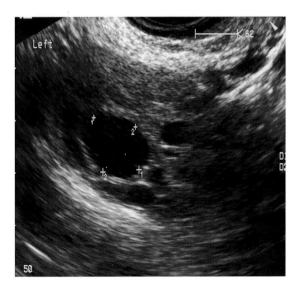

Fig. 11.2 **A dominant follicle on transvaginal ultrasound scan.**

Hormonal changes   Associated with follicular maturation, there is a progressive increase in the production of oestrogen (mainly oestradiol) by the granulosa cells of the developing follicle. This reaches a peak 18 hours prior to ovulation. As the oestrogen level rises the release of both gonadotrophins is suppressed (negative feedback) which serves to prevent hyperstimulation of the ovary and the maturation of multiple follicles.

The granulosa cells also produce inhibin. This has been implicated as a factor in the restriction of the number of follicles undergoing maturation.

Ovulation

Day 14

Ovulation is associated with rapid enlargement of the follicle followed by protrusion from the surface of the ovarian cortex and rupture of the follicle with extrusion of the oocyte and adherent cumulus oophorus (Fig. 11.3). Some women can identify the time of ovulation because they experience a short-lived pain in one or other iliac fossa. Ultrasound studies have shown that this pain – known as 'mittelschmerz' – actually occurs just before follicular rupture.

Hormonal changes   The final rise in oestradiol concentration is thought to be responsible for the subsequent mid-cycle surge of LH and to a lesser extent of FSH – positive feedback. Immediately before ovulation there is a precipitous fall in oestradiol levels and an increase in progesterone production. Ovulation follows within 18 hours of the mid-cycle surge of LH.

Luteal phase

Days 15–28

The remainder of the follicle which is retained in the ovary is penetrated by capillaries and fibroblasts from the theca. The granulosa cells undergo luteinization and these structures collectively form the corpus luteum (Fig. 11.4). This is the major source of the sex steroid hormones, oestrogen and progesterone, secreted by the ovary in the postovulatory phase.

Establishment of the corpus luteum results in a marked increase in progesterone secretion and a secondary rise in oestradiol levels. Both these hormones are produced from the same precursors (Fig. 10.9).

During the luteal phase gonadotrophin levels reach a nadir and remain low until the regression of the corpus luteum which occurs at days 26–28. If conception and implantation occur, the corpus luteum does not regress because it is maintained by gonadotrophin secreted by the trophoblast. If, however, conception and implantation have not occurred successfully, the corpus luteum regresses and menstruation ensues. The consequent

Gynaecology

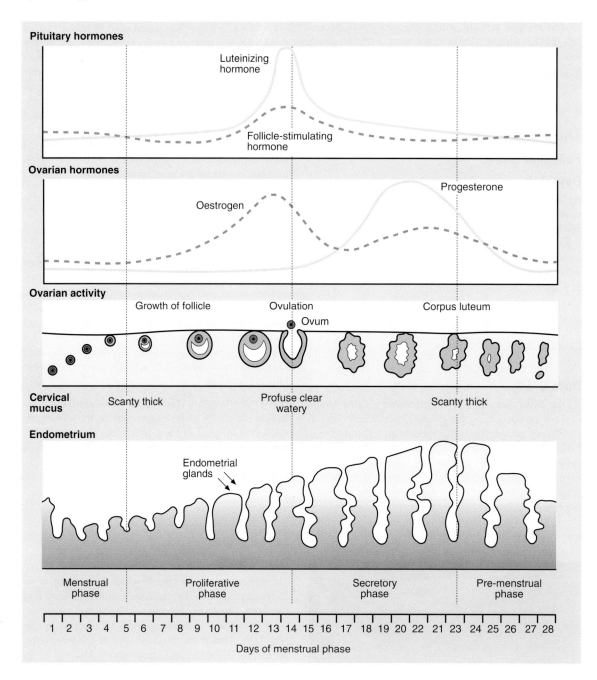

Pituitary hormones

Luteinizing hormone

Follicle-stimulating hormone

Ovarian hormones

Oestrogen

Progesterone

Ovarian activity

Growth of follicle   Ovulation   Corpus luteum

Ovum

Cervical mucus

Scanty thick   Profuse clear watery   Scanty thick

Endometrium

Endometrial glands

| Menstrual phase | Proliferative phase | Secretory phase | Pre-menstrual phase |

1 2 3 4 5 6 7 8 9 10 11 12 13 14 15 16 17 18 19 20 22 21 23 24 25 26 27 28

Days of menstrual phase

Fig. 11.3 **Schematic diagram of ovulation.**

fall in the levels of steroid hormones allows the gonadotrophin levels to rise and initiate the next cycle.

The uterine cycle

The cyclical production of steroid hormones by the ovary induces important changes in the uterus. These involve the endometrium and cervical mucus.

The endometrium

The endometrium is composed of two layers: a superficial layer which is shed in the course of menstruation; and a basal layer which does not take part in this process, but regenerates the superficial layer during the subsequent cycle.

The junction between these layers is marked by a change in the character of the arterioles supplying the endometrium. The portion traversing the basal endo-

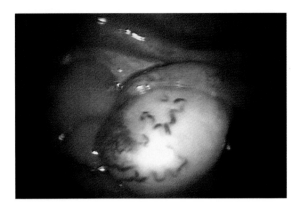

Fig. 11.4 **Laparoscopic view of corpus luteum.**

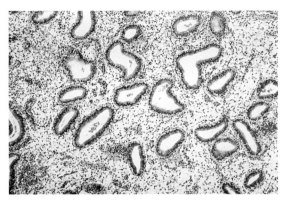

Fig. 11.6 **Secretory endometrium.**

metrium is straight, but thereafter its course becomes convoluted, giving rise to the spiral section of the arteriole. This anatomical configuration assumes importance in the physiological shedding of the superficial layers of the endometrium.

Proliferative phase

During the follicular phase in the ovary the endometrium is exposed to oestrogen secretion. At the end of menstruation regeneration rapidly occurs. At this stage – the 'proliferative' phase – the glands are tubular and arranged in a regular pattern, parallel to each other, and contain little secretion (Fig. 11.5).

Secretory phase

After ovulation, progesterone production induces secretory changes in the endometrial glands (Fig. 11.6). This is first evident as the appearance of secretory vacuoles in the glandular epithelium below the nuclei. This swiftly progresses to secretion of material into the lumen of the glands, which become tortuous and their margins appear serrated.

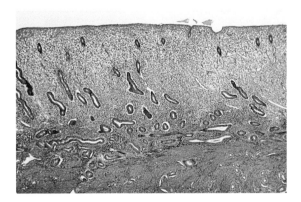

Fig. 11.5 **Proliferative endometrium.**

Menstrual phase

Normally the luteal phase lasts for 14 days, at the end of which regression of the corpus luteum is associated with a decline in ovarian oestrogen and progesterone production. This fall is followed by intense spasmodic contraction of the spiral section of the endometrial arterioles, giving rise to ischaemic necrosis, shedding of the superficial layer of the endometrium, and bleeding.

The vasospasm appears to be due to local production of prostaglandins. Prostaglandins may also account for the increased uterine contractions at the time of the menstrual flow. The failure of menstrual blood to clot has been ascribed to the presence of local fibrinolytic activity in the endometrial blood vessels which reaches a peak at the time of menstruation.

Cervical mucus

In the female there is direct continuity between the lower genital tract and the peritoneal cavity. This continuity is essential to allow spermatozoa access to the ova, as fertilization occurs in the fallopian tubes. It does, however, expose the woman to the risk of ascending infection. Nature has countered this hazard by using the cervical mucus as a barrier, the permeability of which varies during the menstrual cycle.

- Early in the follicular phase the cervical mucus is viscid and impermeable.
- Later in the follicular phase the increasing oestrogen levels induce changes in the composition of the mucus. The water content increases progressively so that just before ovulation occurs the mucus has become watery and is easily penetrated by the spermatozoa. This change is described by the term 'spinnbarkheit'.
- After ovulation the progesterone secreted by the corpus luteum counteracts the effect of the oestrogen, and the mucus again becomes impermeable, while the cervical os contracts.

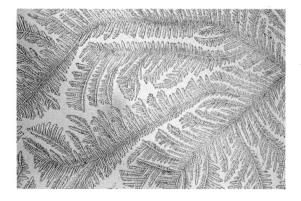

Fig. 11.7 **Cervical mucus – ferning.**

These changes can be monitored by the woman herself, if she is trying to achieve conception, or if she is using the 'rhythm method' of contraception. In the clinic the changes can be monitored by examining cervical mucus under the low power of a microscope. A fern-like pattern increases in parallel with the circulating oestrogen level and is maximal just before ovulation (Fig. 11.7), after which it gradually disappears.

Other cyclical changes

Although the purpose of the cyclical changes in ovarian hormones is to affect the genital tract, these hormones circulate throughout the body and can affect other organs.

Basal body temperature

A rise in basal body temperature of approximately 1°F or 0.5°C occurs following ovulation and is sustained until the onset of menstruation. This is due to the thermogenic effect of progesterone acting at hypothalamic level. Should conception occur the elevation in basal body temperature is maintained throughout pregnancy. A similar effect can be induced by the administration of progestagens.

Breast changes

The human mammary gland is very sensitive to oestrogen and progesterone. Breast swelling is often the first sign of puberty, in response to the small increase in ovarian oestrogen. Oestrogen and progesterone act synergistically on the breast and during the normal cycle breast swelling occurs in the luteal phase, apparently in response to increasing progesterone levels. The swelling is probably due to vascular changes and is not due to changes in the glandular tissue. It can cause discomfort to some women, and is not abolished by the oral contraceptive pill.

Psychological changes

Some women notice changes in mood during the menstrual cycle, with an increase in emotional lability in the late luteal phase. Such changes may be directly due to falling levels of progesterone, although mood changes are not always closely synchronized with hormonal fluctuations. The dividing line between normal cyclical changes and the premenstrual syndrome is unclear (see Ch. 22).

Key points

- At the start of the cycle, levels of FSH and LH are relatively high and these stimulate the development of 10–20 follicles. A dominant follicle matures, secreting oestrogen, and the remainder undergo atresia. As the oestrogen level rises the release of both gonadotrophins is suppressed (negative feedback) which serves to prevent hyperstimulation of the ovary and the maturation of multiple follicles.

- The very high pre-ovulatory oestradiol level stimulates a positive feedback mid-cycle surge of LH and FSH, which in turn stimulate ovulation. The remainder of the matured follicle forms the corpus luteum, a major source of progesterone.

- If conception and implantation occur, the corpus luteum is maintained by gonadotrophin secreted by the trophoblast. If, however, conception and implantation have not occurred successfully, the corpus luteum regresses, the levels of steroid hormones fall, gonadotrophin levels rise and menstruation ensues.

12

Amenorrhoea

Amenorrhoea may be defined as the failure of menstruation to occur at the expected time.

It may be considered in two categories:

1. Primary amenorrhoea – when menstruation has never occurred
2. Secondary amenorrhoea – when established menstruation ceases.

Primary amenorrhoea

Definition

Most girls will start to menstruate before the age of 15. If menstruation has not occurred by this age, patients may be considered in two groups depending on the presence or absence of secondary sexual characteristics. If there has been no secondary sexual development, the problem is delayed puberty (p. 108). If secondary sexual characteristics are otherwise normal, it is referred to as primary amenorrhoea (Table 12.1).

Primary amenorrhoea is most commonly caused by an imperforate hymen. The menstrual blood is retained within the vagina (a haematocolpos) and this often causes cyclical lower abdominal pain. Inspection of the vulva reveals a distended hymenal membrane through which dark blood may be seen, and treatment by incision, usually under anaesthesia, is all that is required (Fig. 12.1a,b). Much more rarely, there may be a horizontal vaginal septum, or even no uterus at all (see p. 111). An ultrasound scan may be useful.

The next most common cause is physiological delay, in other words the development is normal but there is an inherent delay in the onset of menstruation (see also p. 109). There is often a family history of the same problem with the mother. A progestogen challenge test is useful to identify constitutional menstrual delay. A progestogen (e.g. norethisterone) is given orally for 5 days, and withdrawal should lead to a vaginal bleed. If such a bleed occurs, it is reasonable to offer reassurance that spontaneous menstruation is likely to resume.

Low body weight and exercise, as discussed in Chapter 9, are also associated with primary amenorrhoea. The other causes listed in Table 12.1 are rare, although a few are outlined under the 'secondary amenorrhoea' discussion below.

Table 12.1
Causes of primary amenorrhoea

System	Problem	Incidence
Chromosomal	XO – Turner's syndrome	Rare
	XY – testicular feminization	Rare
	– 5-alpha-reductase deficiency	Rare
	XX/XY – true hermaphrodite	Rare
Hypothalamic	Physiological delay	Common
	Weight loss/anorexia/ heavy exercise	Common
	Isolated gonadotrophin-releasing hormone deficiency	Rare
	Congenital CNS defects	Rare
	Intracranial tumours	Rare
Pituitary	Partial/total hypopituitarism	Rare
	Hyperprolactinaemia	Rare
	Pituitary adenoma	Rare
	Empty sella syndrome	Rare
	Trauma/surgery	Rare
Ovarian	True agenesis	Rare
	Premature ovarian failure	Rare
	Radiation/chemotherapy/ autoimmune	Rare
	Polycystic ovaries	Rare
	Virilizing ovarian tumours	Rare
Other endocrine	Primary hypothyroidism	Rare
	Adrenal hyperplasia	Rare
	Adrenal tumour	Rare
Uterine/ vaginal	Imperforate hymen	Not uncommon
	Uterovaginal agenesis	Rare

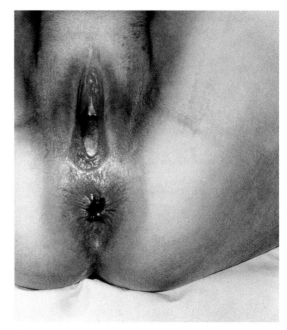

(a)

Secondary amenorrhoea

Secondary amenorrhoea means the cessation of established menstruation. It is defined as no menstruation for 6 months (or more than three times the previous cycle length) in the absence of pregnancy. A full list of causes is given in Table 12.2, but the commonest are weight loss, polycystic ovary syndrome (PCOS) and hyperprolactinaemia. The more common conditions are discussed below.

Causes

Physiological

The commonest causes of amenorrhoea during the reproductive phase of life are physiological – pregnancy and lactation. Pregnancy should therefore be excluded in all sexually active women presenting with amenorrhoea.

The high postpartum level of prolactin associated with suckling suppresses ovulation and gives rise to lactational amenorrhoea. The mechanism is probably

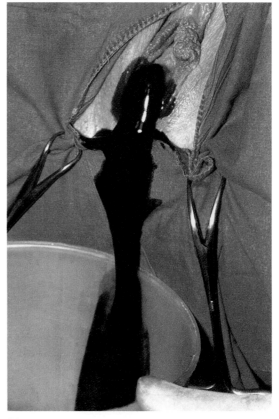

(b)

Fig. 12.1 **Imperforate hymen (a) before and (b) after incision.**

Table 12.2
Causes of secondary amenorrhoea

System	Problem	Incidence
Physiological	Pregnancy	Common
	Lactation	Common
	Menopause	Common
Hypothalamic	Weight loss/anorexia	Common
	Heavy exercise	Common
	Stress	Common
Pituitary	Hyperprolactinaemia	Uncommon
	Partial/total hypopituitarism	Rare
	Trauma/surgery	Rare
Ovarian	Polycystic ovary syndrome	Common
	Premature ovarian failure	Uncommon
	Surgery/radiotherapy/ chemotherapy	Uncommon
	Resistant ovary syndrome	Rare
	Virilizing ovarian tumours	Rare
Other endocrine	Primary hypothyroidism	Rare
	Adrenal hyperplasia	Rare
	Adrenal tumour	Rare
Uterine/vaginal	Surgery – hysterectomy	Common
	Endometrial ablation	Common
	Progestogen intrauterine device	Common
	Asherman's syndrome	Rare

related to reduced gonadotrophin-releasing hormone (GnRH) production as a result of changes in the sensitivity of the hypothalamic–pituitary axis to oestrogen. Amenorrhoea usually persists throughout the time that the infant is fully breast-fed but with the introduction of supplementary feeding, and therefore reduction in the frequency of suckling, prolactin levels fall and ovarian activity is resumed. This hypo-oestrogenic state may lead to atrophic vaginitis, and occasionally to coital problems.

Hypothalamic

Hypothalamic amenorrhoea ('hypogonadotrophic hypogonadism') is frequently associated with stress – for example, leaving home for higher education – and in such cases the condition usually resolves spontaneously. Physical stress in the form of athletic training, or even jogging, can also result in suppression of the hypothalamo–pituitary–ovarian axis. There are low levels of pituitary gonadotrophins in association with low levels of prolactin and oestrogen.

If hypothalamic amenorrhoea is not related to low body weight (see below), treatment will depend on whether or not the woman wants to conceive. If pregnancy is not desired, oestrogen replacement therapy is advisable, and is best given in the form of the oral contraceptive pill. If the woman wishes to become

pregnant, ovulation may be induced with pulsatile GnRH therapy or exogenous gonadotrophins (p. 142).

The hypothalamus is also sensitive to changes in body weight and weight loss, even to only 10–15% below the ideal, may be associated with amenorrhoea. Anorexia nervosa should be considered. Restoration of the body weight results in the return of ovulatory function, although there may be a significant time interval between the attainment of the ideal body weight and the resumption of ovarian activity. Ovulation induction therapy is not recommended prior to the restoration of body weight, as pregnancy, if it occurs, carries an increased perinatal mortality.

Pituitary

Prolactin stimulates mammary development and subsequent lactation. The secretion of prolactin, a polypeptide hormone produced by the lactotrophs of the anterior pituitary, is inhibited by dopamine from the hypothalamus. High levels of prolactin, which may be either physiological (during lactation) or pathological (see below), in turn suppress ovarian activity by interfering with the secretion of gonadotrophins.

Mildly elevated prolactin levels are common and can be due to stress (e.g. of venepuncture). Sustained higher levels can result in amenorrhoea and galactorrhoea unrelated to pregnancy. Galactorrhoea occurs in < 50% of those with hyperprolactinaemia, and < 50% of those with galactorrhoea have an elevated prolactin level. The causes of hyperprolactinaemia are given in Box 12.1.

Box 12.1

CAUSES OF HYPERPROLACTINAEMIA

Pituitary adenoma
- Microadenomas
- Macroadenomas

Secondary to other causes
- Primary hypothyroidism
- Chronic renal failure
- Stalk compression
- PCOS
- Drugs (phenothiazines, haloperidol, metoclopramide, cimetidine, methyldopa, antihistamines and morphine)

Idiopathic

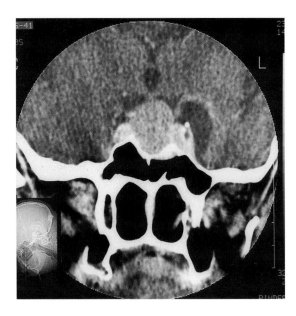

Fig. 12.2 **CT scan of a pituitary macroadenoma.**

Adenomas occur in the lateral wings of the anterior pituitary and are usually soft and discrete with a pseudo-capsule of compressed tissue (Fig. 12.2). If the prolactin is more than 1000 mU/l then imaging with CT or (ideally) MRI should be carried out. A microadenoma is less than 10 mm in diameter and a macroadenoma more than 10 mm. Visual fields should be checked as optic chiasma compression may lead to bitemporal hemianopia. One-third of adenomas regress spontaneously and less than 5% of microadenomas become macroadenomas. Serum levels correlate well with tumour size, so that if the tumour is relatively large and the prolactin level only modestly elevated, then pituitary stalk compression from a non-secreting macroadenoma or other tumour is possible (e.g. a craniopharyngioma). It is possible that idiopathic hyperprolactinaemia may be caused by microadenomas which are too small to be picked up by MRI scan.

All patients should have pituitary imaging before treatment. This treatment is usually with a dopamine agonist, either bromocriptine or cabergoline, which suppresses the prolactin level and also induces regression of the prolactinoma. Transnasal trans-sphenoidal microsurgical excision of an adenoma is only rarely required.

Ovarian

Premature ovarian failure
Ovarian failure normally occurs around the age of 50. The term 'premature ovarian failure' is usually used to describe cessation of ovarian function before the age of 40. As in the natural menopause, failure is usually due to inadequate numbers of primordial follicles in the ovaries.

It occurs in 1% of women and may be due to surgery, viral infections (e.g. mumps), cytotoxic drugs or radiotherapy. It may also be idiopathic and is occasionally associated with chromosomal abnormality (XO mosaics or XXX). A low oestrogen level, very high follicle-stimulating hormone (FSH) and the absence of any menstrual activity are poor prognostic signs for recovery. Pregnancy by in vitro fertilization (IVF) with donor oocytes may be possible. There is an association with other autoimmune disorders. Hormone replacement therapy is required to relieve postmenopausal symptoms and minimize the risk of osteoporosis.

Polycystic ovary syndrome (PCOS)
Polycystic ovary syndrome is associated with menstrual disturbance, and is the most common form of anovulatory infertility. There is good evidence for the hypothesis that decreased peripheral insulin sensitivity, exacerbated by obesity, leads to hyperinsulinaemia. The high insulin then stimulates theca-cell androgen production in the ovary and has an adverse effect on the lipid profile. The aetiology of the condition is unknown, but recent evidence suggests that the principal underlying disorder is one of insulin resistance, with the resultant hyperinsulinaemia stimulating excess ovarian androgen production. Associated with the prevalent insulin resistance, there is a characteristic dyslipidaemia and a predisposition to non-insulin-dependent diabetes and cardiovascular disease in later life. PCOS may therefore be considered to be a systemic metabolic condition rather one primarily of gynaecological origin (Fig. 12.3).

The diagnosis of PCOS is imprecise. The quoted incidence ranges widely from 0.5–25%. It was previously diagnosed clinically based on the presence of some or all of the following signs or symptoms: oligomenorrhoea or amenorrhoea (present in 80%), anovulatory infertility (74%), hirsutism (69%), and central obesity (49%). It seems more appropriate, however, to define the condition in terms of the ovarian appearance at ultrasound. The typical appearance is of bilaterally enlarged ovaries with multiple peripherally situated cysts 'like a ring of pearls' in a dense stroma (Fig. 12.4). The cysts are usually less than 10 mm in size. Biochemical changes also occur. The testosterone level may be elevated and the luteinizing hormone (LH) is usually significantly higher than the FSH.

Treatment depends on whether the presenting problem has been menstrual irregularity, hirsutism or infertility. The combined oral contraceptive pill has been used to regulate the menses but, while it reduces androgen levels, it exacerbates insulin resistance and may be

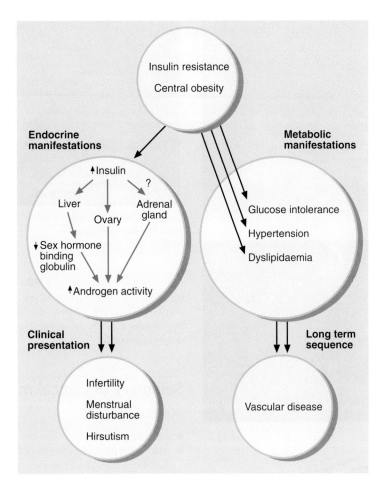

Fig. 12.3 **Pathogenesis of polycystic ovary syndrome.** Polycystic ovary syndrome can be considered to be a disorder primarily of insulin resistance, with the resultant hyperinsulinaemia stimulating excess ovarian androgen production. There may also be dyslipidaemia and a predisposition to later non-insulin-dependent diabetes and cardiovascular disease.

relatively contraindicated in obese women. Hirsutism may be treated with the combined oral contraceptive pill or cyproterone acetate and clomifene is useful for anovulatory infertility (p. 141). Laparoscopic laser or diathermy to the ovary may also give short-term benefits for those with ovulatory problems, but only when the patient is clomifene resistant.

The corner-stone to management, however, is weight reduction, which reduces insulin resistance, corrects the hormone imbalance and promotes ovulation. Recent work has been directed towards the use of insulin-sensitizing agents (e.g. metformin) and this therapeutic option shows considerable promise in the management of anovulation.

Long term there is an increased risk of cardiovascular disease, non-insulin-dependent diabetes mellitus, endometrial hyperplasia, endometrial carcinoma and breast carcinoma. Individuals may gain benefit from early screening for cardiovascular risk factors, particularly hypertension and glucose intolerance.

Virilizing tumours of the ovary

These rare tumours are often small, and may be particularly suspected when amenorrhoea is associated with virilization. Investigation shows plasma testosterone levels elevated above the female range and treatment is with surgical excision (Fig. 12.5).

Other endocrine causes

These are rare. Women with thyrotoxicosis may have amenorrhoea. Primary hypothyroidism is also associated with amenorrhoea, as thyrotrophin-releasing hormone stimulates prolactin secretion. The most common of the rare adrenal problems is late-onset congenital adrenal hyperplasia. This is usually due to a deficiency of the enzyme 21-hydroxylase (Fig. 10.9), and treatment with a low dose of corticosteroids is usually sufficient to re-establish ovulatory function by suppressing adrenal function. Androgen-secreting adrenal tumours can also occur.

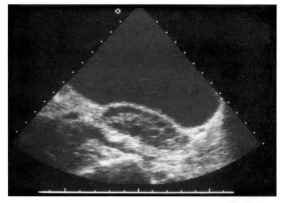

(a)

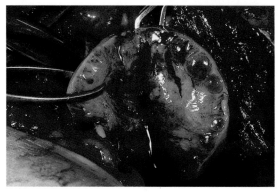

(b)

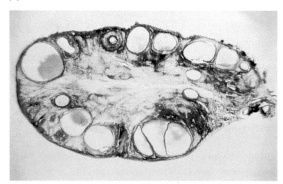

(c)

Fig. 12.4 **Polycystic ovaries.** These are classically bilaterally enlarged with multiple peripherally situated cysts 'like a ring of pearls' in a dense stroma: **(a)** ultrasound scan; **(b)** surgical dissection; **(c)** pathological preparation.

Uterine

Excessive uterine curettage – usually at the time of miscarriage, termination of pregnancy or secondary postpartum haemorrhage – may remove the basal layer of the endometrium and result in the formation of uterine adhesions (synechiae), a condition known as

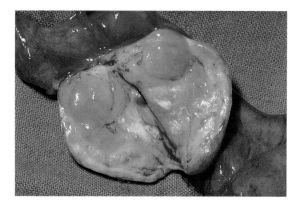

Fig. 12.5 **Hilar cell tumour.**

Asherman's syndrome (Fig. 12.6). It may rarely also result from severe postpartum infection. Treatment involves breaking down the adhesions through a hysteroscope with or without inserting an IUCD to deter reformation.

Summary of clinical management

Initial management:

- Exclude pregnancy.
- Ask about perimenopausal symptoms (e.g. flushings, vaginal dryness).
- Take a history including weight changes, drugs, medical disorders and thyroid symptoms.
- Carry out an examination looking particularly at height, weight, visual fields and the presence of hirsutism or virilization. Also carry out a pelvic examination, unless this is contraindicated.

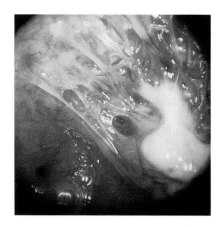

Fig. 12.6 **Rarely, adhesions can form within the uterine cavity.** If so severe that they obstruct the menstrual flow the condition is referred to as Asherman's syndrome.

Table 12.3
Further management based on test results

Ultrasound scan	A scan showing multiple (> 8) small, peripherally placed follicular ovarian cysts surrounded by a thickened echodense stroma confirms the diagnosis of polycystic ovary syndrome. The diagnosis is supported by an LH : FSH ratio > 3 and a testosterone level > 3 mmol/l	If pregnancy desired, clomifene or gonadotrophins. If pregnancy not desired, consider the combined oral contraceptive pill
Elevated PL level	If PL > 800 mU/l on at least two occasions, the diagnosis is hyperprolactinaemia	Arrange imaging of the pituitary. Treat with dopamine antagonist
Elevated FSH	If FSH > 30 U/l, repeat 6 weeks later. If still elevated and the patient > 40 years old, the patient is menopausal. If less than 40, the diagnosis is premature ovarian failure	Consider HRT. Pregnancy with oocyte donation is possible
Abnormal TFTs	If the TFTs are abnormal, treat as appropriate	

FSH, follicle-stimulating hormone; HRT, hormone replacement therapy; LH, luteinizing hormone; PL, prolactin; TFTs thyroid function tests

- Check serum for LH, FSH, prolactin, testosterone, thyroxine and thyroid-stimulating hormone (TSH).
- Arrange a transvaginal ultrasound scan looking for polycystic ovaries.
- Review with the results (Table 12.3).

If the tests listed in Table 12.3 are normal consider the following causes:

- weight loss
- depression, emotional disturbance and extreme exercise
- Asherman's syndrome
- idiopathic amenorrhoea.

In the majority of patients who present with secondary amenorrhoea, investigations will fail to demonstrate any significant endocrine abnormality – idiopathic amenorrhoea. It is probable that there is a disturbance of the normal feedback mechanisms of control. Undue sensitivity of the hypothalamus and pituitary to the negative feedback suppression of endogenous oestrogen may result in impaired gonadotrophin secretion which is inadequate to stimulate follicular development, and results in cycle initiation failure. Those requiring ovulation usually respond well to an anti-oestrogen such as clomifene (p. 141).

Key points

- The commonest causes of primary amenorrhoea (when menstruation has never occurred) are physiological delay, weight loss, heavy exercise and an imperforate hymen.

- Secondary amenorrhoea is said to have occurred when established menstruation ceases. Outwith pregnancy, lactation and the menopause, the commonest causes are the polycystic ovary syndrome, stress, weight loss and hyperprolactinaemia.

- Polycystic ovary syndrome is a systemic metabolic condition associated with decreased peripheral insulin sensitivity and hyperinsulinaemia.

Epidemiology

Infertility is an extremely common problem that affects approximately 1 in 6 couples at some stage in their lives. The cause may be related to a problem with the man, woman or both. In view of the intimate nature of the problem, there can be few conditions that cause such personal distress and embarrassment. However, effective treatment is now available to help an increasing proportion of these couples.

Definitions

Infertility can be defined as the inability of the couple to conceive within a year or two of beginning regular unprotected sexual intercourse. A couple can have primary infertility – no previous pregnancies within the relationship – or secondary infertility, where the couple have had at least one pregnancy.

Infertility is rarely absolute, and most couples have a degree of subfertility. Around 80% of the normal fertile population will conceive within 1 year, and 92% by the end of 2 years. Cumulative pregnancy rates and live birth rates are the terms used to express the chance of conception within a given time interval. Figure 13.1 illustrates the cumulative pregnancy rate for the normal fertile population.

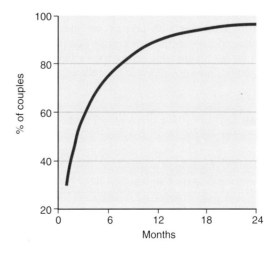

Fig. 13.1 **Cumulative pregnancy rates in the normal fertile population.**

Gynaecology

Fecundability is the percentage of women exposed to the risk of a pregnancy for one menstrual cycle who will produce a live-born infant (normal range – 15–28%). Fecundability usually diminishes slightly with each passing month of not conceiving.

Age and fertility

Normal fertility declines as the woman's age increases. A woman is born with a finite store of oocytes, around one or two million. This falls to approximately 400 000 at puberty, and by the time the menopause is reached the number of oocytes has fallen to below 1000. During her reproductive life a woman will release only 500 mature oocytes – a form of pre-conceptual natural selection – while the remaining oocytes undergo atresia or apoptosis. The rate of oocyte loss is relatively constant throughout early life until around the age of 37 years, when the rate of loss accelerates. At the menopause, which occurs at an average age of 51, there are no functioning oocytes.

There is strong evidence that the decline in fertility is directly related to the declining oocyte population and the eggs' inherent quality. There is a small, but noticeable, fall in monthly fecundity rates from the age of 31 years, a more pronounced decrease from the age of 37 years, and a very steep decline over the age of 40 years. In addition, there is a substantial increase in spontaneous miscarriage rates with age, and a substantially higher risk of having a genetically abnormal child. Although older men are less fertile, the effect of age in men is far less pronounced than with women.

Incidence

The prevalence of infertility in the community is around 14% of couples, just over half with secondary infertility and the remainder with primary infertility. There has been an increase in the demand for infertility services over the last two decades, although the actual prevalence of infertility does not appear to have altered significantly.

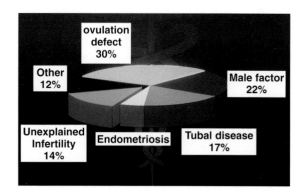

Fig. 13.2 **Causes of infertility (based on a sample of 5129 couples).** (From Taylor & Collins 1992, with permission.)

Causes

The causes of infertility can be classified simply, as outlined in Figure 13.2. In some couples more than one problem can be identified.

Diagnosis

The diagnosis of infertility is a process of exclusion, identifying those patients where the cause is clear, those in whom there is a possible cause, and those in whom the cause is essentially unexplained. The aim of investigation should be to reach a diagnosis as soon as possible, using only tests that are of proven value.

History and examination

Factors that provide clues to the aetiology are outlined in Tables 13.1 and 13.2. Other important factors to be noted are the woman's age and the duration of infertility – generally, the longer the period of infertility the worse the prognosis. The order in which the investigations are performed varies depending on whether the couple has primary or secondary infertility, with an earlier

Table 13.1
Examination of the woman

Examination	Reason
Height and weight for body mass index (BMI)	High or low BMI associated with lower fertility
Body hair distribution	Hyperandrogenism
Galactorrhoea	Hyperprolactinaemia
Uterine structural abnormalities	May be associated with infertility
Fixed or tender uterus	Endometriosis or pelvic inflammatory disease associated with tubal damage

Table 13.2
Examination of the man

Examination	Reason
Scrotum	Varicocele
Size (volume) of the testes	Small testes associated with oligospermia
Position of the testes	Undescended testes
Prostate	Chronic infection

assessment of tubal patency in the latter. Early assessment is also indicated if a specific abnormality is suspected from the history, and for an older patient.

Examination of the woman

Height and weight should be recorded and used to calculate the body mass index (BMI), using the formula: weight (kg)/height (m)^2. The normal range is between 19 and 25. A change of weight of greater than 10% in the preceding year may cause a disturbance of the menstrual pattern and anovulation. A body mass index at either extreme is detrimental to fertility (see later).

Increased body hair is associated with hyperandrogenism, most commonly because of polycystic ovary syndrome. Breast examination may demonstrate galactorrhoea, which is associated with hyperprolactinaemia. Pelvic examination is important to look for signs of structural abnormalities, infection, and pathological processes such as endometriosis or pelvic inflammatory disease.

Examination of the man

Examination of the man is not essential in the absence of any relevant history. If, however, the semen analysis is abnormal, examination of the genitalia is helpful looking specifically at size (volume), consistency and position of the testes, the outline of the epididymis (for the presence of the vas deferens) and finally the scrotum for any evidence of swellings. Examination of the prostate can be omitted unless there is evidence of chronic infection.

Investigations and their interpretation

The investigations should be arranged in a logical manner with reference to the history, along with appropriate general health screening (Box 13.1). Additional tests may be necessary, depending on the clinical circumstances (Box 13.2).

Box 13.1

BASELINE INVESTIGATIONS

Female
- Early follicular phase LH, FSH, oestradiol
- Rubella (to vaccinate if negative)
- Luteal progesterone level (to assess ovulation)
- Test of tubal patency (laparoscopy, HyCoSy, or hysterosalpingogram)

Male
- Semen analysis × 2

Box 13.2

ADDITIONAL INVESTIGATIONS

Female
- Pelvic ultrasound scan for ovarian morphology and uterine abnormalities
- Salpingoscopy or falloposcopy for intraluminal tubal adhesions
- Hysteroscopy for intrauterine anomalies
- Prolactin and thyroid function tests with oligo–amenorrhoea
- Testosterone and sex hormone binding globulin (SHBG) if hirsute

Male
- Sperm function tests (see text) if baseline test is consistently abnormal
- Mixed agglutination reaction (MAR) test or immunobead test for antisperm antibodies
- FSH, LH, testosterone if low sperm count (raised FSH if testicular failure, low if central nervous system cause)
- Transrectal ultrasound for suspected abnormalities of the seminal vesicles and prostate

---

Male factors
Classification

Male factor infertility can be a problem of sperm production, sperm function, or sperm delivery. Sperm production may be completely absent (azoospermia) in, for example, testicular failure. More commonly a patient may present with a reduced count of sperm of normal appearance (oligospermia). Additionally, a high proportion of the sperm may be poorly motile, lacking the normal forward progressive movement (asthenospermia), or may appear morphologically defective (teratospermia) with abnormalities of the head, midpiece or tail.

Normal sperm function is more difficult to demonstrate, but may be suggested by a positive postcoital test (see later), or an ability of sperm to penetrate mucus in vitro or to swim through culture medium. Infection, characterized by leucospermia, or antisperm antibodies, both of which can be associated with agglutination, can affect sperm function.

Problems with sperm delivery may be caused by absence or blockage of the vas deferens or epididymis. It may also be related to impotence, premature ejaculation, or a physical inability to have normal sexual intercourse.

Semen analysis

This provides information about spermatogenesis and sperm delivery, but gives little information about sperm function. The World Health Organization (WHO) has produced a normal range of values for semen (Table 13.3). The values, however, are empirical and do not reflect a cut-off point below which pregnancy will not occur. Only in the 5% of patients that present with azoospermia can an absolute male cause be confirmed. Even if the sperm density is less than 5 million/ml, 19% will father a child, compared to a pregnancy rate of 43% in women whose partners have a count greater than 5 million/ml. A similar picture exists when the other variables, motility and morphology, are considered. Only when motility is below 20% and morphology falls below 15%, does the basic semen analysis have

any significant predictive value. In conclusion, the basic semen analysis (with the exception of azoospermia) is of little prognostic value unless sperm values are very low.

A man's sperm count varies considerably, and in the presence of one abnormal result a second count should be arranged. As spermatogenesis takes approximately 3 months to complete, the samples ought to be produced at least 3 months apart. Samples should be produced by masturbation or after intercourse into a non-lubricated condom after a period of abstinence of between 3–5 days. The sample should be analysed in an accredited laboratory, with careful assessment of morphology using strict definitions of abnormality (Kruger criteria), as morphology is also closely associated with the sperm's ability to fertilize.

Tests of sperm function

These can be in vivo, such as the postcoital test, or in vitro, for example sperm penetration tests into cervical mucus substitutes, or an assessment of sperms' ability to swim through a physiological culture medium. Other tests, such as the ability of the sperm to enter a zona pellucida-free hamster egg (SPA), or to bind to an isolated zona pellucida (HZA) have been employed, but are not used in routine clinical practice. Computerized assessment of sperm motility patterns has been shown to correlate well with the ability of sperm to fertilize oocytes in an in vitro setting.

The postcoital test involves asking the couple to have sexual intercourse timed to the woman's mid-cycle. Then, 6–12 hours later, a sample of endocervical mucus is taken, looking for the presence or absence of sperm. Some studies have shown a positive correlation between the finding of motile sperm in the mucus and the chance of subsequent pregnancy. The use of this test, however, is controversial, as other studies have shown that the finding of a positive or negative result does not alter the chance or timing of a pregnancy. As a result most centres have abandoned this procedure.

Antibodies can develop against sperm. These can be serum (IgG) or bound (IgA), and attach principally to the tail, midpiece or head of the sperm. Tests used to detect antisperm antibodies include the mixed agglutination reaction (MAR) test, and the immunobead test. Levels of greater than 50% are thought to significantly affect fertility.

Female factors
Ovulation

Ovulation is an 'all or nothing' phenomenon, with usually one oocyte released per ovulatory cycle. Interestingly, an inherited propensity for twins is borne down the female line, and is caused by a tendency of these women to release two oocytes.

Table 13.3
WHO criteria for semen analysis

Volume	> 2 ml
pH	7–8
Concentration	$> 20 \times 10^6$/ml
Motility	> 50% forward > 25% with rapid linear progress
Morphology	> 15% normal
Alive	> 50%
Antisperm antibodies (MAR test)	Negative
White cell count	$< 1 \times 10^6$/ml

Causes of anovulation

Ovarian failure   This is found in about 50% of patients with primary amenorrhoea, and 15% of those presenting with secondary amenorrhoea. Most patients with primary amenorrhoea will have an established diagnosis before presenting to an infertility clinic. The cause may be genetic, e.g. Turner's syndrome (45XO), or autoimmune. In those presenting with secondary amenorrhoea and ovarian failure there may be an obvious cause, such as previous ovarian surgery, abdominal radiotherapy or chemotherapy. There will also be a proportion of patients in whom no reason can be identified – idiopathic premature menopause.

Weight-related anovulation   Weight plays an important part in the control of ovulation. A minimum degree of body fat (generally thought to be around 22% of body weight) is needed to maintain ovulatory cycles. Substantial weight loss leads to the disappearance of the normal 24-hour secretory pattern of luteinizing hormone-releasing hormone (LHRH), which reverts to the nocturnal pattern seen in pubescent girls. As a result the ovaries develop a multifollicular appearance on ultrasound. Severe exercise can, by increasing the muscle bulk and decreasing the body fat, have the same effect, and it is not uncommon for women athletes or ballerinas to have amenorrhoea. Excessive weight can also have an adverse effect on ovulation. This probably results from excess oestrone, generated in the adipose tissue from androgens, interfering with the normal feedback mechanism to the pituitary gland.

Polycystic ovary syndrome   50% of patients presenting with anovulatory infertility will have polycystic ovary syndrome (PCOS) – see Chapter 12.

Luteinized unruptured follicle syndrome   In certain patients the oocyte may be retained following the luteinizing hormone (LH) surge, the so-called 'luteinized unruptured follicle syndrome' (LUF). Repeated pelvic ultrasound scans fail to show the expected collapse of the follicle at ovulation, and the follicle persists into the luteal phase. As no longitudinal studies have shown this to be a persistent finding in the same patient, however, there is a question mark over its relevance to fertility.

Hyperprolactinaemia   Hyperprolactinaemia is found in 10–15% of cases of secondary amenorrhoea. About one-third of these patients will have galactorrhoea, and occasionally there may be some evidence of visual impairment (bitemporal hemianopia) due to pressure on the optic chiasma from pituitary adenoma.

Tests of ovulation

There is only one true test that proves ovulation has occurred, and that is pregnancy. However, there are a number of investigations that imply that ovulation has taken place:

- History: over 90% of women with regular menstrual cycles will ovulate spontaneously.
- LH kits.
- Mid-luteal phase progesterone is the most commonly used test of ovulation. A luteal phase progesterone value of greater than 28 nmol/l is found in conception cycles, and as a result this value is generally regarded as evidence of satisfactory ovulation. However, it is important to time the blood sample carefully – between 7 and 10 days before the next menstrual period. This can only be determined with some knowledge of the length of the patient's normal menstrual cycle.

Other tests   Less commonly employed tests include serial ultrasound scans to monitor the growth, and subsequent disappearance, of a Graafian follicle. A luteal phase endometrial biopsy looking for appropriately timed secretory changes is no longer considered of value. Basal body temperature was previously considered to be of value as there is a rise of 0.5°C if ovulation has occurred (due to progesterone) but in practice this is now rarely used.

Further investigations

Pelvic ultrasound is very useful in defining the ovarian morphology. Serum testosterone measurement is necessary if there is evidence of hirsutism, to exclude more sinister disorders such as androgen-secreting tumours of the ovary or adrenal gland. A progestogen challenge test may be useful in patients with a history of amenorrhoea and normal follicle-stimulating hormone (FSH) and prolactin. It is used to determine whether the patient is clinically oestrogenized. This acts as a guide to what would be the most appropriate medication to use to induce ovulation. Medroxyprogesterone acetate, 5 mg daily for 5 days, is usually sufficient to induce a withdrawal bleed. If the bleeding is normal the patient is well oestrogenized, whereas if it is absent or scanty the patient is relatively poorly oestrogenized. Direct measurement of serum oestradiol may also be carried out.

Tubal patency

Classification

The fallopian tube can be blocked distally – at the fimbrial end – or, less commonly, at the proximal end – the cornu. In addition, the tubo-ovarian relationship may be disrupted by peritubal adhesions. Fimbrial disease has varying degrees of severity:

- agglutination of the fimbria to produce a narrowed opening – known as a phimosis
- complete agglutination to form a hydrosalpinx.

Gynaecology

In addition, tubal damage can also involve the endo-salpinx, with intraluminal adhesions and flattening of the mucosal folds. Microsurgery to relieve tubal blockage, therefore, may not restore tubal function.

The important features for fertility prognosis appear to be:

- degree of dilatation of the fallopian tube
- extent of the fibrosis of the wall of the tube
- damage to the endosalpinx.

Tests of tubal patency

Diagnostic laparoscopy is the 'gold standard' investigation. It provides a direct view of the pelvic organs. Methylthioninium chloride (methylene blue) dye is inserted through a cannula in the cervix to demonstrate tubal patency. Hysteroscopy is often carried out at the same time, looking at the uterine cavity. The diagnostic laparoscopy requires admission to hospital, usually as a day case, and a general anaesthetic. As such it is the most invasive and expensive investigation performed on the woman. For this reason, some doctors prefer to use a hysterosalpingogram as a first-line assessment.

Hysterosalpingography (HSG) involves inserting an instrument, with a watertight seal, into the cervix and passing radio-opaque fluid into the uterine cavity and fallopian tubes, demonstrating their outline (Fig. 13.3a,b). The test is performed under X-ray control on an outpatient basis. If the HSG is normal, the diagnosis can be relied upon in 97% of cases. However, if the HSG is abnormal, the diagnosis can only be relied upon in 34% of cases (false positive rate 66%), and a laparoscopy is required to confirm the nature of the abnormality.

Salpingoscopy More detailed investigation of the interior of the fallopian tube is now possible but is only really necessary if the question of tubal surgery is raised. A fine telescope, called a salpingoscope, can be passed down an operating laparoscope and inserted into the ampullary portion of the fallopian tube. Approximately 50% of patients with macroscopically damaged fallopian tubes will have fine intratubal adhesions. If present these adhesions adversely affect the outcome of surgery.

Falloposcopy More recently, advances in fibreoptics have allowed the development of a very fine instrument, a falloposcope, with a diameter less than 1 mm, which can be inserted into the fallopian tube via the uterine cavity. Falloposcopy appears to be effective in detecting tubal pathology, and can be performed on an outpatient basis. The equipment is fragile and expensive, however, and its use is limited to a small number of centres, mainly as a research tool.

Hysterosalpingo-contrast sonography (HyCoSy) This technique involves a standard pelvic ultrasound scan at which galactose-containing ultrasound contrast medium is inserted into the uterine cavity, outlining any abnormalities such as submucosal fibroids and endometrial polyps, before passing down the fallopian tubes to confirm tubal patency. The technique offers a similar level of diagnostic accuracy to HSG.

It is important to note that all of these techniques are useful in demonstrating patency, but none is capable of assessing tubal function.

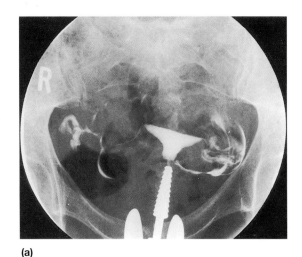

(a)

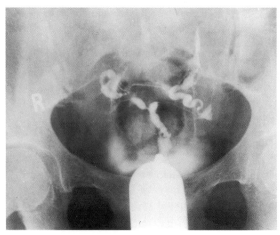

(b)

Fig. 13.3 **Hysterosalpingography of (a) normal and (b) abnormal uteri.** In (b) the radio-opaque dye does not leak from the fallopian tubes, thus indicating a blockage.

Treatment

Approximately 22% of couples with infertility conceive spontaneously during investigation or while awaiting treatment. For those in whom investigations reveal no true cause, many will require nothing more than a careful explanation of their chances of conception. However, age and length of infertility must be taken into account when adopting such a conservative approach. Before considering active treatment the couple should be counselled about general health matters such as smoking, alcohol intake, and diet. Where the diagnosis is clear, specific treatments can be employed.

Anovulation

There are various ways of inducing ovulation, depending on the underlying cause. Successful ovulation-induction treatment should be continued for long enough to give the optimum chance for conception – generally 12 months.

Hyperprolactinaemia is treated with a dopamine agonist, either bromocriptine or cabergoline (Ch. 12).

Excess or decreased body weight should be treated by diet. Although ovulation can generally be induced by exogenous gonadotrophins, this should be avoided, particularly if the patient is underweight, as there is an increased risk of pregnancy complications such as miscarriage or premature labour. Patients with moderate obesity often show resistance to treatment with clomifene citrate and gonadotrophins, requiring much higher doses to induce ovulation.

Anovulation in oestrogenized patients

Most of these patients have polycystic ovary syndrome (85% of patients presenting with oligo–amenorrhoea and 25% of those with amenorrhoea). First-line treatment in this condition is oral anti-oestrogen therapy, usually with clomifene citrate.

Clomifene citrate, a derivative of the weak non-steroidal oestrogen triphenylethylene, is formulated as a mixture of two isomers, enclomifene and zuclomifene, the former being the important isomer for ovulation induction. Its mode of action is to increase the plasma FSH concentration, mainly by competitively blocking the negative feedback effects of endogenous oestradiol on the hypothalamus. FSH is the principal hormone needed for follicular recruitment and development.

Initially a dose of 25–50 mg for 5 days is given at the beginning of a cycle (days 2–6). If there is no response, the dose is increased to a maximum of 100 mg daily for 5 days. Rarely, in obese patients, the dose may be increased to 150 mg daily for 5 days. In monitoring the response to treatment with clomifene, serum progesterone will not indicate whether more than one follicle has developed and serial ultrasound scans of follicular growth may be more useful.

Ovulation can be achieved successfully in approximately 80% of cycles, with cumulative pregnancy rates of up to 81% after 12 months' treatment. Unfortunately, there is a disappointingly high miscarriage rate in patients treated for PCOS, perhaps related to the high background LH. There is an increased risk of multiple pregnancy (7% twins; 1% triplets or greater) mostly confined to patients with PCOS.

Side-effects while using clomifene citrate are uncommon, the most frequent being:

- hot flushes (11%)
- pelvic discomfort (7%)
- nausea (2%)
- breast discomfort (2%).

These are rarely severes, and simple explanation and reassurance are all that is required. More significant problems include visual disturbances (1.5%) and cholestatic jaundice (rare). In both these situations the drug should be discontinued and not used again. Some women do not respond to oral ovulation-induction agents such as clomifene. These patients require treatment with exogenous gonadotrophins.

Exogenous gonadotrophins are derived from two sources: extracted from postmenopausal women's urine or, more recently, created in vitro by genetically engineered mammalian cells. Although the original urinary-derived gonadotrophins contained an equal mixture of FSH and LH (75 IU per ampoule), refinement of the extraction techniques has resulted in highly purified FSH compounds (greater than 99% of protein content is FSH). The recombinant genetically engineered FSH preparations attain similar levels of purity.

All these medications require parenteral administration, by either subcutaneous or intramuscular injection. Around 4% of women undergoing gonadotrophin treatment will develop ovarian hyperstimulation syndrome and this will be severe in 0.5%. The incidence of multiple pregnancy with gonadotrophin treatment is around 20%. The aim is to achieve development of a single follicle using a low-dose regimen, starting at one ampoule (75 IU) daily for 10 days, and then increasing the dose, if necessary, by small increments until satisfactory follicular growth occurs. Response is monitored by ovarian ultrasound, sometimes combined with serum oestradiol measurement.

When the Graafian follicle reaches maturity, ovulation is induced by administering human chorionic gonadotrophin (hCG) (5000 IU). This replaces the normal LH surge. Gonadotrophin therapy is highly successful in restoring normal fertility in patients with hypothalamic amenorrhoea (see below) but patients with PCOS resistant to clomifene are less successfully treated; they are more prone to multifollicular development, have a lower chance of pregnancy, a higher rate of miscarriage and, if the patient does conceive, there is a much greater chance of a multiple pregnancy.

If standard ovulation induction treatment fails in patients with PCOS, laparoscopic ovarian diathermy can be tried. The ovarian capsule is pierced four times for 5 seconds with a needle point diathermy. Although both ovaries are usually treated, recent evidence suggests that only one ovary needs puncturing. Encouraging results have been reported, with spontaneous ovulation returning in up to 71% of cycles, without the risk of hyperstimulation or multiple pregnancy. In patients where spontaneous ovulation does not occur, most become more responsive to clomifene or gonadotrophin therapy. Unfortunately, the effect is time-limited, with chronic anovulation returning in 50% of patients within 2 years. There is also a risk of iatrogenic adhesion formation.

Recent evidence suggests that metformin, an oral antidiabetic drug, which works by increasing peripheral utilization of glucose in the presence of endogenous insulin, may be of value in helping induce ovulation in obese patients with PCOS.

Anovulation in oestrogen-deficient women

Women who have a low FSH, normal prolactin, and either a low serum oestradiol or a negative progestogen withdrawal test (hypogonadotrophic hypogonadism) need exogenous gonadotrophins (see above) or pulsatile LHRH treatment. Exogenous gonadotrophin treatment in this group of patients is less prone to side-effects such as multiple pregnancy but nevertheless careful monitoring as described above is necessary.

Pulsatile LHRH treatment is an alternative to gonadotrophin therapy in patients with hypothalamic disorders of gonadotrophin regulation. Pulsatile doses of LHRH are given either intravenously or subcutaneously at intervals of 60–90 minutes using a small pump. Ovulation occurs in about 90% of cycles, restoring normal fertility rates. This treatment minimizes the risk of multiple follicular development and, as a result, there is a lower risk of multiple pregnancy (10%). Patients with PCOS respond poorly to this treatment with ovulation rates of around 40% and pregnancy rates of < 10%.

Tubal disease

There are two treatments for tubal disease: surgery and in vitro fertilization (IVF). IVF is described later in this chapter.

Tubal surgery

In the past, surgery has been the principal treatment for occlusive tubal disease but as the results of IVF have improved, it is performed less frequently.

Selection of patients

Patients for tubal surgery need to be carefully selected taking into consideration:

- patient's age
- site and extent of the tubal damage
- other factors that might influence fertility.

As with other treatments, age has a profound effect on the outcome, and IVF may be better for older patients. Distal tubal occlusion carries the worst prognosis, and surgery should be reserved only for cases in whom damage is relatively minor. Women with a moderate to severe distal abnormality, and those with bipolar tubal disease (damage at more than one site on the same tube) have a very poor prognosis and require IVF. However, with limited proximal damage, pregnancy rates of close to 50% have been quoted from tubal surgery.

Techniques

Conventionally tubal surgery has been performed by laparotomy, through a Pfannenstiel incision, with microsurgical techniques used to restore tubal patency. However, most tubal surgery is now performed laparoscopically. Even completely occluded tubes have been opened successfully laparoscopically using either a CO_2 laser, or electrodiathermy. In skilled hands the results compare very favourably with conventional tubal surgery using an operating microscope.

More recently, selective salpingography (passing a fine catheter through the uterus and along the fallopian tube under X-ray control) has been used successfully to treat some patients with proximal obstruction caused by a plug of amorphous debris.

Risks of tubal surgery

Patients who have had tubal surgery have a tenfold increased risk of having an ectopic pregnancy. They should be advised that when they do conceive, they should have an ultrasound scan performed at 6 weeks' gestation to confirm the site of the pregnancy.

Endometriosis

Endometriosis is discussed in Chapter 21. There is no evidence that treating minimal and mild peritoneal endometriosis with drugs improves the chance of conception. Indeed, medical treatment of endometriosis involves creating anovulation for up to 6 months, and this delays the patient from trying for a family. However, there is some limited evidence to suggest that surgery to ablate the endometriotic lesions, and to divide adhesions that may have formed from endometriosis, increases the chance of conception. The ablation by diathermy or laser can often be performed at the time of the diagnostic laparoscopy.

If the endometriosis involves the ovary or the fallopian tube, surgical treatment appears to be beneficial, correcting the anatomical defect. The results of surgery, even where the endometriosis is quite severe, appear to be quite encouraging. However, if pregnancy does not occur within 9–10 months, it is reasonable to consider IVF.

Male factor problems

Azoospermia and a raised serum FSH

Azoospermia and raised serum FSH signify spermatogenic failure (non-obstructive azoospermia). This can be confirmed by testicular biopsy. Occasionally, islands of spermatogenesis can be identified and sperm can be extracted from a testicular biopsy, and used for intracytoplasmic sperm injection as part of IVF treatment (see later). In most cases, however, the option likely to give the couple the best chance of a live birth is donor insemination.

Donor insemination (DI)

Men who donate sperm do so for altruistic reasons. Donors, to date, have been anonymous, although there are strong arguments for a change in practice to identified donors. All potential donors are carefully screened for a family history of medical conditions that could be passed to future children and, of course, for infection, particularly with HIV. For the latter reason, semen is frozen in straws and quarantined for a minimum of 6 months. The donor is screened again for infection at the end of this period, and only if this second screen is negative is the sperm used for treatment. The need to freeze sperm reduces the pregnancy rates, as frozen sperm is not as effective as fresh sperm.

Semen is inserted into the woman's cervix – or if appropriately prepared, into the uterus (see below) – at the time of ovulation. Ovulation is usually predicted by serial pelvic ultrasound scans or by the detection of the LH surge using a urinary assay. The chance of conception in the first cycle of treatment is 18.8%, falling rapidly to around 6% per cycle for the next 12 months.

Azoospermia and a normal FSH

Azoospermia in the presence of a normal FSH signifies a block of the vas deferens or epididymis. The most common group of men in this category are those who have had a vasectomy. Using microsurgical techniques the vas can be re-anastamosed (vasovasostomy) or attached to the epididymis (vasoepididymostomy), depending on the site of the obstruction. Although good anatomical results can be achieved, pregnancy rates are often disappointing, partly because the build-up of pressure distal to the obstruction may have damaged the delicate epididymis, and partly because antisperm antibodies may have formed. The time from the original

vasectomy to the reversal procedure provides a useful guide to prognosis. Pregnancy rates are halved in the partners of men where the gap between the vasectomy and reversal is greater than 10 years (rates of 60% and 30% respectively in good hands). Another useful prognostic indicator is the finding of sperm in the vas fluid distal to the obstruction, with pregnancy rates of 80% and 72% for vasovasostomy and vasoepididymostomy respectively. If no sperm are seen in the vas fluid the outlook following surgery is bleak.

Men in whom spermatogenesis is normal, but surgery is not possible, may be suitable for epididymal sperm aspiration in combination with in vitro fertilization and intracytoplasmic sperm injection (ICSI). The sperm can be obtained under local anaesthesia by placing a needle percutaneously into the epididymis, or using more conventional microsurgical techniques under a general anaesthetic. As the sperm sample is usually of poor quality, direct intracytoplasmic sperm injection (ICSI) into the oocytes is necessary (see below).

A significant proportion of men who have congenital absence of the vas (CAV) have been found to have a variant of cystic fibrosis. They have compound heterogenicity, where each chromosome 7 carries a different mutation at the site of the transmembrane conductance regulator gene, which is responsible for cystic fibrosis. These couples therefore need careful screening for the common cystic fibrosis mutations. If his partner is found to be a carrier of one of the same mutations, there would be a 1 : 4 chance of their children having classical cystic fibrosis.

Hypogonadotrophic hypogonadism

Hypogonadotrophic hypogonadism can be treated successfully with exogenous gonadotrophins, FSH and hCG, or by using the LHRH infusion pump.

Idiopathic oligospermia

This is the most common diagnosis. A wide range of oral treatments have been employed: clomifene citrate or tamoxifen, mesterolone, kallikrein and even large doses of vitamin C. Although some studies have shown that the anti-oestrogens can increase the sperm count, there is no firm evidence that the use of any oral medication can improve conception rates. The mainstay of treatment, therefore, is in vitro fertilization using sperm prepared in culture medium. In some men the sperm concentration is so low that standard IVF is not possible, and fertilization can only be achieved by intracytoplasmic sperm injection (see below).

Varicocele

There is ultrasound evidence of a varicocele in 15% of the male population. Surgery to correct the defect is not justified in the absence of symptoms and with a normal semen analysis. If the sperm count is low there is evidence that it can be improved. This is not, however, translated into a better conception rate.

Unexplained infertility

If no cause can be found and couples have been trying for less than 3 years there is little evidence that medical intervention will improve their chances of conception. If infertility is longer than 3 years, the chance of spontaneous conception declines (Fig. 13.4) and evidence demonstrates that medical intervention can improve pregnancy rates. The simplest treatment is oral clomifene citrate, which is generally given during days 2–6 of the menstrual cycle. Although it is commonly given for up to 6 months, the improvement in pregnancy rates is questionable. If this simple treatment fails the only alternative is assisted conception.

Assisted conception

'Assisted conception' techniques are those in which gametes, either sperm or eggs, are manipulated to improve the chance of conception (Table 13.4).

Intrauterine insemination (IUI)

Sperm is prepared in culture medium, separating the seminal fluid, poorly motile sperm and other cellular debris in the ejaculate, and producing a clean sample of highly motile sperm. This is then placed directly into the uterine cavity via a fine plastic catheter.

This technique was developed for patients with 'unexplained' infertility or where there was thought to be a cervical cause. However, there are no studies to show that IUI alone is any better than natural intercourse for these conditions. Its use is limited to cases of sexual dysfunction where intercourse is not feasible.

Generally, IUI is used in conjunction with 'super-ovulation'. This involves giving the woman ovulation-induction agents such as clomifene citrate with or without gonadotrophins to stimulate the production of up to three mature follicles. When the follicles reach an appropriate size, ovulation is induced with hCG, and the prepared sperm is inserted into the uterine cavity. This appears to increase the likelihood of a pregnancy by greater than 2.6 times per cycle.

In vitro fertilization (IVF)

The term 'in vitro fertilization' refers to the mixing of sperm and egg outside the body.

History

The technique was pioneered in the 1970s by Patrick Steptoe and Professor Robert Edwards, initially in Oldham and then at Bourn Hall, Cambridge. The first pregnancy, an ectopic, was established in 1976 but it was not until 1978 that the first baby, Louise Brown, was born. Although this first success was based on the single oocyte developed during a normal ovulatory cycle, it

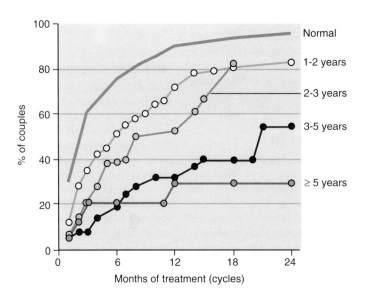

Fig. 13.4 **Spontaneous pregnancy rates with increasing duration of unexplained infertility.** (From Hull et al, *British Medical Journal* 1985, with permission.)

Table 13.4
Assisted conception techniques

Name	Technique	Advantages	Disadvantages
Superovulation with intrauterine insemination (IUI)	Mild ovarian stimulation. Prepared sperm injected through the cervix	2.6-fold increase in pregnancy rate for those with unexplained infertility	Risk of multiple pregnancy
In vitro fertilization (IVF)	Ovaries superovulated, eggs retrieved and mixed with sperm before transcervical transfer to the uterus	Effective for a number of indications, including 'unexplained' infertility	Risks of superovulation, and multiple pregnancy Expensive
Gamete intrafallopian tube transfer (GIFT)	Similar stimulation to IVF, but gametes implanted laparoscopically into the fallopian tube	Effective for 'unexplained' infertility	More invasive than IVF; not suitable for tubal factor infertility (rarely used) Multiple pregnancy Expensive
Zygote intrafallopian tube transfer (ZIFT)	Similar to IVF, but fertilized zygotes transferred laparoscopically into the fallopian tube	Effective for a number of indications, including 'unexplained' infertility	More invasive than IVF; not suitable for tubal factor infertility (rarely used) Multiple pregnancy Expensive
Intracytoplasmic sperm injection (ICSI)	Stimulation and oocyte retrieval as for IVF, but sperm injected directly into the oocyte	Can be used to treat the majority of male factor infertility	Risks of superovulation and multiple pregnancy Some question marks over safety of offspring, increased proportion of children with chromosomal defects Expensive

soon became clear that a higher pregnancy rate could be achieved if a greater number of oocytes were obtained by superovulation.

Indications

In vitro fertilization was originally developed for patients with tubal disease. However, the indications for IVF have expanded enormously:

- male factor infertility
- severe endometriosis
- failed ovulation induction
- long history of 'unexplained' infertility
- pre-implantation diagnosis for genetic disease
- surrogacy
- egg donation.

Technique

Hormonal regimen
The aim of the treatment is to recruit, or rescue, a cohort of antral stage follicles, and support their growth through to maturity. This is achieved by administration of exogenous FSH, given by intramuscular or subcutaneous injection. Although there are two principal pituitary gonadotrophins involved in oocyte development, FSH and LH, only a relatively small background level

of LH is needed. Most commercially available FSH-containing compounds are rich in FSH, with little or no LH component. They are manufactured either by extraction and purification from human postmenopausal urine, or using recombinant DNA technology. In addition most modern protocols use some form of pituitary suppression, either a gonadotrophin-releasing hormone (GnRH) agonist or an antagonist, principally to block an inappropriate LH surge. As the release of LH is blocked, hCG, which has a similar action, is used as a substitute, given approximately 36 hours before oocyte recovery.

Oocyte collection
During superovulation treatment, each ovary enlarges to the size of a tennis ball and they generally lie within 1 cm of the posterior fornix (Fig. 13.5). This allows the oocytes to be collected using a needle passed through the vaginal vault, guided by a vaginal ultrasound probe, with the woman heavily sedated. The oocytes, with their cumulus cell mass, are identified easily (Fig. 13.6) and after removal are placed in an incubator.

Fertilization and incubation
On the morning of oocyte retrieval the man collects a sperm sample by masturbation. After preparation in culture medium the sperm are added to the test tubes containing the oocytes. The tubes are inspected 16 hours later for the characteristic signs of fertilization, the

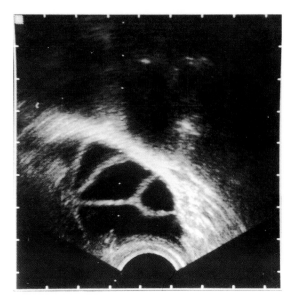

Fig. 13.5 **Vaginal ultrasound illustrating superovulated ovary at egg collection.**

presence of a male and female pronucleus (see Fig. 13.7). The pronucleate embryos are returned to the incubator for a further 24 or 48 hours, with surplus embryos being frozen at this stage.

Embryo transfer

In most situations, a maximum of two embryos are transferred to the uterus using a small plastic catheter, at either the 4- or 8-cell stage, 48 or 72 hours respectively after the oocyte collection (Fig. 13.8a,b). The actual number of embryos transferred will depend on the patient's wishes, her age, and the perceived risk of a multiple pregnancy.

Luteal support

As the pituitary gland has been desensitized, the luteal phase has to be supported with exogenous hCG or progesterone suppositories for 14 days, until the result of the pregnancy test is known.

Results

In the UK in the year 2000 there were 12 051 cycles of IVF and 9322 cycles of ICSI, resulting in 2861 and 2246 live births respectively – live birth rates of 23.7% and 24.1% respectively.

Interpreting success rates

There is considerable variation in success rates from clinic to clinic, depending on the clinic's experience, and the balance of patients treated. In the UK, the Human Fertilisation and Embryology Authority (see below), using the wealth of data at their disposal have produced

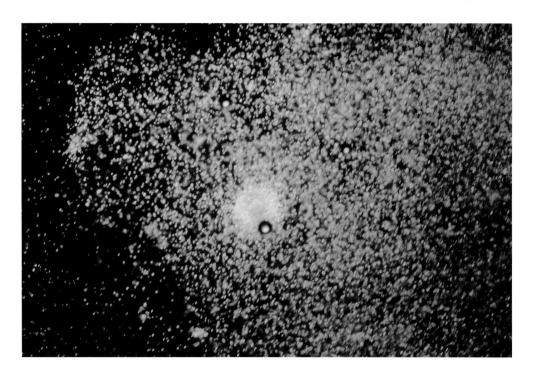

Fig. 13.6 **Oocyte–cumulus cell complex identified at egg collection.**

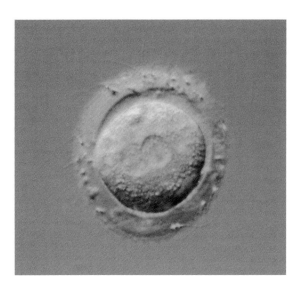

Fig. 13.7 **Fertilized egg showing male and female pronucleus.**

a patient guide providing valuable information on outcomes in each clinic licensed for IVF. The most significant factor in determining an individual couple's chance of success is the woman's age, with a dramatic fall in pregnancy rates as age advances (Fig. 13.9 and Box 13.3). Women over the age of 37 years appear to do less well, and over the age of 40 the 'take-home' baby rate is only around 5%.

The live birth rates quoted represent the chance of success in a single cycle. The first cycle of treatment gives the patient the best chance of success, but the pregnancy rate in subsequent cycles is similar. It is difficult to obtain accurate cumulative pregnancy rates following IVF treatment, although rates between 60–70% after six attempts have been reported. The cause of infertility does not appear to significantly affect the pregnancy rate after IVF.

Embryo freezing

Many patients have a number of 'spare' embryos left over after the initial treatment. These can be frozen in liquid nitrogen and replaced during a subsequent natural or artificial cycle to give a further chance of a pregnancy. Only two-thirds of frozen embryos survive the thaw process. The live birth rate following frozen embryo transfer in 2000 was 13.8%.

Gamete intrafallopian tube transfer (GIFT)

This also involves the use of superovulation using the same protocols as described above for IVF, and oocyte collection by vaginal ultrasound. Thereafter the two techniques differ. With GIFT, the best three oocytes are selected and a laparoscopy is performed. The fallopian tube is cannulated and the selected oocytes, along with approximately 100 000 sperm, are returned to the tube. Fertilization then occurs in the fallopian tube.

Success rates of up to 36% per treatment cycle have been quoted, but GIFT is only applicable to those patients who have 'unexplained' infertility. As it involves a

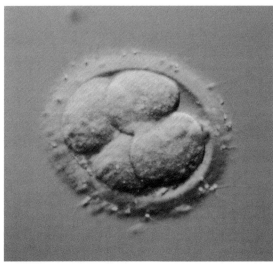

(a)

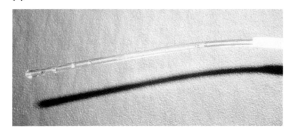

(b)

Fig. 13.8 **Embryo transfer. (a)** 4-cell embryo ready for transfer to the uterus. **(b)** Loaded embryo transfer catheter.

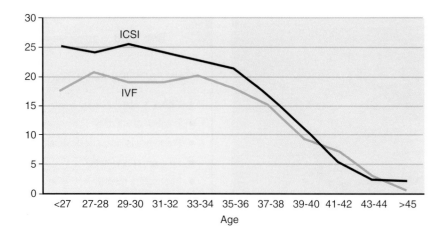

Fig. 13.9 **Live birth rates by age of woman.** ICSI, intracytoplasmic sperm injection; IVF, in vitro fertilization.

general anaesthetic and laparoscopy it is more invasive than conventional IVF and very few centres now practise this technique. The only true indication is for those couples who cannot accept IVF on religious grounds.

Zygote intrafallopian tube transfer (ZIFT)

This is a combination of IVF and GIFT. The first part of the treatment is identical to IVF, but instead of replacing the embryos in the uterus, they are replaced, at laparoscopy, in the fallopian tube. Again this treatment is more invasive than conventional IVF and is generally only used if difficulties are encountered transferring the embryos through the cervix.

Intracytoplasmic sperm injection (ICSI)

This exciting technique, developed in Brussels by Professor Andre Van Steirteghem and colleagues, has revolutionized our ability to treat male infertility. The indications for ICSI are outlined in Box 13.4. If there are no sperm in the ejaculate and none in the epididymis, sperm can still be retrieved from testicular biopsies in a significant proportion (approximately 50%) of men. Sometimes multiple testicular biopsies are required to find areas of active spermatogenesis.

Technique

Oocytes are collected in the standard IVF fashion, and then prepared for ICSI by removing their surrounding cumulus cells. A smooth-ended glass pipette is used to hold the oocyte still, while a sharp ultrafine pipette pierces the egg and deposits one sperm along with a tiny amount of culture medium. Prior to injection the selected sperm needs to be immobilized to avoid damaging the delicate structure of the oocyte.

Results

The pregnancy outcome following ICSI is comparable to that of conventional IVF (live birth rate of 24.1% per cycle), although slightly lower pregnancy rates are reported in the more severe cases where testicular-derived sperm is required. ICSI is a more invasive procedure and some uncontrolled reports have suggested slightly increased rates of genetic and developmental defects. Furthermore, there is clear evidence that a proportion of male infertility has a genetic basis, and by performing ICSI the abnormality may be passed on to the next generation. The true risk will only become evident in time as our understanding of the causes of impaired spermatogenesis become clearer, and the children born following ICSI are followed through to adulthood.

Box 13.4

INDICATIONS FOR ICSI

- Microepididymal sperm aspiration (MESA)
  - congenital absence of the vas deferens
  - obstructive azoospermia:
    post-infection
    iatrogenic

- < 500 000 motile sperm in the ejaculate

- < 5% morphologically normal sperm

- Repeated IVF failed fertilization

Egg donation

Patients with primary ovarian failure can only be treated by oocyte donation (Box 13.5). This treatment is also increasingly being used for patients who appear to have an oocyte problem identified by repeated IVF failure. Another indication for egg donation (or for donor insemination) is genetic disease. Egg donors are in short supply and are generally women who, for altruistic reasons, wish to donate their eggs. Egg donation is much more complicated than sperm donation, as the donors have to undergo IVF treatment as far as the stage of oocyte collection. Some centres offer an 'egg sharing' programme, whereby an infertility patient who cannot afford treatment agrees to go through an IVF cycle but donate half her eggs to a recipient who will fund both patients' treatment. This concept clearly raises ethical and moral concerns, although early research suggests that both parties benefit to equal effect.

Results

This is a very successful treatment, with pregnancy rates generally higher than conventional IVF, and maintained even in women over the age of 40. This illustrates the fact that the quality of the oocyte is the most significant factor in the age-related decline of fertility.

Host surrogacy

Some women have functional ovaries but no uterus, due either to a congenital abnormality or previous hysterectomy. Such a patient could undergo IVF treatment, with the embryos then being transferred to another woman (a 'host surrogate') whose uterus has been suitably prepared by hormone treatment. The host will carry the pregnancy and then return the baby to the commissioning couple after delivery. According to English law the 'mother' is the woman who delivers the child. Therefore the commissioning couple have to adopt the child, even though it is genetically theirs.

Pre-implantation genetic diagnosis (PGD)

Couples who have a history of repeated pregnancy failure for genetic disease, or have had a child with a specific genetic abnormality may benefit from PGD. The couples undergo a conventional IVF treatment cycle, generally using ICSI as the means of fertilization. The embryos are left until day 3, by which stage they have divided to the 6- to 8-cell stage. One or two blastomeres (embryonic cells) are removed and analysed for either specific chromosomal abnormalities using fluorescent in situ hybridization (FISH), or a specific gene defect by polymerase chain reaction (PCR). Unaffected embryos can now be replaced in the usual manner. This allows the couple to potentially start a pregnancy knowing that the child is healthy.

Results

The overall chance of success is slightly lower than for conventional IVF, but greater than 20% per treatment cycle.

Side-effects of assisted conception

Multiple pregnancy occurs in 28% of pregnancies after IVF. Approximately 24% are twin pregnancies and the remaining 4% are triplet pregnancies. To try to prevent triplet pregnancies, the law in the UK dictates that only in exceptional cases can more than two embryos be transferred.

Ovarian hyperstimulation is a condition where the ovaries over-respond to the gonadotrophin injections.

- More than 30 follicles may start to mature, resulting in ovarian enlargement and abdominal discomfort.
- Very high concentrations of oestradiol and progesterone make the patient feel nauseated.
- If the condition is severe, protein-rich ascites can accumulate, and more rarely pleural effusion may result. (This is akin to Meig's syndrome.)
- The sudden shift in fluid can result in hypovolaemia, with resulting renal and thrombotic problems. The condition can be fatal.

The incidence of severe hyperstimulation is small (< 1%) and it only occurs if the hCG injection is given. Patients with polycystic ovaries are the most vulnerable. Treatment is supportive with fluid replacement, generally with protein-rich fluids rather than simple crystalloid solutions. Serum electrolytes need careful monitoring because hyperkalaemia and/or hyponatraemia can develop. Hyperstimulation usually occurs in patients

---

Box 13.5

INDICATIONS FOR EGG DONATION

- Premature ovarian failure
- Gonadal dysgenesis
- Iatrogenic – surgery, radiation and chemotherapy
- Carriers of genetic disease
- Failed IVF – poor response, inaccessible ovaries, repeated failure to fertilize
- Recurrent miscarriage

who conceive and can last throughout the early first trimester. If the patient fails to conceive, the condition is self-limiting and will resolve spontaneously.

Fetal abnormality   Out of a total of 7397 babies born following IVF/ICSI treatment in the UK in 1998, there were 95 babies with developmental defects and syndromes, 7 with chromosomal defects (predominantly Down's syndrome), and 88 with congenital abnormalities, giving a congenital abnormality rate of 1.1% (IVF) and 1.6% (ICSI) respectively, almost identical to that in the general population.

The UK Human Fertilisation and Embryology Act

This Act, passed by the UK Parliament in 1990, brought about the formation of a regulatory body, known as the Human Fertilisation and Embryology Authority (HFEA). It regulates research on human embryos, the storage of gametes and embryos, and the use in infertility treatment of donated gametes and of embryos produced outside the body. The HFEA came into operation in August 1991, with the principal aim of ensuring that human embryos and gametes are used responsibly and that infertile patients are not exploited. Assisted conception treatment can only be performed in a centre licensed by the HFEA. This license is renewed on an annual basis.

All patients who donate gametes (either sperm or eggs) or receive assisted conception treatment have to be registered with the HFEA. The outcome of treatment is also recorded. The HFEA also requires all patients considering assisted conception to be offered counselling by a trained counsellor. Paramount in the HFEA's philosophy is the welfare of the potential child.

Key points

- Infertility is defined as inability to conceive after 2 years of regular unprotected coitus. It affects approximately 1 in 6 of couples.

- The three commonest causes are ovulatory problems, semen abnormalities or blockage of fallopian tubes. Other causes include coital difficulties, cervical mucus hostility or endometriosis.

- Investigation involves semen analysis, tests of ovulation (mid-luteal phase progesterone, or ultrasound monitoring) and tests for tubal patency (diagnostic laparoscopy or hysterosalpingography).

- Treatment of anovulation may include anti-oestrogens (particularly clomifene), pulsatile LHRH or exogenous gonadotrophins (which require careful monitoring).

- ICSI offers hope to men with variable sperm counts. Donor insemination (DI) is another option.

14

Contraception and sterilization

Introduction

Over the last 70 years the global population has tripled from 2 billion to over 6 billion and it is estimated to reach 9 billion in the next 50 years (Fig. 14.1). The current 'ecological footprint', the productive area of earth necessary to support the lifestyle of an individual, is approximately double the level that is sustainable long term. Currently, half the world's population does not have enough food to eat and this situation is likely to deteriorate. The number of people experiencing water shortages is likely to rise from the current level of around 500 million to 3 billion by 2050 and water tables under some cities in China, Latin America, and south Asia are falling by over a metre a year. Contraception is clearly important.

Contraception also has the potential to make a contribution to maternal and child survival. It has been estimated that family planning could save the lives of 3 million children a year by helping women to space births at least 2 years apart, and to bear children during their healthiest reproductive years. When women have the ability to space their births, they are better able to recover from nutritional depletion, blood loss and reproductive-system damage, allowing them to have healthier babies. Babies born less than 2 years after their sibling are more likely to have lower birth weights and are more vulnerable to infection. Many women in the developing world would like to space or limit their births, but do not have access to family planning information or services.

Family planning programmes also help prevent the spread of HIV infection and other sexually transmitted diseases. Half of all new HIV infections in the developing world are among women and nearly 10% are among infants and children.

The provision of appropriate contraception is arguably, therefore, the most important branch of medicine today. A wide variety of effective contraceptive methods are available but there are no 'ideal' contraceptives and choice must be based on the advantages and disadvantages of each method. These will be discussed in more detail in this chapter, but Table 14.1 summarizes the main side-effects, risks and failure rate of each method. In addition, it should be noted that not all methods are suitable for every person and selected suitability criteria are outlined in Table 14.2.

Defining 'contraceptive failure' is not easy as it depends on the population studied: studies on a young

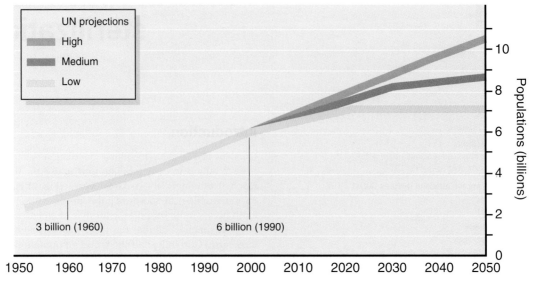

Source: United Nations 1988. *World Population Prospects (The 1998 Revision)*

Fig. 14.1 **Global population growth, actual and projected.**

Table 14.1
Chief side-effects and dangers, and risks of death of selected family planning methods

Method	Side-effects	Serious dangers	Risk of death	Failure rate per 100 woman years
Spermicides	Vaginal and urinary tract infections, allergy	None	None measurable	
Cervical cap, diaphragm, sponge	Vaginal and urinary tract infections	Toxic shock syndrome	None measurable	1.0–15
Condoms (male, latex)	None	Anaphylactic reaction	None measurable	4.0–5.5
Combined oral contraceptives	Nausea, weight gain, dizziness, spotting, breast tenderness, chloasma, decreased libido	Cardiovascular complications, depression, hepatic adenomas, possible increased risk of breast and cervical cancers	Non-smokers aged < 35: 1/200 000 Non smokers aged 35+: 1/28 600 Heavy smokers aged <35: 1/5300 Heavy smokers aged 35+: 1/700	0.1–1.0
Progestogen-only oral contraceptives	Headaches, irregular bleeding, androgenic effects		None measurable	0.3–3.0
Emergency contraception (hormonal)	Nausea, vomiting, headaches, breast tenderness	None	None measurable	
Injectables	Cycle changes, weight gain, headaches, changes in lipid profile, breast tenderness	Depression, allergic reaction, possible bone loss	None measurable	0.1–1.2
IUD (copper)	Increased menstrual cramping, spotting and bleeding	PID following insertion, uterine perforation, iron deficiency anaemia	1:10 000 000	0.5–2.0

Table 14.1   (*cont.*)

Method	Side-effects	Serious dangers	Risk of death	Failure rate per 100 woman years
Implants	Tenderness at implant site, cycle changes, alopecia, weight gain, breast tenderness	Infection at implant site, depression, removal complications	None measurable	0
Female sterilization	Pain at incision site, possible regret that method is permanent	Infection at surgical site, anaesthesia complications, ectopic pregnancy	Laparoscopic tubal ligation: 1/38 500 Hysterectomy: 1/1600	0.13
Male sterilization	Pain at incision site, possible regret that method is permanent	Infection at surgical site, anaesthesia complications	Vasectomy: 1/1 000 000	0.02

PID, pelvic inflammatory disease

Table 14.2
Medical eligibility criteria for selected family planning methods (WHO)

Condition	Combined oral	Combined injectable	Progestogen-only oral	Depot progestogens	Subdermal implants	Copper IUD	Levonorgestrel IUD
Age <20	1	1	1	1–2	1	2	2
Age ≥40	2	2	1	1-2	1	1	1
Smoking	2–4	2–3	1	1	1	1	1
Obesity	2	2	1	2	2	1	2
Multiple risk factors for arterial cardiovascular disease	3–4	3–4	2	3	2	1	2
History of venous thromboembolic disease	4	4	2	2	2	1	2
Migraine with focal neurological symptoms	2–3	2–3	1–2	2	2	1	2
HIV positive	1	1	1	1	1	3	3
Non-vascular disease diabetes	2	2	2	2	2	1	2
Diabetes with vascular disease or of > 20 years' duration	3–4	3–4	2	3	2	1	2
History of cholestasis	2–3	2	1–2	1–2	1–2	1	1–2
Cancer of cervix	2	2	1	2	2	2–4	2–4
Cancer of breast	3–4	3–4	3–4	3–4	3–4	1	3–4
Cancer of ovary	1	1	1	1	1	2–3	2–3
Pelvic inflammatory disease	1	1	1	1	1	2–4	2–4

Classification categories:
1. A condition for which there is no restriction for the use of the contraceptive method
2. A condition where the advantages of using the method generally outweigh the theoretical or proven risks
3. A condition where the theoretical or proven risks usually outweigh the advantages of using the method
4. A condition which represents an unacceptable health risk if the contraceptive method is used.

population will suggest a higher failure rate than in an older group as fertility is higher in younger people. Failure rates will also be higher in those who have sex more frequently, but appear lower if the population studied has couples who would be unable to conceive even without contraception. Caution is therefore required in interpreting precise figures. The illustrative failure rates quoted in Table 14.1 refer to 'method' failure, in other words the inherent risk of failure providing the method is used correctly. It is quantified in the units 'per 100 woman years', that is to say the number of women who would become pregnant if 100 of them used that method of contraception for 1 year (or 50 women for 2 years and so forth). 'User' failure is said to occur when a given method is not used correctly.

Hormonal contraception is discussed first, followed by intrauterine devices, barrier methods, 'natural' contraception, emergency contraception and finally sterilization.

Hormonal methods

Combined oestrogen–progestogen pills

These preparations, sometimes referred to simply as 'the pill', contain oestrogen, and a progestogen, and are given for 3 weeks out of every 4. They work primarily by inhibiting ovulation, but also by making cervical mucus less favourable to sperm penetration and by rendering the endometrium more atrophic. Although attention has been frequently drawn to potential risks (see Table 14.1 and below), these should be seen in the context of the potential benefits (Box 14.1), which include protective effects against ovarian and endometrial cancers. The combined oral contraceptive (COC)

pill is also useful in the treatment of dysmenorrhoea, menorrhagia and endometriosis.

Each COC pill contains an oestrogen, usually ethinylestradiol, and a progestogen. The progestogens are considered in two groups: the second-generation preparations, like levonorgestrel and norethisterone, and the third-generation progestogens, desogestrel and gestodene. The third-generation progestogens were introduced as they had fewer adverse lipid effects than earlier preparations. Subsequent data, however, showed that they also carried a slightly greater risk of venous thromboembolic disease and the decision about whether a second- or third-generation preparation is appropriate depends on an individual's risk factors.

Contraindications to the COC

All risks should be considered in perspective (Fig. 14.2). Absolute contraindications to the COC are uncommon in women requiring contraception, but as death in users over 35 years of age is eight times more common in smokers than non-smokers, it is recommended that either the COC, or the smoking, should be stopped at this age. Hypertension increases the risk of stroke in pill users and is also a contraindication. Low-risk non-smokers may continue the COC until the age of 50 years.

Drug interactions

Most anticonvulsants have some enzyme-inducing properties which will accelerate the hepatic breakdown of contraceptive steroids. The options are to increase the dose, perhaps even by taking two pills per day, or to reduce the pill-free interval from 7 to 4 days.

Most broad-spectrum antibiotics alter the bowel flora, reducing the recirculation of oestrogens and therefore reducing the effectiveness of the pill for around 3 weeks after use. Other methods of contraception should be used over this time. For those on long-term antibiotics, the cautionary time is still only 3 weeks as bowel flora is restored relatively quickly despite ongoing treatment. A few antibiotics, particularly rifampicin and the antifungal griseofulvin, also cause enzyme induction.

Prescribing

The aim is to achieve good contraception and cycle control with as low a dose of oestrogen and progestogen as possible. The course of COC pills is usually commenced on the first day of the menstrual cycle. Most packs contain 21 active tablets and a withdrawal bleed usually occurs in the 7-day pill-free interval between successive packs. Some preparations are available with 7 placebo tablets to substitute for the pill-free interval. Other formulations contain active tablets with two or three different ratios of oestrogen and progestogen.

Box 14.1

BENEFITS OF THE COMBINED ORAL CONTRACEPTIVE PILL

- High efficacy
- Easily reversible
- High convenience
- Generally well tolerated systemically
- Reduction in menstrual disorders
- Reduction in functional ovarian cysts
- Less pelvic inflammatory disease
- Less benign breast disease
- Reduction in incidence of endometrial and ovarian carcinoma

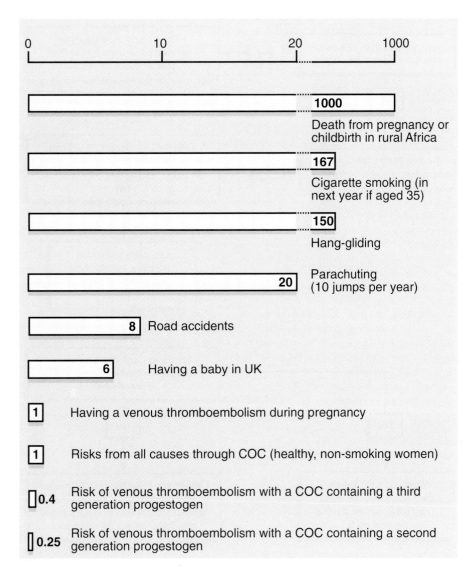

Fig. 14.2 **Risks of the combined oral contraceptive pill compared to other risks in life.**

Such biphasic and triphasic pills aim to mimic the steroid ratios of the natural ovarian cycle, but although they may allow an overall reduction in progestogen dose, there are few other advantages. Failure most commonly results from forgotten pills. The '7 day rules' should be followed if such circumstances arise (Fig. 14.3).

Follow-up

Follow-up should ideally be carried out to a set plan, for example at 3 months initially, then 6-monthly for the first 2 years and annually thereafter. The most important aspect of these visits is to check the blood pressure, which may rise even years after the start of treatment. Any rise may be judged as a relative contraindication but levels persistently greater than 160/95 mmHg warrant a change of contraceptive method. The pill should also be stopped prior to elective surgery, if immobile, or if jaundice occurs. Follow-up visits are also an opportunity to carry out other well women screening.

Progestogen-only contraceptives

Progestogen-only contraceptives were developed to minimize the side-effects attributed to the oestrogen component of the COC pill. This is less of a problem than previously as the oestrogen component of most current preparations is relatively low. Progestogen-only contraceptives are available in oral, injectable and implant form. Their main action is to thicken cervical

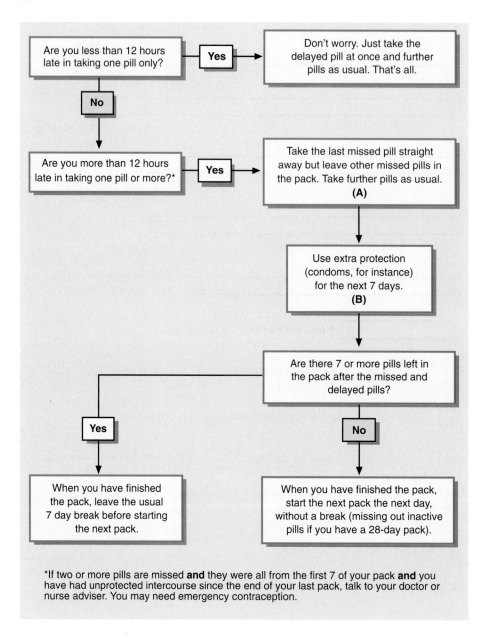

Fig. 14.3 **Flow chart for missed combined oral contraceptive pills.**

mucus, thereby limiting sperm penetration, but they also act to suppress the endometrium and in some instances inhibit ovulation.

Most progestogen-only methods are associated with a disturbance of the menstrual cycle which may range from occasional 'spotting' to menstrual irregularity and even daily loss. Some patients become amenorrhoeic. These features are most noticeable with depot injectables but can occur to some extent with all progestogen-only methods. Other side-effects are uncommon, but include bloating, weight gain, weight loss, acne, hirsutism and headaches.

The effect of enzyme-inducing drugs on the metabolism of progestogens is similar to that for oestrogens, and progestogen-only pills are not suitable in patients using these drugs long term. The 12-weekly depot preparation, Depo-Provera, should be given 8-weekly in those taking these enzyme-inducing drugs.

Progestogen-only pills (POP)

These are the so-called 'everyday' or 'mini-' pills. Although suitable for most patients they are often offered as an alternative where the combined pill is inappropriate, e.g. lactating mothers, smokers, older women, and those with mild hypertension, diabetes mellitus or migraine. POP pills are taken every day without a pill-free interval or break for menstruation and there is a slightly higher method failure rate than with the combined pill (Table 14.1). They have the disadvantage that they must also be taken at the same time every day (to within 3 hours).

Progestogen-only injectable preparations

The most widely used preparation is medroxyprogesterone acetate 150 mg (Depo-Provera) which is given every 12 weeks and has the advantage of a long duration of action. The menstrual effects described above may be particularly marked, however, and any other side-effects may persist for at least as long as the contraceptive effect. When this contraceptive method is discontinued, the return of fertility may be delayed beyond the 12-week time-scale, with an average of around 7–8 months. A minority of users experience weight gain.

Progestogen-only subdermal implants

These are available in different forms in different parts of the world, and are sold in the UK as a single subdermal capsule known as Implanon (Fig. 14.4). This is made from a non-biodegradable polymer, about the size of a matchstick, which contains an active slow-release progestogen formulation and it is marketed for 3-year use. Menstrual side-effects are common, however, and specific training is required for insertion and removal. A previous preparation, Norplant, has been withdrawn from the UK market.

Progestogen-releasing intrauterine devices
(Fig. 14.5a–d)
A levonorgestrel-impregnated intrauterine contraceptive device marketed in the UK as the Mirena, offers a highly

effective and again rapidly reversible contraceptive method (Fig. 14.5a). It acts locally within the uterus to prevent proliferation of the endometrium, and reduces menstrual loss by an average of 90% after 3 months' treatment. Initial worsening of menstrual symptoms is common and intermenstrual bleeding occurs frequently, but these problems often settle 5 or 6 months after insertion. 20% of women experience complete amenorrhoea. Systemic side-effects of skin problems and mastalgia are rare. Although it is licensed for 5-year use in most countries, there is good evidence that it remains effective in the treatment of menstrual dysfunction for up to 7 or 8 years.

Copper-bearing intrauterine devices (IUDs)

This is the most commonly used reversible form of contraception worldwide, with over a 100 million users, many of them in China. Its main advantage is convenience, and there is virtually no chance of user-failure. The presence of a foreign body within the uterine cavity exerts a contraceptive effect by a number of mechanisms:

- interfering with the passage of sperm through the uterine cavity
- interfering with the fertilization process within the tube
- rendering the oocyte less capable of being fertilized
- reducing the chances of a fertilized egg implanting in the endometrium, probably as the result of local inflammation.

Although the last of these mechanisms may also occur with hormonal methods of contraception, the IUD has attracted criticism from those who regard the prevention of implantation as morally equivalent to abortion. The main mechanism of action, however, is thought to be in preventing fertilization.

Most IUDs (Fig. 14.5b–d) carry metallic copper, which enhances the contraceptive effect. As the copper surface may break down, or become coated with protein or calcium deposits, it is necessary for an IUD to be removed and refitted every 3–10 years depending on the device. Most are probably effective for at least 5 years and there is good evidence that if an IUD is inserted after the age of 40 years, it may be left in situ until after the menopause.

Insertion

Correct technique minimizes pain and reduces the risks of perforation, infection and expulsion. Syncope occasionally occurs and resuscitation facilities should

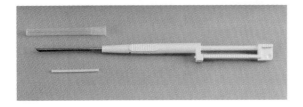

Fig. 14.4 **Implanon.** (Courtesy of Organon Laboratories Ltd.)

Gynaecology

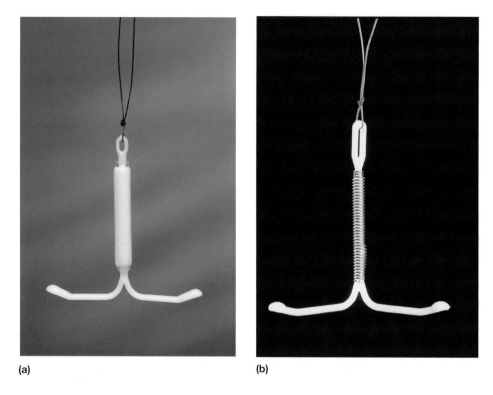

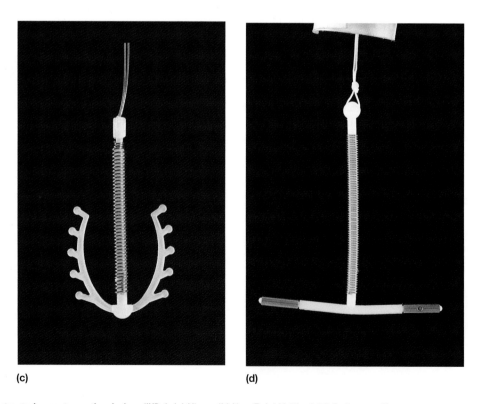

Fig. 14.5 **Intrauterine contraceptive devices (IUDs). (a)** Mirena; **(b)** Nova T; **(c)** Multiload; **(d)** Orythogynae T.

with endometrial shedding, and typically the menstrual period is prolonged with a few days 'building up' and a few 'tailing off.' This increased loss is in contrast to the Mirena mentioned above. Intermenstrual bleeding, with or without pain, often occurs during the first few months of use and a watery vaginal or mucus discharge is common. 15% of women request removal of the device before 1 year because of persistent prolonged or irregular bleeding, or because of pain.

Uterine perforation

This is a rare complication, probably occurring after no more than 1 per 1000 insertions. Most perforations occur at the time of insertion, but a delayed form of 'migration' is recognized to occur. Immediate perforation may be detected because of acute pain or it may be detected later if pregnancy occurs. Most commonly, however, it is identified following the investigation of 'missing threads'. When the threads are found to be missing the first step is to check by ultrasound scan whether the device is in the uterine cavity. Providing it is, no further action is required, although a variety of manoeuvres may be required when it is time for the device to be changed (Fig. 14.6a). If the IUD is not in the uterine cavity, an abdominal X-ray is used to decide whether it has been expelled or is in the peritoneal cavity (Fig. 14.6b). Abdominally sited copper IUDs may cause dense adhesion formation and should be removed by laparoscopy or laparotomy.

be available. Contraindications should be excluded (Box 14.2), and care taken to ensure that the woman is not pregnant.

Complications
Bleeding, pain and discharge

Copper IUDs are associated with an increase in menstrual loss, probably because of mechanical interference

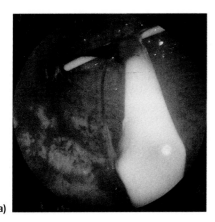

(a)

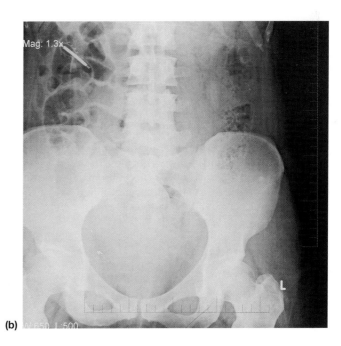

(b)

Fig. 14.6 **Missing threads may simply be in the uterine cavity (a) or the IUD may either have fallen out or no longer be within the uterus.** In **(b)**, the IUD has perforated the uterus and attached itself to the omentum.

Pelvic infection

Infection may be introduced at the time of insertion despite aseptic technique, and usually leads to symptoms within the first few weeks of use. Thereafter, the risk of pelvic inflammatory disease (PID) is no greater with IUD use than in someone using no contraception. The risk of infection is higher than in barrier or hormonal method users, however, as these methods exert a protective effect against infection. As the risk of acquiring pelvic inflammatory disease with an IUD is proportional to the number of sexual partners, an IUD is most suitable for women in a stable relationship and should be used with caution in younger women and those with a high number of sexual partners. The risk of introducing infection can be minimized by screening prior to insertion.

The cervical smears of IUD users occasionally reveal actinomyces-like organisms. Treatment is not required if there are no symptoms. If the patient is symptomatic (pain, discharge, intermenstrual bleeding) the coil should be removed and sent for culture to exclude this organism.

Expulsion

Most expulsions occur during the first few months after insertion and sometimes result from the IUD being placed too low in the uterine cavity. A user should be advised to check the presence of the IUD thread by digital examination after each period as spontaneous expulsion may occur unnoticed, particularly during menstruation. Providing she is able to do this, regular check-up visits are not required.

Pregnancy

An IUD-failure pregnancy is rare, but if it occurs, the chance of having an ectopic pregnancy is higher than in those without a device. It is of note, however, that an IUD user is less likely to conceive an ectopic pregnancy than a woman using no contraception. If the pregnancy is intrauterine there is a considerable increase in the risk of spontaneous miscarriage and preterm labour (Fig. 14.7). Removal of the IUD reduces these risks and should be carried out as soon as is practical providing the threads are easily seen. If not, no attempt at retrieval should be made.

Barrier methods

Barrier methods of contraception block the passage of sperm from the male partner to the oocyte, and an extensive array of barriers have been used. They offer advantages in terms of safety and reversibility, but their efficacy depends critically on quality of use. The failure rates are relatively low when they are used consistently and correctly by well-motivated couples.

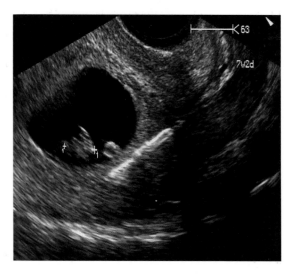

Fig. 14.7 **Ultrasound scan of 7-week fetus with an IUD visible low in the uterine cavity.**

Male condom

The first condoms described historically were used for decoration and later for protection against disease – Fallopio, for example, an Italian anatomist, described the use of a linen sheath to protect against syphilis. With the development of vulcanized rubber and then liquid latex, condoms became widely available as a method of contraception. The use of barrier methods fell in the 1960s with the introduction of hormonal contraceptive methods, but increased again with the recognition that they offered protection against sexually transmitted infections (STIs), particularly HIV. They can be used in addition to other methods of contraception for this protective benefit.

Condoms are available in a variety of shapes, colours and even flavours and with or without spermicide. They must be unrolled over the erect penis before there is any genital contact. Difficulties may occur when air is not excluded from the teat, or when trying to put them on inside out, or if snagging with fingernails occurs, and the condom should be held onto the penis during withdrawal from the vagina to avoid leakage of semen. The standard size available in a particular country may not meet the requirements of all men; a condom that is too large may roll off during intercourse. Where condoms are the intended sole primary method of contraception it is important to inform the user about emergency contraception (see below).

Female condoms

The female condom is a polyurethane sheath, its open end attached to a flexible polyurethane ring which sits at the vaginal entrance (Fig. 14.8). It is marketed in the UK as the Femidom and, like the male condom,

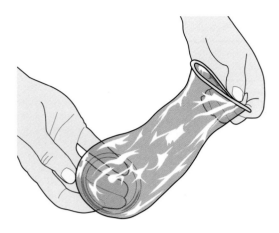

Fig. 14.8 **Female condom.**

also offers protection against sexually transmitted infections. Initial adverse responses to female condoms have become less as couples have become more familiar with their use.

Female occlusive diaphragms and caps

These require a relatively high degree of user motivation, and failure rates are comparable to those seen with the male condom. They are divided into two groups: the diaphragm and those that cover the cervix (Fig. 14.9).

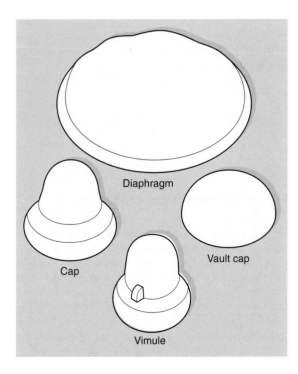

Fig. 14.9 **Female barrier methods of contraception.** D, diaphragm; Va, vault cap; Vi, vimule; C, cervical cap.

The diaphragm

This consists of a soft latex dome, the edge of which contains a supporting metal spring to exert a slight pressure on the vaginal walls. It is inserted to lie diagonally across the vagina between the back of the symphysis pubis and the posterior fornix, but it does not form a complete barrier between the upper and lower vagina. An important key to its use is that it holds spermicidal cream in contact with the cervical mucus. Like the male condom it must be in place before genital contact occurs but it can be left in place during a number of coital events. It should not be removed for 6 hours after the last intercourse and retention for more than 24 hours is not recommended.

A user needs to be taught insertion and removal techniques and particularly to check that the diaphragm actually covers the cervix with no obvious gaps around the rim. Size requirements will change, particularly after childbirth and when approaching the menopause. This type of contraceptive is unlikely to be suitable in those with a prolapse.

Cervical caps, vault caps and the vimule

Cervical and vault caps and the vimule depend on suction to hold the cap over the cervix or the vaginal vault. Again, they are best used with a spermicide and are available in a range of sizes. The techniques for insertion and removal need to be carefully taught.

Spermicides

Spermicidal preparations are usually used in conjunction with other methods, particularly the barriers described above. Nonoxynol-9 is the most commonly used substance but recent work suggests that it may increase the possibility of HIV transmission, possibly because of local genital toxicity.

'Natural' contraception

These methods are referred to as 'natural' because they do not involve the use of pharmacological or mechanical agents.

The rhythm method or periodic abstinence   This is the only method of contraception sanctioned by the Roman Catholic Church. It requires the restriction of intercourse to those days of the menstrual cycle on which conception is least likely. During the fertile period cervical mucus is clear, watery (i.e. of low viscosity) and is easily stretched into strands (spinnbarkeit). In the non-fertile period it is viscous. This knowledge, used in combination with a mid-cycle core temperature rise (0.5–1°C)

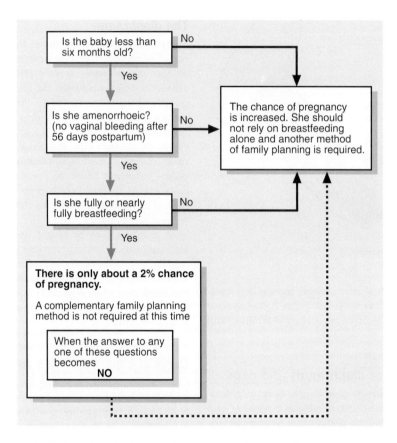

Fig. 14.10 **Use of lactational amenorrhoea during the first 6 months postpartum.**

and awareness that the fertile period is 6 days before to 2 days after ovulation, has a low failure rate in well-motivated couples.

Breast-feeding   Full unsupplemented breast-feeding in which the mother is amenorrhoeic is highly effective in the first 6 postnatal months. Another method of contraception should be introduced if menses occur (bleeding before 56 days can be ignored), or with the introduction of weaning, or after 6 months (Fig. 14.10).

Coitus interruptus or withdrawal   This relies on the removal of the penis from the vagina before ejaculation. Even when this is achieved, spermatozoa may enter the vagina before orgasm and ejaculation. This technique is unreliable and may cause considerable levels of dissatisfaction for both partners.

Emergency contraception

Emergency contraception can be used:

- after unprotected intercourse
- after 'accidents' with a barrier method (e.g. burst condom or diaphragm removed too early)
- if one or more combined pills has been missed at the beginning or end of a packet, or three or more missed at other times
- if more than three progestogen-only pills have been missed.

Two methods are currently available: hormonal and the IUD.

Hormonal emergency contraception

Formerly referred to as the 'morning after pill', this method can be used up to 72 hours after unprotected intercourse but is more successful the earlier it is taken. The pills inhibit or delay ovulation and prevent 75% of pregnancies which would have occurred that cycle. The next 'period' may be early, on time or late, and barrier contraception should be used until then. In those who do become pregnant despite treatment there is no evidence of teratogenic problems. The traditional oestrogen–progestogen combination of the 'Yuzpe' method has been superseded by a progestogen-only preparation which is more effective and has fewer side-effects.

Non-hormonal emergency contraception

An IUD can be inserted up to 5 days after the estimated day of ovulation (which may be more than 5 days after intercourse) and has an almost 100% success rate in preventing pregnancy in that cycle. In practice it may be difficult to estimate the day of ovulation and it is reasonable to limit IUD use to those who have had intercourse within the previous 5 days. The patient may choose whether to continue with the IUD as a primary method of contraception.

Sterilization

It has been estimated that 150 million women worldwide have chosen sterilization as their method of contraception. Preoperative counselling details are outlined below and these details must be recorded in the notes:

- irreversibility and alternative methods of contraception (10% regret their decision at 18 months and 1% seek reversal, especially those who are single and younger)
- failure rates and, in women, the risk of ectopic pregnancy
- a woman should be aware that if laparoscopy is unsuccessful or if there are complications, it might be necessary to perform a laparotomy under the same anaesthetic
- after sterilization in men, it is necessary to wait until two clear semen specimens have been obtained before other contraception is stopped and this may take months; in women, it is necessary to continue with alternative contraception until the next menstrual period.

Female sterilization

This can be performed by laparotomy, at caesarean section or, more radically, by hysterectomy. It is much more usually carried out, however, laparoscopically using one of a number of different devices such as Filshie clips, Hulka clips, Falope rings or diathermy, to occlude the tubes. Of these, clips are considered by most to have the lowest failure rate.

Male sterilization

Vasectomy can be performed on an outpatient basis under local anaesthesia. Bruising and haematoma formation are not uncommon. The evidence suggests that the incidence of testicular cancer is not increased, although a possible association with prostate cancer cannot be excluded.

Key points

- Worldwide, contraceptive provision is important but is affected by cultural, political and financial problems.
- Efficacy of contraception is measured by failure rate expressed as pregnancies per 100 woman years.
- Hormonal methods include the combined oral contraceptive pill, which contains oestrogen and a progestogen. The combined pill is contraindicated in those with significant cardiovascular risk factors and those with specified risk factors for venous thromboembolic disease.
- Progestogen-only contraception can be given in the form of pills, injections, implants, or coating an IUD or vaginal ring.
- Barrier methods help to prevent STIs. Condoms are widely available. Female barrier methods include the female condom, the diaphragm and cervical caps. Barriers are most effective when combined with spermicides.
- 'Natural' contraception is acceptable to the Roman Catholic Church. Efficacy is improved by the use of temperature charts, self-examination and ovulation prediction kits.
- Emergency contraception comprises either a progestogen preparation which can be used up to 72 hours after unprotected intercourse, or an IUD, which may be used up to 5 days after unprotected intercourse.

15

Miscarriage and ectopic pregnancy

Miscarriage

Miscarriage is relatively common, occurring in approximately 25% of all pregnancies. As it is so upsetting for the parents, the utmost sensitivity is required, even at very early gestations. Clinical management should be founded on two important principles:

1. The most extreme care must be taken not to advise uterine evacuation if there is any possibility of fetal viability. It should not be assumed that the pregnancy is non-viable simply because the gestation does not agree with the expected dates.
2. There should be a low threshold of suspicion for ectopic pregnancy. The absence of an ectopic pregnancy on ultrasound scanning does not mean that there is no ectopic pregnancy.

Miscarriage includes a wide range of clinical and pathological conditions and accurate definition is important.

Definitions
Miscarriage

Miscarriage can be defined according to the gestation or the weight of the fetus. The World Health Organization definition is 'the expulsion from its mother of an embryo or fetus weighing 500 g or less' (500 g is approximately the 50th centile for 20 weeks' gestation). Note that the word 'abortion' has connotations of induced abortion (Ch. 16) and should not be used for miscarriage.

In the UK any pregnancy loss before 24 weeks is regarded as a miscarriage, and any fetus born dead at or after 24 weeks of gestation is registered as a stillbirth. If a fetus shows signs of life after delivery at any gestation, however, the loss can be considered to be a live birth and subsequent neonatal death. There is therefore a discrepancy between the legal definition used in the UK and the internationally accepted definition. Because of the rapid advances in neonatal intensive care and the survival of babies born at 23 weeks, most modern epidemiological studies follow the WHO guideline and confine the definition to losses occurring before 20 weeks.

Miscarriage has traditionally been classified in a clinical way:

- *threatened:* vaginal bleeding and an ongoing pregnancy
- *inevitable:* the cervix begins to dilate

165

- *incomplete:* passage of some, but not all, of the products of conception
- *complete:* all products of conception have been expelled from the uterus
- *missed (silent):* where the fetus has died in utero before 20 weeks but has not been expelled
- *anembryonic pregnancy:* a variety of 'missed' miscarriage in which embryonic development fails at a very early stage in the pregnancy; the sac continues to develop, but there are no fetal parts evident on ultrasound scan
- *septic:* a complication of incomplete miscarriage, when intrauterine infection occurs
- *recurrent:* the somewhat arbitrary definition of three or more consecutive miscarriages.

The term 'blighted ovum', formerly used to describe an anembryonic pregnancy, is considered offensive by some and should not be used. 'Silent miscarriage', 'delayed miscarriage' or 'early fetal demise' are more appropriate.

Incidence

The miscarriage ratio (the number of miscarriages divided by the total number of pregnancies in a population) is probably around 10–25%. This risk is highest early in pregnancy and falls as the pregnancy advances. The quoted ratio, however, refers to clinically recognized pregnancies and it is possible for the embryo to die before any obvious signs of pregnancy have appeared. Evidence from very early human chorionic gonadotrophin (hCG) assays, and from assisted conception units, suggests that rates of such very early miscarriage may be as high as 50–60%.

The incidence of miscarriage has been shown to increase with maternal age, rising by a factor of 10 after the age of 40 years compared to before 35 years. Overall, however, when the fetus is found to be viable on ultrasound scan the chance of a successful outcome is high.

Recurrence risk

This knowledge is important for parental counselling. While a few women have a specific recurring cause (such as uterine abnormality) which excludes them from general risk estimation, it is reasonable to reassure the couple that the outlook for future pregnancies is good. A woman who has had three consecutive miscarriages still has a 60–75% chance of a successful fourth pregnancy.

Aetiology

Firm evidence about the causes of miscarriage is scant and there is a real danger of confusing association with cause. There are, however, a number of known conditions causing both sporadic and recurrent miscarriage.

Fetal chromosomal abnormalities

About half of all clinically recognized first trimester losses are chromosomally abnormal, with 50% of these being autosomal trisomy, 20% 45XO monosomy, 20% polyploidy, and 10% with various other abnormalities.

In second trimester miscarriage, the incidence of chromosomal abnormality is lower at about 20% overall. Attempts to confirm the presence of chromosomal abnormality in a particular instance are often unsuccessful owing to failure of culture.

Endocrine factors

Patients with polycystic ovary syndrome have an increased incidence of both sporadic and recurrent miscarriage and although this has been attributed to high circulating levels of luteinizing hormone in the follicular phase of the cycle, there is no evidence of any effective therapy. Inadequate luteal function has been reported in association with recurrent miscarriage in 20–60% of cases. Again, there is no evidence to support the use of artificial progestogens and there is the additional problem that they may carry significant androgenic side-effects.

In those with diabetes mellitus who have poor control around the time of conception, the incidence of miscarriage is high at around 45%, possibly for teratogenic reasons. Those whose control is good are no more likely to have a miscarriage than those who do not have diabetes. There is no clear association between thyroid dysfunction and miscarriage.

Immunological causes

Recent advances in reproductive immunology have revealed both autoimmune and alloimmune associations with miscarriage.

Autoimmune disease

Approximately 15% of women who are investigated for recurrent miscarriage (three or more consecutive pregnancy losses) are found to be positive for either lupus anticoagulant, antiphospholipid antibodies or both. Untreated, they have a subsequent rate of fetal loss approaching 90%. There is now some evidence that giving low-dose aspirin (75 mg daily) from the time of the first positive pregnancy test until delivery results in an approximately 70% incidence of live births. These antibodies are also associated with arterial and venous thrombosis, fetal growth restriction, pre-eclampsia and thrombocytopenia, and this should be borne in mind for later pregnancy management. Lupus anticoagulant is not synonymous with systemic lupus erythematosus

(SLE). It is present in only 5–15% of patients with SLE and occurs more commonly in isolation.

Alloimmune disease

Immunological tolerance of pregnancy is partly related to the special properties of the fetomaternal interface:

- the lack of classic major histocompatibility antigen from the trophoblastic cells of chorionic villi
- the presence of antigens, encoded by paternal genes, which are thought to stimulate production of 'blocking' antibodies.

This process is complex and it has been suggested that some miscarriages may result from maternal immunological rejection of fetal trophoblast cells. Attempts to immunize women against paternally derived antigens have been unsuccessful.

Uterine anomalies

Structural uterine anomalies, such as bicornuate or septate uteri, may cause miscarriage in a few instances, particularly if the loss has occurred in the second trimester. Uterine fibroids may also interfere with early pregnancy growth, but the extent to which they cause miscarriage is difficult to determine because of other associated factors such as age, hormonal dysfunction and subfertility.

Infections

Any serious maternal infection causing high fever at any time in pregnancy may adversely affect the fetus and lead to pregnancy loss. There are also a number of specific maternal infections, however, which may precipitate miscarriage. Viruses, such as rubella and cytomegalovirus, have the ability to cross the placenta and affect the placenta and fetus. Such congenital infection in early pregnancy may lead to miscarriage, as well as to later fetal abnormality and neonatal illness (p. 348). Malaria, trypanosomiasis, *Chlamydia trachomatis*, mycoplasma, *Listeria monocytogenes* and syphilis have also all been implicated in early pregnancy loss.

Environmental pollutants

Cigarette smoking, both active and passive, and high alcohol consumption have been shown to be associated with higher rates of sporadic and recurrent miscarriage.

Unexplained

At least 50% of miscarriages, either sporadic or recurrent, have no identifiable cause.

Clinical presentation and management

Presentation

There is usually a history of bleeding per vaginam (p.v.) and lower abdominal pain, and the passage of tissue is sometimes reported (Fig. 15.1). The bleeding can be life-threateningly severe, requiring urgent and aggressive resuscitation, or there may be only the smallest of brown spotting.

Occasionally there may be no symptoms at all and an empty gestational sac, or fetal pole with absent fetal

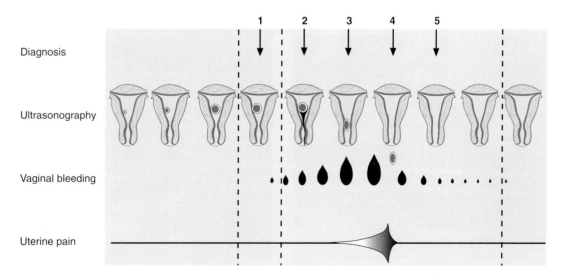

Fig. 15.1 **Clinical and ultrasound features of a miscarriage.** 1. Ultrasound may show fetal heart activity, or the pregnancy may appear non-viable. 2. Vaginal bleeding and pain begin. 3. The cervical os is open – an inevitable miscarriage. 4. The gestational sac is extruded. 5. Pain and bleeding usually settle rapidly.

Table 15.1
The first 9 weeks

Days	Weeks	Clinical features	Scan features
0	0	Menses	
7	1		
14	2	Conception	
21	3		
28	4	Pregnancy test positive (menses due)	Empty uterus
	5		Gestational sac (hCG > 2000)
	6	Nausea Breast tenderness	Yolk sac, fetal heartbeat on transvaginal scan Fetal pole 4 mm
	7		Fetal pole 10 mm
	8		Fetal heartbeat on transabdominal scan Fetal pole 14 mm
	9		Fetal pole 22 mm

heartbeat, may be found at a routine booking scan. It is not possible to make consistently reliable diagnoses based on clinical examination alone, and management is based on ultrasound scan (USS) findings. This management relies on an understanding of the normal ultrasound findings (Table 15.1).

Viable intrauterine pregnancy

The prognosis is good and the parents can be offered reasonable reassurance (Fig. 15.2).

Empty gestational sac

If there is an empty gestational sac greater than 25 mm maximum in diameter the pregnancy is very likely to be non-viable (Fig. 15.3). If a pregnancy test was positive more than 3 weeks previously, the gestation is likely to be at least 6+ weeks and a fetal pole would always be expected on transvaginal (TV) ultrasound scanning. If the first positive pregnancy test was less than 3 weeks previously, however, conservative management is most appropriate, with a repeat scan in at least 10 days.

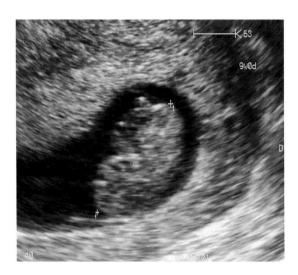

Fig. 15.2 **An intrauterine 22 mm fetal pole, consistent with 9 weeks' gestation.** Fetal heart activity was seen.

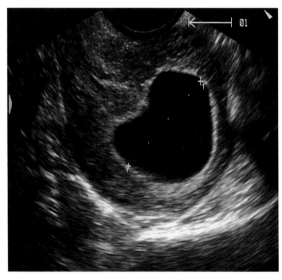

Fig. 15.3 **An empty gestational sac at 8 weeks' gestation.** This pregnancy was an anembryonic, sometimes referred to as a 'silent', miscarriage.

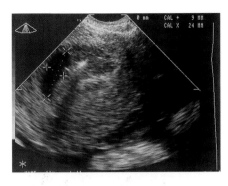

Fig. 15.4 **A pseudosac and intrauterine contraceptive device in the presence of an ectopic pregnancy.**

Although this will add anxious waiting time for the mother, it is preferable to arranging a uterine evacuation on a potentially viable pregnancy.

A true gestational sac should be differentiated from a 'pseudosac' (Fig. 15.4). This is caused by fluid secreted under the hCG stimulation of an ectopic pregnancy, and it lacks the 'double decidual ring' outline seen with a true sac (Figs 15.3 and 15.5).

Fetal pole with no fetal heartbeat

A fetal heartbeat is usually seen on a TV scan if the fetal pole is more than 2–3 mm, but will always be seen by 6 mm (Fig. 15.5). A similar cut-off of 15 mm is appropriate for a transabdominal scan. If there is any doubt, re-scanning should be arranged in 7–10 days. If con-

firmed to be non-viable, the choice is between surgical uterine evacuation, medical uterine evacuation and conservative management.

Empty uterus

Either there has been a complete miscarriage (tissue may have been passed), or the pregnancy is very early (e.g. < 5 weeks), or there is an ectopic pregnancy. Ectopic pregnancy must be excluded. An intrauterine sac will usually be seen on TV scan if the hCG is > 1000 IU, and its absence raises the possibility of an ectopic pregnancy. Serum levels of hCG should double in 48 hours if the pregnancy is viable and intrauterine; less suggests an ectopic pregnancy (although by using this method in isolation 15% of intrauterine pregnancies would be diagnosed as ectopics and 13% of ectopics as intrauterine). If the level doubles and the patient remains well, the ultrasound scan should be repeated in 1 week to ensure that the pregnancy is ongoing. If less than doubling, steady, or only slightly reduced, a laparoscopy should be considered to exclude ectopic pregnancy.

Retained products

Evacuation of retained products of conception (ERPOC) has become the established management for miscarriage with retained products. For those with heavy bleeding this remains appropriate, although it is occasionally possible to remove retained products from the cervical os at speculum examination and save the need for further intervention. While ERPOC may still be offered to those with little bleeding there is evidence that if the diameter of retained products is small (e.g. less than 40 mm) ERPOC may not be necessary. The patient may be reviewed in 2 weeks and re-scanned, at which about 20% will still have retained products. This group may then be offered ERPOC. All should be advised to return before 2 weeks if there is heavy bleeding, pain or fever. An additional option is to give mifepristone and misoprostol for a 'medical' evacuation of retained products.

Adnexal mass suggestive of an ectopic pregnancy

Possible adnexal findings with an ectopic pregnancy are of a sac (30% – Fig. 15.6), a sac containing a yolk sac (15%) and a sac with a fetal pole and fetal heartbeat (15%). The absence of adnexal findings on USS therefore *does not exclude an ectopic pregnancy and clinical findings and hCG levels should be taken into account.*

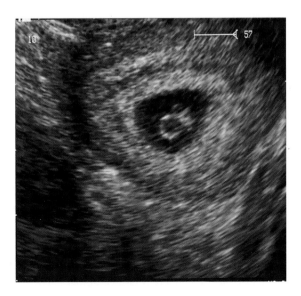

Fig. 15.5 **Intrauterine gestational scan containing a 6 mm fetal pole with a yolk sac.** There was no fetal heart activity on transvaginal scan. Note the double decidual ring consistent with intrauterine pregnancy.

Hydatidiform mole

See page 285.

Gynaecology

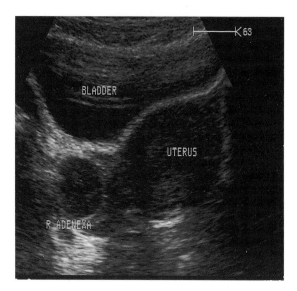

Fig. 15.6 **The sac of a right-sided tubal ectopic pregnancy.**

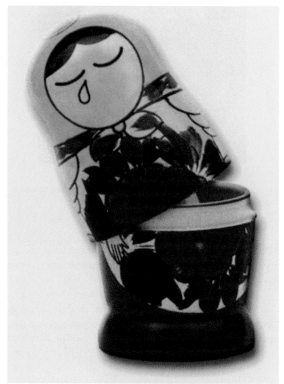

Fig. 15.7 **Logo of The Miscarriage Association with permission.**

Rhesus isoimmunization

Rhesus isoimmunization may occur in rhesus negative women who have lost a rhesus positive fetus (p. 387). As there is no convenient way of assessing fetal blood group in miscarriage, all rhesus negative women should be offered anti-D immunoglobulin if appropriate:

- *Confirmed miscarriage:* anti-D should be given to all non-sensitized Rh negative women who miscarry after 12 weeks, whether complete or incomplete, and to those who miscarry below 12 weeks when the uterus is evacuated (either surgically or medically).
- *Threatened miscarriage:* anti-D should be given to all non-sensitized Rh negative women with threatened miscarriage after 12 weeks. Routine administration of anti-D is not required below 12 weeks when the fetus is viable, unless the bleeding is heavy or associated with abdominal pain. If there is clinical doubt then anti-D should be given.

After the miscarriage

There has been a bereavement and the parents have lost 'a baby'. They should be reassured that they did nothing which might have caused the miscarriage and given time to grieve. There is no medical indication to wait before trying again, but they may request contraception for personal reasons. There is often further upset around the date the baby would have been born. Support groups, such as The Miscarriage Association (www.miscarriageassociation.org.uk), may be of help (Fig. 15.7).

Septic abortion

This is rare unless after illegal terminations with inadequate asepsis, and therefore obviously more common in countries with anti-abortion policies. There is usually pyrexia, tachycardia, malaise, abdominal pain, marked tenderness and a purulent vaginal loss. Endotoxic shock may develop and there is a significant mortality. Usual organisms are Gram-negative bacteria, streptococci (haemolytic and anaerobic) and other anaerobes (e.g. *Bacteroides*).

Recurrent spontaneous miscarriage

This is the consecutive loss of three or more fetuses weighing < 500 g (incidence 0.5–1%). Investigation is based on the principles discussed above and includes:

- *Karyotype* from both parents. The incidence of chromosomal abnormality in this group, usually a balanced reciprocal or Robertsonian translocation, is around 3–5% and the finding of such an abnormality should prompt genetic referral.
- Maternal blood for *lupus anticoagulant* and *anticardiolipin antibodies.*
- *Thrombophilia screen.* Retrospective studies have indicated an increased incidence of thrombophilic defects in those with recurrent miscarriage (activated protein C resistance, antithrombin III deficiency, protein C deficiency, and protein S deficiency, and possibly hyperhomocystinaemia).

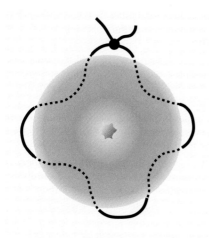

Fig. 15.8 **A cervical suture.**

Evidence for effective treatment in this group is lacking.

• Possible *hysterosalpingogram* and/or *pelvic ultrasound scan* (uterus and ovaries) to look for uterine abnormalities. It is very difficult to estimate the significance of anatomical abnormalities, and great caution is required before undertaking significant surgical procedures.

In those with recurrent mid-trimester loss, the possibility of cervical incompetence should be considered. Inserting a cervical suture may be of benefit, but at the risk of infection developing after insertion (Fig. 15.8). Transabdominal cerclage has also been used, but is not

without considerable risk and should be considered a subspecialist procedure.

Where no specific abnormalities are found, counselling and reassurance are the mainstays of successful management: 60–75% of women who have suffered three consecutive miscarriages will have a successful pregnancy at their next attempt. The use of unproven treatments should be resisted.

Ectopic pregnancy

This refers to any non-intrauterine pregnancy. Although ectopic pregnancies may be ovarian, cervical or intra-abdominal, the vast majority are tubal (Fig. 15.9). The incidence of tubal ectopic pregnancy is 1 : 200–400 pregnancies, with 50% occurring in the ampulla, 28% in the isthmus and the rest either fimbrial or interstitial. There may be a history of a previous ectopic pregnancy, previous surgery, pelvic infection, endometriosis or IVF, but 50% occur in those with no predisposing risk factors.

Clinical features

Clinical features range from no symptoms at all, to right, left or bilateral lower abdominal pain, p.v. bleeding, intra-abdominal haemorrhage (peritonism and shoulder tip pain) and collapse. Pelvic examinations should be gentle to avoid tubal rupture. Undiagnosed intra-abdominal pregnancies have progressed to term to be delivered by caesarean section.

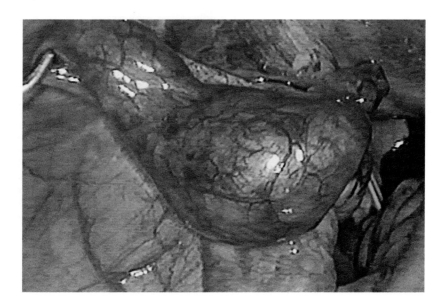

Fig. 15.9 **An ampullary ectopic pregnancy.**

Investigations

Ultrasound is useful in demonstrating an intrauterine pregnancy. As noted above, a gestational sac may be confused with a pseudosac (due to fluid in the thickened endometrium) which is seen in 20% of ectopic pregnancies and which lacks the echogenic ring of a gestational sac (Figs 15.3 and 15.5). A true sac is usually smooth with a double rim, eccentrically placed and may contain a yolk sac. Adnexal features are discussed on page 169.

Management

This depends on the overall clinical picture, the scan result and the hCG:

- If the patient is collapsed, shocked and has a positive pregnancy test, *two* i.v. lines should be set up and the patient crossmatched for 6 units of red cell concentrate. The circulating volume should be rapidly restored with colloid or crystalloid and afterwards, if necessary, O negative or un-crossmatched group-specific blood. An urgent laparotomy is required.
- If there is a positive pregnancy test with clinical signs of an ectopic (pelvic tenderness, cervical excitation, shoulder tip pain) and an empty uterus on TV ultrasound, a diagnostic laparoscopy should be carried out.
- If there is a positive pregnancy test, an empty uterus and no clinical signs, a quantitative hCG should be checked. If >1000 IU following TV scan or > 6500 IU following transabdominal (TA) scan, a laparoscopy should be considered, as an intrauterine sac is usually seen above these levels. Otherwise, the hCG level should be rechecked after at least 48 hours as above. If less than doubling, or steady, or only slightly reduced a laparoscopy may be required to exclude ectopic pregnancy.
- If the hCG levels are falling rapidly the pregnancy (whether intrauterine or ectopic) is aborting. If the patient is well, conservative management is often appropriate, with further hCG checks to ensure that the level continues to fall. Laparoscopy may be warranted if symptoms develop.

Treatment

Surgical treatment may be carried out laparoscopically or at laparotomy. Laparotomy is preferred if there is significant haemodynamic compromise. Although laparoscopy has the advantage over laparotomy of shorter hospital stay and quicker recovery time, subsequent reproductive outcome is similar.

The surgery can be either by salpingectomy (removal of the tube), or salpingostomy. Salpingostomy requires a linear incision to be made over the ectopic using

unipolar needlepoint diathermy (Fig. 15.10a). The ectopic is then removed, and the tube left to close spontaneously (Fig. 15.10b). Salpingostomy carries an approximately 60% subsequent intrauterine pregnancy rate with an ectopic rate of 15%. With salpingectomy, the intrauterine pregnancy rate is around 40% with a 10% ectopic rate. Salpingectomy is indicated in the presence of uncontrollable bleeding, recurrent ectopic in the same tube, a severely damaged tube or when childbearing is complete. If the tube is conserved it is essential to ensure that the hCG is falling; if it is not falling there is likely to be residual trophoblast. The hCG should fall to 25% of the pretreatment level within 4 days of surgery (average time to undetectable is 4 weeks).

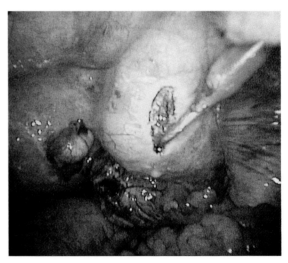

(a)

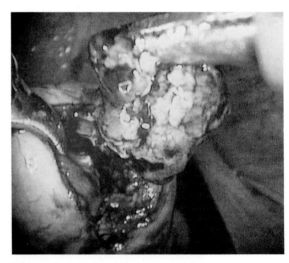

(b)

Fig. 15.10 **Laparoscopic salpingostomy. (a)** A linear incision is made laparoscopically through the tube using monopolar high-frequency current. **(b)** The products of conception are removed using forceps.

With a fimbrial ectopic it might also be possible to 'milk' the pregnancy from the tube at laparotomy.

There is growing interest in medical management of ectopic pregnancy, particularly with giving methotrexate i.m., providing the patient is haemodynamically stable and the ectopic is relatively small.

As there is a significant association between chlamydial infection and ectopic pregnancy, it is important to check the appropriate swabs.

Conclusion

For most miscarriages, whether sporadic or recurrent, no specific cause can be found. Competent management of the acute episode and timely investigation of patients with recurrent miscarriage are the mainstays of treatment.

Ectopic pregnancy is a potentially life-threatening condition and a high index of suspicion is required.

Key points

- Miscarriage is the loss of a pregnancy before 24 weeks' gestation. The World Health Organization definition is 'the expulsion from the mother of a fetus or embryo weighing 500 g of less'.

- There are few successful interventions for preventing miscarriage and management is centred on accurate diagnosis, counselling, and minimizing complications.

- Extreme care must be taken not to advise uterine evacuation if there is any possibility of viability. It should not be assumed that the pregnancy is non-viable simply because the gestation does not agree with the expected dates.

- There should also be a low threshold of suspicion for ectopic pregnancy. The absence of an ectopic pregnancy on ultrasound does not mean that there is no ectopic pregnancy.

16

Therapeutic abortion

Introduction

Termination of unwanted pregnancies, or abortion, has been carried out for thousands of years. Both Aristotle and Hippocrates favoured its selective use, and yet its provision in a legal, medically supervised, and safe framework is still one of the most contentious issues in medicine. Strictly speaking, the term 'termination' is used here to refer to any pregnancy induced at < 24 weeks' gestation (UK) or with a fetal weight of < 500 g but as fetal survival has been achieved below these parameters, the definitions are debatable. The term 'abortion' here refers to 'induced abortion', and the expression 'miscarriage' is reserved for spontaneous loss.

Many people have an opinion, often strongly held, about abortion. Those who are pro-abortion argue they are 'pro-choice' and believe in the right for individuals to make their own decisions. They focus on the potential problems of bringing an unwanted baby into the world, and of the surrounding social difficulties they might face. Those who are anti-abortion, 'pro-life', argue that the fetus is more than just part of the mother, but a life in itself and should be protected as such, even to the extent of limiting the mother's own actions. The advantages and disadvantages are outlined in Box 16.1

Box 16.1

ADVANTAGES AND DISADVANTAGES OF ABORTION

Advantages

- Medically available abortion reduces the incidence of illegal abortions and their complications (particularly sepsis and uterine perforation).

- It provides an opportunity to screen for STIs, discuss contraception and support the patient through difficult circumstances.

- Births of unwanted children are reduced.

Disadvantages

- There may be moral, ethical and religious objections.

- Abortion may be inappropriately looked upon as a form of contraception.

and the moral and philosophical debate is discussed further in Chapter 3.

Worldwide, unsafe abortion is a major public health issue. At least 20 million women undergo unsafe abortion each year and over 60 000 women die as a result, with many others suffering chronic morbidities and disabilities. The mortality from an appropriately conducted abortion, on the other hand, is minimal, and the morbidity small.

The abortion rate is much higher in those countries with limited access to contraception. Where abortion is permitted by the law, the large majority of abortions (typically > 90%) take place before the end of the 12th week of pregnancy.

Legal issues

Some countries have made legal provision for abortion. It is legal in Great Britain for example, under the Abortion Act 1967, amended by the Human Fertilisation and Embryology Act 1991 (Table 16.1). Two doctors are required to sign a form, and if a doctor does not wish to sign, he or she has a duty to refer to another doctor who would. There is also a duty to treat complications in an emergency situation. Great Britain has similar family planning provision to The Netherlands but for social and cultural reasons contraception is less widely used. Overall abortion rates in Britain are higher than in The Netherlands, although still lower than in many developed countries. In young women, however, they are among the highest in Europe.

In practice, section 'C' can be interpreted in such a way as to support termination of pregnancy 'on request'. It is argued that continuing an unwanted pregnancy might be injurious to the mother's mental health as the risk of psychiatric morbidity, in general, is greater after delivery of a baby than after an abortion.

Table 16.1
Circumstances under which an abortion may be carried out under the Abortion Act 1967 (amended by the Human Fertilisation and Embryology Act 1991)

A   To save the mother's life
B   To prevent grave permanent injury to the mother's physical or mental health
C   If < 24 weeks, to avoid injury to the physical or mental health of the mother
D   If < 24 weeks, to avoid injury to the physical or mental health of the existing child(ren)
E   If the child is likely to be severely physically or mentally handicapped

Counselling

It is necessary to ensure that a woman seeking abortion not only has legal grounds but is also certain that termination of pregnancy is the option most suitable for her. Counselling should be non-directive; in other words the woman should be helped to come to her own decision rather than accept the view of the counsellor.

In this counselling, many areas may need to be explored. It is often helpful to start by acknowledging that this is a difficult situation, e.g. 'This must have been a very difficult week or two for you,' and then follow with an open question, 'Tell me what all has been happening.' It is important to find out the patient's own views and to ensure that she is not being forced into having the abortion against her will. If the person is present with a parent or partner, it may be useful to see the patient alone for at least part of the time.

It is also important to find out whether the baby's father knows about the pregnancy, how they get on together, who else knows and what they all feel. The counsellor should try to explore how the woman might cope afterwards, or how she would feel if they went ahead with the pregnancy. Plans for future children, whether they have considered adoption, and subsequent contraception are all also important.

The woman should be aware that there is a possibility, albeit rare, that infection after termination may lead to tubal occlusion and secondary infertility. There is also a small procedure failure rate and either a clinical follow-up or pregnancy test 2–6 weeks post-abortion is important (note that a pregnancy test may remain positive for up to 4 weeks despite successful termination). It is important to either screen for and treat any infections (including chlamydia), or treat all patients prophylactically, e.g. with metronidazole and azithromycin.

Methods of abortion

It is important to confirm that the woman is pregnant and to establish the gestation either clinically or preferably by ultrasound scan. Blood should be sent for grouping and antibody testing, and anti-D should be given to rhesus negative women after termination.

A considerable variety of medical and surgical methods of abortion have been used in the past, including intra-amniotic hypertonic saline or urea, hysterotomy and hysterectomy. Two main methods, however, predominate now. Options (if available) should be explained and the woman given the choice as outlined below:

- *Less than 12 weeks:* suction termination or medical termination (Box 16.2)
- *More than 12 weeks:* medical termination, or dilatation and evacuation.

Box 16.2

PROS AND CONS OF MEDICAL VS SURGICAL TERMINATION < 12 WEEKS

- Medical termination avoids a general anaesthetic.
- There is probably little to choose in terms of the infection risk, pain, post-procedure bleeding and subsequent fertility.
- Those that choose either method are usually satisfied with their choice.
- Medical may be more effective at earlier gestations and surgical more effective closer to 12 weeks.

Surgical termination

Misoprostol pessaries are given 4 hours prior to the operation to soften the cervix and to minimize trauma from the dilatation, particularly if the woman is young or at a gestation of more than 10 weeks. Evacuation of the uterus is usually carried out under general anaesthetic, although local anaesthesia is an option, and cervical dilators are used to dilate the cervical os. A rigid or flexible suction curette is then used to aspirate the fetus and placenta (Figs 16.1 and 16.2). It is important to check and document that definite products of conception have been seen to be coming away at the time of surgery.

After 12–14 weeks' gestation fetal parts cannot be aspirated, but with adequate dilatation they can be morcellated with forceps and removed piecemeal from the uterus. Morcellating a fetus in this way is unpleasant and few doctors are willing to undertake the procedure.

Medical termination

First trimester

Mifepristone, an anti-progesterone, is given orally and the patient admitted to hospital 36–48 hours later for a prostaglandin or misoprostol pessary. 80% of patients will pass products of conception in the following 4 hours, and this should be confirmed by clinical inspection and before discharge. Overall 94% will abort spontaneously and most will bleed for a total of 10 days. Follow-up should be arranged at 2 weeks to ensure that bleeding has settled and to confirm complete abortion

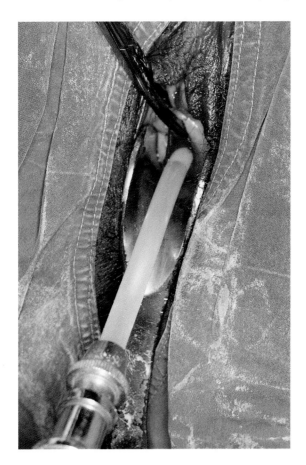

Fig. 16.1 **Surgical termination of pregnancy at 10 weeks' gestation.**

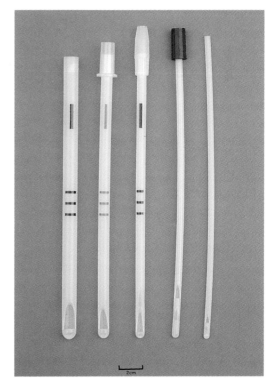

Fig. 16.2 **A selection of suction curettes for surgical pregnancy termination.**

by bimanual examination or ultrasound scan. Retained products can almost always be managed conservatively unless bleeding is particularly heavy, and less than 5% require uterine evacuation.

Second trimester

Oral mifepristone and vaginal prostaglandins or misoprostol are given as above. Further prostaglandin pessaries are inserted 6-hourly to a maximum of 24 hours or alternatively oral misoprostol is given 3-hourly. Nearly all patients will have aborted by 24 hours, with a mean of 8 hours. During this time analgesia and sympathetic emotional support are required. It is important to ensure that the placenta appears complete and that the uterus is well contracted on bimanual examination. Approximately 6% will require a uterine evacuation.

Risks of termination

Although early termination of pregnancy is a relatively safe procedure, there are risks and these generally increase with advancing gestation. The first possibility is of failure to terminate the pregnancy, particularly when suction termination is carried out at an early stage. With suction termination, there is also a risk of uterine perforation and damage to the abdominal viscera, as well as the possibility of the longer-term consequences of cervical trauma and subsequent cervical incompetence. Postoperative pelvic infection may occur with either method and, although rare, may lead to tubal occlusion. With pregnancy termination overall, however, there seems to be little statistical impact on the successful outcome of subsequent pregnancies.

> ### Key points
>
> - Unsafe abortion is a major worldwide public health issue.
> - There is vocal public support for both 'pro-life' and 'pro-choice' viewpoints.
> - All women requesting termination of pregnancy must be adequately counselled, and the other options of proceeding with pregnancy or considering adoption should be discussed.
> - Pregnancy may be terminated medically or surgically. After 12–14 weeks it is usually necessary to use medical means.

17

Sexual problems

Introduction

It is important for any doctor to be able to take a sexual history and to have some idea of how sexual problems are managed. Understanding the physiology of the normal sexual response will allow the doctor to help many of the simpler sexual problems. This is still true even in our age of apparent openness about sex.

Scientific investigation of the normal sexual response is necessary to our understanding, but because of society's disapproval few scientists have chosen to work in this area until recently. Early workers were:

- Sigmund Freud (1856–1939), an Austrian doctor, was the founder of psychoanalysis and the first to recognize the importance of childhood influences on sexuality. His studies were on patients rather than normal subjects.
- Havelock Ellis (1859–1939) studied medicine at St Thomas's Hospital, London. His seven-volume *Studies in the Psychology of Sex* (1897–1928) caused controversy but was the first detached treatment of the subject.
- Alfred Kinsey (1894–1956), an American zoologist, became director of Indiana University's Institute for Sex Research in 1942. To investigate 'normal' sexual experience, 18 500 Americans were interviewed. *Sexual Behaviour in the Human Male* was published in 1948, and *Sexual Behaviour in the Human Female* in 1953.
- Masters and Johnson: William Masters (b. 1915), a doctor, and Virginia Johnson (b. 1925), a psychologist, working at Washington University, St Louis, carried out the first direct observations on sexual activity under laboratory conditions. *Human Sexual Response* appeared in 1966, and *Human Sexual Inadequacy* in 1970.

Normal sexual response

The normal human sexual response can be regarded as having five phases: desire, arousal, orgasm, resolution and the refractory phase (Fig. 17.1).

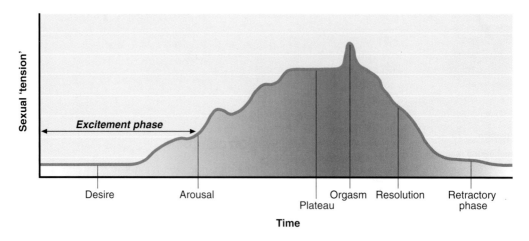

Fig. 17.1 **The normal sexual response.**

Desire

Sexual desire refers to the general level of interest in sexuality. It is modulated by hormones – hence the change in sexual interest at puberty. The main modulator in both sexes is testosterone.

Arousal

This phase has three components: central arousal, genital response, and peripheral arousal.

Central arousal

This refers to the response to sexual stimuli, which may be visual or tactile or may result from internal imagery or from a relationship. These stimuli act through the cerebral cortex (Fig. 17.2). The areas of the brain involved in sexual arousal are thought to be in the limbic system. There are thought to be excitatory centres with endorphins as the neurotransmitter, and inhibitory centres, linked to the centres for pain and fear.

Genital response

The spinal pathways leading to the genitalia are not precisely known but appear to be near the spinothalamic pathways for pain and temperature. Genital responses are due to vasocongestion and neuromuscular changes. Arteriolar dilatation is probably controlled by the parasympathetic sacral outflow at S2, 3 and 4 via the nervi erigentes. Thoracic sympathetic outflow also plays a part. The local neurotransmitters involved include vasoactive intestinal polypeptide (VIP), a potent vasodilator found in the penis and vagina.

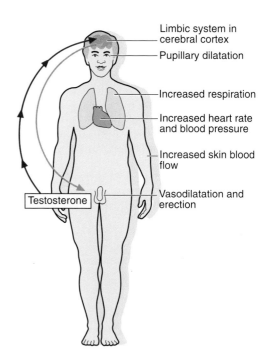

Fig. 17.2 **Control of sexual activity.**

In the male, engorgement of the corpora cavernosa is due mainly to arteriolar dilatation and probably a reduction in the venous outflow (Fig. 17.3). The scrotum tightens due to contraction of the dartos muscle and the testes are elevated due to contraction of the cremaster muscle.

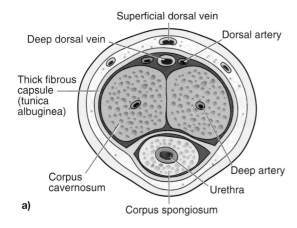

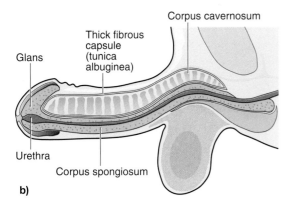

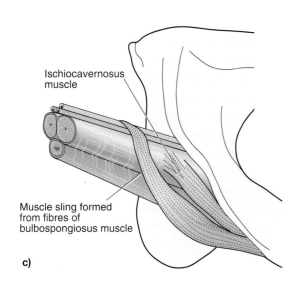

Fig. 17.3 **The penis. (a)** Cross-section showing erectile spaces and principal blood vessels. **(b)** Erectile tissues. Each crus of the corpora cavernosa is inserted into the pubic bone. **(c)** Muscles.

In the female, there is engorgement of the venous plexus surrounding the lower part of the vagina, and of the erectile bulbs of the vestibule on either side of the introitus (Fig. 17.4). There is reddening and pouting of the labia minora. The clitoris becomes erect and later is said to retract against the symphysis pubis.

The vagina becomes lubricated by a transudate as the blood supply to the vaginal wall increases. This fluid is not the product of mucous glands: beads of fluid appear all over the vaginal wall. Mucous secretion from the cervix makes relatively little contribution to vaginal lubrication (which is therefore usually unaffected by hysterectomy). Secretion from Bartholin's glands, formerly thought to be mainly responsible for lubrication, is only moderate in amount and occurs relatively late during arousal.

The uterus becomes engorged, increases in size, and rises in the pelvis. The upper part of the vagina 'balloons' and there may be slow irregular contractions of the lower third of the vagina.

In both sexes but particularly in the male, the genital response interacts with the central response, so that arousal becomes self-amplifying.

Peripheral arousal

Sexual arousal causes:

- a rise in systolic and diastolic blood pressure (which may only be transient)
- general flushing of the skin
- change in heart rate (either an increase or a decrease)
- respiratory changes
- pupillary dilatation.

Plateau phase

When arousal is complete, there may be a 'plateau' phase during which the couple prolong the pleasure of intercourse before orgasm. If this continues too long, however, coitus may become painful for one or both partners.

Orgasm

Orgasm involves genital, muscular and sensory changes as well as cardiovascular and respiratory responses.

In the male

First there is smooth muscle contraction of the epididymis, vas deferens, seminal vesicle, prostate and ampulla, propelling seminal and prostatic fluid into the urethral bulb. Then the male becomes aware that orgasm is imminent and ejaculation usually follows within a few seconds. The internal bladder sphincter remains shut

Gynaecology

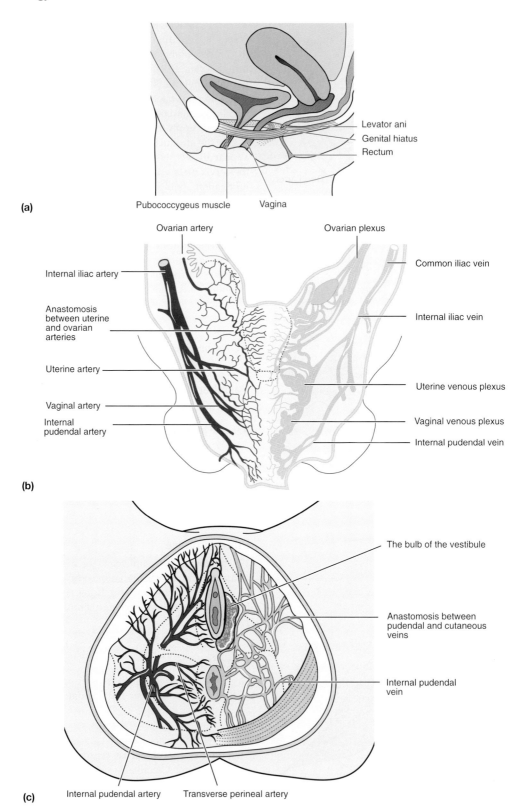

(a)

Levator ani
Genital hiatus
Rectum

Pubococcygeus muscle   Vagina

(b)

Ovarian artery   Ovarian plexus

Internal iliac artery   Common iliac vein

Anastomosis
between uterine
and ovarian
arteries   Internal iliac vein

Uterine artery

Vaginal artery   Uterine venous plexus

Internal
pudendal artery   Vaginal venous plexus
                                                    Internal pudendal vein

(c)

The bulb of the vestibule

Anastomosis between
pudendal and cutaneous
veins

Internal pudendal
vein

Internal pudendal artery   Transverse perineal artery

Fig. 17.4 **Female reproductive organs. (a)** The muscular supports of the vagina. This shows the sling of muscle fibres that surround the urethra, vagina and rectum, running from the pubic bone to the coccyx. The levator plate formed by these fibres supports the rectum and vagina in its non-aroused horizontal position. **(b)** Arteries and veins supplying the female reproductive organs. **(c)** Blood vessels of the pelvic floor showing the rich arterial and venous networks surrounding the vaginal opening.

but the external sphincter relaxes and semen is propelled along the urethra by rhythmic contractions of the bulbospongiosus and ischiocavernosus muscles.

In the female

A few seconds after the onset of the subjective experience of orgasm there is a spasm of the muscles surrounding the lower third of the vagina (the 'orgasmic platform') followed by a series of rhythmic contractions, usually five to eight in number. Uterine contractions may also occur.

In both sexes

There is contraction of rectus abdominis, pelvic thrusting, contraction of the anal sphincter and sometimes carpopedal spasm. Systolic and diastolic blood pressure rises by at least 25 mmHg, and hyperventilation occurs. There is a feeling of intense pleasure and an alteration of consciousness to a variable degree.

Resolution

The events of arousal are gradually reversed. In men there is a moderate immediate loss of erection followed by a slower complete reversal. In women, if no orgasm has occurred pelvic congestion may take hours to resolve and may be uncomfortable. In both sexes there is a subjective feeling of relaxation, though its duration may differ between the man and the woman.

Refractory phase

There follows an interval during which further stimulation does not produce a response. In men this varies from minutes in young men to many hours in older men. Some women do not experience a refractory period but only a minority of women (14% according to Kinsey) can have multiple orgasms.

The effect of age

Normal sexual behaviour differs from couple to couple. It also alters with age and with the evolution of a sexual relationship. Patients may present with problems due to difficulties in adjusting to the change from one phase to the next phase of a relationship.

Adolescence

An adolescent usually has a high capacity for sexual arousal and a need to find out whether he or she is sexually attractive. Alongside the need to learn about sexual behaviour there is emotional vulnerability. Unsatisfactory sexual experience at this time can set the scene for continuing problems later. Young women in their late teens are at high risk of unwanted pregnancy due to uncertainty about contraceptive needs.

The couple

The early months of a relationship may be characterized by frequent sex but a couple need to learn quickly how to establish good communication and to adjust their sexual behaviour to each other's needs. Otherwise, dysfunctional patterns may develop; for example, of premature ejaculation, or of the man continually making inappropriate sexual advances and being rebuffed.

Early parenthood

The time taken for sexual interest to return after childbirth is variable and in some women can be a year or more. Problems may be due to a painful episiotomy or postnatal depression but more commonly are due to tiredness and the difficulty of coping with the demands of the new baby.

Middle age

When the novelty of a sexual relationship has worn off, sexual activity becomes less frequent and this may cause anxieties. Couples may feel they 'ought' to be having sex more often. Stresses at work for both partners may combine with social commitments to make it difficult to relax together. In the years before the menopause women often have menstrual problems. After the menopause there may be a reduction in sexual interest or a problem with vaginal dryness; these can usually be corrected by hormone replacement therapy. One partner may no longer find the other physically attractive, or may be increasingly put off by what he or she considers irritating characteristics.

Old age

Loss of erectile capacity increases with age and may also be due to physical disease (Fig. 17.5). Couples used to an active sex life may find these changes difficult to accept and men may seek treatment to restore their youthful abilities.

The functions of sex

It is important to remember how much people differ from one another and, how wide the range of normality may be.

Reproduction

Now that the average number of children per family is around two, reproductive sex is often limited to a short

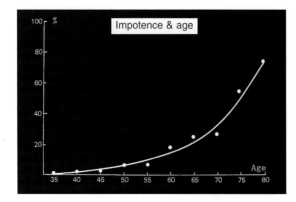

Fig. 17.5 **Impotence increases with age.** (From Bancroft 1989, with permission. Data from Kinsey et al 1948.)

interval in a couple's relationship. Couples who have had a problem with infertility may find that it causes difficulty with their sex life, or conversely may find that after they achieve pregnancy it is difficult to have sex for pleasure only.

Pleasure

Though sex is readily associated in people's minds with pleasure, the many taboos that surround it make purely 'recreational' sex more often a fantasy than a reality.

Pair-bonding

Enjoying sex means lowering one's defences, and sharing this experience strengthens the bond between the partners. People who have had to build particularly strong defences – for example, after emotional abuse in childhood – may have difficulty in relinquishing them.

Asserting masculinity or femininity

People may use sexual activity to reassure themselves about their sexuality. This is normal in adolescence but for some people the pattern continues or recurs at times of stress.

Bolstering self-esteem

Satisfactory sex improves a person's self-esteem and unsatisfactory sex has the opposite effect. People who have had an unsatisfactory sexual relationship may hurry straight into another one to try to re-establish their confidence, often with the opposite result.

Achieving power

Some people see the sexual relationship in terms of dominance and submission. This can apply to coitus itself or to the power to allow or deny access to sex.

Expressing hostility

For many people anger is incompatible with sexual arousal but for some people anger enhances arousal and aggressive sex may be used to express anger. Rape or sexual assault may have more to do with aggression than with sex.

Reducing anxiety or tension

The use of orgasm to relieve tension applies particularly to people who habitually masturbate. They may do so more often at times of stress. A person who has got used to relieving sexual tension by masturbation may have difficulty adjusting to a shared sex life after marriage.

Risk taking

The risks of sexual activity range from fear of discovery to contracting HIV infection. For some people, an element of risk adds to their pleasure.

Material gain

Prostitution is the most obvious form of sex for gain, and is often the result of poverty. Marriage, even nowadays, may also be a way of using sex to buy security.

History-taking

Some sexual problems may present disguised as another symptom such as pelvic pain, or are discovered apparently fortuitously, for example when a routine enquiry is made about contraception. It is inappropriate to take a detailed sexual history from every patient whatever their complaint but it is reasonable, particularly in a gynaecological clinic, to ask one or two questions about sex as a matter for routine; for example 'Do you have any trouble with intercourse?' or, if appropriate, 'Is this symptom worse after intercourse?' For some patients this will not be necessary but for others it will be a chance to mention a sex problem. An evasive reply may suggest that all is not well. Obtaining accurate information requires skill and practice.

Elucidating a sexual problem relies mainly on the history, though useful information may be obtained from examination or investigation. The interviewer must be comfortable with the subject as the patient is likely to be embarrassed by talking about a sexual problem. A sympathetic but matter-of-fact approach may help to reduce this embarrassment. The vocabulary used must also be appropriate, using words that avoid on the one hand being too technical and on the other hand appearing too crude.

It is usually helpful to see both partners but not necessarily together on the first occasion. A patient may be more frank if interviewed alone, but the partner may give quite a different version of the history. When treatment is planned, however, both partners should ideally be involved.

The history needs to be thorough but, if too intrusive, it may be off-putting. If a topic seems painful the subject can be changed and then returned to later. Sometimes more than one interview is necessary, with sensitive topics being explored on the second occasion after a rapport has been built up. A detailed account of a specific instance may be more helpful than asking general questions. For example, if the patient is asked 'How often do you have intercourse?' the reply is likely to be a vague guess which depends partly on what the patient thinks is expected (e.g. 'About twice a week'). It may be better to ask 'When did you last have intercourse?', and then, if the couple's last attempt was unsatisfactory, to ask in detail about what went wrong. Open-ended questions should also be used; for example 'How did you feel when that happened?'

Many patients, especially if talking about their sexual problem for the first time, find it difficult to put their feelings into words. It may be helpful to offer the occasional summing-up: 'What I think you're saying is that ...'. The patient will usually give a clearly positive response if the doctor has summed up the situation correctly. If the patient's response is more guarded the doctor should be cautious about the conclusions drawn.

Sex problems

Problems with sex include sexual variations and sexual dysfunction.

Sexual variations

Only a minority of patients requesting treatment are homosexual or have problems of deviant sexuality.

Homosexuality

Homosexual behaviour has been tolerated or approved of in many primitive societies but widely rejected in western societies. Male homosexual acts were illegal in England until 1967 and 'gay' men are still discriminated against; for example homosexuality is illegal in the armed forces. Kinsey reported that 30% of men had experienced orgasm during a homosexual encounter at least once, but only about 3% were exclusively homosexual, with another 3% having extensive homosexual experience. The incidence of female homosexuality is much lower, with 6% of women having at least one homosexual experience, 2% having significant experience and 1% being exclusively homosexual.

Problems encountered by homosexual people are of two types: (1) sexual dysfunction or (2) dissatisfaction with their sexual orientation. Fear of an unsympathetic

response may inhibit them from seeking treatment for dysfunction. Prejudice by their family or by society often adds to their problems.

Transsexuality

A transsexual is a man or woman who believes himself or herself to be of the opposite gender in spite of his or her anatomy. Transsexuals are likely to seek medical help to alter their bodies to be consistent with their psychological gender. There are a number of 'gender identity clinics' in various parts of the world, which provide specialist services for transsexuals using the combined expertise of psychologists, psychiatrists, endocrinologists and surgeons.

Transvestism

A transvestite is someone who enjoys dressing in the clothes of the opposite gender. This group includes transsexuals and some homosexuals but also people (mainly men) who enjoy cross-dressing without the wish to change sex, and men who obtain sexual gratification from wearing women's clothes. A high proportion of the latter groups are married and parents: they may be referred to a specialist clinic because of the strain that their behaviour is putting on their relationship.

Sadomasochism

Moderate pain inflicted during sexual arousal (e.g. as a 'love bite') was enjoyed by 50% of subjects in Kinsey's study. Ritualized dominance and submission are enjoyed by a small number of people, almost entirely male, most of whom can switch between dominant and submissive roles. Submission may be a way of avoiding responsibility if sex is associated with guilt. Such people rarely request treatment.

Fetishism

Particular parts of the body, articles of clothing (e.g. shoes) or materials (e.g. nowadays, rubber or plastic) can become objects of sexual gratification. Fetishism hardly ever occurs in women. These men rarely request treatment.

Sexual dysfunction

Sexual dysfunction may be due to psychological or relationship problems or may have a medical or surgical cause. It is so common as to be almost physiological. Not everyone with sexual dysfunction considers that they have a problem. In one survey of married couples, nearly 66% of the women reported some degree of difficulty with arousal and 40% of the men reported problems, mainly premature ejaculation. In another study, only one-third of anorgasmic women considered themselves to have a problem.

The incidence of dysfunction varies with age. Kinsey reported that 50% of women had not experienced orgasm by their late teens: by the age of around 35 the proportion was 10%. Permanent erectile impotence becomes more common with age (Fig. 17.5), the incidence rising from about 2% at age 40 to about 25% at 70 and 75% at 80, according to Kinsey's survey. This does not necessarily cause a problem if the woman's interest in sex has also decreased with age.

The common disorders of sexual function can be classified according to the physiological stages described early in this chapter:

- impaired desire (diminished libido in both sexes)
- disorders of arousal (erectile dysfunction in men, vaginismus in women)
- disorders of orgasm (premature ejaculation in men, anorgasmia, usually in women)
- dyspareunia (mainly in women).

The causes of sexual dysfunction can be classified into pathological or psychological factors but it is unhelpful to make a sharp distinction between the two as they often coexist. For example, painful intercourse due to a physical cause such as a herpetic lesion may lead to secondary anxiety in both partners. On the other hand, anxiety due to sexual abuse in childhood may lead to pelvic congestion or spasm of the pelvic floor muscles. Treatment often needs to be directed towards physical and psychological causes at the same time.

A list of pathological causes of sexual dysfunction is given in Box 17.1. These causes are more common in older people. More commonly, however, the cause of sexual dysfunction is due to psychological factors. These can be classified as in Box 17.2.

Female sexual dysfunction

Impaired desire

This is the commonest symptom presenting to specialist sexual medicine clinics although it is not such a frequent symptom in routine gynaecology clinics. The woman complains that she is just not interested in sex. Such 'loss of libido' may be primary or secondary. The unhelpful and offensive term 'frigidity' is no longer used.

Primary

Some women have never felt interested in sex and in these cases there is usually impairment of arousal and orgasm as well. The underlying cause is often in an upbringing in which sex was regarded as dirty. The woman may choose a partner who also has an apparently low sex drive.

Box 17.1

PATHOLOGICAL CAUSES OF SEXUAL DYSFUNCTION

Medical disorders

- Acute and chronic illness
- Psychiatric illness
- Cancer – especially gynaecological
- Neurological problems, e.g. spinal cord injuries, multiple sclerosis, neuropathy
- Endocrine, e.g. diabetes
- Cardiovascular, e.g. myocardial infarction
- Respiratory
- Arthritic
- Renal, e.g. dialysis
- Gynaecological, e.g. vaginitis

Surgical procedures

- Mastectomy
- Colostomy
- Gynaecological – oophorectomy, episiotomy, vaginal repair
- Amputation

Drug effects

- Anticholinergics
- Anticonvulsants
- Antihypertensives
- Anti-inflammatories
- Hormones
- Hypnotics and sedatives
- Major tranquillizers
- Alcohol
- Opiates

Secondary

More commonly, loss of libido follows an interval of apparently normal sex drive, during the woman's teens or early 20s, or early in the relationship with her partner. Loss of interest in sex may occur after childbirth, when both parents (particularly the woman) devote all their attention to the baby, often nowadays combining motherhood with a return to the woman's

Box 17.2

PSYCHOLOGICAL FACTORS IN SEXUAL DYSFUNCTION

Remote
- Repressed family attitudes to sex
- Poor sex education
- Sexual or physical trauma

Precipitant
- Psychiatric illness
- Childbirth
- Infidelity
- Partner's dysfunction
- Relationship problem – may be cause or effect

Maintaining
- Anxiety
- Poor communication
- Lack of foreplay
- Depression
- Poor information

communication between the partners. A specific cause, such as childhood abuse, may require specialist referral, e.g. for psychotherapeutic counselling. Hormone therapy is appropriate for postmenopausal women but not for those who still have a normal menstrual cycle.

Orgasmic dysfunction

Inability to achieve orgasm is usually associated with lack of interest in sex, but sometimes can be an isolated symptom in a woman who has an otherwise satisfactory sex drive and is able to experience normal arousal.

Primary

As noted above, Kinsey reported that 10% of women had never achieved orgasm by the age of 35, and other studies indicate that up to a third of women are dissatisfied in some way with their orgasmic ability. Only a small proportion of these will seek medical treatment.

Inability to achieve orgasm despite adequate arousal may be due to inexperience of the woman or her partner or unrealistic expectations, e.g. reading erotic fiction may have led the couple to believe that orgasm occurs automatically on penetration. Sometime the cause is more deep-seated; because of childhood repression the woman is unable to let go her defences. Psychological counselling may be helpful.

Secondary

Secondary orgasmic dysfunction follows an interval of adequate sexual functioning. It is usually associated with reduced desire or arousal as discussed in the previous section.

Situational orgasmic dysfunction

Some women can achieve orgasm through masturbation but not coitus, or with one partner and not with another.

Vaginismus

Vaginismus is involuntary spasm of the pelvic floor muscles and perineal muscles, provoked by attempted penetration. It is also provoked by vaginal examination or by attempts to insert a tampon or the woman's own finger into the vagina. When severe, the conditioned reflex includes spasm of the adductor muscles of the thighs.

Primary vaginismus

In most cases the problem is primary vaginismus and is discovered during the first attempt at intercourse. It may be due to apprehension that intercourse will be painful or due simply to failure to control the pelvic

paid employment. If there has been postnatal depression this will exacerbate the problem.

Other causes include:

- depression
- bereavement
- the menopause
- gynaecological investigation, e.g. for an abnormal cervical smear; hysterectomy causes loss of libido in only a few instances, and more commonly improves a woman's sex life
- loss of self-esteem (e.g. problems at work).

Sometimes the secondary loss of libido has no obvious specific cause. A woman who has suffered sexual or physical abuse in childhood, or who has had a sexually repressed upbringing, may go through a phase of normal or increased sexual activity in her teens and 20s and then present with loss of libido due to the long-term effects of her childhood experiences.

Often the man reacts to the woman's loss of interest by making persistent sexual demands and then, after some years, giving up approaching her for sex. Loss of desire is often due to a problem with the relationship, and counselling will be directed towards improving

musculature. Persistent attempts at penetration cause more pain and a 'vicious circle' is set up, reinforcing the vaginismus.

Primary vaginismus may also be due to more deep-seated psychological problems, such as an unwillingness to accept sexual maturity, or sexual repression in childhood.

Secondary vaginismus

Vaginismus may also follow a physically painful experience, such as a sexual assault, an obstetric problem at delivery or an insensitive vaginal examination.

The vulva and vagina should be examined for any painful lesion, though in most cases no such cause will be found. In a few cases examination will reveal a firm intact hymen and this may require dilatation under anaesthesia. This is necessary in only a small minority of cases.

Most cases of primary and secondary vaginismus respond well to simple treatment, involving training in relaxation and the use of vaginal dilators. The woman should be helped to relax completely: she should let her head rest on the pillow and vaginal examination should not be attempted until the adductor muscles of the thighs have fully relaxed. The woman is then taught to insert a small vaginal dilator: such patients need a combination of gentleness and encouragement to overcome their apprehension. Once she is comfortable about inserting the small dilator regularly she can progress to gradually larger sizes. During treatment she is also taught pelvic floor exercises, which help her to gain control of the muscles. It may take several weeks or months before full control is achieved.

Attempts at intercourse should be discouraged until she is able to insert the larger sized vaginal dilators. In some cases it then becomes apparent that the husband has a problem with erectile dysfunction but in most instances satisfactory intercourse follows. An alternative to vaginal dilators is for the woman to use her own finger and then for the partner to insert one and then two fingers into the vagina. In most instances which present to the clinic, however, the couple are reluctant to do this and prefer the dilators. If primary vaginismus is due to more deep-seated problems, treatment may take many months and the prognosis is less good. Psychotherapy may be appropriate in these cases.

Dyspareunia

Pain on intercourse is the commonest sexual problem presenting to the routine gynaecology clinic. It is usually classified into superficial and deep dyspareunia, but it is not always possible to make a clear distinction between the two (Box 17.3). With superficial dyspareunia, there is a pain at the vaginal introitus on attempted penetration, often making full intercourse impossible.

Box 17.3

CAUSES OF DYSPAREUNIA

Superficial dyspareunia
- Infection, e.g. candida, herpes
- Atrophic change, particularly after the menopause
- Vulval dystrophy
- Vaginismus

Deep dyspareunia
- Endometriosis
- Pelvic inflammatory disease
- Bowel dysfunction
- Pelvic mass
- 'Unexplained' pelvic pain

In deep dyspareunia there is pain in the pelvis on deep penetration. Bimanual examination may reveal a specific area of tenderness, e.g. on moving the cervix or on palpating the posterior fornix, the rectum or one or other lateral fornix. Sometimes, however, the tenderness is more general and a specific site cannot be identified.

Examination of the vulva may reveal the inflammatory appearance of candidal infection, the lesions of herpes or the presence of atrophy or dystrophy. Careful examination may be necessary to reveal the localized inflammation of vestibulitis. Vulval and vaginal swabs should be taken for microbiological examination and treatment given if appropriate. If no cause is found for what appears to be superficial dyspareunia, it may be necessary to consider the causes of deep dyspareunia.

Deep dyspareunia is often associated with other symptoms such as dysmenorrhoea or persistent pelvic pain. The history should include questions about bowel habit. Bowel dysfunction is not uncommon and can be treated with a high-fibre diet. The timing of the pain in relation to the cycle should also be noted – it may occur just before ovulation or menstruation. Bimanual examination may reveal a pelvic mass.

The finding of a retroverted uterus is unlikely to be significant, as uterine retroversion is common. Occasionally, however, a sharply retroverted uterus can be the only site of tenderness. High vaginal and cervical swabs should be taken if there is any suspicion of pelvic infection. In most cases laparoscopy is necessary to diagnose or exclude endometriosis or pelvic inflammatory disease.

When a specific cause is identified the appropriate treatment is given. If laparoscopy is negative a high-fibre diet may help even in the absence of obvious bowel symptoms. If no cause is found and the deep dyspareunia is not associated with other symptoms, the problem may be due to too little foreplay leading to inadequate arousal and insufficient relaxation of the upper vagina. The couple should try allowing more time for arousal, and may be advised to avoid positions (such as the woman sitting on top of the man) in which penetration is particularly deep.

If deep dyspareunia is associated with 'unexplained pelvic pain' treatment can be difficult and may require a combination of endocrine manipulation and psychological support.

Male sexual dysfunction

Male sexual dysfunction can be classified as impairment of desire, erection or ejaculation. There is considerable overlap between these disorders.

Impaired desire

In the male, libido is dependent on normal testosterone levels, and serum testosterone should be checked in men complaining of lack of libido. If the level is normal, testosterone supplements are unlikely to help.

As noted above, male libido diminishes with age. This is not simply due to falling testosterone levels. Older men may seek treatment because they are unwilling to accept this physiological change.

There is an assumption among many men that the male should always be ready for sex. There is also a widespread expectation that medications exist which can increase libido. Male patients are often unwilling or unable to change a busy lifestyle which leaves little time for sex.

Erectile dysfunction

Inability to achieve or maintain a satisfactory erection ('impotence') is the commonest sex problem among men. It may be associated with impaired desire but desire usually is normal. Indeed, the anxiety provoked by the erectile dysfunction may increase his awareness of sexual stimuli.

Erectile dysfunction is usually due to psychological factors but it is important to investigate possible physical causes. If a physical cause is found it may indicate a general disease and it may be treatable. The patient may not accept a diagnosis of a psychological cause until possible physical causes have been excluded (Box 17.4).

In addition to a full sexual history, the man should be asked about the duration of the problem, whether it is primary or secondary, and whether it is situational (i.e. does he get 'early morning' erections, or can he get an erection by masturbation but not with his partner).

Box 17.4

PHYSICAL CAUSES OF ERECTILE FAILURE

Endocrine disorders
- Disorders causing reduced plasma testosterone may cause erectile failure, but these usually cause loss of libido as well.
- Diabetes may cause impotence. The incidence of erectile failure at age 50 is 40% among diabetic men, and only 5% among non-diabetic men. The mechanism may be either diabetic neuropathy or vascular disease.

Neurological disorders
- Multiple sclerosis may cause erectile failure.
- Spinal injury causes erectile failure but after the initial phase of 'spinal shock', reflex erectile ability may return if the sacral segments of the spinal cord are intact.

Vascular disorders
- There is a decline in sexual activity after myocardial infarction and, interestingly, before a heart attack.
- Hypertension, when untreated, is also associated with erectile dysfunction.

Drugs
- Antihypertensives, particularly methyldopa may cause erectile failure. Beta-blockers are less likely to cause erectile failure, though it can occur idiosyncratically.

Psychiatric illness
- Severe depression causes loss of sexual interest in over 60% of cases.

Surgery
- Prostatectomy need not cause impotence, particularly if it is by the transurethral or retropubic route. Perineal prostatectomy for cancer is a more radical operation and usually causes erectile failure.

Physiological
- Ageing reduces the frequency of erections. Some men may also fail to understand the refractory period, and may have unrealistic expectations of how soon erection can recur after orgasm.

Enquiry should be made about symptoms of general disease, including those listed above; for example, does exercise bring on claudication?

Clinical examination should include a check for signs of systemic disease. The genitalia should be examined for abnormalities of the penis (such as hypospadias) or abnormally small testes. Serum testosterone should be checked as a matter of routine and, if it is low, serum sent for follicle-stimulating hormone (FSH) and prolactin assay.

Drug treatment is now often used in addition to, or instead of, psychosexual counselling. Therapeutic options include:

- Sildenafil (Viagra). Penile erection is due to relaxation of the smooth muscle around the cavernosal vascular spaces, allowing them to fill with blood. This is under the control of the autonomic nervous system, mediated by cyclic guanosine monophophate (cGMP). Sildenafil is taken orally and acts as an enhancer of erection by blocking breakdown of cGMP. It works best in psychogenic erectile failure and milder organic problems in which the success rate is $\approx 85\%$. Side-effects are mild and transient and include flushing, dyspepsia, headache and disturbance to colour vision. It must not be used with nitrates, as it may lead to a potentially life-threatening profound drop in blood pressure.
- Alprostadil (PGE_1). This drug also relaxes cavernosal smooth muscle but has to be injected directly into the corpora cavernosa. It is more effective than sildenafil in erectile failure due to more severe organic problems. It is also available as a urethral pellet (MUSE) but this is much less effective.
- Other treatments used include vacuum devices (Fig. 17.6) and penile implants, the latter only where no other treatment has been effective.

Ejaculatory dysfunction

The most common type of ejaculatory dysfunction is premature ejaculation. Retarded ejaculation is much less common and may be associated with other psychological problems. Painful ejaculation is relatively rare.

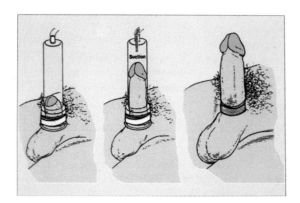

Fig. 17.6 **The use of a vacuum device to manage impotence.**

Premature ejaculation is normal in early sexual experiences. It is difficult to define, and the best guide is if the man feels he has insufficient control to satisfy himself and his partner. Sometimes ejaculation occurs before penetration or within a few seconds of penetration. The cause of premature ejaculation is usually psychological, with anxiety increasing each time the problem occurs.

Treatment requires the cooperation of the partner and it is difficult to help a man who presents for treatment without his partner's knowledge. If the couple have a good relationship, they can be instructed in the 'stop–start' technique, in which the partner manually stimulates the penis until orgasm is near, when he signals her to stop. Practice with this technique helps to build a feeling of control. The 'squeeze' technique – firm pressure at the level of the frenulum – may also help to retard ejaculation.

Treatment of sexual problems

The treatment of sexual problems can be divided into two categories:

- counselling, which should be within the scope of a general practitioner
- sex therapy, which requires specialist training.

Counselling

Some problems can be helped by a single consultation or a few consultations. Simple counselling may include the following.

Permission giving

A patient may become very anxious about some activity, such as masturbation, and may be helped to know that it is normal. Simply talking about sexual matters in a matter-of-fact way is helpful to many patients who feel they are unique in experiencing difficulties.

Limited information

An explanation of normal anatomy or physiology may also be helpful. He or she may be reassured by an examination, which shows that the genitalia are normal. The clinician may also recommend a book which explains sexual matters.

Advice

Commonsense advice on sexual technique may be helpful. In spite of the apparent openness about sexual matters in many countries, many people do not seem to understand the importance of foreplay, the pleasures of non-penetrative sex, or the fact that the positions adopted during intercourse can be varied. Many couples, with both partners leading busy lives, seem to expect to be able to 'switch on' sexual activity during the brief interlude when it is convenient, and sensible advice about making time for each other may be helpful.

Sex therapy

Some problems are resistant to simple counselling and require specialist referral. Specialist treatment usually involves an average of about 12 sessions. About two-thirds of couples benefit from specialist therapy; vaginismus and premature ejaculation respond particularly well but results are less good for reduced desire. The components of therapy are a graduated behavioural programme and counselling.

Graduated behavioural programme

This involves first banning attempts at intercourse or touching the breasts or genitalia. 'Sensate focus' then follows, in which the partners make time to touch each other's bodies, tell each other what feels enjoyable, and relax without feeling pressure to have sex. The third stage is to touch the genital areas, though the ban on intercourse remains. After that stage, the couple progress to 'vaginal containment', which means penetration without movement, and then to intercourse including movement within the vagina.

Counselling

The graduated behavioural programme usually takes several months, and while the couple are proceeding through it they attend regularly for counselling. The counsellor may help the couple to reconsider their attitudes to sexual matters, and may discuss the feelings they have for sex and for each other. Counselling also involves permission-giving, education, reassurance, summing up feelings that the couple may not have recognized, and reinforcing positive aspects of the relationship.

Conclusion

Sexual problems cause much unhappiness and may present to any clinician. Some can be treated easily with simple advice; others need more prolonged specialist treatment. A few never respond to treatment. The main aim for a young doctor is to be able to discuss the subject comfortably. This is not easy, particularly when the patient is older than the doctor but still expects advice because the doctor has a medical degree. With sexual problems, more than with many aspects of medicine, the learning curve is long. When treatment is successful, however, patients are very grateful and it can be very gratifying to be able to help so much, merely by listening and talking to them.

Key points

- Sexual problems are important and history-taking requires considerable skill. The problems may present directly or in the guise of another condition or may be discovered coincidentally.

- Normal sexual response has five phases: desire (general sexual interest), arousal (which involves central and genital responses), orgasm, resolution and a refractory phase during which further arousal does not occur.

- Sexual response varies with age and with different phases of a relationship.

- Sex has several functions in addition to reproduction, e.g. the strengthening of the pair bond.

- Commonest male problems include erectile failure and premature ejaculation.

- Commonest female problems include loss of libido, orgasmic dysfunction and vaginismus.

- Causes of sexual dysfunction may be physical, medical or psychological. Psychological factors include predisposing factors (e.g. poor sex education or childhood abuse). Dysfunction is also more likely after childbirth, or if there has been infidelity, anxiety or poor communication.

- Treatment involves counselling and education, hormonal therapy, and relaxation exercises. Sometimes couple, group or psychotherapy is required.

Female genital infections

Introduction

Genital infections in females can be caused by sexually transmitted infections (STIs) such as *Chlamydia trachomatis* or human papillomavirus, or by infections such as bacterial vaginosis and *Candida albicans* which are not sexually transmitted. There has been a dramatic change in the pattern of infections over the past 30–40 years. In the UK there was a decline in syphilis following the end of the Second World War, and in gonorrhoea from the 1970s, until the 1990s. However, during this time there was an increase in chlamydia, herpes, wart virus and human immunodeficiency virus (HIV) infections. Since the mid-1990s the downward trend in the bacterial STIs has reversed, and viral STIs have continued to increase. Cases of asymptomatic HIV infection have risen by 24% in the past 10 years within the UK. Between 1995 and 1999 cases of chlamydia infection increased by 76%, gonorrhoea by 55% and infectious syphilis by 54%. These rises have been highest among women aged 15–19 years, and have continued despite advances in diagnosis and treatment. Among the factors believed responsible for the increases are changes in sexual behaviour, particularly the use of non-barrier contraceptives, the emergence of drug-resistant strains, symptomless carriers, a highly mobile population, lack of public education, and the reluctance of some patients to seek treatment.

The World Health Organization (WHO) estimated that in 1995 there were over 333 million cases of the four major curable STIs in adults aged 15–49 throughout the world. These were due to 12.2 million cases of syphilis, 62.2 million of gonorrhoea, 89.1 million of chlamydia and 167.2 million of trichomoniasis. It estimated that 90% of these infections were in developing countries. The WHO and Joint United Nations Programme on HIV/AIDS (UNAIDS) estimated that in 2001 40 million adults and children were living with HIV/AIDS worldwide, and that 20 million had already died. About 95% live in developing countries, with two-thirds estimated to be in Africa, and one-quarter in Asia.

Many of the STIs can cause long-term morbidity, particularly in females. Untreated, some infections can lead to infertility or cause miscarriage, premature birth, or infection of the newborn. Prompt diagnosis and appropriate management is crucial in reducing these complications. The infections likely to cause long-term morbidity are the sexually transmitted infections such as *Chlamydia trachomatis.* Unfortunately they are often

Gynaecology

asymptomatic until complications arise, so the greatest aid in the diagnosis of such infections is probably to suspect they may be present and test for them.

Certain demographic features increase the likelihood of someone having an STI. These are: age under 25 years; lack of barrier contraception use; being single, separated or divorced; and having an occupation involving staying away from home. Also women undergoing termination of pregnancy (TOP) and those with an infection such as genital warts are at increased risk of STIs. In reality these factors are surrogate markers of sexual activity and rates of partner change, which are what mainly determine the risk of transmission and acquisition of an STI. To be able to accurately assess someone's risk of having an STI, therefore, it is necessary to be able to take a good sexual history.

Sexual history

A woman who is complaining of genital symptoms expects to be asked questions related to this. She will not be offended as long as the questions are appropriate and asked in a sensitive and non-judgemental manner. Choice of words, appropriate facial expressions and body language in the questioner are extremely important. As many of the questions are personal, it is very important to consider where such histories are taken; they should only be taken in a situation where others cannot overhear the conversation. Remember that curtains on wards and in outpatient clinics are not soundproof and such a setting would be most inappropriate for taking a sexual history.

The history-taking should start by asking about the presenting complaint. The woman should be asked if she has any vaginal discharge, dysuria, vulval lumps or ulcers, or lower abdominal pain. Supplementary questions about these symptoms are given below. She should then be asked about her gynaecological history. The final part should be the sexual history in order to assess the risk of STIs. The questions that need to be asked are:

The woman's most recent sexual exposure:

- How long ago was it?
- Was this with a regular or casual partner?
- If a regular partner, how long has the relationship been?
- What kind of contraception/protection was used?
- If condoms were used, were they used consistently and properly, and have there been any recent breakages?
- Has the sexual partner got any genital symptoms?

The woman's previous sexual partner:

- How long ago is it since she had sex with a different partner? If within the past few months the same details as above need to be obtained.

- How many different partners have there been over the past few months?

Remember the sexual partners may not necessarily be of the opposite sex. If the woman has not volunteered the sex of her partner it is important that she is sensitively, but directly, asked this.

Supplementary questions about risk of exposure to HIV infection should also be asked:

- Has the woman ever injected drugs?
- Are any male partners known to be bisexual, injecting drug users, or from areas of the world with high HIV levels such as sub-Saharan Africa and Asia?

Examination for genital infections

Clinical symptoms are not helpful at indicating the site of infection, or in indicating which infection is likely to be present. Examination and microbiological testing should therefore be performed. It is again important to consider the setting in which an examination is performed. It should be in a private room and the woman should be provided with a gown to cover the areas not being examined. It is essential that all males have a chaperone when examining a woman's genital tract and it is good practice for females to also have a chaperone present. The procedure should be explained to the woman prior to the examination. Simple considerations, such as making sure the patient is in a comfortable position and warming the speculum, will usually result in a more cooperative patient. This will allow a thorough examination with properly taken swabs. Lubricant jelly should not be used on the speculum as this can inhibit the growth of some bacterial infections. The speculum should be lubricated by warm water.

The woman should be in the lithotomy position, and there should be a good light source behind the examiner. The following genital examination should be performed:

- Inspect the pubic hair and surrounding skin for pubic lice and any skin rashes.
- Palpate the inguinal region for lymphadenopathy.
- Inspect the labia majora and minora, clitoris, introitus, perineum and perianal area for warts, ulcers, erythema or excoriation.
- Inspect the urethral meatus and Skene's and Bartholin's glands for any discharge or swelling.
- Insert a bivalve speculum into the vagina.
- Inspect the vaginal walls for erythema, discharge, warts, ulcers.
- Inspect the cervix for discharge, erythema, contact bleeding, ulcers or raised lesions.
- Perform a bimanual pelvic examination to assess size and any tenderness of the uterus, cervical motion tenderness, adnexal tenderness or masses.

Taking swabs for genital infections

During the examination, specimens for microbiological tests should be obtained. It is important that swabs are performed adequately and that the specimen is placed in the appropriate culture or transport medium. For urethral and endocervical specimens cellular material needs to be obtained. To take a urethral specimen a fine swab should be gently inserted into the urethral opening. It should be rotated and then placed in the medium. For an endocervical sample the swab should be inserted about 1 cm into the endocervical canal and it should be rotated vigorously for several seconds and placed in the medium. To reduce costs on microbiological tests, the urethral and endocervical samples for gonorrhoea and chlamydia can both be placed in the same container and processed together.

In order to correctly diagnose a female genital infection the following should be performed:

- A urethral culture for gonorrhoea placed in Amies, Stuart's or similar transport medium.
- A first-pass urine sample for chlamydia DNA amplification testing, or if only enzyme immunoassay (EIA) is available, a urethral sample placed in the EIA kit container.
- Observe the vaginal discharge to see if it has the homogeneous, white appearance typical of bacterial vaginosis.
- Swab the lateral vaginal walls and the pool of discharge in the posterior fornix. Smear some of the discharge onto a glass slide and allow to air dry (for Gram staining by the laboratory for clue cells, pseudohyphae and spores). Place the swab in Amies, Stuart's or similar transport medium for *Candida* and *Trichomonas vaginalis* culture.
- Test the pH of the vaginal discharge either by touching the swab used to take the vaginal specimen onto narrow-range pH paper, or the paper can be pressed against the lateral vaginal walls with sponge holders. It is important that cervical secretions are avoided for this as cervical mucus has a pH of 7 and any contamination will give a falsely high reading.
- A vaginal amine whiff test by mixing a loop of vaginal discharge with 10% potassium hydroxide on a glass slide; smell the mixture immediately for the transient fishy odour.
- Any vaginal secretions should be wiped from the cervix.
- An endocervical culture for gonorrhoea placed in Amies, Stuart's or similar transport medium with the urethral swab.
- An endocervical sample for chlamydia DNA amplification testing or EIA if only that is available, placed with the urethral sample.
- A blood sample for syphilis serology

- A blood sample for hepatitis B testing if the woman or any of her sexual partners are from areas of high hepatitis B prevalence (e.g. sub-Sarahan Africa or Asia), followed by hepatitis B immunization if the test is negative.
- A blood sample for hepatitis B and C testing if the woman or any of her sexual partners have ever injected drugs, followed by hepatitis B immunization if the test is negative.
- A blood sample for HIV testing if the patient gives informed consent.
- If vesicles, ulcers or fissures are seen, a sample for herpes culture should be taken from the base of the lesion and sent to the laboratory in viral transport medium.

Symptoms associated with genital infections

None

Unfortunately many of the more serious infections may cause no symptoms in females. About 80% of women with chlamydia, 50% with gonorrhoea, 65% with pelvic inflammatory disease (PID), 30% with genital warts, and 50% with genital herpes have no symptoms. In such circumstances, the only way to detect these infections is by examining and testing for them.

Vaginal discharge

An increase in vaginal discharge may be due to a number of infective and non-infective conditions (Table 18.1). The physiological discharge can only be diagnosed after negative swabs have excluded the infective causes.

Questions that help discriminate between the various causes are:

- Does the discharge have an offensive odour?
- Is there any vulval itching or soreness?
- Are there any other symptoms such as dysuria, intermenstrual or postcoital bleeding, abdominal pain?

Table 18.1
Causes of vaginal discharge

Vaginal infections	Bacterial vaginosis
	Candida albicans
	Trichomonas vaginalis
Cervical infections	*Chlamydia trachomatis*
	Neisseria gonorrhoeae
Physiological discharge	Cervical ectopy
Other causes	Retained tampon
	Retained products of conception

Table 18.2
Causes of dysuria

Acute bacterial cystitis	Coliform bacteria *Staphylococcus saprophyticus*
Urethritis	*Chlamydia trachomatis* *Neisseria gonorrhoeae*
Vulvitis	Genital herpes Candida infection *Trichomonas vaginalis* Vulval dermatological conditions

Dysuria

Dysuria is usually due to acute bacterial cystitis, urethritis or vulvitis (Table 18.2).

Questions that help distinguish between the causes are:

- Is the dysuria external, i.e. is it as the urine comes into contact with the vulval mucosa?
- Is there any urinary frequency, nocturia, or haematuria?
- Is there any vaginal discharge, postcoital or intermenstrual bleeding or abdominal pain?
- Are there any vulval sores or itching?

Vulval lumps

Raised lesions on the vulva can be due to infections, or anatomical variants. Genital warts are by far the most common cause of vulval lumps (Table 18.3).

Questions that help distinguish between the causes are:

- Are the lumps painful?
- How many are there?
- How long have they been present?
- Are there any other symptoms such as dysuria, intermenstrual or postcoital bleeding, abdominal pain?

Table 18.3
Causes of vulval lumps

Viral infections	Genital warts Molluscum contagiosum Vulval intraepithelial neoplasia and vulval cancer
Bacterial infections	Syphilitic condylomata lata Skene's or Bartholin abscesses due to *Chlamydia trachomatis* or *Neisseria gonorrhoeae*
Anatomical variants	Sebaceous glands Vulval papillae
Other	Sebaceous cysts

Table 18.4
Vulval ulcers – types

Infective	Genital herpes Syphilis
Non-infective	Aphthous ulcers Behçet's syndrome

Vulval ulcers

Infective lesions are the most common cause of vulval ulcers, with genital herpes being the main infection in the UK (Table 18.4).

Questions that help distinguish between the causes are:

- Are the ulcers painful?
- How many are there?
- How long have they been present?
- Are there any other symptoms such as dysuria, intermenstrual or postcoital bleeding, abdominal pain?

Lower abdominal pain

Lower abdominal pain can be caused by a number of differing conditions (Table 18.5). Infective causes are particularly common in young (under 25 years) sexually active women.

Questions that help distinguish between the causes are:

- Is there any vaginal discharge, postcoital or intermenstrual bleeding or deep dyspareunia?
- When was her LMP, what contraception has she been using, and is there any possibility of her being pregnant?
- Has she any dysuria, urinary frequency, nocturia or haematuria?

Table 18.5

Causes of lower abdominal pain

Uterus	Endometritis due to *Chlamydia trachomatis*, *Neisseria gonorrhoeae* or bacterial vaginosis Endometriosis
Fallopian tubes	Salpingitis due to *Chlamydia trachomatis* and/or *Neisseria gonorrhoeae* Ectopic pregnancy
Ovary	Torsion of, or haemorrhage into, an ovarian cyst
Urinary tract	Cystitis
Bowel	Acute appendicitis Irritable bowel syndrome

- Has she any nausea, vomiting, diarrhoea or constipation?

Specific infections

Chlamydia trachomatis

Background information

- *C. trachomatis* is the most frequently seen bacterial STI, affecting at least 3–5% of sexually active women in the UK, and as many as 14% of those aged under 20 years.
- It can cause infertility, so is considered to be a serious public health issue.
- Screening for, and treating, asymptomatic chlamydia reduces the rate of pelvic inflammatory disease.

Symptoms and signs

- The cervix is the primary site of infection, but the urethra is also infected in about 50%.
- Approximately 80% of women with chlamydia are asymptomatic.
- If symptoms are present they are usually non-specific such as increased vaginal discharge and dysuria.
- Lower abdominal pain and intermenstrual bleeding may be present if the infection has spread beyond the cervix.
- On examination there may be mucopurulent cervicitis (Fig. 18.1) and/or contact bleeding (Fig. 18.2), but the cervix may also look normal.

Diagnosis

- Enzyme immunoassay (EIA) is the most commonly used method of diagnosis at present. This has low

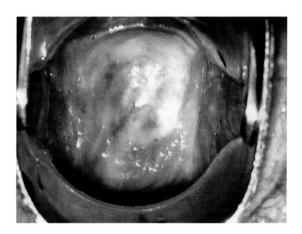

Fig. 18.1 **Mucopurulent cervicitis.** This may be a feature of infection with *C. trachomatis*. The cervix, however, can look normal.

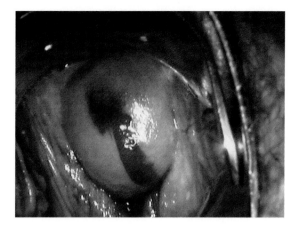

Fig. 18.2 **Contact bleeding.** This can occur for a number of reasons, one of which is *C. trachomatis* infection.

sensitivity of only 60–70%, so if it is used it is important to recognize that a significant number of infected women may be missed.
- Detection rates can be increased to over 90% by using a DNA amplification test such as the polymerase chain reaction (PCR).

Treatment and management

- Uncomplicated chlamydia infection can be treated with:
  - doxycycline 100 mg twice daily for 1 week, or
  - azithromycin 1 g as a single dose.
- Pregnant and lactating women can be treated with:
  - erythromycin 500 mg twice daily for 14 days.
- Patients should abstain from sex until they and their partner(s) have completed treatment. Partner notification (contact tracing) is an essential part of management to prevent reinfection.
- All patients should be seen after treatment to check that medication has been completed, that there has been sexual abstinence, and that the partner(s) has been treated. If all of these have occurred, test of cure is not necessary, unless erythromycin has been prescribed (as it has a lower cure rate).

Complications

- *C. trachomatis* can spread beyond the lower genital tract causing Skene's and Bartholin's gland abscesses, endometritis, salpingitis, and perihepatitis. It may therefore lead to tubal damage, predisposing to tubal pregnancies and tubal infertility.
- At least 8–10% of women with chlamydia develop symptomatic ascending infection, but the figure overall is higher as some women have asymptomatic upper genital tract infection.

- In pregnancy it can cause miscarriage, preterm birth, postpartum infection and neonatal infection.
- In genetically susceptible people reactive arthritis can occur (Reiter's syndrome).
- It increases a woman's risk of acquiring HIV infection three- to fourfold.
- Recent studies have linked chlamydia infection and cervical cancer.

Neisseria gonorrhoeae
Background information

- Gonococcal infections are less common than chlamydial, but there has been a rise in cases in women aged 15–19 years over the past few years.
- It is sexually acquired in adults.

Symptoms and signs

- The cervix is the primary site of infection, but the urethra is also infected in 70–90%.
- About 50% of women with gonorrhoea have no symptoms.
- The most common symptoms are increased vaginal discharge, dysuria, and postcoital bleeding.
- Lower abdominal pain and intermenstrual bleeding may also be present if the infection has spread beyond the cervix.
- On examination there may be a purulent (Fig. 18.3) or mucopurulent cervicitis and/or contact bleeding, but again the cervix may look normal.

Diagnosis

Culture of *N. gonorrhoeae* is the main method of diagnosis.

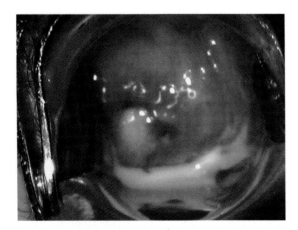

Fig. 18.3 **Purulent cervicitis.** The cervix is the primary site of infection in 90% of cases of gonococcal infection, and a purulent discharge may be seen.

Treatment and management

- Uncomplicated gonorrhoea can be treated with:
  - ciprofloxacin 500 mg single oral dose, or
  - ofloxacin 400 mg single oral dose, or
  - ampicillin 3 g plus probenecid 1 g single oral dose (if the antibiotic sensitivity confirms susceptibility to penicillin), or
  - ceftriaxone 250 mg i.m. single dose.
- Pregnant and lactating women can be treated with:
  - ceftriaxone 250 mg i.m. single dose, or
  - cefotaxime 500 mg i.m. single dose, or
  - ampicillin 3 g orally plus probenecid 1 g (if the antibiotic sensitivity confirms susceptibility to penicillin).
- About 40% of females with gonorrhoea also have *Chlamydia trachomatis* infection, so they should be tested for and/or treated for chlamydial infection.
- Patients should abstain from sex until they and their partner(s) have completed treatment. Partner notification (contact tracing) is an essential part of management to prevent reinfection.
- All patients should be seen after treatment to check that medication has been completed, that there has been sexual abstinence, and that the partner(s) has been treated and to repeat the swabs to check the infection has cleared.

Complications

- *N. gonorrhoeae* can spread beyond the lower genital tract causing Skene's, and Bartholin's gland abscesses, endometritis, salpingitis, and perihepatitis.
- Consequently it can cause tubal pregnancies and tubal infertility.
- About 10–20% of women with acute gonococcal infection will develop salpingitis.
- In pregnancy it can cause miscarriage, preterm birth, postpartum infection and neonatal infection.
- Rarely gonococcal septicaemia can occur and present as an acute arthritis/dermatitis syndrome (disseminated gonococcal infection).
- It increases a woman's risk of acquiring HIV infection four- to fivefold.

Pelvic inflammatory disease (PID)
Background information

- PID results when infections ascend from the cervix or vagina into the upper genital tract. It includes endometritis, salpingitis, tubo-ovarian abscess and pelvic peritonitis.
- The main causes are *C. trachomatis* and *N. gonorrhoeae*, but *Mycoplasma hominis* and anaerobes are frequently also found. Sometimes in women

with laparoscopically proven PID no bacterial cause is found.

- Cases of chlamydial PID reported from STI clinics within the UK doubled between 1995 and 1999, being most common in women under 25 years.
- The true incidence is unknown because about two-thirds of cases are asymptomatic.

Symptoms and signs

- Clinical symptoms and signs vary from none to very severe.
- The onset of symptoms often occurs in the first part of the menstrual cycle.
- Women with chlamydial PID usually have clinically milder disease than women with gonococcal PID.
- Lower abdominal pain is the most common symptom, with increased vaginal discharge, irregular bleeding, deep dyspareunia and dysuria also present in some women.
- The cervix may have a mucopurulent discharge with contact bleeding, indicative of cervicitis.
- Adnexal and cervical motion tenderness on bimanual examination is the most common sign, but pyrexia and a palpable adnexal mass may also be present.

Diagnosis

- No specific symptoms, signs or laboratory tests are diagnostic of PID. Non-specific tests of inflammation such as the ESR, white cell count and acute phase reactants may be raised.
- Laparoscopy, with microbiological specimens from the upper and lower genital tract, is considered the 'gold standard' for diagnosis, but this is not always available in clinical practice.
- The diagnosis is often made on clinical findings (presence of lower abdominal pain, increased vaginal discharge, cervical motion and adnexal tenderness on bimanual examination) and swabs taken only from the lower genital tract. The advantages are that this is quicker, cheaper, and non-invasive, unlike laparoscopy, but it is less accurate with specificity of only 65–70%.
- Clinical symptoms and signs do not accurately predict the extent of tubal disease found at laparoscopy.
- A pregnancy test should be performed on all women suspected of having PID, to exclude the rare possibility of an ectopic pregnancy.

Treatment and management

- The woman should be admitted if there is diagnostic uncertainty, severe symptoms or signs, or failure to respond to oral therapy.

- Prompt diagnosis and early treatment reduce the risk of tubal damage, so empirical treatment should be started before microbiology results are known.
- The antibiotic regimen should cover the main bacterial causes and take into account local sensitivity patterns.
- Intravenous therapy for the first few days is recommended in women with severe clinical disease.
- Recommended regimens are:
  - cefoxitin 2 g i.v. three times daily plus doxycycline 100 mg (i.v. or oral) twice daily plus metronidazole 400 mg (i.v. or oral) twice daily for 14 days, or
  - ofloxacin 400 mg (i.v. or oral) twice daily plus metronidazole 400 mg (i.v. or oral) for 14 days, or
  - ceftriaxone 250 mg i.m. single dose, or cefoxitin 2 g i.m. single dose with probenecid 1 g single oral dose plus doxycycline 100 mg (i.v. or oral) twice daily plus metronidazole 400 mg (i.v. or oral) twice daily for 14 days.
- Appropriate analgesia should be given.
- Patients should abstain from sex until they and their partner(s) have completed treatment. Partner notification (contact tracing) is an essential part of management to prevent reinfection.
- Women with moderate or severe clinical findings should be reviewed after 2–3 days to ensure they are improving. Lack of response to treatment requires further investigation, intravenous therapy and/or surgical intervention.
- All patients should be seen after treatment to check their clinical response, and that medication has been completed, that there has been sexual abstinence, and that the partner(s) has been treated. Repeat testing of initially positive swabs is recommended.

Complications

- The main complications from PID are due to tubal damage.
- Tubal infertility occurs in 10–12% of women after one episode of PID, 20–30% after two episodes, and 50–60% after three or more episodes. Increasing severity of infection also increases the risk of tubal infertility.
- The risk of ectopic pregnancy is increased six- to tenfold, with higher rates in women with several episodes, and increasing severity, of PID.
- Abdominal or pelvic pain for longer than 6 months occurs in 18% of women. The severity is related to the number of episodes of PID and the extent of pelvic adhesions. Women with a past history of PID are five to ten times more likely to need hospital admission and hysterectomy.
- About a third of women have repeated infections. This may be due to relapse of infection because of

inadequate treatment, reinfection from an untreated partner, post-infection tubal damage, or further acquisition of STIs.

- In 5–15% of women with salpingitis, the infection spreads from the pelvis to the liver capsule causing perihepatitis (Fitz-Hugh–Curtis syndrome).

Bacterial vaginosis (BV)
Background information

- BV is due to an overgrowth of anaerobic bacteria, genital mycoplasmas and *Gardnerella vaginalis* (all of which can be present in small numbers in the vagina).
- It is not sexually acquired, so sexual partners do not need to be treated.
- It is the most common cause of vaginal discharge in women of reproductive age.
- It is found in 9% of women in general practice, in 15% of pregnant women, and 20–25% of women undergoing termination of pregnancy.

Symptoms and signs

- About 50% of women with BV are asymptomatic.
- If symptoms are present they are mainly increased vaginal discharge and fishy odour. The odour is often worse after sexual intercourse and during menstruation.
- On examination the discharge is milky white and adherent to the vaginal walls, and may be frothy (Fig. 18.4). There is no inflammation of the vulva or vagina.

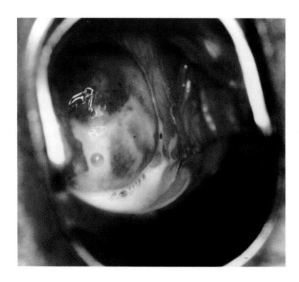

Fig. 18.4 **Bacterial vaginosis.** BV is due to an overgrowth of anaerobic bacteria, genital mycoplasmas and *Gardnerella vaginalis*. The discharge is milky white, adherent to the vaginal walls, and may be frothy.

Diagnosis

- A clinical diagnosis of BV can be made using Amsel's criteria. Three of the following should be present: the typical thin homogeneous discharge on examination; vaginal pH greater than 4.5; amine odour after adding 10% potassium hydroxide to the vaginal fluid (the whiff test); clue cells on microscopy (at least 20% of all epithelial cells). These are epithelial cells covered with bacteria that are 'clues' to the diagnosis. Menses, semen, and infection with *T. vaginalis* can also give a raised pH and positive amine test.
- A Gram-stained vaginal smear has good sensitivity and specificity for the diagnosis of BV.
- Culture of vaginal secretions has no place in the diagnosis of BV. 30–50% of women are colonized with *G. vaginalis*, anaerobes and mycoplasmas, as part of their normal vaginal flora.

Treatment and management

- Treatment is recommended in all women with symptoms, those undergoing gynaecological surgery (including TOP), and pregnant women with a previous preterm birth.
- Recommended treatments are:
  - metronidazole 400 mg orally twice daily for 5–7 days
  - metronidazole 2 g orally single dose
  - metronidazole 0.75% vaginal gel, 5 g daily for 5 days
  - clindamycin 2% vaginal cream, 5 g daily for 7 days.

Complications

- BV increases vaginal cuff cellulitis following hysterectomy, postpartum endometritis following caesarean section and post-abortal pelvic inflammatory disease (PID) after surgical termination of pregnancy.
- In pregnancy it may increase the risk of late miscarriage and preterm birth.
- It increases a woman's risk of acquiring HIV infection two- to threefold.

Candida infections
Background information

- 75% of all women get at least one episode of symptomatic candida in their lifetime.
- About 20% of asymptomatic women have vaginal colonization with candida. Increased rates of colonization (30–40%) are found in pregnancy and uncontrolled diabetes.

- Recognized predisposing factors that are associated with symptomatic candida are pregnancy, diabetes, immunosuppression, antimicrobial therapy, and vulval irritation/trauma.
- It is not sexually acquired, so sexual partners do not need to be treated.

Symptoms and signs

- The most common symptom is vulval itching, which is present in nearly all symptomatic women. Thick, white vaginal discharge, vulval burning, external dysuria, and superficial dyspareunia may also be present.
- On examination vulval erythema, fissuring and oedema may be present. There may be the typical white plaques on the vaginal walls (Fig. 18.5), but the discharge may be minimal.

Diagnosis

Culture is the most sensitive method of diagnosis.

Treatment and management

There are a number of effective intravaginal and oral antifungal agents available such as:

- Topical treatments:
  - clotrimazole pessaries for 1, 3, or 6 nights
  - econazole pessaries for 1 or 3 nights
  - miconazole pessaries for 1 or 14 nights.
- Oral treatments (should not be used during pregnancy):
  - fluconazole 150 mg single dose
  - itraconazole 200 mg twice daily for 1 day.

Complications

There are no known long-term complications from candida infections.

Trichomonas vaginalis (TV)
Background information

- TV is relatively rare in the UK, but in other parts of the world, e.g. Africa and Asia, it remains a major cause of vaginal discharge.
- It is sexually transmitted and only infects the urogenital tract.

Symptoms and signs

- It may be asymptomatic in 10–50% of women.
- The most common symptom is vaginal discharge, with a malodour. There may also be vulval pruritus, external dysuria and dyspareunia.
- On examination there may be vulval erythema and excoriation, and the purulent discharge may be visible on the vulva. The vaginal mucosa is often inflamed, with a yellow or grey discharge.

Diagnosis

Culture is the most sensitive method of diagnosis.

Treatment and management

- The recommended treatment is:
  - metronidazole 2 g single oral dose.
- 30% of women with TV have gonorrhoea and/or chlamydia, so they should be tested for other STIs.
- Patients should abstain from sex until they and their partner(s) have completed treatment. Partner notification (contact tracing) is an essential part of management to prevent reinfection.

Complications

- TV in pregnancy is associated with low birth weight and preterm delivery.
- TV increases a woman's risk of acquiring HIV infection.

Genital warts
Background information

- Genital warts are painless, benign, epithelial tumours caused by human papillomavirus (HPV) types 6 and 11.
- They are highly infectious; two-thirds of sexual partners will develop warts.

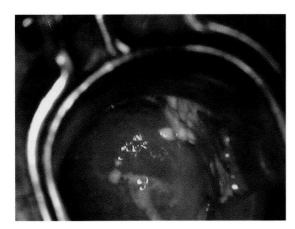

Fig. 18.5 **Candida infection.** Although candida may present with these 'typical' white plaques, the discharge is sometimes minimal.

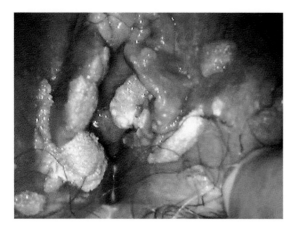

Fig. 18.6 **Flesh-coloured papules characteristic of warts.** They may be single, but are usually multiple, and can spread onto the labia, perineum, and perianal area.

- They have a long incubation period; on average 3 months, but can extend to years.
- They are the commonest viral STI in the UK.
- A cohort study of women in the USA reported an incidence of 0.8% per annum.

Symptoms and signs

- Genital warts are painless, so in women they may be asymptomatic.
- If symptomatic it is usual that the woman has felt the vulval lumps.
- On examination the flesh-coloured papules can be seen around the introital opening. They can spread onto the labia, perineum, and perianal area. They may be single but are usually multiple (Fig. 18.6).
- On the mucous membranes they are usually soft and cauliflower-like (condylomata acuminata).
- On the drier surfaces they are harder and keratinized.

Diagnosis

- They are diagnosed by their clinical appearances.
- Atypical lesions should be biopsied, particularly in older women, as premalignant and malignant lesions can look similar.

Treatment and management

- No single treatment is suitable for all warts.
- Multiple, soft warts (condylomata acuminata) can be treated with podophyllotoxin solution or cream. It acts as a cytotoxic agent and is therefore contraindicated in pregnancy.
- Fewer, or keratinized warts, are better treated with an ablative therapy such as cryotherapy,

trichloroacetic acid, curettage or electrocautery. All of these can be used in pregnancy.
- Imiquimod cream works by stimulating local cell-mediated immunity resulting in clearance of the warts. It can be used on both soft and keratinized warts, but should also not be used in pregnancy.
- All treatments can have recurrence rates of up to 25%, because of residual subclinical viral infection.
- Women with genital warts often have more serious STIs such as chlamydia, and should be tested for other STIs.
- Sexual partners should be advised to be examined for genital warts and tested for other STIs.
- There is evidence that condoms reduce the spread of HPV so patients should be advised to use condoms until their warts have cleared.

Complications

- Complications from HPV 6 and 11 are rare.
- Vertical transmission can occur, but it is rare.
- HPV 6 and 11 are not associated with cervical cancer.
- The main morbidity of genital warts is psychological because of the length of time it may take for them to clear.

Genital herpes
Background information

- Genital herpes can be caused by herpes simplex virus (HSV) type 1 or 2.
- Cases have increased sixfold between 1972 and 1994 in the UK. HSV-2 antibodies are found in 7.6% of blood donors, but less than 50% give a clinical history of herpes, suggesting that many people have subclinical infection.
- Cases due to HSV type 1 are increasing, particularly in young women.
- It is initially an acute vesicular/ulcerating eruption, frequently followed by recurring lesions.
- HSV ascends the peripheral sensory nerves into the dorsal root ganglion where latent infection develops. This can reactivate, giving recurrent lesions. These are not always noticeable; asymptomatic, subclinical, viral shedding can occur. However, all of these reactivated episodes are potentially infectious.

Symptoms and signs
Primary infection

- This is the first-ever exposure to either HSV-1 or 2. It can cause vulval soreness and external dysuria, but it can also be asymptomatic. As the symptoms are non-specific it may be misdiagnosed as either a urinary tract infection or candida.

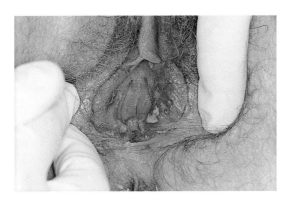

Fig. 18.7 **Primary herpes.** Multiple painful superficial ulcers are present.

- On examination there are multiple painful superficial ulcers (Fig. 18.7). Tender inguinal lymphadenopathy is also usually present.

Non-primary, first-episode genital herpes

This occurs in people with previous oro-labial HSV-1 who then acquire genital HSV-2 infection. There is some cross-protection from this prior infection, resulting in a milder illness than in primary infection. These non-primary infections are more likely to be asymptomatic than are primary infections.

Recurrent herpes

- These episodes may be asymptomatic (subclinical shedding). If symptoms are present they are usually milder than in first infections. They may be preceded by a prodrome of tingling, itching or pain in the area.
- On examination there are usually just a few ulcers confined to a small area.
- 90% of people with HSV-2 infection and 60% with HSV-1 will develop recurrences within the first year. The average number of recurrences is two per year but a few patients get more frequent recurrences. Long-term studies show that symptomatic recurrences gradually decrease with time.

Diagnosis

Viral culture for herpes simplex virus is the main method of diagnosis.

Treatment and management

Primary and first-episode genital herpes

- Antiviral drugs reduce the severity and duration of the symptoms. They do not prevent latency so have no effect on future recurrences.

- Recommended regimens are:
  - aciclovir 200 mg five times daily for 5 days
  - famciclovir 250 mg three times daily for 5 days
  - valaciclovir 500 mg twice daily for 5 days
  - aciclovir can be used in pregnancy and breast-feeding.
- Analgesia and saline bathing are recommended. Patients can be advised to pass urine in a bath of warm water, to ease external dysuria.
- Testing for other STIs should be performed, but this can wait until the vulval ulcers have healed, when it will be more comfortable to insert a vaginal speculum.
- The natural history of HSV infection should be explained, covering recurrences, subclinical viral shedding, the potential for sexual transmission and treatments that are available.

Recurrent genital herpes

- Recurrences are self-limiting and can often be managed with supportive therapy.
- When recurrences are infrequent but severe, episodic antiviral therapy, started early, will reduce the duration and severity of an attack, but will not reduce the number of recurrences. The patient should initiate this at home as soon as a recurrence is noticed.
- Episodic regimens are:
  - aciclovir 200 mg five times a day for 5 days
  - famciclovir 125 mg twice daily for 5 days
  - valaciclovir 500 mg twice daily for 5 days.
- Suppressive therapy can be used to reduce frequent recurrences, such as in those with more than six recurrences in a year.
- Suppressive treatment regimens are:
  - aciclovir 400 mg twice daily
  - famciclovir 250 mg twice daily
  - valaciclovir 500 mg once daily.
- This is usually prescribed for 6–12 months after which about 20% of patients will have fewer recurrences. It may be restarted if frequent recurrences persist.
- Patients should be advised to avoid sexual contact during the prodrome and recurrence, as this is when the risk of transmission is highest. It should be explained that there is a low risk of transmission even when they have no obvious recurrence, because of subclinical viral shedding. Condoms may reduce this risk.

Complications

- Women who acquire primary genital herpes during pregnancy, particularly in the third trimester, may transmit the infection to the baby at the time of delivery. The risk of perinatal transmission with recurrent HSV is low.

Gynaecology

- Genital herpes increases the acquisition and transmission of HIV two- to threefold.
- Many people with recurrent HSV infection develop psychological problems and fear rejection by sexual partners.
- Aseptic meningitis and autonomic neuropathy can occasionally occur with primary infection, even leading to urinary retention.
- Rarely the infection can disseminate, causing a life-threatening condition. This is more likely in the immunocompromised and in pregnancy.

Syphilis

Background information

- Before the mid-1990s, cases of infectious syphilis in women were so rare in the UK that the value of antenatal screening for syphilis was being questioned. Throughout the 1990s there were several outbreaks of infectious syphilis and some cases in women were only detected through antenatal screening.
- Syphilis is caused by the spirochaete, *Treponema pallidum*.
- It is sexually transmitted in adults.

Symptoms and signs

- Syphilis can be asymptomatic, and identified on screening serology such as in antenatal testing.
- There are several stages of symptomatic syphilis infection.
- *Primary syphilis.* About 3 weeks after exposure a chancre appears. This is usually a single, painless ulcer with rolled indurated edges, which usually goes unnoticed in women. Even without treatment it heals spontaneously. Syphilis serology may still be negative at this stage of infection.
- *Secondary syphilis.* After several weeks a generalized illness develops with fever, malaise, and skin and mucosal rashes. The rash is present on the trunk, limbs, palms and soles. Wart-like moist papules occur on the vulva (condylomata lata). Even if untreated, these symptoms and signs resolve after 3–12 weeks. Syphilis serology is strongly positive at this stage of infection.
- *Late syphilis.* Up to 40% of untreated patients will develop symptomatic late syphilis with neurosyphilis, cardiovascular syphilis or gummata.

Diagnosis

- Syphilis can be diagnosed by serological testing.
- The initial test is likely to be an enzyme immunoassay (EIA), but if positive the Venereal Disease Research Laboratory (VDRL) test or rapid plasma reagin (RPR) test, and *Treponema pallidum* haemagglutination (TPHA) test and fluorescent treponemal antibody absorption (FTA-abs) test should be performed.

Treatment and management

- The treatment of all stages of syphilis requires long courses of antibiotics, and long-term follow-up.
- This should be undertaken by a department of genitourinary medicine.

Complications

- Without adequate treatment, complications of late syphilis can occur.
- Syphilis in pregnancy can cause miscarriage and stillbirth, and can be transmitted to the infant, causing congenital syphilis.

Human immunodeficiency virus infection

Background information

- HIV infection can be transmitted by contact with body fluids (either sexually, or through needles or blood transfusion) and by vertical transmission from mother to baby.
- It was estimated that 33 500 people were living with HIV in the UK in 2000, but that 30% were unaware of their infection.
- Antenatal testing for HIV infection is now routinely performed in the UK.
- Without antiretroviral therapy there is progressive reduction in cell-mediated immune function, resulting in susceptibility to opportunistic infections (when the CD4 count drops below $200 \times 10^9/l$), after a median time of 10 years, and death.
- Antiretroviral therapy with three or more drugs has dramatically improved morbidity and mortality from HIV.

Symptoms and signs

- Most people with HIV infection have no symptoms in the first few years of infection.
- There may be a mild systemic illness with fever, malaise and rash at the time of seroconversion 6–12 weeks after infection. This is rarely recognized as being HIV related.
- As the immune function is starting to deteriorate infections such as oral candida, and herpes zoster may occur.
- Women with HIV infection get more frequent episodes of vaginal candida and HSV recurrences.

- Opportunistic infections and HIV-related malignancies can present in many different ways.

Diagnosis

- Serology for evidence of antibodies to HIV is the method of diagnosis.
- Patients should be aware that they are having an HIV test and should have given informed consent for it.

Treatment and management

- Patients should have their CD4 count (this measures cell-mediated immune function) and HIV viral load (this measures the level of viral replication) performed about every 3 months.
- No treatment is needed if the immune function is normal.
- Antiretroviral therapy with three or more drugs should be started when the CD4 count drops to between $250–350 \times 10^9/\mathrm{l}$.

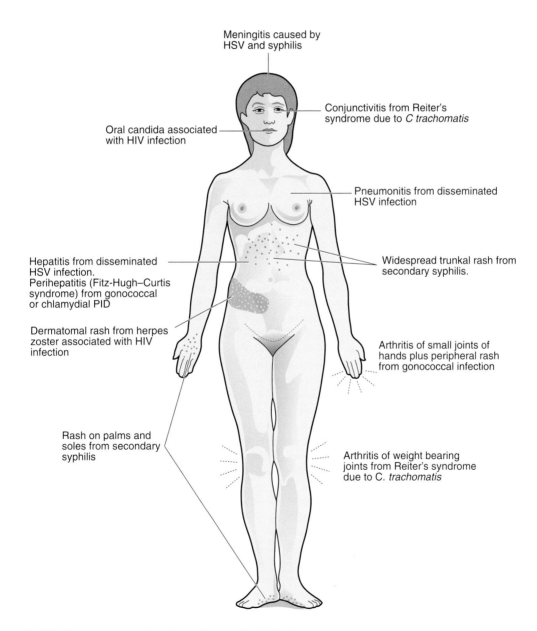

Meningitis caused by HSV and syphilis

Conjunctivitis from Reiter's syndrome due to *C trachomatis*

Oral candida associated with HIV infection

Pneumonitis from disseminated HSV infection

Hepatitis from disseminated HSV infection.
Perihepatitis (Fitz-Hugh–Curtis syndrome) from gonococcal or chlamydial PID

Widespread trunkal rash from secondary syphilis.

Dermatomal rash from herpes zoster associated with HIV infection

Arthritis of small joints of hands plus peripheral rash from gonococcal infection

Rash on palms and soles from secondary syphilis

Arthritis of weight bearing joints from Reiter's syndrome due to C. *trachomatis*

Fig. 18.8 **Systemic presentations of sexually transmitted infections.**

Gynaecology

- If the CD4 count is below $200 \times 10^9/l$ prophylaxis to *Pneumocystis carinii* pneumonia should be given.

Complications

- Without treatment there is increasing damage to the cell-mediated immunity, leading to susceptibility to opportunistic infections and eventually death.
- Treating the pregnant woman with triple antiretroviral therapy, delivery by caesarean section, and avoiding breast-feeding can reduce vertical transmission. Rates of transmission are now as low as 1–2%.

Systemic presentations of sexually transmitted infections

STIs do not always present with genital symptoms or signs. Many can cause systemic infections, which produce symptoms and signs in other systems of the body. HIV almost always presents in this way. It is not within the scope of this chapter to cover all the presentations of HIV-related opportunistic infections and malignancies, but the common early presentations are shown in Figure 18.8.

Key points

- Sexually transmitted infections in females are often asymptomatic. If symptoms or signs are present they are usually non-specific.

- High rates of STIs are found in sexually active women aged less than 20 years.

- Sexually transmitted infections often coexist; screen for other infections if one is diagnosed.

- The management of STIs, but particularly chlamydia, gonorrhoea and PID, includes treatment of the sexual partners and advice about abstinence from sex until the patient and partner(s) have completed treatment, in order to prevent reinfection.

19

Menorrhagia and dysmenorrhoea

Although heavy periods (menorrhagia) and painful periods (dysmenorrhoea) often occur together, they are considered here separately for clarity.

Menorrhagia

The mean menstrual blood loss in the healthy European population is approximately 40 ml with 70% lost in the first 48 hours. Menorrhagia is defined subjectively as heavy cyclical menstrual bleeding over several consecutive menstrual cycles. Objective menorrhagia, which occurs in around 10% of the population, is taken as menstrual blood loss in excess of 80 ml per month, and 60% of these develop anaemia. Menorrhagia is the most common cause of iron-deficiency anaemia in women in the developed world.

It is not surprising that menstrual problems are becoming more prevalent, since women experience more periods in their lifetime than did their predecessors 100 years ago (approximately 400 periods vs 40). This is because women have fewer children and breast-feed less. Menorrhagia is therefore a significant problem, and is one of the main reasons for which women seek medical advice in the UK. Only 50% of women who complain of excessive heavy bleeding, however, actually suffer from objective menorrhagia.

The medical and surgical treatment is also a significant burden to health-service resources. Menorrhagia is a common indication for hysterectomy, with 1 in 5 women in the UK having their uterus removed by the age of 55 years. In one-half of these cases, the uterus is pathologically normal. Although a commonly performed procedure, hysterectomy is a major surgical procedure and its use needs to be balanced against the potential associated mortality and morbidity.

Causes of menorrhagia

The causes are summarized in Table 19.1.

Table 19.1
The main causes of menorrhagia

Uterine pathology	Common
Dysfunctional uterine bleeding (DUB)	Very common
Medical disorders, including clotting defects	Very rare

Uterine pathology

Menorrhagia is associated with both benign pathology (e.g. uterine fibroids, endometrial polyps, adenomyosis, pelvic infection) and, more rarely, malignant pathology (e.g. endometrial cancer). Over half of those women with a menstrual blood loss more than 200 ml will have fibroids.

Endometrial polyps are common benign localized growths of the endometrium. They consist of a fibrous tissue core covered by columnar epithelium, and it is believed that they arise as a result of disordered cycles of apoptosis and regrowth of endometrium. Although their relationship to menorrhagia is unclear, it is likely that intrauterine endometrial polyps do increase the likelihood of heavy bleeding (Fig. 19.1). It is unlikely however that small endocervical polyps detected at the time of a routine cervical smear cause the same effect. Malignant change is considered to be rare.

Uterine fibroids (leiomyomas) are benign tumours of myometrium. They are well-circumscribed whorls of smooth muscle cells with collagen. They may be single or multiple and vary enormously in size from microscopic growths to tumours that weigh as much as 40 kg (Fig. 19.2). They are present in approximately 20% of women of reproductive age and many are asymptomatic. They are more common in women of Afro-Caribbean origin. When symptoms do occur, they are often related to the site and size of the fibroid. Submucosal fibroids project into the uterine cavity, intramural fibroids are contained within the wall of the uterus and subserosal fibroids project from the surface of the uterus. Cervical fibroids arise from the cervix (Fig. 19.3). Common presenting symptoms are menstrual dysfunction, infertility, miscarriage, dyspareunia or pelvic discomfort. The mechanism by which fibroids adversely affect reproduction is unclear, but may be related to distortion of the uterine cavity affecting implantation or due to fibroids causing disturbance of

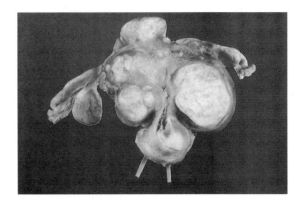

Fig. 19.2 **Pathology specimen showing multiple uterine fibroids.**

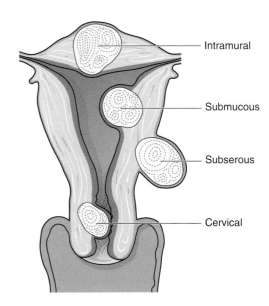

Fig. 19.3 **Sites of fibroids throughout the uterus.**

uterine blood flow. Fibroids may also present because of pressure effects on surrounding organs, such as frequency of micturition as a result of pressure on the bladder, or even hydronephrosis due to ureteric compression. Growth of fibroids is mediated by sex steroids, particularly oestrogen, and they therefore grow during pregnancy and shrink after the menopause. Occasionally during pregnancy, necrosis of the fibroid ('red degeneration') leads to acute abdominal pain. The incidence of malignant change (leiomyosarcoma) in fibroids is considered to be extremely low (0.1%).

Dysfunctional uterine bleeding (DUB)

DUB is said to be the cause for menorrhagia in the absence of recognizable pelvic pathology, complications of pregnancy or systemic disease. It is thus a diagnosis of exclusion. Some clinicians further classify DUB as

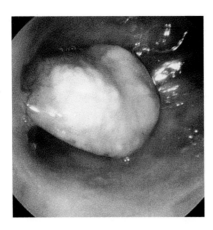

Fig. 19.1 **Hysteroscopic view of intrauterine polyp.** (Courtesy of Karl Storz Endoscopy (UK) Ltd.)

'anovulatory DUB' or 'ovulatory DUB', although clinically this is not an important distinction as treatment is the same in both cases. Ovulatory DUB may be used to refer to excessive ovulatory or 'idiopathic' bleeding whereas anovulatory DUB may be used to refer to bleeding associated with anovulatory cycles. In a normal ovulatory cycle, bleeding occurs in response to withdrawal of progesterone. In the absence of progesterone, oestrogen is able to act unopposed on the endometrium resulting in uncontrolled proliferation. Eventually, bleeding will occur because the endometrial height cannot be sustained by continuing levels of oestrogen. This 'anovulatory' bleeding is classically irregular and painless, whereas 'ovulatory' bleeding is regular and associated with cramping pain. It is possible that a lack of specific factors, perhaps prostaglandins (which are normally synthesized in response to progesterone), may account for the painless nature of anovulatory bleeding. Anovulatory DUB commonly occurs around the extremes of reproductive life (menarche and menopause). The definition of DUB is understood to include both ovulatory and anovulatory bleeding.

Medical disorders and clotting defects

Very rarely, menorrhagia is associated with such medical problems as thyroid disease (both hypo- and hyperthyroidism), hepatic disease and renal disease (although the majority of those with end-stage renal failure are amenorrhoeic).

Certain coagulation abnormalities (e.g. von Willebrand's disease) and platelet defects (e.g. thrombocytopenia) are associated with an increased risk of menorrhagia. There also seems to be an occasional association between menorrhagia and those on heparin and warfarin treatment.

Assessment of menorrhagia

History

The number of sanitary towels used, duration of bleeding, or passage of clots has been shown to have little or no correlation with actual blood lost. However, complaints of 'flooding' (leakage of heavy blood loss onto clothing) or having to use 'double sanitary protection' (pad and tampon) to prevent leakage of blood onto clothes are indicative of heavy menstrual loss. Similarly, severity of bleeding can be assessed by determining the impact it has on the individuals' quality of life. It is important therefore, to ask about the degree of disability experienced, such as time lost from work, or becoming housebound during menses owing to fear of social embarrassment from an episode of flooding in public.

The patient should also be questioned about symptoms suggestive of anaemia. A history of irregular bleeding, dyspareunia, pelvic pain, intermenstrual or postcoital bleeding may raise the suspicion of underlying pathology. A history suggestive of systemic disease such as thyroid disorder or a clotting abnormality would signal that further investigation for such causes would be required. The patient should also be questioned about risk factors for endometrial cancer such as use of unopposed oestrogen, tamoxifen use, polycystic ovary syndrome and family history of endometrial or colon cancer. It is also important to establish if the patient has a history of thromboembolism, as many medical treatments for menorrhagia are hormonal and thus their use may be contraindicated.

Examination

The patient should be examined for signs suggestive of anaemia. An abdominal, bimanual and speculum examination should be performed. An enlarged bulky uterus suggests uterine fibroids, and tenderness suggests endometriosis, pelvic inflammatory disease or adenomyosis.

Investigations

Full blood count to exclude anaemia, with iron supplementation offered if required. Thyroid function tests and tests of coagulation should only be performed if there are features suggestive of this in the history. No other endocrine tests are necessary.

Ultrasound   A pelvic ultrasound scan should be performed if history or examination suggests structural uterine pathology, or if it is not possible to assess the uterus clinically because of obesity. The site and size of abnormalities such as fibroids can be determined, together with assessment of the ovaries (Fig. 19.4).

Endometrial assessment should be performed in all women > 40 years, or younger women with persistent menorrhagia, irregular bleeding, or for whom there are risk factors for endometrial cancer. This can take the form of an endometrial biopsy or a hysteroscopy, both of which can be carried out either as an outpatient or inpatient (Fig. 19.5 and p. 267).

A cervical smear should be taken if one is due, or if the cervix looks clinically suspicious.

Treatment of causes of menorrhagia

Focal uterine pathology

Benign intrauterine polyps may be removed under general anaesthetic by polypectomy or using hysteroscopic techniques such as laser or resection. If malignant pathology is detected, then this should be treated as appropriate.

Fibroids may be treated medically or surgically.

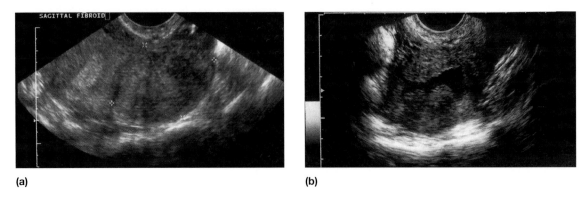

(a)   **(b)**

Fig. 19.4 **Uterine fibroids. (a)** A large intramural fibroid. **(b)** Two submucous fibroids projecting into the cavity of the uterus, which contains a small amount of fluid (saline infusion ultrasound scan).

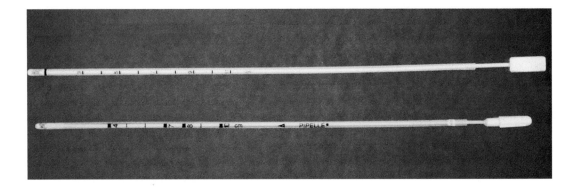

Fig. 19.5 **Two varieties of endometrial samplers.**

Medical

Unfortunately the symptoms caused by fibroids respond poorly to medical treatments such as those used in the treatment of DUB (see below). Since growth of fibroids is hormone dependent, gonadotrophin-releasing hormone (GnRH) analogues (which result in hypo-oestrogenism) may be used to cause fibroid shrinkage. GnRH analogues are derivatives of natural GnRH, but peptide substitutions give the agonists greater potency and longer activity. Depot injection of the GnRH analogue, however, leads to pituitary downregulation with hypo-oestrogenism, as the constant level of GnRH masks the natural pulsatile levels. Fibroids shrink by approximately 50% over 3 months of treatment but regrowth occurs on cessation of treatment. During treatment, hypo-oestrogenism can result in symptoms such as hot flushes and also bone loss. In view of concern about osteoporosis, use of GnRH analogues is limited to short-term use (< 6 months). For longer treatment periods, additional hormone replacement therapy ('add-back') is required to minimize the risk of osteoporosis.

Surgical

Hysteroscopic resection of small submucous fibroids may be possible. Some studies have suggested that this can lead to improved fertility and relief of menstrual problems.

If a patient wishes to conserve her fertility then myomectomy is an option. This involves incision of the pseudocapsule of the fibroid, enucleation of the bulk of the tumour and closure of the resulting defect. The operation is usually performed as an open abdominal procedure, although some use laparoscopic techniques. Myomectomy is associated with a similar degree of morbidity to that of hysterectomy. There is a risk of haemorrhage (due to the vascularity of fibroids) and the small possibility that an emergency hysterectomy may need to be performed during surgery to arrest uncontrollable bleeding. Furthermore there is a risk of adhesion formation which could compromise fertility (as a result of tubal obstruction) and the possibility that residual seedling fibroids may grow and lead to recurrence of fibroids. GnRH agonists may be used preoperatively to shrink the fibroids, with associated decreased blood loss. However, agonists can change the consistency of the fibroids and thus render it more difficult to separate them from the surrounding myometrium.

Uterine artery embolization, performed by interventional radiologists, is a relatively new technique. It involves interruption of the blood supply to the fibroid by blocking the uterine arteries with coils or foam de-livered through a catheter placed in the femoral artery. The healthy myometrium revascularizes immediately, owing to the development of collateral circulations from vaginal and ovarian vessels. Fibroids, however, do not appear to revascularize and shrink by about 50%, a reduction which appears to be sustained. Pain following occlusion of the vessels is often severe and usually requires opiate analgesia. Potential complica-tions include infection, fibroid expulsion, and the effects of exposure of the ovaries to ionizing radiation. Deaths, though rare, have occurred. This treatment is not currently recommended for women wishing to preserve their fertility.

If childbearing is complete and the patient is expe-riencing severe symptoms as a result of her fibroids, then hysterectomy may be considered (see below).

Dysfunctional uterine bleeding

In the vast majority of cases, no specific cause is found and the diagnosis is, by definition, DUB. The following treatments may be considered.

Medical treatment

Prostaglandin synthesis inhibitors   Non-steroidal anti-inflammatory drugs (NSAIDs) reduce menstrual blood loss by around 25%, possibly by reducing endometrial prostaglandin concentrations. The NSAID most com-monly used for treatment of menorrhagia is mefenamic acid, although side-effects include gastrointestinal complaints, dizziness and headache. These drugs are also of benefit for treating dysmenorrhoea.

Antifibrinolytics such as tranexamic acid work by inhibiting plasminogen activator, thereby reducing the fibrinolytic activity, which has been shown to be greater in women with menorrhagia. This increases clot forma-tion in the spiral arterioles and reduces menstrual loss. Tranexamic acid, if taken during menses, can reduce blood loss by around 50%. Gastrointestinal side-effects, nausea and tinnitus can occur. The drug should not be taken by women who are predisposed to thromboembolism.

The combined oral contraceptive pill reduces blood loss by approximately 50%. Its mechanism for doing so is thought to be due to suppressive effects on the endo-metrium. There is no age restriction on use of the combined oral contraceptive in women at low risk (see p. 153).

Systemic progestogens   Administration of the oral progestogen norethisterone (5 mg three times per day) from day 5 of the menstrual cycle for 21 days has been shown to reduce menstrual blood loss by 80%.

The mechanism of action is thought to be by inhibition of ovulation and by direct suppression of the endo-metrium. If the depot injectable progestogen (medroxy-progesterone acetate) is administered for long enough, amenorrhoea can result. During initial months of use, however, bleeding can be unpredictable and heavy. Side-effects of progestogens include nausea, bloating, headache, breast tenderness, weight gain and acne.

Intrauterine progestogens   The levonorgestrel intra-uterine system (LNG-IUS; i.e. the Mirena) delivers progestogen directly to the uterus (Fig. 19.6). It is a highly effective reversible method of contraception and can stay in place for up to 5 years. After 12 months, menstrual blood loss is reduced by around 95%. The main problem with the LNG-IUS is the high incidence of irregular bleeding, particularly within the first 3–6 months after insertion.

GnRH analogues   Amenorrhoea occurs as a result of pituitary downregulation and thus inhibition of ovarian activity. Women may experience problems, however, associated with the resultant hypo-oestrogenism – particularly hot flushes and vaginal dryness. With pro-longed use (> 6 months), there is also the likelihood of loss of bone mineral density. GnRH analogues are thus usually reserved for short-term use only.

Danazol   This is a synthetic androgen with anti-oestrogenic and antiprogestogenic activity. It inhibits pituitary gonadotrophins and has a direct suppressive effect on the endometrium. It was originally introduced for the treatment of endometriosis but causes a signifi-cant reduction in menstrual blood loss. A high incidence of adverse androgenic effects, however, particularly hirsutism, acne, weight gain and breast atrophy, have limited its use.

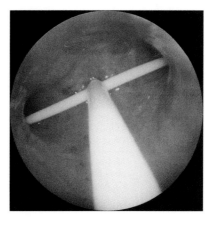

Fig. 19.6 **An intrauterine progestogen-releasing system in the uterus.** (Courtesy of Karl Storz Endoscopy (UK) Ltd.)

Surgical treatment

Endometrial ablation Using a number of different techniques it is possible to destroy most or all of the endometrium, thereby lessening menstrual flow or even occasionally stopping it altogether. Since endometrium regenerates from the basal layer it is essential to ablate to the endo–myometrial border. Endometrial ablation offers a safer method of symptom control, much shorter hospital stay, and shorter recovery period than hysterectomy. Some techniques involve a hysteroscopic procedure under general anaesthesia during which the endometrium is treated under direct visualization. The endometrium may be destroyed by laser ablation (with an Nd-YAG laser), resected (using a cutting loop 'resectoscope') or electrically coagulated using an electric roller-ball. Non-hysteroscopic procedures include ablation with a heated balloon, electrocautery and destruction through microwave energy (Fig. 19.7). These latter procedures may carry fewer risks than the hysteroscopic resections and some can be performed under local anaesthesia.

The success rates of the different ablative techniques are similar. Ablation is successful at relieving the majority of symptoms in 80% of cases. In 20% of these cases there is amenorrhoea but, for the rest, lighter menstrual flow is the norm. In the unsuccessful cases, it may be worth considering a repeat procedure. Complications are rare but include uterine perforation, hyponatraemia (as a consequence of excessive absorption of irrigation fluid), haemorrhage and infection. Pregnancy is contraindicated after an ablation procedure.

Hysterectomy This is the only treatment that will guarantee amenorrhoea and it can be performed by the abdominal or vaginal route. Abdominal hysterectomy involves a laparotomy incision, which is either trans-

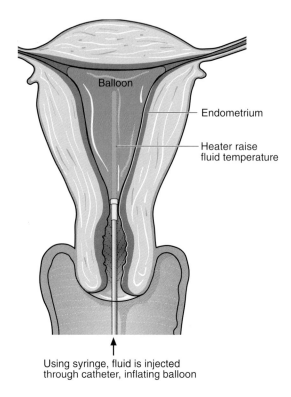

Fig. 19.7 **A thermal balloon.**

verse or longitudinal. A vaginal hysterectomy involves an incision through the vaginal wall. The choice between the two procedures depends on the size of the uterus, the degree of uterine descent, the wish to remove the ovaries (difficult by the vaginal route), and the skills and preferences of the surgeon (Table 19.2). Complications of hysterectomy include haemorrhage, bowel trauma, damage to the urinary tract, infection,

Table 19.2
Pros and cons of different hysterectomy methods

	Pros	Cons
Total abdominal hysterectomy (TAH)	Cervix is removed, therefore no further smears or risk of cervical malignancy (particularly suitable for those with a history of abnormal cytology) Good access to ovaries	Increased surgical morbidity Conservation of the cervix may be associated with better sexual function
Subtotal abdominal hysterectomy	Fewer complications than TAH (↓bleeding, ↓infection, ↓bladder injury, ↓ureteric damage) Good access to ovaries	Risk of cervical cancer remains as before

Vaginal hysterectomy	May be lower incidence of bladder and bowel injury in straightforward cases (compared to abdominal hysterectomy)
	 No potentially painful abdominal wound
		There is only limited ovarian access
		 Is contraindicated with:
		    Large uterus
		    Restricted uterine mobility
		    Limited vaginal space
		    Adnexal pathology
		    Cervix flush with vagina

postoperative thromboembolism and risk of vaginal prolapse in later years. The complication rate for abdominal hysterectomy may be greater than for vaginal hysterectomy. In addition, women having a vaginal procedure recover more quickly from the operation and are able to go home sooner.

For women with DUB, who are undergoing an abdominal hysterectomy and who have a history of normal cervical cytology, there is the choice of having a 'subtotal' hysterectomy. This involves removing the body of the uterus but leaving the cervix in situ. The advantages of a subtotal compared to a 'total' hysterectomy are that the operation is quicker, with less risk of damage to structures surrounding the cervix (bowel and urinary tract) (Fig. 19.8). There are also reported but unproven advantages of less disruption to bowel, bladder and sexual functioning postoperatively. If the cervix is left, the surgeon must be careful to remove any residual endometrium in the cervical canal at the time of surgery. This is to minimize the small risk that menses would continue from the small amount of endometrium

in the canal. The disadvantages of a subtotal hysterectomy are that the woman must continue to have her regular cervical smear tests. The risk of cervical cancer arising in the stump of cervix is extremely small (< 0.1%) providing that cervical cytology had been normal prior to the operation.

Whether to remove ovaries at abdominal hysterectomy depend on the patient's wishes, her age, her family history of breast or ovarian carcinoma and her plans for HRT. In someone who is 50 years old, it is unlikely that there will be much further ovarian function (average age of menopause 51), and bilateral salpingo-oophorectomy will significantly reduce the incidence of later ovarian carcinoma. Residual ovaries may also occasionally cause chronic pain or dyspareunia if adherent to the posterior fornix. In someone who is 40, however, a further 10 years of ovarian oestrogen secretion may be expected. It is unclear whether HRT is as effective in terms of long-term prophylaxis as endogenous oestrogens. It may therefore be appropriate to discuss routine oophorectomy in those over 45 and ovarian conservation in those under 45. The decision must remain, however, a very individualized consideration.

Medical disorders and clotting defects

In these cases, referral should be made to the appropriate physician/haematologist to institute further investigation and treatment of the underlying condition.

Dysmenorrhoea

Excessive menstrual pain (dysmenorrhoea) is a significant clinical problem. It is characteristically a cramping lower abdominal pain, which may radiate to the lower back and legs and may be associated with gastrointestinal symptoms or malaise. It has been estimated that dysmenorrhoea affects 30–50% of menstruating women. It is also one of the most frequent causes of absenteeism from school and of days off work. As with menorrhagia, dysmenorrhoea may be idiopathic (primary dysmenorrhoea) or due to pelvic pathology (secondary dysmenorrhoea).

Primary dysmenorrhoea

This generally begins with the onset of ovulatory cycles, typically within the first 2 years of the menarche. Pain is usually most severe on the day of menstruation or the day preceding this. There is good evidence that prostaglandins are involved in the aetiology. Studies have shown that there are higher concentrations of PGE_2 and $PGF_{2\alpha}$ in the menstrual fluid of women who suffer from dysmenorrhoea. $PGF_{2\alpha}$ increases the contractility of the myometrium and can lead to the dysmenorrhoea pain.

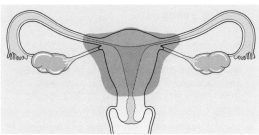

a) Subtotal hysterectomy

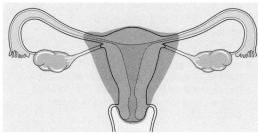

b) Total hysterectomy

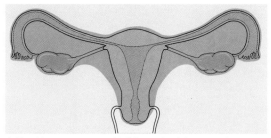

c) Total hysterectomy with bilateral salpingo-oophorectomy

Fig. 19.8 **Types of hysterectomy. (a)** Subtotal. **(b)** Total. **(c)** Total with bilateral salpingo-oophorectomy.

Gynaecology

Management of primary dysmenorrhoea

Pelvic examination may not be helpful in primary dysmenorrhoea (although this is essential for secondary dysmenorrhoea). Discussion and reassurance are an essential part of the management. Often the pain may be exacerbated by fear that there is a serious underlying disorder, and reassurance may lessen the symptoms. If dysmenorrhoea is unresponsive to standard medical therapy (see below), then consideration should be given to the possibility of underlying pathology and appropriate investigation instituted.

Treatment

Prostaglandin synthesis inhibitors   NSAIDs reduce the uterine production of $PGF_{2\alpha}$ and thus dysmenorrhoea. Most NSAIDs have been shown to be effective treatments, but mefenamic acid or ibuprofen are preferred in view of their favourable efficacy and safety profiles.

Combined oral contraceptive pill Suppression of ovulation with the combined contraceptive pill is highly effective in reducing the severity of dysmenorrhoea.

Depot progestogens   The injectable progestogen-only contraceptive suppresses ovulation and thus may be a useful treatment in alleviating dysmenorrhoea.

Levonorgestrel intrauterine system (LNG-IUS)   In addition to reducing menstrual blood loss, the LNG-IUS is effective at reducing dysmenorrhoea. Insertion of the device may, however, be difficult in those who have not been pregnant.

Secondary dysmenorrhoea

This is, by definition, associated with pelvic pathology. It usually has its onset many years after the menarche. Common associated pathologies are endometriosis, adenomyosis, pelvic infection and fibroids. It may also be associated with the presence of an intrauterine contraceptive device. In contrast, however, the LNG-IUS is associated with reduced dysmenorrhoea.

Management of secondary dysmenorrhoea

Women who have no other complaints but dysmenorrhoea and who have no abnormalities on abdominal, pelvic or speculum examination, may be safely treated without further investigation. Swabs from the genital tract, however, are helpful to exclude active pelvic infection particularly *Chlamydia trachomatis*. If pelvic masses such as fibroids are suspected then a pelvic ultrasound may be helpful. A laparoscopy is indicated if endometriosis or pelvic inflammatory disease is suspected, or for those women in whom standard medical therapy has been ineffective.

Treatment of secondary dysmenorrhoea

Treatment is dependent on the underlying pathology.

Key points

- Menorrhagia (heavy periods) can be classified as being related to structural uterine pathology (e.g. fibroids) or as dysfunctional uterine bleeding (DUB), i.e. no identifiable structural cause. Very rarely, menorrhagia may be secondary to some specific medical disorders, including clotting defects.

- Medical treatment for DUB includes prostaglandin synthesis inhibitors, antifibrinolytics, the combined contraceptive pill, systemic progestogens, intrauterine progestogens, GnRH analogues and danazol. Endometrial ablation and hysterectomy are the two surgical options.

- Dysmenorrhoea may be idiopathic (primary dysmenorrhoea) or due to pelvic pathology (secondary dysmenorrhoea). Treatment is with prostaglandin synthesis inhibitors, the combined contraceptive pill, and depot or intrauterine progestogens.

20

Pelvic pain

Introduction

Physiological pelvic pain with menstruation or childbirth is almost universal, but many women will present with pelvic pain for other reasons. This is most commonly acute pelvic pain – for example with appendicitis, a miscarriage or an ectopic pregnancy – but the pain may also be chronic, lasting for months or years.

With acute pain there is usually a well-defined pathological cause which either resolves spontaneously or can be effectively treated. Chronic pain, on the other hand, can be a more challenging problem. There may be no identifiable cause despite extensive investigations, and treatment can therefore be more difficult to plan.

In this chapter, pelvic pain is considered under the two headings of 'acute' and 'chronic' (Boxes 20.1 and 20.2), although it is important to note that there is significant overlap between the two groups. Although

---

Box 20.1

CAUSES OF ACUTE PELVIC PAIN

Gynaecological
- Ectopic pregnancy
- Miscarriage
- Acute pelvic infection
- Ovarian cysts

Gastrointestinal
- Appendicitis
- Constipation
- Diverticular disease
- Irritable bowel syndrome

Urinary tract
- Urinary tract infection
- Calculus

Other causes
- Musculoskeletal

Box 20.2

CAUSES OF CHRONIC PELVIC PAIN

Gynaecological
- Endometriosis
- Adenomyosis
- Chronic pelvic infection
- Ovarian cysts

Gastrointestinal
- Adhesions
- Appendicitis
- Constipation
- Diverticular disease
- Irritable bowel syndrome

Urinary tract
- Urinary tract infection
- Calculus

Other causes
- Musculoskeletal
- Degenerative joint disease
- Symphysalgia
- Low back pain
- Psychological

we will focus on the gynaecological causes of pelvic pain, the non-gynaecological causes are also important and it is for this reason that a multidisciplinary approach, particularly for those women with chronic pelvic pain, is important.

Pain

Pain is a subjective phenomenon. Many of the factors affecting pain are centrally mediated such that pelvic pain is often made worse by psychological, psychiatric or social distress. Unlike external organs such as the skin, which contains pain sensors, the organs within the peritoneal cavity (the viscera) are sensitive to inflammation, chemicals and stretching or distortion caused by specific stimuli, for example adhesions or gaseous distension. The sensitivity of different organs to varying stimuli is an important factor influencing pelvic pain: the cervix and uterus are relatively insensitive, for example, whereas the fallopian tubes are conversely exquisitely sensitive. Crushing of the bowel is associated with minimal discomfort whereas stretching and distension cause severe pain. Unlike cutaneous painful stimuli, localization of visceral pain is often very difficult.

History-taking and examination are centrally important to the diagnosis and management of all women with pelvic pain and these are dealt with first. Investigation and management of acute and chronic pain are then considered under separate subheadings, and finally there is a short section about clinical attitudes to chronic pelvic pain.

History

The history is arguably the most important factor in determining how quickly the diagnosis is reached and appropriate treatment instigated. The importance of this cannot be over-emphasized.

Gynaecological history-taking is described in Chapter 8. Particular attention should be given to the time of onset of the pain, the characteristics, radiation, duration, severity, exacerbating and relieving factors, cyclicity and analgesic requirements. Associated symptoms of gastrointestinal, urological or musculoskeletal origin should be sought. It is also important to take a detailed menstrual history, in particular the frequency and character of vaginal bleeding, any intermenstrual bleeding or vaginal discharge and their relationship to the pain. Ectopic pregnancy can occur without recognizable amenorrhoea.

A sexual history may be of help, particularly details of any superficial or deep dyspareunia, contraception and sexually transmitted infections. There may be a family history of gynaecological disorders, for example endometriosis or ovarian cancer. A smear history should be recorded with particular emphasis on any abnormal cytology.

With chronic pain, there is often value in detailing a family and social history including marital or relationship problems, pressure at work, financial worries and childhood or adolescent problems such as sexual abuse. Listening is a centrally important facet of the history-taking which may in itself be therapeutic for many women, particularly those with chronic pain. It is useful to ask some open-ended questions such as: 'What do you think the cause of your pain might be?' and 'How is the pain affecting your life?' to give the patient an opportunity to tell you about aspects of the problem which might not be apparent from a more systematic history.

Examination

Observation of the woman's general demeanour is important when assessing the severity of pain. Eye-witness accounts from other health professionals and friends or family may also be helpful. The temperature, pulse and blood pressure should be recorded.

Abdominal examination should include inspection for distension or masses, palpation for tenderness, rebound and guarding, and abdominal auscultation if gastrointestinal obstruction or ileus is suspected. Permission should then be sought to perform a gentle vaginal and rectal examination. Inspection of the vulva and vagina at speculum examination may reveal abnormal discharge (suggestive of infection) or bleeding. Following inspection of the cervix a high vaginal swab, endocervical swab and a cervical smear may be appropriate.

A bimanual examination may reveal uterine or adnexal enlargement suggestive of a pelvic mass, fibroids or an ovarian cyst. Cervical excitation (pain associated with gentle displacement of the cervix) is associated with ectopic pregnancy and pelvic infection. Tenderness or pain elicited by bimanual palpation of the pelvic organs themselves is suggestive of an on-going inflammatory process which may be infective (e.g. chlamydia) or non infective (e.g. endometriosis). A fixed immobile uterus suggests multiple adhesions from whatever cause and nodularity within the uterosacral ligaments (sometimes palpable only by combined rectovaginal examination) can be a feature of endometriosis.

Acute pelvic pain

There are many causes of acute pelvic pain, but the most important gynaecological conditions are ectopic pregnancy, miscarriage, pelvic inflammatory disease and torsion or rupture of ovarian cysts (Box 20.1). The history and examination should particularly include the date of the last period, the date of any pregnancy tests, and symptoms suggesting pelvic infections. If the patient is shocked on admission an immediate pregnancy test should be carried out to exclude ectopic pregnancy, with consideration given to an urgent laparotomy if the result is positive. If the test is positive and the patient is not shocked, an ultrasound scan will be helpful to decide between ectopic pregnancy and miscarriage. If the pregnancy test is negative a high vaginal swab, endocervical swab and full blood count should be checked looking for evidence of infection. An ultrasound scan is helpful in identifying ovarian cysts, but non-gynaecological causes of pain should not be forgotten in the rush to identify gynaecological pathology.

Whilst the results of investigations are awaited it is important to continue monitoring pulse, blood pressure and temperature, and to provide adequate analgesia. The patient and her family should be kept up to date with results, including a realistic estimate of when these results will be available. If the diagnosis is unclear and the pain is not resolving, a diagnostic laparoscopy may be warranted.

The management of ectopic pregnancy, miscarriage, pelvic inflammatory disease and ovarian cysts is discussed in the appropriate chapters. An innocent cause of pain not mentioned above is that experienced mid-cycle with ovulation – so-called 'mittelschmerz'. This pain is usually sudden in onset, can occasionally be quite severe and, if persistent each cycle, will respond to treatment with the combined oral contraceptive (which suppresses ovulation).

Effective communication and collaboration between specialists is fundamental in acute pelvic pain management, and an essential requirement if optimal care is to be provided.

Chronic pelvic pain

It is estimated that in the USA the healthcare costs associated with chronic pelvic pain are in excess of $2000 million per annum. These costs do not take into consideration the disability and suffering associated with this condition, and the loss of earnings to both the individual and employer. Chronic pelvic pain can lead to loss of employment, family and marital discord, divorce, medical misadventures and litigation.

The definition of chronic pelvic pain is somewhat arbitrary, but can be defined as pain persisting for at least 3 months continuously, or for 6 months intermittently (for example the cyclical pain of severe dysmenorrhoea or the recurrent pain of dyspareunia). To warrant the specific diagnosis of 'chronic pelvic pain syndrome', the pain should be severe enough to cause a functional disability, to require medical or surgical intervention, and to have an adverse effect upon the individual's (and often her family's) quality of life. A comparison between acute and chronic pelvic pain is shown in Table 20.1.

The management of chronic pelvic pain is particularly challenging as there are so many possible causes and contributory factors (Box 20.2). The importance of a careful history once again cannot be overestimated and, even if the patient has been seen by yourself or other clinicians previously, it can often be surprisingly useful to return to the history afresh. An association with dysmenorrhoea, dyspareunia, irregular menstruation, abnormal vaginal discharge and infertility may all be helpful in suggesting an underlying gynaecological

Table 20.1
Comparison of acute and chronic pelvic pain

Acute	Chronic
Well-defined onset	Ill-defined onset
Short duration	Unpredictable duration
Rest often helpful	Rest usually not helpful
Variable intensity	Persistent
Anxiety common	Depression common
Disease symptom	May not be possible to identify an underlying disease process

problem. Altered bowel habit, excess flatulence or flatus, constipation or diarrhoea, on the other hand, point to a gastrointestinal problem, particularly irritable bowel syndrome. Psychiatric, urological and musculoskeletal causes of chronic pain are further possibilities.

More than a third of women with chronic pelvic pain, however, do not have an identifiable biological cause despite extensive investigations. It is therefore important to plan which investigations are necessary, carry them out and then *call a halt to any further investigations if no pathology is identified*. In gynaecology, such investigation often involves a diagnostic laparoscopy. Further management then depends on whether a pathological cause has been identified or not, and this is considered below. Again there is some overlap between the two groups.

Identifiable pathological cause for the pain

Endometriosis

The commonest gynaecological cause of chronic pelvic pain is endometriosis (Ch. 21). Despite its recognized symptom complex the average time to diagnosis is around 7 years. Endometriosis is often associated with adenomyosis, but it is only possible to make the diagnosis of adenomyosis after pathological examination of the uterus post-hysterectomy.

GnRH (gonadotrophin-releasing hormone) analogue therapy is one of the most effective and commonly used pharmacological interventions for endometriosis, but the associated menopausal symptoms may exacerbate any depression. Vaginal dryness may also exacerbate dyspareunia. These symptoms are usually very much less if hormone replacement therapy (HRT) is given at the same time (so-called 'add-back' therapy). As endometriosis and adenomyosis are difficult to treat effectively long term, a high proportion of women will ultimately request a hysterectomy, often at a relatively young age. Although this gives a 95% chance of cure, it will result in a premature surgical menopause if a bilateral salpingo-oophorectomy is carried out at the same time.

When managing patients with endometriosis it is easy to focus on the treatment of the disease itself and forget to consider the psychosocial consequences. Many of these women become depressed as a consequence of the pelvic pain and the ineffectiveness or inadequacy of treatment options. Antidepressant therapy is often required in addition to the specific hormonal or surgical interventions. Further, the dyspareunia may affect the patient's sexual relationship culminating in marital disharmony, particularly if the partner is unaware of the nature of the problem.

Pelvic infection

Chronic pelvic infection is associated with a high incidence of tubal damage, and consequently an increased incidence of ectopic pregnancy or infertility (Ch. 18). It may be due to relapse of infection because of inadequate treatment, reinfection from an untreated partner, post-infection tubal damage, or further acquisition of sexually transmitted infections. The severity of the problem is related to the number of episodes of pelvic inflammatory disease and the extent of pelvic adhesions. Women with a past history of pelvic inflammatory disease are five to ten times more likely to be admitted to hospital and to undergo hysterectomy than those without.

Ovarian cysts

The majority of ovarian cysts are benign, particularly those presenting with acute pain (Ch. 26). Pain may occur because of torsion, cyst rupture or bleeding occurring into a cyst. Management depends an the particular clinical situation.

Other causes

If investigations are negative and there remains significant diagnostic doubt about whether a pain is gynaecological or not, it may be worth considering a 3-month trial of ovarian suppression with a GnRH analogue or a progestogen. A dramatic reduction of symptoms following suppression with recurrence after treatment suggests a true gynaecological cause, including the possibility of adenomyosis, and there is evidence that hysterectomy will lead to long-term improvement in around three-quarters of this responding group. Many, however, may not wish or be suitable for such radical surgery, and others will be no better despite the suppression.

No identifiable pathological cause for the pain

Once again, it may be worth re-exploring the history from the beginning. This is an area of clinical medicine where communication skills are of paramount importance. Listening to the patient, asking 'open-ended' non-directional questions, ensuring adequate consultation time and building up a rapport to discover the concerns and priorities of the patient are centrally important when devising an investigation and treatment strategy for women with this condition. The issues that arise most frequently are the need to know the cause of the pain and the effect of the pain on quality of life, employment, relationships and fertility. A history of pelvic pain is associated with an increased incidence of psychosexual trauma either as a child or later in life.

Treating a patient with chronic pelvic pain without a specific diagnosis is particularly difficult because of the uncertainty for both the clinician and patient, and the problems that this then causes in choosing therapeutic interventions. The first step has to be that both the clinician and patient have to accept the 'chronic pelvic pain syndrome' as a disease entity in its own right and then devise strategies to relieve the physical, psychological and social distress that this causes.

Management options range from psychosocial, analgesia management, hormonal treatments and complementary therapies. Communication with the patient should include sharing of information, honest and realistic discussion of the pros and cons of various investigation and treatment options and the likelihood of there being a beneficial outcome. The patient must be centrally involved in all decisions and be given realistic expectations. It may also be helpful to involve a partner or friend in the decision-making process.

Encouragement to lead as normal a life as possible whilst investigation and treatment are instigated is also acknowledged to be very important in the likelihood of making a full recovery. This would include encouraging a return to work, increasing exercise, maintaining a healthy diet, avoiding the inappropriate use of analgesia and looking for alternatives to analgesia where possible. Complementary therapies such as reflexology, homeopathy and acupuncture may be helpful and should be encouraged if they are available and the patient is willing to pursue these alternatives.

A multidisciplinary team approach should ideally include expertise in gastroenterology, neurology, psychiatry and psychology. Specific psychological approaches to the management of chronic pelvic pain, with input from psychologists and liaison psychiatrists, may be helpful to many women. These approaches include behavioural therapy, cognitive behavioural therapy, group therapy and pharmacological therapy. Pharmacological therapy (e.g. antidepressants and anxiolytics) may be particularly valuable for those individuals who have become secondarily depressed as a consequence of their chronic pain. Amitriptyline is commonly used as it works both centrally as an antidepressant and peripherally to reduce the passage of painful nerve impulses to central receptors.

Clinical attitudes to chronic pelvic pain

One of the problems associated with chronic pelvic pain is that many clinicians become frustrated and sceptical when dealing with such patients. A natural response following extensive investigations is to say that they can find 'nothing wrong' and that the problem is being imagined. The likely response from the patient is one of anger and distress such that the 'doctor–patient' relationship breaks down.

Another approach adopted by some clinicians is to continue with further investigations, many of which are irrelevant and inappropriate, simply to placate the patient and to 'buy time' in the hope that the cause of the problem will resolve spontaneously. The investigations themselves may result in harm or distress, making things worse rather than better. Polypharmacy is another risk, starting with simple analgesics and gradually increasing to the use of opiates. This often leads to tolerance and addiction, and may ultimately make it more difficult for patients to rationalize and cope with their pain. The addition of hormonal therapies or antispasmodic treatments for irritable bowel syndrome, however, may be justifiable in some patients.

Finally there is the possibility that the patient may have an inappropriate surgical operation, particularly a hysterectomy and oophorectomy. Whilst this may be appropriate for women who have a clearly defined gynaecological cause for their chronic pain, or for those who respond well to ovarian suppression, it often proves unhelpful and may result in even greater morbidity, particularly for those who experience complications or become prematurely menopausal as a consequence of bilateral oophorectomy.

These 'medical misadventures' often result in distrust between the patient and clinician. Patients lose faith and appear to become uncooperative by failing to comply with the investigations or treatments ordered by the doctor, adding weight to the doctor's suspicion that there is not actually anything wrong with the patient, and that the pain is psychological in origin. The patient may then be referred from one doctor to another for second or third opinions and from department to department. Unsurprisingly, given these scenarios, litigation is becoming increasingly common and the healthcare and legal costs can be astronomical.

Gynaecology

Key points

- Acute and chronic pelvic pain have numerous, occasionally overlapping, causes (Boxes 20.1 and 20.2).

- In treating acute pelvic pain it is important to exclude ectopic pregnancy and miscarriage, and to consider acute pelvic infection and problems with ovarian cysts. There are also important non-gynaecological causes of acute pain, particularly appendicitis.

- While the commonest causes of chronic pelvic pain are endometriosis and chronic pelvic infection, over a third will have no identifiable pathology. It is important to call a halt to unnecessary investigations, accept the 'chronic pelvic pain syndrome' as a disease entity in its own right and then devise strategies to relieve the physical, psychological and social distress that this causes.

The risks of medical misadventure associated with chronic pelvic pain can be minimized by adopting a sympathetic and caring multidisciplinary approach, or by referral to healthcare professionals with a special interest and expertise in managing this condition.

21

Endometriosis

Introduction

Although endometriosis is a common condition, our knowledge about it is incomplete. Debate remains about its origins, pathological features, diagnosis, prognosis and treatment.

The term 'endometriosis' refers to tissue resembling the endometrium which is lying outside the endometrial cavity. It usually lies within the peritoneal cavity and predominantly in the pelvis, commonly on the uterosacral ligaments behind the uterus (Fig. 21.1). Rarely, it can also be found in distant sites such as the umbilicus, abdominal scars, perineal scars and even the pleural cavity and nasal mucosa. Like the true endometrium it responds to cyclical hormonal changes and it bleeds at menstruation. Such bleeding may cause problems.

'Adenomyosis' occurs when there is endometrial tissue within the myometrium of the uterus. This tissue may provoke fibrosis, leading to uterine enlargement and associated heavy menses. It is difficult to diagnose clinically and is usually only apparent retrospectively, with histological examination of the uterus after hysterectomy. It is commonly considered to be a separate entity from endometriosis, occurring in a different population and having a different aetiology.

Incidence

Endometriosis occurs in approximately 1–2% of women of reproductive age, but among infertile women the incidence may be 20 times greater. As it is oestrogen dependent, it is rare postmenopausally, but recurrence has been associated with the use of hormone replacement therapy.

Aetiology

The precise aetiology of endometriosis remains unclear, with no single explanation reliably explaining all its features.

Sampson's 'implantation' theory postulates that endometrial fragments flow retrogradely along the fallopian tube during menstruation, 'seeding' themselves on the pelvic peritoneum. In support of this theory is the fact that it is sometimes possible to see blood flowing from the fimbrial end of the fallopian tube if a

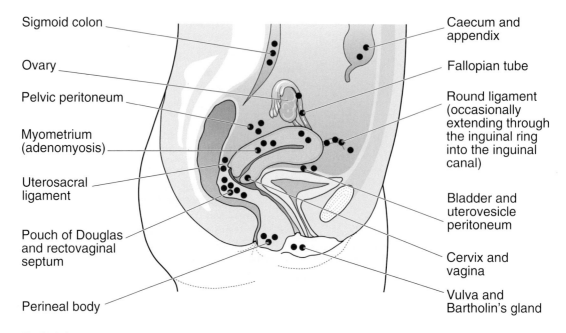

Fig. 21.1 **Common sites for endometriotic deposits in the pelvis.**

laparoscopy is carried out during menstruation. Seeding is also observed onto scars such as after hysterectomy, or on perineal scars after delivery and there is some animal research in which endometrial tissue has been surgically implanted directly onto the peritoneum.

This theory, however, cannot be the only mechanism of endometriosis formation as endometriosis has been reported in women with congenitally obstructed fallopian tubes. Meyer's 'coelomic metaplasia' theory proposes that cells of the original coelomic membrane transform to endometrial cells by metaplasia, possibly as a result of hormonal stimulation or inflammatory irritation. This could explain the presence of endometriosis in nearly all the distant sites, although it is also possible that spread from the uterus to these distant sites occurs by venous or lymphatic microembolism.

In some instances, the presence of endometriosis may be explained by neoplasia. This is particularly so in the ovary where a solitary ovarian endometrioma is sometimes included in the classification of ovarian neoplasia as the benign counterpart of endometrioid carcinoma.

The question remains as to why endometriosis becomes established in some, but not all, women and it is possible that there is some genetic or immunological predisposition to account for such wide variation.

Clinical presentation

In most instances, clinical presentation occurs because of pelvic disease. Endometriosis is the commonest

cause of secondary dysmenorrhoea. There is usually a continuous, non-spasmodic pain, which is worse immediately before and during the first day of the period, and colicky dysmenorrhoea may also occur in association with heavy menstrual loss and the passage of clots. In addition, there may be dyspareunia which may relate to endometriotic deposits in the pouch of Douglas or to ovarian endometriomata. Some patients also complain of continuous, lower abdominal pain that is not specifically related to their cycle or to sexual activity.

One of the puzzles regarding endometriosis is the lack of correlation between the severity of these symptoms and the extent of the disease. Extensive deposits leading to the obliteration of the pouch of Douglas and involving the ovaries, fallopian tubes and other pelvic organs, may be completely asymptomatic and, conversely, patients with lesions only a few millimetres across may be debilitated by pain.

Menstrual disturbances may be associated with endometriosis, and in particular with adenomyosis. Where there is also significant ovarian involvement, the menstrual cycle may become erratic. Rarely, postcoital bleeding is experienced in the presence of endometriosis involving the ectocervix, or where deposits in the pouch of Douglas penetrate into the posterior fornix.

Endometriosis in distant sites is rare but may generate local symptoms, such as cyclical epistaxes with nasal deposits, or catamenial pneumothoraces with pleural deposits. Monthly rectal bleeding may occur if the bowel mucosa is affected.

Examination

The clinical diagnosis of endometriosis is aided by findings of:

- thickened pelvic ligaments, particularly the uterosacral ligaments, which may be nodular like a 'string of beads'
- a fixed retroverted uterus
- uterine or ovarian enlargement if these organs are involved.

There may also be tenderness in the lateral and posterior fornices and with pressure on the uterosacral ligaments. Attempts to move the uterus may also provoke pain. This pain often resembles the presenting symptom, particularly when this was dyspareunia.

None of these features is pathognomonic of endometriosis and conversely their absence does not exclude the disease. There are many other causes of pelvic pain, including irritable bowel syndrome or recurrent urinary infection, which can confuse the differential diagnosis. In particular, chronic conditions such as pelvic inflammatory disease and pelvic venous congestion mimic many endometriotic features. Laparoscopy is therefore necessary to make the diagnosis.

Endometriosis and infertility

Endometriosis is not uncommonly diagnosed in women who are undergoing laparoscopic investigations for infertility, but who do not have specific symptoms. Although endometriosis and infertility are associated more commonly than can be explained by chance, the exact mechanism of their interrelationship is uncertain (Table 21.1).

While it is recognized that severe disease can cause infertility by forming periovarian and peritubular

Table 21.1
Possible mechanisms by which endometriosis may reduce fertility

System	Mechanism
Coital function	Dyspareunia, leading to reduced frequency of coitus
Sperm function	Inactivation of spermatozoa by antibodies Phagocytosis of spermatozoa by macrophages
Tubal function	Fimbrial damage Reduced tubal motility with prostaglandins
Ovarian function	Anovulation Luteinized unruptured follicle syndrome (LUFS) (see text) Luteolysis caused by prostaglandin $F_{2\alpha}$ Altered release of gonadotrophins

adhesions and by destroying ovarian tissue, the association between mild endometriosis and infertility is less clear. Theoretically, high prostaglandin output from endometriotic tissue could impede tubal motility, or the spermatozoa may be affected by adverse immunological factors.

Another possibility is that infertility caused by some unrelated factor may predispose to endometriosis simply because, in the absence of pregnancy and lactational amenorrhoea, there will have been more periods. Other theories suggest that both endometriosis and infertility are manifestations of a third problem. Pelvic inflammatory disease for example, even if too mild to cause tubal obstruction and observable tubal distortion, may cause endosalpingeal damage leading to infertility, and also predispose to endometrial implantation in the peritoneum.

A final explanation is an association with the luteinized unruptured follicle syndrome (LUFS) in which follicular development proceeds along apparently normal lines, but oocyte release does not occur. The follicular granulosa cells undergo luteal change as if ovulation had occurred. As endometriosis is more common in this condition, it has been proposed that failure to release follicular fluid mid-cycle may result in a preferential environment for endometriosis to become established.

Investigation

It is virtually impossible for a firm diagnosis to be reached on clinical grounds alone (with the very rare exception of cyclical symptoms associated with superficial lesions). Laparoscopy has therefore become the standard diagnostic method. Active endometriotic lesions are classically described as 'chocolate cysts' if large or 'burnt match heads' if small. Inactive lesions look like scars. The degree to which laparoscopic visualization alone may be adequate, however, has been questioned (see Box 21.1).

Little is known about the rate of progression of low-grade endometriosis, but a proportion of untreated patients may deteriorate over as little as 6 months. The prompt return of symptoms after treatment, seen in many patients, may represent re-extension of uneradicated residual disease.

It is impossible to guarantee a cure after treatment. Routine repeat laparoscopy after completion of treatment, therefore, has limited prognostic value and is probably best reserved for those patients with recurrent symptoms.

Management

Medical treatment is most useful for symptomatic relief, but is of no value for the treatment of endometriosis

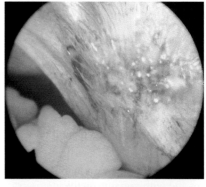

(a)

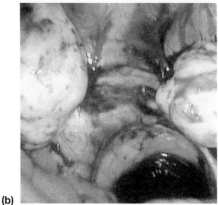

(b)

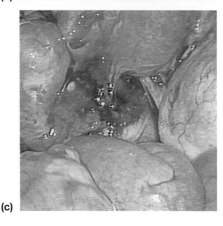

(c)

Box 21.1

LAPAROSCOPIC AND HISTOLOGICAL APPEARANCES

- Haemosiderin deposits covered with peritoneum resemble the classical appearance of endometriosis, but may arise from local haemorrhage of any origin. The typical chocolate-coloured cysts contained within the ovary, for example, need not be caused by endometriosis, and histological examination often shows that these have arisen from haemorrhage into a follicular or corpus luteum cyst.

- A wide range of subtle peritoneal changes, such as clear 'sago' blisters, glandular papillae, white opacified patches, red flame-like lesions and circular peritoneal defects may prove on biopsy to be a result of endometriosis (Fig. 21.2).

- Even more perplexing is the finding that normal peritoneum, when biopsied and studied with scanning electron microscopy, may contain cells of endometrial type. These may be more common in patients with proven disease elsewhere, but can also be found in apparently normal women.

- As many as 52% of patients with pelvic pain, but no visible peritoneal deposits of endometriosis, have been found on histological examination to harbour lesions deep in the uterosacral ligaments.

Fig. 21.2 **Peritoneal appearances of endometriosis.** Laparoscopic views show **(a)** clear blisters ('sago' granules), 'blood blisters', yellow brown patches, 'powder burns', atypical vascularity and telangiectasia; **(b)** bilateral endometriomas; **(c)** severe endometriosis with adhesions. (Parts (b) and (c) courtesy of Karl Storz Endoscopy (UK) Ltd.)

---

in patients wishing to conceive. Treatment is usually limited to between 3 and 6 months. Surgical treatment may be conservative, with laser or diathermy ablation, or radical, involving hysterectomy and oophorectomy.

Medical

All therapies suppress ovulation, and conception is therefore unlikely with good compliance. Nonetheless it is still advisable for patients to use barrier methods of contraception, unless using the combined oral contraceptive as their treatment method. To avoid inadvertent administration during pregnancy, all therapies should be initiated within the first 3 days of the start of a menstrual period.

For symptomatic endometriosis, continuous progestogen therapy (e.g. medroxyprogesterone acetate 10 mg t.i.d. for 90 days) is most cost-effective, has fewer side-effects and is more suitable for long-term use compared with more expensive alternatives. Progestogens have a direct action on the endometrial target tissue by binding to progestogen receptors. This produces decidualization of the endometrial tissue which then leads to subsequent necrosis. The combined oral contraceptive pill is also an appropriate alternative.

Second-line drugs are the gonadotrophin-releasing hormone (GnRH) analogues, which can be administered by nasal spray or implants (e.g. nafarelin, buserelin, goserelin or leuproelin acetate), and the orally administered androgen danazol. GnRH analogues bind to GnRH receptors in the pituitary, initially stimulating gonadotrophin release but rapidly desensitizing the pituitary to GnRH stimulation, thereby in turn suppressing gonadotrophin release and hence ovarian steroid secretion. The profound hypo-oestrogenic state produced not only affects endometrial tissue but causes side-effects mimicking the climacteric. Danazol combines androgenic activity with anti-oestrogenic and antiprogestogenic activity, and it inhibits pituitary gonadotrophins. It has a relatively high incidence of androgenic and perimenopausal side-effects.

Choice will depend on the side-effect profile; for example overweight women or those tending towards hirsutism would do better with a GnRH analogue. Underweight women or those particularly at risk of bone loss should be prescribed danazol. Danazol is unlikely to be satisfactory for women already experiencing weight gain or bloating with a progestogen or the combined oral contraceptive. Therapy for both should be restricted to 3–6 months.

Failure of symptom relief if amenorrhoea has been induced implies that the problem is unlikely to be due to endometriosis and is an indication for a review of the diagnosis. It is not necessary to achieve complete amenorrhoea if patients have a good symptomatic response, provided that spotting or bleeding is acceptable to the patient.

Surgical treatment

When continued fertility is required, conservative surgery is appropriate. This is usually carried out laparoscopically and includes diathermy destruction or laser vaporization of endometriosis deposits. It may bring about symptom relief and has a role in subfertile women (see below).

Hysterectomy with bilateral oophorectomy for women who have completed their childbearing is usually curative. Hormone replacement will be needed and, while this may activate residual disease, the possibility may be minimized by using some form of combined preparation rather than an oestrogen-only form.

Fertility treatment

There is no evidence that medical treatment of endometriosis is of any value in the management of subfertility. Surgical ablation of minimal and mild endometriosis does improve fertility, but whether surgery has a role in moderate and severe endometriosis is less clear. Surgical treatment of large ovarian endometriotic cysts probably enhances spontaneous pregnancy rates and will improve transvaginal access if IVF is considered. In cases of moderate and severe endometriosis, assisted reproduction techniques should be considered as an alternative to surgery, or following unsuccessful surgery.

Complications, prognosis and long-term sequelae

Depending upon the severity of the disease, adhesions and fibrosis may distort bowel, bladder, ureters and other neighbouring viscera, leading to chronic problems with these systems. The physical and psychological morbidity from long-term pain can be immense.

Key points

- Endometriosis is caused by endometrium-like tissue outside the uterine cavity. Endometrium-like tissue growing within the uterine wall is referred to as adenomyosis, and may be a different pathological entity.

- Endometriosis may be caused by the seeding of endometrial cells when menstrual fluid spills retrogradely along the fallopian tubes. Other possible aetiological mechanisms are coelomic metaplasia and venous or lymphatic spread.

- Clinical endometriosis affects 1–2% of women, but the incidence is higher among women with subfertility. Symptoms include secondary dysmenorrhoea, dyspareunia, lower abdominal pain and menorrhagia. There may be ovarian enlargement, thickening of uterosacral ligaments, fixed retroversion of the uterus and tenderness on pelvic examination.

- Diagnosis usually requires laparoscopy.

- Medical management is by progestogens, the combined oral contraceptive pill, danazol or GnRH analogues. Surgical management may involve laparoscopic laser ablation of deposits, open surgery with local resection, or hysterectomy with or without bilateral oophorectomy.

22

Premenstrual syndrome

Introduction

Premenstrual syndrome (PMS) can be defined as a regular pattern of symptoms occurring in the time before menstruation, with a lessening of symptoms soon after the start of bleeding. PMS is said to be severe if it impairs work, relationships, or usual activities. Some observers note that as many as 95% of women suffer mild symptoms, and between 5% and 10% of women have symptoms severe enough to disrupt their lives in the 2 weeks leading up to the start of menstruation.

Women's experiences of PMS are so varied that it is difficult to classify these symptoms into categories, and a precise diagnosis may therefore be difficult. Over 150 symptoms have been attributed to PMS, but particularly:

- abdominal bloatedness
- breast tenderness (cyclical mastalgia)
- headaches
- oedema
- mood changes.

Aetiology

The aetiology of PMS remains unknown. Many hypotheses have considered whether there might be abnormal levels of specific hormones, and research has focused on progesterone, oestrogen, adrenocortico-trophic hormone, vasopressin, luteinizing hormone, prolactin and thyroid-stimulating hormone. There is no consistent evidence that any of these are abnormal in PMS, but there are suggestions that it is the changing patterns of hormone levels, rather than the absolute levels, which is important. Other suggestions are that there may be an abnormality in levels of neuro-transmitter function, particularly serotonin, and this is discussed further under 'Management' below.

Clinical presentation

As there are no specific biochemical tests for PMS the diagnosis is dependent on a prospective charting of symptoms to confirm that there is a true exacerbation in the luteal phase when compared to the follicular phase of the cycle (Fig. 22.1). There are numerous specific criteria, many of them research tools which are not

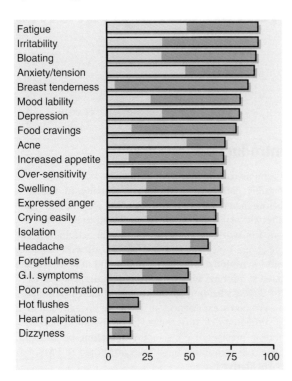

Fig. 22.1 **Incidence (percent of cycles) with which individual symptoms were reported in the follicular phase of the cycle (open bars) and luteal phase of the cycle (entire bars) in 170 women.** GI, gastrointestinal.

necessarily always applied strictly to clinical practice. An example of one of these is shown in Box 22.1.

Differential diagnosis

Symptoms that are worse other than premenstrually are not attributable to PMS. Other conditions, such as endometritis, migraine headaches, depression and anxiety disorders are exacerbated premenstrually, but again should not be confused with the more specific diagnosis of PMS. Perimenopausal mood changes are usually non-cyclical and consideration may be given to checking a serum follicle-stimulating hormone (FSH) level. A normal FSH level does not exclude the menopause, but the investigation may be of particular value in those who have had a hysterectomy with ovarian conservation.

The breast pain of PMS is usually cyclical, bilateral and poorly localized, and 'lumpiness' is common. By contrast, non-cyclical breast pain is precisely localized and rarely bilateral.

In those with abdominal swelling, it is important to consider intra-abdominal pathology such as ovarian cyst or ascites. The abdominal bloating of PMS is rapidly relieved by the onset of menstruation, perhaps owing to the relaxing effect of prostaglandins on smooth muscle or to comparative stasis of the gut in response to morphine-like endorphins. Hypothyroidism and anaemia should be considered in those complaining predominantly of tiredness.

Management

Women with mild PMS do not usually need medical treatment and may be helped by reassurance and counselling. General health measures such as improved diet, increased exercise, self-relaxation, and reducing smoking and drinking might be helpful. Some women find self-help groups supportive, while others choose yoga or hypnosis. Treatment can be aimed at the symptoms, or at a hypothesized underlying cause.

Symptomatic treatment

A number of symptomatic treatments are in use, although the evidence supporting their effectiveness is limited. Those with premenstrual bloatedness can be treated in the same way as those with irritable bowel syndrome, and those with oedema may respond to a diuretic. Breast tenderness can also be treated with diuretics, as well as with bromocriptine or low-dose danazol. Headaches may respond to simple analgesics or to treatments reserved for those with migraine. Mood changes are considered in more detail below.

Treatment aimed at the hypothesized underlying cause

A wide variety of medical treatments have been considered, many of which are still in current use. Close scrutiny, however, reveals that only a limited number of these are of proven value and the treatment modalities are classified this way in Box 22.2. The 'probably effective' group consists of treatments demonstrated to be effective by good-sized trials, usually randomized placebo-controlled trials. The use of a placebo arm is particularly important in PMS research, as most placebo treatments demonstrate symptom improvements of

---

Box 22.2

CLASSIFICATION OF POSSIBLE TREATMENTS FOR PMS BASED ON EFFECTIVENESS

Probably effective
- SSRIs
- Suppression of ovulation
- Oophorectomy

May be effective
- Diet
- Exercise
- Psychological approaches
- Vitamin B_6
- Complementary therapy

Probably not effective
- Progesterone
- Evening primrose oil
- Vitamin E

---

around 30%. Treatments classified as 'probably not effective' have also been examined in well-conducted studies, and no significant benefit has been demonstrated over placebo. The 'may be effective' group include therapies in which studies have been inconclusive, often because of small patient numbers. The three groups will be considered in more detail below.

Probably not effective

Progesterone or progestogens

The rationale for the use of progesterone or progestogens in the management of premenstrual syndrome is based on the unsubstantiated premise that there is a progesterone deficiency. The hypothesis is that, with insufficient progesterone, unopposed oestrogens cause water retention and some of the other reported symptoms. Although initial data suggest there to be abnormal concentrations of metabolites of progesterone (pregnenolone and allopregnenolone), there is no consistent evidence that low concentrations of progesterone are found in women with the premenstrual syndrome. Furthermore, randomized trials do not suggest any useful clinical benefit.

Evening primrose oil

The hypothesis is that there is a deficiency in essential fatty acids, particularly gamolenic acid, leading to low levels of prostaglandin E_1 and therefore premenstrual symptoms.

Evening primrose oil contains essential fatty acids, including gamolenic acid, and is available in many countries without a prescription. It is heavily promoted as an effective treatment for a range of conditions including PMS and it appears to have minimal side-effects. It is, however, an expensive treatment and trials demonstrate only very marginal, if any, clinical improvement in PMS symptoms.

Vitamin E

Vitamin E is advocated by some for the treatment of benign breast disease and, in those treated with vitamin E for breast problems, it has been noted that there is some improvement in premenstrual symptoms as well. Further studies looking at this association, however, have been unsupportive.

May be effective

Diet

The usual recommendations are for a reduction in salt, sugar, alcohol and caffeine, and an increase in carbohydrates. It is suggested that the increased carbohydrate intake increases serotonergic activity, which in turn improves symptoms. As the trials in this area are small it is difficult to draw firm conclusions.

Gynaecology

Exercise

Aerobic activity leads to increased endorphin levels which are recognized to improve mood, and several studies suggest there may be some benefit in the treatment of PMS.

Psychological approach

Techniques aimed at reducing stress may be beneficial. Cognitive behavioural therapy which encourages relaxation, and the use of 'coping skills', may also be helpful. Research studies, however, have involved only small numbers of patients and are inconclusive.

Vitamin B_6 (pyridoxine)

It has been suggested that treatment with pyridoxine, the active form of which is a co-enzyme in amino acid metabolism, may act by correcting some deficiency within the hypothalamus. Pyridoxine is particularly involved in the metabolism of dopamine and serotonin, low levels of which lead to high levels of prolactin and aldosterone, possibly explaining the fluid retention experienced in PMS. It may also account for some of the psychological symptoms attributable to alterations in neurotransmitter levels.

Vitamin B_6 is taken daily, and this can be on a continuous basis or simply during the second half of the menstrual cycle. While any conclusion about effectiveness is limited by the low quality of some of the trials, results suggest that it may be of some benefit in treating premenstrual symptoms and premenstrual depression.

Complementary therapy

Studies have explored the use of homeopathy, dietary supplementation, relaxation, massage, reflexology, chiropractic and biofeedback. While there were some positive findings, there is no compelling evidence to support any of these therapies.

Probably effective

Selective serotonin reuptake inhibitors

PMS presents with symptoms similar to those of anxiety and depression and this association has resulted in treatment with a variety of antidepressants. Clomipramine, a tricyclic inhibitor of serotonin and noradrenaline reuptake, is significantly more effective than placebo at symptom reduction.

Reduced platelet uptake of serotonin and reduced levels in the blood of women with PMS during the luteal phase have been used to infer a role for selective serotonin reuptake inhibitors (SSRIs) in PMS treatment.

Meta-analysis shows that SSRIs are effective, with around 60% of those with severe PMS reporting a reduction in physical and behavioural symptoms compared to around 30% of controls. This effectiveness is often apparent after only one or two cycles. Side-effects of insomnia, gastrointestinal disturbances and fatigue, however, are sometimes problematical but usually acceptable at the recommended low dose. Intermittent use in the luteal phase may be as effective as continuous daily dosing.

Ovarian suppression

The use of the combined oral contraceptive pill for the treatment of PMS is controversial. Some work suggests an improvement in symptoms, whereas other work suggests that those with PMS experience symptom exacerbation. Depot medroxyprogesterone may also be helpful.

Gonadotrophin-releasing hormone (GnRH) analogues are a highly effective way of suppressing ovarian function, and are therefore a highly effective treatment for severe refractory PMS. As oestrogen is suppressed to postmenopausal levels, however, the PMS symptoms may be replaced by menopausal ones including hot flushes. These in turn can be minimized with the use of continuous combined 'add-back' hormone replacement therapy. Treatment with GnRH analogues cannot be continued long term, however, because of the risks of osteoporosis and other side-effects associated with a premature menopause. GnRH analogues are also expensive.

Bilateral oophorectomy

This is also a highly effective treatment for PMS. It is, however, a surgical procedure and therefore not without significant short-term surgical risks, even if carried out laparoscopically. There are also the longer-term risks of premature menopause as with the GnRH analogues, particularly if compliance with subsequent HRT is poor. This surgical option is therefore only suitable for those very likely to benefit from it, as suggested by a definite response to a GnRH analogue, and only in those who have completed their family. It is also reasonable not to opt for this procedure if the natural menopause is likely to be occurring relatively soon, and also not to consider the operation in someone too young.

Individual management strategy

Given the large numbers of treatments advocated it can be difficult to find a practical way through them.

As PMS is usually a chronic condition, at least up until the menopause, it is important to consider the side-effect profile of treatments that may be used over many years. Once the diagnosis is clear, it seems sensible to try those treatments with no significant side-effects, initially diet, regular aerobic exercise and techniques aimed at stress reduction. A significant proportion of patients will benefit from these three tried together, and drug therapy can then be considered for those who are no better.

An SSRI is the most appropriate first-line drug, used initially for the second half of the cycle and then throughout the cycle if there is no improvement over the first two or three cycles. The next stage is ovarian suppression with a GnRH analogue. Successful symptom improvement, however, leaves a dilemma as continuous treatment is not appropriate for reasons of both side-effects and cost. Ongoing suppression with medroxyprogesterone acetate 3-monthly i.m. (which may be associated with significant side-effects), or surgical oophorectomy are the main subsequent options to be considered.

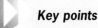

Key points

- Premenstrual syndrome (PMS) can be defined as a regular pattern of symptoms occurring in the time before menstruation, with a lessening of symptoms soon after the start of bleeding.

- The aetiology of the condition is poorly understood, and diagnosis is dependent on prospectively charting the symptoms to confirm that there is a true cyclical variation.

- Only a limited number of advocated treatments are of proven value and these are listed in Box 22.2. Initial treatment could include diet, regular aerobic exercise and techniques aimed at stress reduction. An SSRI is the most appropriate first-line drug and, if unsuccessful, it may be appropriate to institute a trial of ovarian suppression. Long-term suppression with medroxyprogesterone acetate or surgical oophorectomy is considered to be a last resort.

The menopause and hormone replacement therapy

Introduction

Human female fertility terminates relatively abruptly in middle age. This seems to be rather a puzzle as, in evolutionary terms, those genes that 'favour' giving birth to as many offspring as possible would be expected to proliferate. In other words, the genes of mothers who continued giving birth to children for as many years as they could would be expected to be successful. Human children, however, remain dependent on their mothers for many years after birth and, if mothers continued to reproduce until the end of their lives, they would be less able to support the later children to independent maturity. This would be a waste of personal resources without genetic benefit, and would also limit the support such a mother could offer to her grandchildren in whom she has a quarter-part genetic investment.

The flaw in this otherwise reasonable teleological argument (p. 293), however, is that the vast majority of women previously died long before reaching the current average age of menopause, thus diluting the role of longevity in the evolutionary process. The true reasons behind this process of ovarian failure, the menopause, are therefore not yet fully elucidated.

Menopause literally means 'last menstrual period' but the word is often used to cover the physiological changes that occur around this time. The falling levels of oestrogens as ovarian function slowly declines lead to changes in a number of systems, and may give rise to significant symptoms. Although physiological, the menopause has important adverse long-term effects on health (Table 23.1) which can, in part, be offset by the use of hormone replacement therapy (HRT). The pros and cons of this treatment will be discussed in more detail and need to be carefully considered on an individual basis before treatment is started.

Physiology

The perimenopause (or climacteric) may begin months or years before the last menstrual period, and symptoms may continue for years afterwards. The median age at menopause in the UK is 50.8 years. It occurs when the supply of oocytes becomes exhausted. A newborn girl has over half a million oocytes in her ovaries: one-third of these disappear before puberty and most of the remainder are lost during reproductive

233

Gynaecology

Table 23.1
The consequences of oestrogen deficiency

Short-term problems	Vasomotor (85% of women)	Headaches Hot flushes Night sweats Palpitations Insomnia
	Psychological	Irritability Poor concentration Poor short-term memory Depression Lethargy Loss of libido/ self-confidence Generalized aches
Intermediate problems	Urogenital	Urethral symptoms Uterine prolapse Stress/urge incontinence Dyspareunia Atrophic vaginitis/vulvitis
	Cutaneous/ connective tissue	Vaginal dryness Dry skin Dry hair Brittle nails
Long-term problems (> 50% of women)	Arterial	Cardiovascular disease Cerebrovascular disease
	Skeletal	Osteoporosis

Sources: National Osteoporosis Society 1994; Oldenhave A et al 1993, *American Journal of Obstetrics and Gynecology* 168: 772–780

life. In each menstrual cycle some 20 or 30 primordial follicles begin to develop and most become atretic. As only about 400 cycles occur during an average woman's lifetime, most oocytes are lost spontaneously through ageing rather than through ovulation.

In premenopausal women, oestradiol is produced by the granulosa cells of the developing follicle but as the menopause approaches, this production is reduced. The proportion of anovulatory menstrual cycles increases and progesterone production declines. Pituitary production of follicle-stimulating hormone (FSH) and luteinizing hormone (LH) rises because of diminishing negative feedback from oestrogen, but other pituitary hormones are not affected. Serum levels of FSH over 30 IU/l can be used clinically to clarify the diagnosis of menopause (see below). The relationship of the last period to the rise in FSH is not constant, and gonadotrophin levels may be raised for months or years before the menopause itself.

Circulating androstenedione, mainly of adrenal origin, is converted by fat cells into oestrone, a less potent form of oestrogen than oestradiol. After the menopause, this is the predominant circulating oestrogen rather than ovarian oestrogens.

Signs and symptoms (Table 23.1)

Vaginal bleeding

Irregular periods before the menopause are usually the result of anovulatory menstrual cycles and, if irregular bleeding persists, endometrial assessment may be required to exclude the possibility of endometrial carcinoma (p. 267). The menopause itself can be recognized only in retrospect after an arbitrary length of amenorrhoea, usually taken as 6 months or a year. Further vaginal bleeding after this is 'postmenopausal' and endometrial assessment may again be required. Approximately 10% of those with postmenopausal bleeding have a gynaecological malignancy.

Hot flushes

A 'hot flush' is an uncomfortable subjective feeling of warmth in the upper part of the body, usually lasting around 3 minutes. Approximately 50–85% of menopausal women experience such vasomotor symptoms, although only 10–20% seek medical advice. Flushes are sometimes accompanied by nausea, palpitations and sweating, and may be particularly troublesome at night. They are thought to be of hypothalamic origin and may in some way be related to LH release. It is thought that a fall in oestrogen levels affects central alpha-adrenergic systems which in turn affect central thermoregulatory centres and LH-releasing neurons.

About 20% of women begin experiencing flushes while still menstruating regularly. Flushes slowly improve as the body adjusts to the new low oestrogen concentrations, but in approximately 25% of women they continue for more than 5 years. Exogenous oestrogen administration, in the form of HRT, is effective in relieving these symptoms in about 90% of cases.

Genitourinary atrophy

The genital system, urethra and bladder trigone are oestrogen dependent and undergo gradual atrophy after the menopause. Thinning of the vaginal skin may cause dyspareunia and bleeding, and loss of vaginal glycogen causes a rise in pH which can predispose to local infection. Urgency of micturition may result from atrophic change in the trigone. Unlike flushes, these atrophic symptoms may appear years after the menopause and do not improve spontaneously, although they respond well to a short course of local or systemic oestrogen.

Other symptoms

Some studies have suggested that many symptoms, including irritability and lethargy, can be improved by hormone therapy more effectively than by placebo.

Most investigators, however, feel that the symptom of depression is not due directly to oestrogen withdrawal although it has been reported that oestrogen treatment can improve the symptoms of depression. It is possible that this effect may be related to the indirect relief of specific symptoms, such as insomnia caused by night sweats.

Long-term effects

The menopause alters a woman's susceptibility to breast cancer, cardiovascular disease and osteoporosis.

Breast cancer

Although the risk of breast cancer increases with increasing age the rate of increase slows after the menopause. The risk of breast cancer is decreased if the menopause is premature and increased if it occurs late, such that a woman who has had a menopause in her late 50s has double the risk of breast cancer when compared to a woman who has had a menopause in her early 40s.

Cardiovascular disease

A premenopausal woman's risk of developing coronary artery disease is less than one-fifth of that of a man of the same age, a sex difference that has disappeared by the age of 85 years. This has been assumed to indicate that oestrogens protect against vascular disease, but the phenomenon may be due to other risk factors affecting the male and to the fact that high-risk men die before they reach old age.

Studies looking at the effect of postmenopausal oestrogen therapy on cardiovascular disease suggest that unopposed oestrogen treatment may reduce the risk of ischaemic heart disease. More recent studies, however, looking at the incidence of subsequent myocardial infarction in those with pre-existing coronary heart disease who use combined oestrogen–progestogen preparations suggest that this form of HRT may increase the risk of ischaemic heart disease.

Osteoporosis

Bone resorption by osteoclasts is accelerated by the menopause (Fig. 23.1a,b). Oestrogen receptors have been demonstrated on bone cells, and oestrogens have been shown to stimulate osteoblasts directly. Calcitonin and prostaglandins may also be involved as intermediate factors in the link between oestrogen and bone metabolism.

In the first 4 years after the menopause there is an annual loss of 1–3% of bone mass, falling to 0.6% per year after that. This leads to an increased rate of

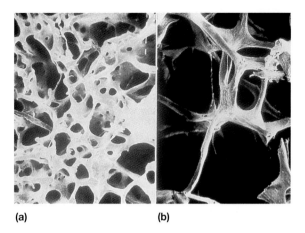

(a) (b)

Fig. 23.1 **Sections of (a) normal and (b) osteoporotic bone.** (From Dempster D et al, 1986, *Journal of Bone and Mineral Research* 1:15–21, with permission.)

fractures, particularly of the distal radius, the vertebral body and the upper femur, and one or more of these fractures will affect 40% of women over 65 years. Wedge compression fractures of the spine, leading to the so-called 'dowager's hump' affect 25% of white women over 60 years (Fig. 23.2), and fractures of the hip have occurred in 20% of women by the age of 90 years. Women who are underweight have a higher risk of osteoporosis because of reduced peripheral conversion of androgens to oestrogen. Women of Afro-Caribbean origin have a smaller risk of osteoporosis than white or Asian women as they have a greater initial bone mass.

Osteoporosis has important consequences for women and for health services. In the UK over 35 000 postmenopausal women suffer femoral fractures every year and 17% of them die in hospital. HRT has a very significant benefit in reducing the incidence of osteoporosis and osteoporotic fractures.

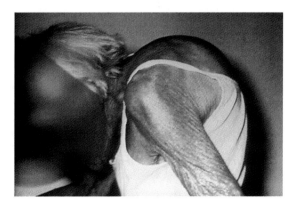

Fig. 23.2 **Severe osteoporosis of the spine.** (Courtesy of Wyeth-Ayerst Laboratories.)

Diagnosis

The menopause may be confused with premenstrual syndrome (PMS), depression, thyroid dysfunction, pregnancy and, rarely, phaeochromocytoma or carcinoid syndrome. Vasomotor symptoms may be caused by calcium antagonists and by antidepressive therapy, especially tricyclics.

The diagnosis of menopause is usually clinical and can only be made in retrospect after 6–12 months of amenorrhoea. If there is clinical confusion there may be some value in checking the serum FSH level which should be > 30 U/l postmenopausally. Perimenopausally the level may be normal and it should be noted that FSH levels peak physiologically in mid-cycle, making it worth rechecking apparently high levels a second time. If there is diagnostic doubt about whether a woman is perimenopausal, especially over 45 years of age, a therapeutic trial of HRT may be considered. Absence of a satisfactory response suggests that symptoms are unrelated to low levels of oestrogen.

Hormonal therapy

Oestrogen supplementation is the basis of replacement therapy, although progestogens may have a small role in relieving vasomotor symptoms. The oestrogens may be systemically administered as daily oral tablets, twice-weekly or weekly transdermal patches, or subcutaneous implants administered every 6–8 months. Daily nasal sprays, skin creams and 3-monthly vaginal rings are also used.

Whatever the route of administration, women who have not undergone hysterectomy should be placed on a regimen which includes a progestogen to minimize the risk of endometrial cancer associated with un-opposed oestrogen therapy. This advice applies also to women who have undergone endometrial resection. Women who have had a hysterectomy do not require a progestogen.

Oral preparations

The oral route may have a more beneficial effect than parenteral therapy on lipid profiles, leading to higher HDL and lower LDL levels, but it is potentially more thrombotic. Tablets may be given as an oestrogen-only preparation for those who have had a hysterectomy, or as a combined oestrogen–progestogen preparation for those who have not. The combined form may be administered cyclically or continuously.

Cyclical preparations, which usually lead to monthly withdrawal bleeds, are used perimenopausally, and the continuous combined preparations, the so called 'no-bleed' HRT, are an option from more than 2 years after the last menstrual period. This continuous com-bined therapy is more convenient for the 80+% who do not suffer unscheduled bleeding, but erratic bleeding beyond the first 6 months of treatment warrants further investigation.

Alternatives to these oestrogen–progesterone prep-arations are tibolone and raloxifene. Tibolone is a syn-thetic steroid with weak oestrogenic, progestogenic and androgenic effects which may be started 2 years after periods have ceased in a similar way to the continuous combined preparations. Raloxifene, a synthetic selective oestrogen-receptor modulator (SERM), has oestrogenic effects on bone and lipid metabolism but has a minimal effect on uterine and breast tissue. It is therefore ineffec-tive for controlling perimenopausal symptoms but it has a useful role in protecting against osteoporosis and it does not cause vaginal bleeding.

Transcutaneous administration

Transdermal patches are available as an unopposed oestrogen form, or as cyclical or continuous oestrogen–progestogen combinations. Skin reactions, ranging from hyperaemia to blisters, affect only a very small percentage of users.

The clinical advantage of transcutaneous administra-tion is that it should avoid gastrointestinal side-effects, and minimize the effects on hepatic production of both lipoproteins and coagulation factors. Patches are usually applied to the buttock, and each patch lasts for between 3–7 days depending on the formulation. This method appears to be as effective as oral preparations in treating symptomatic women and for the prevention of osteoporosis.

Percutaneous oestrogen gels are also available. A measured dose is rubbed into the skin and avoids the prolonged skin contact of patches. The same contra-indications apply as for other unopposed oestrogens.

Subcutaneous implants

Estradiol may be implanted in subcutaneous fat, usually in the lower abdomen, at intervals of no less than 5 or 6 months. The estradiol level does not always fall away to baseline before symptoms recur and there is a risk of tachyphylaxis (persistent symptoms despite ever-increasing estradiol levels) unless strict dose control is observed. Providing that pre-implant estradiol levels are monitored, however, the risk of tachyphylaxis is minimized. Testosterone implants are occasionally used to increase libido, but evidence for their effectiveness is lacking.

Vaginal preparations

These include estradiol tablets, low-dose estradiol-releasing Silastic ring pessaries, estriol vaginal pessaries and vaginal cream. They are all useful in the treatment of atrophic vaginitis.

Risks and side-effects of hormone treatment
General

Nausea and breast tenderness occur in about 5–10% of patients. Uterine bleeding is less common with low-dose regimens and, in general, the lowest dose that controls symptoms should be used. Irregular bleeding should be investigated as appropriate. There is a slight risk of cholelithiasis, and there is a theoretical chance of glucose tolerance impairment.

Endometrial carcinoma

Unopposed therapy (i.e. oestrogen only) increases the incidence of endometrial cancer fourfold, and it should therefore be used only for those who have had a hysterectomy. The incidence is reduced to a relative risk of less than 1.0 with opposed therapy (i.e. with the addition of progesterone for at least 10 days per cycle). The levonorgestrel-releasing intrauterine system (*Mirena*) protects the endometrium effectively when used in conjunction with oestrogen-only HRT in postmenopausal women.

Breast cancer

A link between oestrogen treatment and breast cancer is biologically plausible because of the connection between late menopause and breast cancer as noted above. For those between the age of 50 and 70 years, the incidence of breast carcinoma is increased from a baseline of 45/1000 to 47/1000 after 5 years of oestrogen treatment, 51/1000 after 10 years and 57/1000 after 15 years. There is no increased risk in those who stopped taking HRT more than 5 years previously. It may be that breast cancer diagnosed while on HRT is more curable.

Other cancers

There is no evidence of any adverse effect on other cancers. The oral contraceptive pill reduces the risk of ovarian cancer but there is no evidence that HRT does the same.

Venous thromboembolic disease

There is an increased risk of venous thromboembolic disease in the first year of HRT treatment, with a relative risk of approximately 4.0 in the first 6 months and 3.0 in the second 6 months (baseline risk 1.3/1000/year). There is apparently no increased risk in those taking it beyond 1 year. Routine pretreatment screening for thrombophilia is not recommended but it should be carried out in those with a personal or family history of venous thromboembolic disease.

Contraindications to hormone treatment

Pregnancy, thromboembolic disease and a history of recurrent venous thromboembolism are recognized contraindications to HRT, as are liver disease and undiagnosed vaginal bleeding. Treated hypertension and other cardiovascular risk factors are probably not contraindications.

Use of oestrogen-containing HRT is widely considered to be contraindicated following breast carcinoma (including intraduct carcinoma) and following advanced endometrial carcinoma. There are also theoretical reasons why it should be avoided in those who have had ovarian cancer.

Duration of HRT

When oestrogens are given for vasomotor symptoms they are generally continued for 2 or 3 years and then stopped. Whether to continue therapy beyond this time depends on whether symptoms recur and on a weighing up of the risks of osteoporosis against the potential side-effects of breast cancer and venous thromboembolic disease for that particular individual.

Non-hormonal treatment
Drugs

Vasomotor symptoms may be reduced by clonidine, which acts directly on the hypothalamus, but in practice it is of limited value. Palpitations and tachycardia may be improved by beta-blockers. Sedatives, hypnotics and antidepressants may be helpful in the treatment of non-vasomotor symptoms.

Although oestrogen supplementation is the mainstay for the prevention and treatment of osteoporosis, other therapies may be effective. In elderly women, supplementation with calcium, calcitonin and vitamin D reduces the risk of hip fractures. Moderate exercise may slow the rate of bone loss, though compliance with exercise programmes is often poor.

Psychological support

Some women with menopausal symptoms need only reassurance. Others may have particular stresses at this time of life, such as children leaving home, which may accentuate their perimenopausal symptoms. The marked placebo benefits in various studies show the importance of psychological support and a sympathetic ear.

Key points

- The average age of women experiencing spontaneous menopause is 51.

- The menopause is caused by ovarian failure as the supply of oocytes is depleted. FSH rises as oestrogen production falls and an FSH of >30 IU/l is suggestive of postmenopausal status.

- Cessation of periods is often preceded by irregular bleeding. A vaginal bleed more than 6 months or a year after menopause probably warrants investigation.

- Vasomotor symptoms such as hot flushes affect around two-thirds of women and may continue for more than 5 years after the menopause. Other symptoms include genitourinary atrophy and, possibly, some psychological symptoms.

- Long-term health risks of the menopause include cardiovascular disease and osteoporosis. Fractures of the radius, vertebral body or femoral neck affect 40% of women over the age of 65 years.

- HRT is offered to treat menopausal symptoms and to reduce long term hypo-oestrogenic side-effects. If the woman still has a uterus, opposed HRT (oestrogen and progesterone) is necessary to avoid the risk of endometrial carcinoma. Oral, transcutaneous, and vaginal preparations are available as well as subcutaneous implants.

- Side-effects of HRT include an increased incidence of breast carcinoma and venous thromboembolic disease.

24

Genital prolapse

Introduction

Uterovaginal prolapse may be described as descent of some of the pelvic organs (urethra, bladder, uterus, small bowel and rectum) into the vagina. The structures lying immediately above the vagina are in close proximity to each other and if the integrity of pelvic fascia is disrupted, descent of a single organ seldom occurs in isolation. This becomes important when considering different modalities of treatment and how best to relieve symptoms.

Aetiology

The aetiology of genital prolapse is multifactorial and the main predisposing factors are listed in Box 24.1. In addition, obesity, chronic cough and constipation, which all raise intra-abdominal pressure, can aggravate the condition.

Childbirth

Childbirth results in trauma to the pelvic floor and loss of tissue support to the female pelvic organs. Vaginal delivery, and in particular multiparity, may disrupt the fascia and cause ligament weakening. A prolonged labour, in particular prolonged second stage, a large baby, and perineal trauma have all been implicated in causing direct damage to the fascia and neuromuscular tissue of the pelvic floor.

Box 24.1

FACTORS PREDISPOSING TO GENITAL PROLAPSE

- Childbirth
- Menopause
- Congenital
- Suprapubic surgery for urinary incontinence
- Genetics

Menopause

The menopausal state, characterized by oestrogen deficiency and loss of connective tissue strength, is a causative factor in the development of prolapse. This may be because oestrogen influences collagen formation.

Congenital

Congenital weakness and neurological deficiency of the tissues account for prolapse in a small proportion of patients. Rarely children may be born with prolapse or they may develop significant prolapse during childhood. There may also be anatomical variants that may make certain women more susceptible to prolapse in later life.

Gynaecological surgery

Although surgery is often used to treat prolapse it may be responsible for a small number of cases. Suprapubic surgical procedures for urinary incontinence (e.g. Burch colposuspension) alter the anatomy such that the bladder neck is approximated behind the symphysis pubis. This increases gravitational effects on the pouch of Douglas, prolapse of which leads to enterocele formation.

Genetic

Genetic factors have been implicated in the development of prolapse. It is uncommon, for example, in the African population, possibly related in some way to the different collagen content of tissues.

Classification

The classification of prolapse, and the main symptoms, are summarized in Table 24.1.

Urethrocele/cystocele

A urethrocele is descent of the part of the anterior vaginal wall which is fused to the urethra. This is approximately the first 3–4 cm of the anterior wall superior to the urethral meatus. Any descent of this tissue may alter the urethrovesical angle and disrupt the continence mechanism, predisposing to genuine stress incontinence.

The bladder base lies immediately above this. Descent of this area is termed a cystocele (Fig. 24.1). Urethroceles and cystoceles are often considered together, and when both are present the term cystourethrocele is used.

Uterus and cervix

The cervix occupies the upper third of the vagina and descends when there is uterine prolapse. Uterine prolapse may be described as first, second or third degree (Fig. 24.2):

- First degree – there is descent of the uterus and cervix within the vagina but the cervix does not reach the introitus
- Second degree – descent of the cervix to the level of the introitus
- Third degree – the cervix and uterus protrude out of the vagina.

Procidentia is a term used when the cervix, uterus and vaginal wall have completely prolapsed through the introitus. Exposure of the cervix and vagina outside the introitus may lead to ulceration of the cervix and thickening of the vaginal mucosa.

Rectocele

Weakening of the tissue that lies between the vagina and rectum (rectovaginal fascia) allows the rectum to protrude into the lower posterior vaginal wall causing a rectocele (Fig. 24.3). Laxity of the perineum may also

Table 24.1
Types of genital prolapse

Original position of organs	Prolapse	Symptoms (in addition to the general symptoms of discomfort, dragging, the feeling of a 'lump' and, rarely, coital problems)
Anterior	Urethrocele Cystocele	Urinary symptoms (stress incontinence, urinary frequency)
Central	Cervix/uterus: 1st, 2nd and 3rd degree Procidentia	Bleeding and/or discharge from ulceration in association with procidentia
Posterior	Rectocele Enterocele	Bowel symptoms, particularly the feeling of incomplete evacuation and sometimes having to press the posterior wall backwards to pass stool

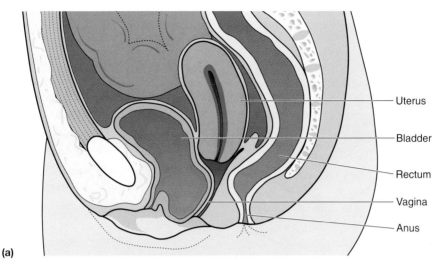

(a)

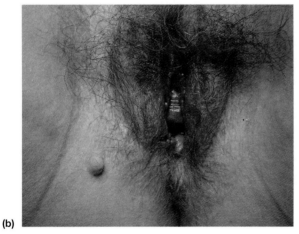

(b)

Fig. 24.1 **Cystocele.**

be present which gives a gaping appearance to the fourchette (the posterior margin of the introitus).

Enterocele

An enterocele is the only type of vaginal prolapse which is truly a hernia (Fig. 24.4). It has a sac, neck and contents. The sac is a protrusion of the peritoneum of the pouch of Douglas and may contain small bowel, or omentum.

Symptoms

Prolapse may be asymptomatic and it may only be detected when patients present for a cervical smear. If symptoms are present, they are usually non-specific but there may be features that are related to a specific type of prolapse (Table 24.1).

Non-specific symptoms may be attributable to the 'stretch effect' on tissues. Patients may describe an uncomfortable dragging feeling or backache that characteristically improves when lying down. Patients may also describe 'something coming down'. Coital difficulties are very uncommon as a presenting symptom.

Anterior wall prolapse may cause urinary symptoms because it involves bladder and urethra. Over 50% of women with genuine stress incontinence have a significant cystourethrocele. Other urinary symptoms such as frequency and urgency may also be present. A large cystocele can cause problems of incomplete emptying of the bladder, and retained urine then predisposes to recurrent urinary tract infections.

Uterine prolapse does not usually present until the patient feels a lump. If there is a procidentia present, then there may be bleeding or discharge from ulceration of the cervix.

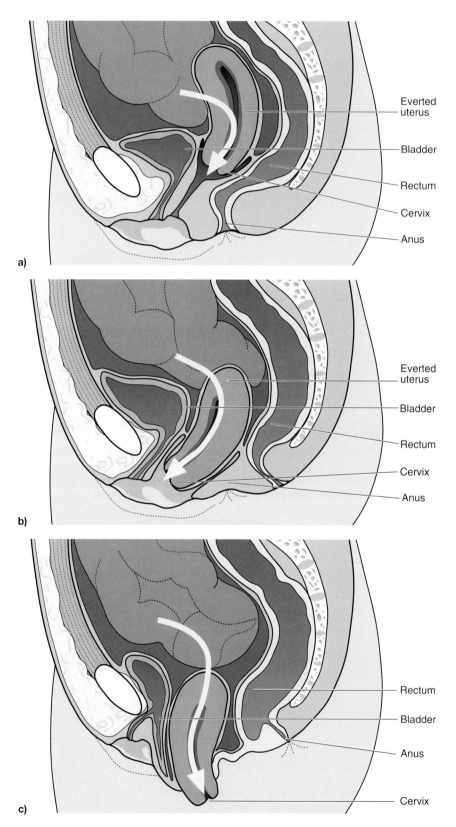

Fig. 24.2 **Uterine prolapse. (a)** First-degree, **(b)** second-degree, and **(c)** third-degree prolapse.

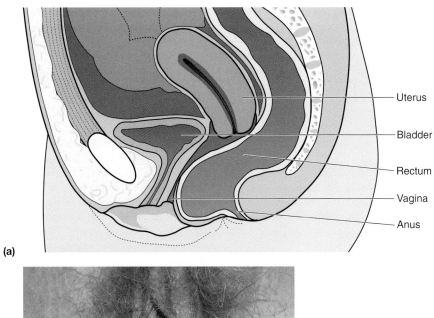

(a)

Uterus

Bladder

Rectum

Vagina

Anus

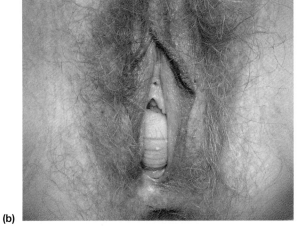

(b)

Fig. 24.3 **Rectocele.**

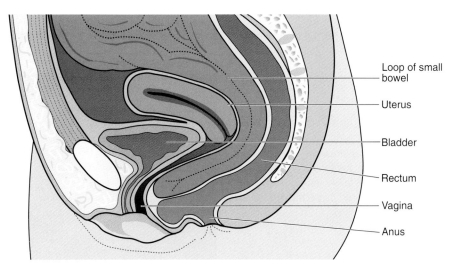

Loop of small
bowel

Uterus

Bladder

Rectum

Vagina

Anus

Fig. 24.4 **Enterocele.**

Bowel symptoms related to a rectocele involve a feeling of incomplete evacuation of the bowel contents. When straining occurs with defecation the rectocele balloons forward and some women need to digitally push the rectocele back to pass stool. Enteroceles usually present as a lump but may be also associated with non-specific lower abdominal discomfort.

Signs

Examination for prolapse forms part of the general gynaecological examination. First, features such as obesity, mobility and general well-being should be noted. Dyspnoea, nicotine-stained fingers, productive cough and abnormal chest signs may all lead to a suspicion of a chronic chest condition.

Next, abdominal examination is carried out focusing particularly on the possibility of a pelvic mass which may be pushing the pelvic organs downwards.

Pelvic examination is then performed, initially with the patient supine. On inspection of the vulva one may note atrophic changes (scanty hair, thinning of the labia). The patient is asked to abduct her legs and strain. By gently parting the labia majora with the thumb and index finger of the left hand, prolapse may be seen appearing at the introitus. Urinary leakage may also be apparent and an assessment of the perineum can also be made. A bimanual examination may then be performed, and may give a useful indication of uterine descent.

Examination in the left lateral, or 'Sims', position can also be helpful. This allows a systematic examination of the entire vagina exerting gentle traction with the speculum on the posterior vaginal wall. Sponge forceps are occasionally used during this examination to reduce a large prolapse to enable the examiner to distinguish the anatomy. The speculum can then be slowly withdrawn along the posterior wall of the vagina and the full extent of any rectocele will come into view.

If a prolapse is not apparent with the patient lying down it may sometimes be necessary to examine the patient in the standing position.

Management

It is a fundamental rule that if prolapse is not causing symptoms and the patient is unaware of it, then one should question whether any treatment is necessary. Simply because a doctor notices laxity within the vagina does not mean that surgery should be performed.

Conservative

Conservative treatment may be considered if a patient does not want, or is not fit enough for, surgery. Conservative measures may also be used for temporary relief before surgery and even as a therapeutic test to see if reduction of the prolapse improves specific symptoms.

Pelvic floor exercises are not effective when prolapse is well established. They do have a role in the treatment of associated urinary incontinence but their main value may be as a prophylactic treatment, particularly postpartum and postoperatively.

Pessaries are commonly used. A ring pessary is an inert plastic ring which is placed in the vagina so that one edge of the ring is behind the symphysis pubis and the other is in the posterior fornix (Figs 24.5 and 24.6). The ring tends to support the uterus and vault of the vagina. It may also help reduce cystocele but it will not reduce a rectocele. Once a ring is fitted, arrangements are usually made to change it every 4–6 months. At this examination, the vagina is inspected thoroughly for atrophic changes and ulceration due to pressure necrosis. Complications from the ring may include urinary symptoms (frequency, infection), vaginal discharge, bleeding or, very rarely, fistula formation (if the ring is neglected). Other types of ring pessary are available, particularly the 'shelf' pessary which has a useful role in procidentia.

If atrophy of the lower genital tract is noted in association with prolapse, a course of oestrogen therapy (commonly administered topically as a cream) may improve vaginal tissue thickness. This may improve some symptoms and if the patient requires surgery, it will make the procedure easier.

Surgery

Most procedures for the treatment of genital prolapse are performed through the vagina, with only a few requiring an abdominal approach. When considering a surgical technique particular attention should be given to preserving the calibre of the vagina if the woman wishes to remain sexually active. This aspect should always be discussed before operation.

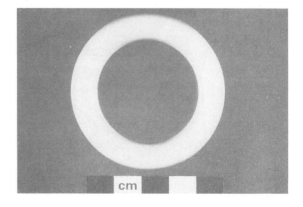

Fig. 24.5 **Ring pessary (50 mm diameter).**

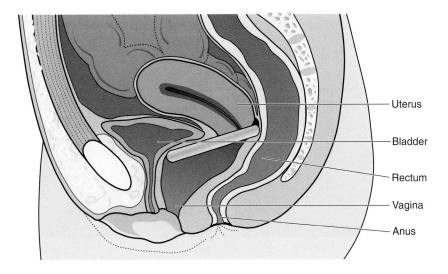

——— Uterus

——— Bladder

——— Rectum

——— Vagina

——— Anus

Fig. 24.6 **Ring pessary in situ.** Note that the anterior vaginal wall is elevated to reduce the cystocele and the uterine prolapse has been corrected.

Anterior vaginal wall – anterior repair (anterior colporrhaphy)

Anterior vaginal wall prolapse may be associated with stress urinary incontinence which may need to be investigated prior to surgery.

The principle of an anterior repair is to make a midline incision through the vaginal skin and to reflect the underlying bladder off the vaginal mucosa. Once this is achieved, lateral supporting sutures are placed into fascia in order to elevate the bladder and bladder neck (Fig. 25.2). The remaining redundant vaginal skin that has been 'ballooning' down is excised, and the vaginal skin is then sutured closed.

Uterine descent – vaginal hysterectomy or Manchester repair

Vaginal hysterectomy is the definitive operation for uterine prolapse. However, one must not presume that just because the uterus is prolapsing, it can be removed vaginally, as it may be too large to remove because of, for example, associated fibroids. One should also consider whether the uterus is being pushed down from a mass above (e.g. advanced ovarian cancer with gross ascites), or whether bowel is likely to be adherent to the uterus (e.g. after previous abdominopelvic surgery, endometriosis or severe infection). Once the uterus is removed it is important that the supporting ligaments are approximated so as to prevent further prolapse of the vaginal vault.

Manchester repair (also called 'Fothergill repair') has a role in treating uterine prolapse, but is less commonly performed than vaginal hysterectomy. The uterosacral ligaments are divided and shortened, the cervix is amputated and the shortened ligaments are approxi-

mated anterior to the cervical stump. The body of the uterus is not removed.

Posterior vaginal wall – posterior repair (posterior colpo-perineorrhaphy)

The principles of a posterior repair are similar to those of an anterior repair. An incision is made in the vaginal wall and the rectum is separated from the vagina (Fig. 24.7). Supporting sutures are placed laterally to reduce the prolapse. The lax vaginal skin is then excised and the incision closed. This operation can be combined with a repair of the perineal body to support the perineum. Again, particular care must be taken not to narrow the vagina and cause problems with dyspareunia.

As the procedure reaches the apex of the rectocele, the surgeon must identify whether or not there is an enterocele present. If one is present the peritoneum must be opened (avoiding bowel injury). The hernial sac must be transfixed and excised, and supporting lateral tissue approximated in order to prevent recurrence.

Total vault prolapse (after hysterectomy)

This condition refers to the complete eversion of the vagina following a hysterectomy (Fig. 24.8). It is effectively a procidentia without the uterus, not unlike a sock that has been turned inside out. The two surgical options are sacrocolpopexy and sacrospinous fixation, both of which serve to maintain coital function.

Sacrocolpopexy

Sacrocolpopexy involves suturing the vaginal vault to the body of the sacrum either directly, or indirectly by using a graft (porcine dermis, Goretex, Marlex)

Gynaecology

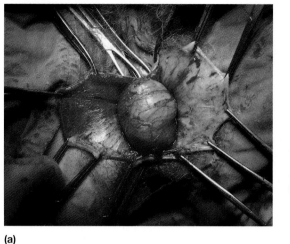

(a)

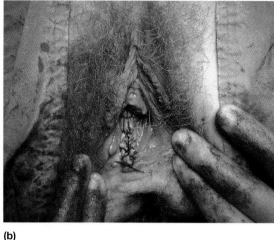

(b)

Fig. 24.7 **Posterior colporrhaphy. (a)** The posterior wall is opened in the midline to expose the rectum. **(b)** The posterior wall is closed after reducing the prolapse.

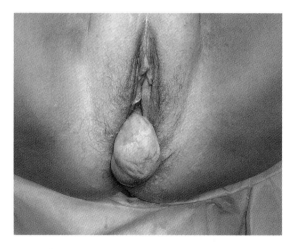

Fig. 24.8 **Vault prolapse.**

interposed between the two structures. The procedure is performed through an abdominal incision but can be carried out laparoscopically.

Sacrospinous fixation
Sacrospinous fixation requires the surgeon to suture the top of the vaginal vault to the sacrospinous ligament. The procedure is performed through the vagina. Complications of the procedure include damage to the sciatic nerve and pudendal vessels.

Key points

- Genital prolapse describes the descent of the pelvic organs (urethra, bladder, uterus, small bowel and rectum) into the vagina.

- It is more common after childbirth, in obese patients, postmenopausal patients and those women with any condition which raises intra-abdominal pressure, such as chronic cough or constipation.

- Prolapse may be classified as anterior compartment defects (urethrocele or cystocele – urethra or bladder respectively); central compartment deficit leading to the prolapse of the uterus (first-, second- or third-degree prolapse); or a posterior compartment deficit (prolapse of the rectum or small bowel – rectocele and enterocele respectively).

- Patients with prolapse may present with a 'something coming down', discomfort, or urinary or bowel symptoms. Asymptomatic prolapse does not usually need to be treated.

- Treatment may be conservative (ring pessaries, pelvic floor exercises) or surgical repair, i.e. repairing the vaginal wall defect or performing vaginal hysterectomy for uterine prolapse. In fit patients the treatment of choice is pelvic floor surgery.

25

Urinary incontinence

Introduction

Urinary incontinence is defined as the condition in which there is involuntary loss of urine which can be objectively demonstrated and which is a social or hygienic problem. It should be noted that the volume of urine lost is not a feature of the definition, but the ability of an independent person to confirm that there is urine loss is essential.

Whilst urinary incontinence is rarely, if ever, a life-threatening condition, it is an important condition in that it is common and it causes significant distress. Various prevalence studies have been reported and it is generally accepted that somewhere between 10 and 20% of the adult female population are incontinent of urine on one or more occasion per month. The prevalence changes little with age until over the age of 75 years when the prevalence of urinary incontinence is between 25 and 50% of women. It is considered that certain conditions predispose to urinary incontinence, including faecal impaction, decreased mobility, confusional states, and the presence of certain drugs including diuretics and hypnotics. There is contradictory evidence on any relationship between incontinence and previous hysterectomy and all that can really be concluded upon this point is that the evidence is inconclusive. Retrospective studies suggest that there is a causal relationship but prospective studies suggests that there is not.

Types of urinary incontinence

The commonest types of urinary incontinence in women are:

- genuine stress incontinence
- overactive bladder
- retention with overflow
- fistula
- congenital abnormalities.

Genuine stress incontinence is the commonest cause of urinary incontinence in adult women. It is the condition in which urine is lost in relationship to raised intra-abdominal pressure in the absence of detrusor activity, such as with coughing, walking or sneezing. The condition is called genuine stress incontinence to distinguish it from the symptom of stress incontinence, as discussed below. Overactive bladder, sometimes termed detrusor instability, unstable bladder, or hyperactive bladder, is the condition in which urine is lost in response to an involuntary detrusor contraction. It is the second commonest cause of urinary incontinence in adult women and may coexist with genuine stress incontinence. Retention with overflow is the female equivalent of the incontinence that occurs in men with an enlarged prostate. It is relatively uncommon in women. A fistula is an abnormal connection between two epithelial surfaces and hence a vesicovaginal fistula or a ureterovaginal fistula may cause incontinence, whilst a urethrovaginal fistula only causes urinary leakage immediately post-micturition. Congenital abnormalities, such as an ectopic ureter, are rare.

Clinical presentation

Lower urinary tract symptoms tend to fall into three groups: incontinence, irritative symptoms, and voiding difficulties. Unfortunately, the symptoms do not always allow for an accurate clinical diagnosis to be made, although they allow for the severity of the condition to be assessed. For instance, a woman who states that she is incontinent and either has to stay at home or has to wear protective garments when she goes out may have a more severe problem than the patient who requires no protection. The difficulty with the symptoms is that different conditions may have similar symptoms.

Stress incontinence, the symptom, is not synonymous with genuine stress incontinence, the condition. The symptom of stress incontinence (incontinence on coughing, laughing, sneezing, running, etc.) is the loss of urine with activity, and whilst most patients with the symptom of stress incontinence will have the condition of genuine stress incontinence, in other women it may represent a loss of urine whilst running to the toilet because of a feeling of intense urgency. Urgency is the irresistible desire to pass urine and urge incontinence is incontinence associated with that desire. The symptoms of urgency and urge incontinence are commonly found in the overactive bladder but a minority of patients with the overactive bladder may complain of the symptom of stress incontinence, although they do not have the condition of stress incontinence, and a minority of patients with genuine stress incontinence may complain of urgency and urge incontinence, even though they do not have an overactive bladder. Nocturnal enuresis, bedwetting, may occur on its own or in conjunction with other complaints, especially those associated with an overactive bladder. The symptoms of voiding difficulty include hesitancy, poor stream, and incomplete bladder emptying.

Whatever the patient's symptoms, it is essential to elicit from her how these symptoms affect her lifestyle. The degree of urgency with which one woman can cope may be devastating for another women, either by virtue of severity, personality, or occupation. The effect upon lifestyle must therefore be documented. It is also important to consider conditions that are more common in women with urinary incontinence, such as prolapse or anorectal symptoms. An accurate drug history is essential; for instance, elderly people taking tricyclic antidepressants may have voiding difficulties. A past history of urinary problems should also be sought. For instance, a woman who perhaps developed a transient episode of acute urinary retention after childbirth or a previous operation is more prone to develop a voiding disorder after surgery for her urinary incontinence than is a woman without such a history.

Unfortunately, clinical examination is of limited value in eliciting the cause of urinary incontinence. Over and above the general examination, however, excoriation of the vulva may indicate a long-standing or severe problem. The condition of genuine stress incontinence may be demonstrated if, upon parting the vulva and asking the woman to give a single sharp cough, urinary incontinence immediately follows, and the presence or absence of a prolapse may affect management options. What is frequently forgotten, yet essential, is some form of neurological examination especially of the nerve roots S2–4.

Despite an accurate history, the clinical diagnosis is only made with accuracy in a limited number of patients. It has been estimated, for instance, that the condition of genuine stress incontinence is only correctly diagnosed on history in approximately 68% of patients, a similar figure being quoted for bladder overactivity. If the patient complains of stress incontinence as her only symptom, then it is very likely that she has genuine stress incontinence. If the patient complains of urgency and urge incontinence as her only symptoms, it is very likely that she has an overactive bladder. If a patient, however, complains of a combination of stress incontinence, urgency and urge incontinence, a not uncommon situation, then it is virtually impossible clinically to decide whether the patient has genuine stress incontinence, an overactive bladder, or both.

Investigations

Given the fact that the bladder may therefore be described as 'an unreliable witness', a range of investigations are available and should be performed under appropriate circumstances. Unless a fistula is being considered, imaging of the urinary tract (by ultrasound or IVU) and/or cystoscopy is rarely helpful in making the diagnosis. The commonest investigations to be considered are:

- examination of midstream specimen of urine
- frequency–volume chart
- filling urodynamic assessment
- voiding urodynamic assessment.

Midstream urine examination

A midstream urine is the most simple of investigations, yet is frequently forgotten in the investigation of urinary incontinence. The presence of microorganisms may indicate infection, which in turn may be a transient and easily treatable cause of lower urinary tract symptoms. Perhaps more important is the presence or absence of white blood cells and red blood cells within the urine. The presence of a sterile pyuria may indicate a chronic bladder or renal infection, such as tuberculosis, whilst the presence of red cells may indicate a bladder tumour. Under such circumstances, of course, cystoscopy and imaging then become appropriate investigations.

Frequency–volume chart

It is often helpful to ask a woman to complete a frequency–volume chart, sometimes referred to as a urinary diary. The information obtained may be of assistance in assessing both cause and severity. For instance, the chart may indicate an abnormally high fluid intake which may be the cause of the urinary tract symptoms. The chart may give a more objective guide as to the presence of urinary frequency and the number of episodes of incontinence. A chart which shows frequent small voided volumes may indicate an overactive bladder. Occasionally, the charts may provide the basis of a discussion between patient and clinician, leading to an alteration in the patient's habits.

Urodynamic assessment

A urodynamic assessment is a study which is able to investigate both the phase of bladder filling and the phase of bladder voiding.

Filling urodynamic assessment

In a filling urodynamic assessment, sometimes termed a cystometrogram, the bladder is filled via a urethral catheter using sterile saline at room temperature and running at approximately 100 ml per minute. At the same time, the detrusor pressure is measured. The detrusor pressure is the pressure within the bladder due to the bladder itself. The bladder is of course an intra-abdominal organ and hence the actual pressure in the bladder will be the sum of the detrusor pressure and the intra-abdominal pressure. The detrusor pressure cannot be measured directly and so a subtraction measurement is obtained by the simultaneous measurement of the total pressure within the bladder (generally with a second smaller urethral catheter) from which the pressure above the pelvic floor (measured with either a vaginal or a rectal catheter) is subtracted.

From the above, it should therefore be clear that if the patient has genuine stress incontinence, leaking urine in the presence of raised intra-abdominal pressure and the absence of detrusor activity, then the total bladder pressure will be raised at the moment of incontinence but the detrusor pressure will be unchanged. Conversely, if the patient has an overactive bladder, the total bladder pressure and the detrusor pressure will both be equally elevated at the time of incontinence.

The disadvantages of a filling cystometrogram are cost, some loss of dignity, and the possible introduction of infection. It is for these reasons that the investigation should be used whenever it is indicated but not necessarily routinely. It is considered that the major indications for a filling cystometrogram are:

1. any patient who complains of the symptom of both stress incontinence and urgency, because a clinical diagnosis cannot be made with any accuracy without the investigation
2. any patient who has failed to respond to seemingly previous appropriate treatment, medical or surgical
3. any patient to be involved in a formal scientific study where the accuracy of diagnosis is important to assess specific outcomes.

Voiding urodynamic assessment

A urodynamic assessment may also be performed during the voiding phase, where the measurements include the total volume voided, the peak flow of urine voided, and the detrusor activity required in order to produce that flow. Thus, the investigation may demonstrate that there must be significant residual urine if, say, the patient was filled with 500 ml but only voided 350 ml. Secondly, the patient who voids by abdominal straining, rather than the creation of detrusor activity, is likely to have a voiding disorder. Thirdly, whilst the peak flow of urine generally exceeds 15 ml/s, a reduced flow may also indicate a voiding disorder.

A voiding study should therefore be performed in all women with voiding symptoms in order to assess the cause of the voiding disorder. Many gynaecologists would also argue that a voiding study should always be performed before any woman undergoes surgery for genuine stress incontinence since some women will have an asymptomatic voiding disorder and the result of surgery may be to create a symptomatic voiding disorder by creating a bladder neck or proximal urethral outlet obstruction.

Special investigations

There are a series of special investigations which are indicated under very specific conditions. The anatomy and mobility of the bladder neck and urethra may be studied with ultrasound, whilst electromyography may be used to assess the integrity of the nerve supply to pelvic musculature.

The mechanism of continence

The mechanism of continence must be understood if the pathophysiology of incontinence is to be understood. In the normal woman, continence is maintained at the level of the bladder neck. If, for instance, a radio-opaque medium were to be placed in the bladder of a normal continent woman and that woman was asked to stand, an X-ray would demonstrate that urine does not flow into the urethra. The concept therefore arose of a so-called proximal urethral sphincter, a mechanism present in the region of the bladder neck and proximal urethra which maintains continence. It was originally considered that this was an arrangement of smooth muscle in the proximal urethra. However, no such sphincter mechanism based upon muscle exists. There is smooth muscle in the proximal urethra but it generally runs in a longitudinal rather than a circular direction and as such could not maintain continence.

It is now considered that the so-called proximal urethral sphincter mechanism is a water-tight seal which maintains the pressure in the urethra greater than the pressure in the bladder. The anatomical basis of that seal is considered to be a series of arteriolovenous anastomoses within the wall of the proximal urethra. These can be demonstrated on histological examination. They allow some degree of turgor pressure to be exerted circumferentially around the urethra which results in the formation of a hermetic seal by keeping the urethra occluded. The effect of any pressure exerted around the periphery of a hollow tube is to occlude that tube. If the pressure is exerted in numerous places around the circumference of the tube, then the tube will simply close. Such is the proximal urethral sphincter.

The situation becomes more complex in that if a pressure study is performed to compare the pressure in the urethra with the pressure within the bladder, then whilst the pressure in the proximal urethra exceeds that in the bladder, the greatest pressure difference exists at the mid-urethra. This is the so-called distal urethral sphincter mechanism. This does have an anatomical basis in muscle in that striated muscle, derived embryologically from levator ani, innervated by spinal roots S2–4 but anatomically discreet from levator ani, is found within the wall of the mid-urethra.

There are further features which aid the above mechanisms. There are supporting tissues around the urethra which maintain the proximal urethra in an intra-abdominal position. The importance of this position is that if the proximal urethra is intra-abdominal, then any pressure rise within the abdomen will be transmitted equally to the bladder and the proximal urethra, and hence the pressure difference will not change and hence continence will be maintained. Weakness or damage to the supporting tissues may therefore predispose to genuine stress incontinence. The supporting tissues are characterized anatomically as the pubourethral ligaments, derived from the fascia of the pelvic floor, and to a lesser degree the pelvic floor musculature, namely levator ani. It has been demonstrated that vaginal delivery, especially the first vaginal delivery, may denervate both the pubourethral ligaments and levator ani, the nerve damage being manifest within the pudendal nerve. Thus, the first vaginal delivery may predispose towards genuine stress incontinence. Secondly, there is the concept of bladder stability. The bladder muscle, the detrusor, should only contract during micturition, whereas it should relax during bladder filling. Such a situation is described as a stable bladder. In women who have an overactive bladder, the detrusor initially relaxes during filling but then contracts involuntarily. Such a situation used to be termed an unstable bladder but is now termed an overactive bladder. If the contraction is modest, then the woman will appreciate the contraction as urinary urgency but if the contraction is strong enough to elevate the pressure in the bladder above that in the urethra, then there will be the symptom of urge incontinence.

Genuine stress incontinence

The definition of genuine stress incontinence has already been given. It clearly requires some degree of weakness of both the proximal and distal sphincter mechanisms and is the commonest form of urinary incontinence in adult women. Whilst no single aetiological factor exists in all women with genuine stress incontinence, there are a series of predisposing factors which may explain the condition. These include:

- pregnancy
- prolapse
- menopause
- collagen disorder
- obesity.

Pregnancy

It has already been noted that vaginal delivery may cause denervation of the pudendal nerve and hence damage to the supporting tissues of the urethra. Moreover, the pudendal nerve in part supplies the distal urethral sphincter. It is demonstrable that the first vaginal delivery is more likely than any subsequent vaginal delivery to cause genuine stress incontinence, and this incontinence may be preventable by elective caesarean section. There is also a transient form of genuine stress incontinence which occurs during pregnancy but is not present outside of pregnancy. The mechanism of this incontinence is a combination of the raised intra-abdominal pressure related to uterine contents together with the smooth-muscle-relaxant effect of progesterone. Thus, some women will complain of genuine stress incontinence during pregnancy but not at other times.

Prolapse

Prolapse is not a cause of genuine stress incontinence but the same pathophysiological abnormality which causes the incontinence may cause prolapse, namely a deficiency of supporting tissues. It may be that anterior vaginal wall prolapse is therefore a surrogate indicator of a predisposition to genuine stress incontinence.

Menopause

Many patients date the onset of their symptoms not from childbirth but from the menopause. There is evidence that the withdrawal of oestrogen reduces the so-called maximal urethral closure pressure; hence the pressure in the urethra, whilst still greater than that in the bladder, is not as great as it used to be. The effect of this pressure reduction is that a smaller rise in intra-abdominal pressure will result in genuine stress incontinence, and hence it is more likely and more common for the woman to leak urine.

Collagen disorder

Collagen is clearly a major component of the pubo-urethral ligaments. There are several different types of collagen present within the body and there is some evidence that there are different types of collagen in different proportions in the pubourethral ligaments of women who become incontinent compared with the pubourethral ligaments of those who do not.

Obesity

It is sometimes stated that obesity is an aetiological factor in genuine stress incontinence. What evidence there is does not support such a conclusion other than in a woman who is morbidly obese.

Treatment

The treatment of genuine stress incontinence may be conservative or surgical, the choice of treatment depending upon the patient's wishes, her wish for further children, the severity of her symptoms, the presence or absence of other pathology, and the efficacy of such treatment.

Conservative treatment

Conservative treatment includes:

- pelvic floor exercises

- the use of vaginal cones
- drugs.

Pelvic floor exercises

Pelvic floor exercises have traditionally been used in the treatment of genuine stress incontinence. The woman is taught to contract her pelvic floor and in doing so will also contract the striated muscle of the distal urethral sphincter. The efficacy of such exercises is well recognized; approximately one-third of women become continent, one-third of women are improved but not continent, and one-third of women are unchanged. Other studies have demonstrated that approximately 50% of women who would have undergone surgery for genuine stress incontinence are so improved by pelvic floor exercises that they no longer wish the surgery. Given that pelvic floor exercises are harmless but surgery is not, it perhaps should be argued that all women should be offered a trial of pelvic floor physiotherapy before undergoing surgery. The technique of pelvic floor physiotherapy has a limited effect upon the outcome in that all of the techniques appear to be relatively similar in efficacy. These techniques may include formal exercises, preferably supervised by a physiotherapist, or electrical stimulation (sometimes termed interferential therapy), or faradic stimulation.

Vaginal cones

There has been a vogue for the use of weighted vaginal cones, each set consisting of some four or five cones of increasing weight. The woman is instructed to place the smallest cone in the vagina, learn to support that cone and when she is able to do so then use a heavier cone. This therapy has the advantage that the woman feels very involved in her own therapy, but it is no more efficacious than pelvic floor exercises.

Drugs

There is evidence that the use of oestrogen, either vaginally or systemically, in postmenopausal women with genuine stress incontinence will result in the restoration of continence to some patients. However, the benefit is immensely modest and it is unlikely that even 10% of women who are postmenopausal with genuine stress incontinence would regain any real degree of continence by the use of oestrogen. There are no drugs in current use which are licensed for the treatment of genuine stress incontinence, although it is possible that alpha-adrenergic agonists, such as phenyl-propanolamine, may become licensed and may help a minority of women in the future.

Surgery

Surgery is the most effective way of curing genuine stress incontinence, and a cure rate in the region of 80–90% can generally be expected from appropriate and properly performed primary surgery. Surgery does not replace the physiological mechanism but rather aims to support the bladder neck and proximal urethra and hence prevent incontinence associated with raised intra-abdominal pressure. There are numerous surgical procedures currently in use, which indicates that none is fully effective. The one most commonly used is the Burch colposuspension.

Burch colposuspension

The Burch colposuspension is a suprapubic procedure in which non-absorbable sutures are placed retro-pubically in order to approximate the paravaginal tissues to the ileopectineal ligament of the pelvic side-wall (Fig. 25.1). The procedure appears to have stood the test of time in that an 80–90% cure rate may be obtained in the short term and a 70% cure rate at 10–15 years.

However, no operation is free of complications and the specific complications of the Burch colposuspension include voiding difficulty. This is only very rarely a long-term voiding dysfunction with the need for long-term clean intermittent self-catheterization, but empha-sizes the need to exclude an asymptomatic voiding disorder urodynamically prior to surgery. Other compli-cations include a predisposition to prolapse, especially rectocele or enterocele, and a transient overactivity of the bladder.

There is a vogue to perform the traditional Burch colposuspension, an open procedure, laparoscopically. The information currently available would suggest that laparoscopic colposuspension may not be as effective as the open procedure but no satisfactory large series with long-term follow-up has yet been published.

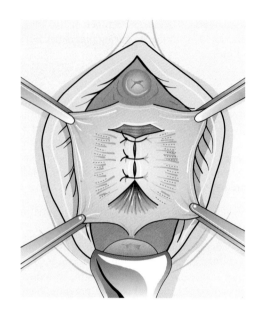

Fig. 25.2 **Anterior colporrhaphy and bladder buttress.** The anterior vaginal wall is opened in the midline and the bladder buttressed by sutures anchored in the fascia either side of the bladder neck.

Anterior repair and bladder buttress

The procedure most commonly performed for genuine stress incontinence prior to colposuspension was an anterior repair and bladder buttress, a vaginal operation in which the pubocervical fascia is approximated underneath the bladder neck and proximal urethra and provides support (Fig. 25.2). Although it is an easier operation to perform than colposuspension, is asso-ciated with fewer complications, and may be better able to treat an anterior vaginal wall coexisting prolapse, the results are more modest than those of colposuspension in both the short and long term. It is a procedure which should generally be reserved for patients who wish a smaller procedure and who are happy to accept a lesser cure rate, perhaps in the region of 65–70% in the short term.

Tension-free vaginal tape

There is a more recent minimally invasive procedure for the use of suburethral slings, the so-called tension-free vaginal tape (TVT), a procedure which is rapidly gaining in popularity (Fig. 25.3). The tape consists of a knitted Prolene mesh inserted transvaginally at the level of the mid-urethra using two trocars. Whilst the short-term results of this procedure are as good as those of any other procedure, it is relatively 'early days' to know the long-term results but it may well be that this procedure is as effective as a colposuspension.

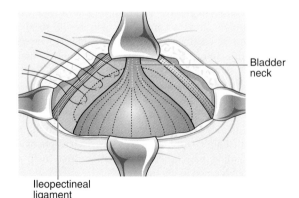

Bladder neck

Ileopectineal ligament

Fig. 25.1 **Burch colposuspension.** The retropubic space is opened and the bladder neck identified. The bladder neck is then suspended from the iliopectineal ligaments by sutures placed in the paravaginal fascia.

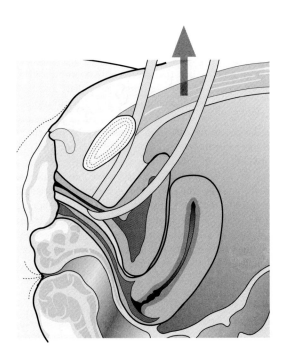

Fig. 25.3 **Tension-free vaginal tape.** A Prolene tape is inserted upwards transvaginally, with the ends of the tape brought out through suprapubic stab incisions. The tape is not sutured abdominally and the bladder neck is therefore supported in a tension-free manner.

Suburethral sling procedure

There will be some women who undergo an appropriate surgical procedure for genuine stress incontinence yet remain incontinent. If it is urodynamically demonstrated that they do indeed have genuine stress incontinence and there is no voiding disorder, then a second procedure may be performed and a so-called suburethral sling procedure is arguably the most appropriate (Fig. 25.4). The sling is placed rather like a hammock between two areas of the abdominal wall, running from the wall to pass underneath the proximal urethra and bladder neck and back towards the abdominal wall. The sling material can be organic (such as rectus fascia) or inorganic (such as Silastic tape). It carries similar efficacy to colposuspension and may also be complicated by either a long-term voiding disorder or transient overactive bladder.

In the group of women who are particularly difficult to treat in that they have undergone numerous previous operations and have a thick scarred fibrosed urethra, the use of injectable substances into the proximal urethra may improve continence. The injections can be performed on a day case basis and the commonest injectables currently in use are based upon bovine collagen or microparticulate silicone. Lastly, if the incontinence is severe enough, despite repeated surgery, the use of an artificial sphincter may be considered in specialist units.

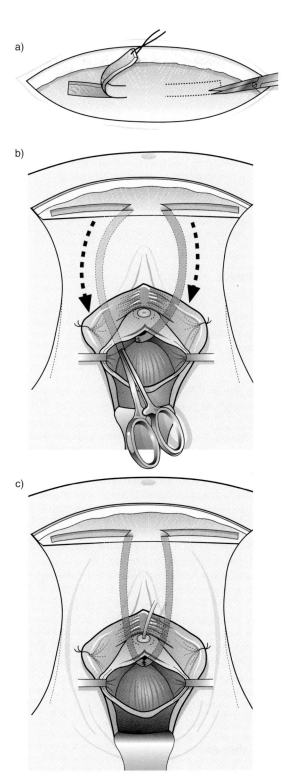

Fig. 25.4 **Urethral sling. (a)** Two strips of rectus sheath are mobilized through an abdominal incision, **(b)** guided downward retropubically into a vaginal incision, and **(c)** sutured together under the bladder neck.

Overactive bladder

The diagnosis and symptoms of an overactive bladder have already been stated. This is the second commonest cause of incontinence in adult women and may be associated with either a history of childhood nocturnal enuresis or indeed with coexisting nocturnal enuresis in adulthood. The aetiology of the condition is uncertain and in the vast majority of women it may actually be a variant upon normal rather than a pathological process. In those patients in whom it is pathological, there may be neuropathy, or outlet obstruction. The neuropathy is generally either an overt or covert neurological disorder, such as multiple sclerosis, or be consequent upon spinal cord trauma. Bladder neck outlet obstruction is unusual in women unless there has been previous surgery for genuine stress incontinence.

Treatment

The treatment options are:

- behavioural therapy
- drug therapy
- surgery.

Behavioural therapy

The principle of behavioural therapy is to re-establish central control of the bladder. Various behavioural interventions have been used including biofeedback and bladder retraining. Whilst they are time consuming, they have a high success rate. For instance, over 80% of women with idiopathic overactive bladder treated with bladder retraining will become continent. The principles of bladder retraining can be summarized as:

- Exclude frequency.
- Explain the unstable bladder to the patient together with the rationale of the intervention.
- Instruct the patient to void, say, every hour and a half during the day. She must not void between these times; she must wait or be incontinent.
- Give praise when the patient achieves the above and then increase the voiding interval by half an hour and keep increasing in half-hourly intervals until the patient is able to reach a voiding interval of some 3–4 hours.
- Drug treatment, as described below, may be used to augment behavioural therapy.

Drug therapy

There is no single drug which is to be considered as the drug of choice for the treatment of the overactive bladder. The general principle of all drug treatment is that the drug has an anticholinergic effect. The neurotransmitter which causes the detrusor to contract is acetylcholine, hence the use of anticholinergic drugs. Unfortunately, these are of limited specificity and hence anticholinergic side-effects, especially dry mouth, blurring of vision, and constipation may occur. Using drug treatment, up to 70% of patients may be expected to have an improvement in their symptoms but up to 15% of patients will unilaterally cease therapy because of side-effects. The commonest drugs in contemporary use are oxybutynin, tolterodine, propiverine, and trospium. Side-effects may be reduced either by the alteration of one agent to a different agent, by adjusting dosage, or by the use of slow-release preparations. Oestrogen may be of limited benefit in reducing frequency and urgency but has no demonstrable effect upon incontinence.

Surgery

For those women with severe overactive bladder which has not responded to conservative treatment, surgery may be considered. The problem, however, is that the surgical procedures are not of an insignificant size. They include bladder denervation procedures, or the attachment of small bowel to the bladder, such as the clam ileocystoplasty.

Voiding disorders

Voiding disorders may present with the symptoms described above (hesitancy, incomplete emptying, poor stream) or even retention with overflow. Generally, these are complications of bladder neck surgery. They may respond to simple treatment with either cholinergic drugs (such as bethanecol) or urethral dilatation. Occasionally, long-term intermittent clean self-catheterization is indicated.

Fistulae

Fistulae may be classified as ureterovaginal, vesicovaginal, urethrovaginal, or a combination thereof. The commonest cause of such a fistula worldwide is neglected childbirth but the commonest cause of such a fistula in the UK is gynaecological surgery, especially following pelvic malignancy when there has been a combination of both surgery and radiotherapy. The classical symptom of a ureterovaginal fistula or a vesicovaginal fistula is of being permanently wet both by day and by night. The fistula may be visible on speculum examination of the vagina and is usually confirmed by either imaging of the renal tract or cystoscopy.

The surgical treatment of a fistula is complex but the surgical principles include:

- Separating the two epithelial surfaces which form the fistula.
- Closure of the two epithelial surfaces separately and without tension.
- Interposition of neutral tissue between the two closed areas, such as a piece of omentum between the bladder and the vagina.
- A prolonged period of drainage either with a urethral catheter for a vesicovaginal fistula or a ureteric stent for a ureterovaginal fistula.

Conclusion

Urinary incontinence is a common condition causing great distress. The diagnosis must be made with accuracy if the appropriate treatment is to be offered. Much treatment can be given in the community or in the outpatient department, but specialized surgical units result in the best success rates for surgical intervention.

Key points

- Urinary incontinence affects 10–20% of the adult female population, at least.

- An accurate history may lead to the diagnosis but in other situations investigation, including urodynamic assessment, is important.

- Genuine stress incontinence may be treated conservatively or surgically.

- An overactive bladder is generally treated conservatively but may occasionally need surgery.

- Voiding disorders, whilst not common, are a cause of urinary symptoms that it is important to recognize.

- Fistulae are rare, generally complicate gynaecological surgery, and their prompt recognition and treatment is highly appreciated by the patients.

26

Ovarian neoplasms

Epidemiology

Ovarian cancer is the most common of the gynae-cological malignancies in most industrialized countries, and the incidence is rising. In the UK there are around 5000 newly diagnosed cases each year and approximately 3700 women annually die of the disease. The overall 5-year survival is around 25%.

Ovarian cancer occurs predominantly in the fifth, sixth and seventh decades of life, with the peak age being around 75 years. There is some evidence that mortality is falling in women under the age of 50 years, raising the possibility that either they have had less exposure to some risk factor or greater exposure to some protective factor.

Natural history

Unlike cervical and endometrial cancer there is no clearly defined preinvasive ovarian lesion. Benign, borderline and invasive tumours are recognized but these are distinct pathological entities and there is little evidence of progression from one to the other (Fig. 26.1). Indeed, there is controversy about whether malignant epithelial tumours, which are the most common, arise from the ovary and then metastasize or arise as multicentric disease de novo. The multicentric theory is supported by the fact that ovarian-like tumours can arise in the peritoneum of women who have previously had both ovaries removed.

Aetiology

It is entirely possible that the different types of ovarian neoplasm have differing aetiologies particularly as germ cell tumours, which account for 25% of ovarian neoplasms, occur in much younger women than do the epithelial tumours.

Reproductive history

Reproductive history is an important determinant of epithelial ovarian cancer risk. Nulliparous women have a higher risk than parous women and the risk is inversely correlated with parity (Fig. 26.2). At present it is not clear if low parity itself predisposes to the disease or if low parity is a consequence of some other

257

Gynaecology

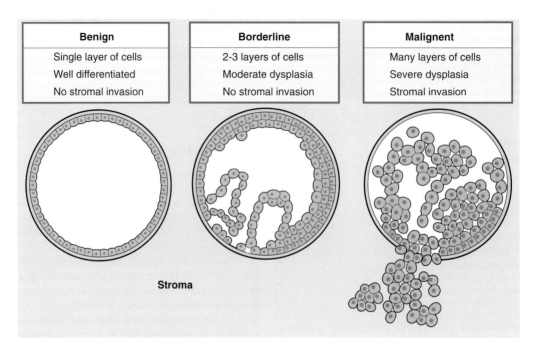

Benign	Borderline	Malignent
Single layer of cells	2-3 layers of cells	Many layers of cells
Well differentiated	Moderate dysplasia	Severe dysplasia
No stromal invasion	No stromal invasion	Stromal invasion

Stroma

Fig. 26.1 **Morphology and behaviour of surface-epithelium-derived neoplasms.**

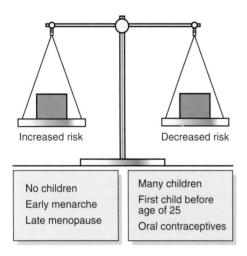

Increased risk — Decreased risk

No children	Many children
Early menarche	First child before age of 25
Late menopause	Oral contraceptives

Fig. 26.2 **Risk factors in ovarian cancer.**

factor associated with ovarian cancer risk. Some evidence suggests that subfertility may be a significant primary risk factor but the causal association and the precise mechanism remain unclear.

Exogenous oestrogens

Oral contraceptives

Overwhelming evidence now exists that women who have used the combined oral contraceptive pill at some stage in the past have a reduced risk of developing ovarian cancer. The longer the use, the lower the risk. It seems that this is a direct effect and not just due to the association between normal fertility (and hence contraceptive use) and lower risk.

Hormone replacement therapy

In postmenopausal women the effect of oestrogen replacement therapy has been investigated because of a reported increased risk in women who received diethyl stilbestrol (a non-steroidal oestrogen) early in life. The balance of evidence, however, suggests that HRT has no effect on ovarian cancer risk.

Repeated (incessant) ovulation

It has been suggested that the more often a woman ovulates, the greater the risk of ovarian carcinoma. The apparently protective effects of both pregnancy and the combined oral contraceptive pill further support this theory. The mechanism is uncertain, but it may be that repeated monthly repair of the ovarian epithelium after ovulation predisposes to malignant change. Despite this plausible theory, however, it is likely that ovarian carcinogenesis is multifactorial.

Pelvic surgery

Hysterectomy, unilateral oophorectomy and sterilization appear to reduce the risk of ovarian cancer. Since ovarian cancer is bilateral in only 25% of cases the beneficial effect of unilateral oophorectomy is not surprising. The effect of hysterectomy with ovarian conservation and the effect of sterilization are more difficult to explain. Possible mechanisms include reduced exposure to an exogenous factor as a result of occlusion of the fallopian tubes or an effect on ovarian function as a consequence of alterations in ovarian perfusion.

Genetic factors

It is now accepted that a genetic predisposition exists in at least a proportion of ovarian cancer cases. Although overall there is a slightly increased risk of ovarian cancer in those with a family history, the risk is small for most categories except for those of early onset, and those with more than one affected relative. If one affected primary relative has ovarian cancer and it was diagnosed when she was less than 50 years old, a woman's risk of developing ovarian cancer is around 5%. If there are two primary relatives under the age of 50 years with the disease, the risk is approximately 25%.

Only 5–10% of cases of ovarian carcinoma, however, have a direct genetic association. Of particular significance in this small group are the breast–ovarian cancer tumour suppressor genes *BRCA1* and *BRCA2*, as these are associated with a 10–50% lifetime risk of developing ovarian carcinoma. Mismatch repair genes associated with cancer of colorectum, endometrium, stomach, urinary tract and small bowel, are also responsible for a small proportion of this hereditary group. Women with such a history may warrant regular screening, and it is reasonable to consider bilateral oophorectomy after completion of their family. Such an operation, however, does not offer complete protection, as discussed above.

Other factors

There has been controversy about the possible role of asbestos and talcum powder in the aetiology of ovarian cancer. Insufficient evidence in the form of case-controlled studies exists to completely dismiss reported associations. Similar problems beset the assessment of smoking, diet and alcohol consumption.

Pathology

Neoplasms can arise from any of the elements that comprise a mature ovary, including its surface serosal or mesothelial elements (Fig. 26.3). A number of simpler themes can be drawn from a wide diversity of tumour types, namely: epithelial tumours, which are by far the most common (70% of primary ovarian tumours); sex cord/stromal tumours; germ cell tumours; and metastatic tumours (Table 26.1). Most of the epithelial

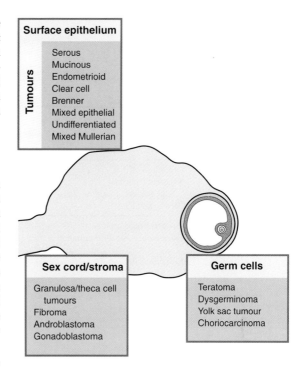

Fig. 26.3 **Ovarian neoplasms arise from three basic tissue components.**

tumour types can be further broadly classified as benign, borderline or malignant.

Borderline tumours

The term 'borderline' is reserved for tumours which display all the characteristics of malignant tumours but show no evidence of invasion. Women with borderline ovarian tumours have a much better prognosis than those with frankly malignant tumours. Nevertheless, long-term survival is by no means as high as might be expected and late recurrence up to 20 years after removal of the primary does occur. Despite lacking the features of invasion these tumours may present at an advanced stage, raising the possibility of multicentric origin.

Epithelial tumours

Serous tumours

Serous tumours are the most common ovarian neoplasm, accounting for almost 50% of ovarian cancers. They also account for 20% of all benign ovarian tumours, and these cases occur primarily in women of reproductive age. Serous cystadenomas are usually unilocular cysts, filled with straw-coloured fluid and of variable size. They are bilateral in 20% of cases. Serous cystadenocarcinomas involve both ovaries in over

Table 26.1
Pathology of ovarian tumours

Borderline		Common	Separate clinical entity; do not invade
Epithelial	Serous	Common	Benign and malignant
	Mucinous	Common	Benign and malignant; associated with pseudomyxoma peritonei
	Endometrioid	Uncommon	Usually malignant
	Clear cell	Uncommon	Usually malignant
	Urothelial like (Brenner)	Uncommon	Rarely malignant
Sex cord/stromal tumours	Granulosa cell	Rare	Low grade; often secrete sex hormones
	Thecoma/fibroma	Rare	Rarely malignant; may secrete sex hormones; Meigs' syndrome
	Sertoli/Leydig	Rare	May secrete sex hormones
Germ cell tumours	No differentiation	Rare	Dysgerminoma; may secrete hCG
	Extra-embryonic differentiation	Rare	Yolk sac tumours (endodermal sinus tumours), malignant ovarian choriocarcinoma
	Embryonic differentiation (teratoma)	Common	Mature teratomas (benign) may contain epithelium, hair, teeth and greasy white sebum; immature (malignant) are rare
Metastases		Common	Especially endometrial, gastrointestinal tract and breast

50% of cases and may have both cystic and solid components. Psammoma bodies, concentrically laminated calcified concretions, are a frequent histological finding.

Mucinous tumours

These comprise 20% of all ovarian tumours and less than 10% are malignant. Benign tumours are usually unilateral and only 20% of malignant tumours are bilateral. Mucinous tumours are usually multiloculated and contain mucinous fluid of variable viscosity. They are generally the largest of the common epithelial tumours. In less than 5% of cases, concomitant pseudo-myxoma peritonei may be present. There is characteristic gelatinous tumour within the peritoneal cavity. It is unclear to what extent pseudomyxoma peritonei truly arises from the ovary rather than from a primary mucinous tumour of the appendix.

Endometrioid tumours

Endometrioid tumours are usually malignant and closely mimic endometrial cancer in histological appearance. In around 30% of cases there is a coexistent second primary in the endometrium.

Clear cell tumours

These are virtually all malignant and may be a variant of endometrioid tumours. They are the most frequent epithelial tumour found in association with ovarian endometriosis.

Urothelial-like tumours

Urothelial-like or Brenner tumours are uncommon, usually unilateral and rarely malignant. They in part comprise epithelium of urothelial type but their main component is ovarian stroma. A rare aggressive variant is the urothelial or transitional cell carcinoma.

Sex cord/stromal tumours

Rare neoplasms, they comprise 5% of all ovarian tumours.

Granulosa cell tumours

These are functional low-grade cancers and account for around 5% of ovarian malignancies. Three-quarters secrete sex hormones, most commonly oestrogen which in turn may lead to precocious pseudopuberty, irregular menstrual bleeding or postmenopausal bleeding, depending on the age of presentation. They tend to recur late but can be monitored with serum oestradiol measurements. Characteristically they contain cells with 'coffee bean' nuclei and 'gland-like' spaces called Call–Exner, bodies, which are pathognomonic.

Thecoma/fibroma tumours

These tumours are usually unilateral and rarely malignant. They contain cells ranging from theca cells to fibroblastic-type cells. Tumours containing the former are oestrogenic although they are less common than granulosa cell tumours. Rarely, ovarian fibromas may present with non-malignant ascites and pleural effusion which resolve after removal of the tumour (Meigs' syndrome).

Sertoli/Leydig cell tumours

These are among the rarest ovarian tumours, accounting for < 1% of ovarian tumours. They occur in young women, the mean age being in the mid-20s. They are almost invariably unilateral and are commonly androgenic, though many are non-functional and only a few are oestrogenic. They contain either Sertoli cells or Leydig cells and in the case of the latter may be accompanied by stroma-derived fibroblasts.

Germ cell tumours

This heterogeneous group of tumours affects mainly children and young women and comprises 20–25% of all ovarian tumours. Around 4% are malignant. They represent the majority of ovarian tumours in children, where around a third are malignant.

Dysgerminoma

Dysgerminoma is the most common malignant germ cell tumour, comprising at least 50% of this group. Nevertheless, it is relatively uncommon and represents only 3% of all ovarian cancers. 75% occur in females aged 10–30 years, the median being 22 years, and it is the most frequently encountered ovarian malignancy in pregnancy. It is also the malignancy most likely to be associated with gonadoblastoma in gonadal dysgenesis. At least 10% are bilateral and there may be a raised serum human chorionic gonadotrophin (hCG) level.

Endodermal sinus or yolk sac tumour

This is the second most common malignant germ cell tumour of the ovary but comprises only 1% of all ovarian cancers. It rarely affects women over 40, the median age being 19 years. Presentation is commonly with a sudden onset of pelvic symptoms and a pelvic mass. Elevated serum levels of alpha-fetoprotein are found with normal hCG levels. Coexistent teratomas are found in 20% of patients.

Choriocarcinoma

These secrete hCG and may present with precocious pseudopuberty. They have a poor prognosis and do not respond well to chemotherapy (unlike uterine trophoblastic disease).

Teratoma

Teratomas characteristically contain elements from all three embryonic germ cell layers and are thought to occur via parthenogenesis, a form of reproduction in which the ovum develops without fertilization. Mature teratomas may contain epithelium, hair, teeth and greasy white sebum, and constitute 20% of all ovarian neoplasms. They are commonest in women in their 20s but account for 50% of ovarian neoplasms in females under 20 years. Malignant change, usually squamous cell, is rare (< 1%) and usually occurs in postmenopausal women.

Immature teratomas are rare, characteristically occurring in children under 15 years of age. Specialized tissue derivatives from a single germ layer are found in 3% of teratomas, notably among those with predominantly thyroid tissue (struma ovarii) and carcinoid tumours.

Metastatic tumours

Secondary tumours in the ovaries are surprisingly common. Cervical cancer only rarely metastasizes to the ovaries but spread from endometrial cancer is far more frequent. Breast cancer may also metastasize to the ovaries, and patients presenting with single or bilateral ovarian masses should be examined carefully to exclude a breast lesion.

Cancers of the gastrointestinal tract also metastasize to the ovary and in the case of gastric cancer give rise to the so-called Krukenberg tumour. This contains mucin-producing 'signet ring' adenocarcinoma cells. Such tumours may elicit a stromal response in the ovary which may result in hormone production so that virilization may be a presenting complaint. In such cases confusion with sex cord/stromal tumours is possible although these, unlike Krukenberg tumours, are usually unilateral.

Spread

Ovarian cancer spreads mainly via the peritoneal cavity, and those that die usually do so from intestinal obstruction and cachexia as a consequence of widespread intraperitoneal disease. Intrahepatic metastases and malignant pleural effusions are seen, and para-aortic lymph node metastases are found in up to 18% of cases where the disease appears otherwise to be confined to the ovary.

Presentation

Occasionally ovarian cancers are diagnosed incidentally during pelvic or abdominal palpation for another reason. This mode of presentation, however, is the exception rather than the rule. In general the symptoms are diverse and non-specific. As a result patients often do not recognize the sinister nature of their

Gynaecology

symptoms, and the disease progresses insidiously until they develop gastrointestinal complications or bowel obstruction secondary to widespread intraperitoneal malignancy.

The varied nature of these symptoms results in many cases being referred to inappropriate specialties for investigation. The most frequent complaint is abdominal distension due either to ascites or masses (Table 26.2). The most common clinical signs are an abdominal or pelvic mass and ascites (Table 26.3).

Table 26.2
Symptoms in ovarian cancer

Symptoms	% of patients
Pain	50–60
Abdominal swelling	50–65
Anorexia	20
Nausea and vomiting	20
Change in bowel habit	5
Weight loss	15
Abnormal vaginal bleeding	15
Frequency	10
Malaise	5
Virilization	Rare
Precocious puberty	Rare

Table 26.3
Signs in ovarian cancer

Sign	% of patients
Abdominal mass	60–70
Pelvic mass	70–80
Ascites	30–40
Pleural effusion	10–15
Hepatomegaly	< 5
Cervical lymphadenopathy	< 5

Box 26.1

SYNDROMES IN OVARIAN CANCER

- Dermatomyositis
- Cerebellar degeneration
- Thrombophlebitis migrans
- Hypoglycaemia
- Hyperamylasaemia
- Cushing's syndrome
- Zollinger–Ellison syndrome

Rarely, patients may present with a paraneoplastic syndrome (Box 26.1). In some cases this is due to ectopic hormone secretion and in the case of cerebellar degeneration it may be due to the production of Purkinje cell antibodies.

Investigation and staging

Having established the possibility of ovarian cancer it is necessary to confirm the diagnosis and establish disease extent (staging). This almost invariably entails a laparotomy and biopsy and is frequently combined with definitive surgical management. Ovarian cancer is staged according to the FIGO system (Table 26.4).

Before laparotomy, blood should be taken for tumour markers (see below) and for routine biochemical and haematological measurements. An intravenous urogram may be helpful in identifying whether both kidneys have normal function and anatomy. An ultra-

Table 26.4
Staging of ovarian cancer

Stage	Definition	5-year survival
I_A	One ovary	
I_B	Both ovaries	60–70% but can
I_C	I_A or I_B with ruptured capsule, tumour on the surface of the capsule, positive peritoneal washings or malignant ascites	be 95% for I_A
II_A	Extension to uterus and tubes	
II_B	Extension to other pelvic tissues, e.g. pelvic nodes, pouch of Douglas	30%
II_C	II_A or II_B with ruptured capsule, positive peritoneal washings or malignant ascites	
III_A	Pelvic tumour with microscopic peritoneal spread	
III_B	Pelvic tumour with peritoneal spread < 2 cm	10%
III_C	Abdominal implants > 2 cm ± positive retroperitoneal or inguinal nodes (Fig. 26.5)	
IV	Liver parenchymal disease. Distant metastases. If pleural effusion, must have malignant cells	10%

sound or CT scan may help differentiate ovarian masses with solid and cystic areas, which are likely to be malignant particularly in older women, from simple ovarian cysts and uterine fibroids. Scanning is also a sensitive method of detecting ascites. A chest X-ray will exclude metastases and pleural effusions.

Tumour markers

Around 80% of malignant ovarian masses are associated with elevated levels of CA125, and this marker may be of value in monitoring the response to therapy and to help identify presymptomatic disease during follow-up. CA125 may also be elevated in the serum of women with benign conditions, such as endometriosis, or where peritoneal trauma has taken place. A positive result therefore, while suggestive of ovarian cancer, is not pathognomonic. Conversely a negative result for tumour markers does not exclude a diagnosis of ovarian cancer.

About 65% of ovarian germ cell tumours produce elevated serum levels of hCG, alpha-fetoprotein or both. These markers can again, if elevated, be very useful in monitoring response to therapy and in detecting tumour recurrence after completion of therapy.

Treatment

Benign tumours

Benign tumours merely require either simple excision or possibly drainage under laparoscopic control. There are problems, however, in deciding whether a cyst is clinically benign or malignant. In general ovarian cysts in young women tend to be benign and the risk of malignancy increases with age. A cyst is often assumed at surgery to be benign if it is unilateral and unilocular with smooth external and internal surfaces and no solid elements (Figs 26.4 and 26.5). Although not conforming to this rule, teratomas are benign and the diagnosis is usually obvious when they are opened after removal.

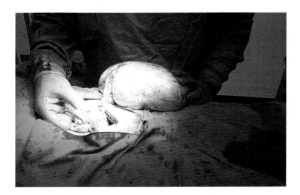

Fig. 26.4 **A unilateral benign cystadenoma.**

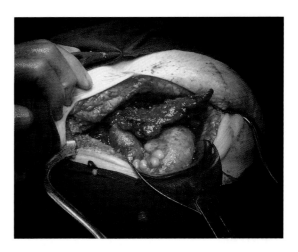

Fig. 26.5 **The omentum in this stage III$_C$ cystadenocarcinoma is almost completely replaced with tumour.** Optimal debulking was not achieved.

Epithelial cancers

The mainstays of treatment for epithelial cancer are radical surgical debulking of the tumour followed by platinum-based chemotherapy (cisplatin or carboplatin). This is given either as a single agent or as a part of a combination which may include one of the taxanes, an extract of the bark of the Pacific Yew tree. Chemotherapy is thought to be appropriate for epithelial tumours if the staging is more than I$_A$, or for those with poorly differentiated I$_A$ disease.

In young women who wish fertility to be preserved, and in whom the disease appears confined to one ovary, it is reasonable to consider conservative surgery. The other ovary and omentum, a common site for metastases, should be biopsied and a thorough inspection made of all peritoneal surfaces. In all other instances an attempt should be made to excise all tumour deposits, since complete removal is associated with a better prognosis. This will usually involve hysterectomy and bilateral oophorectomy, and occasionally includes bowel resection and a defunctioning colostomy.

As the disease presents at a late stage in most cases, complete excision is frequently not possible and surgery is therefore palliative.

Non-epithelial tumours

These tumours frequently occur in young women where preservation of fertility is an important consideration. It is also clear that many of these tumours, especially those of germ cell origin, are exquisitely sensitive to chemotherapy, and radical surgery is therefore inappropriate. Extremely good survival can be achieved with limited surgery and subsequent combination chemotherapy.

Recurrent disease

Most women with advanced epithelial ovarian cancer relapse after primary management. There is considerable potential for palliative therapy in such instances. New chemotherapeutic agents have traditionally been first evaluated in such patients, but if a patient is offered palliative experimental chemotherapy in this way it is vitally important to consider the side-effects as these can considerably impair a patient's quality of life. If relapse occurs more than a year after platinum-based chemotherapy the disease will often respond again and patients may gain useful palliation in this way.

Survival

Overall 5-year survival (all stages) is in the order of 25% (Table 26.4), a figure which has remained unaltered for many years. A better prognosis can be expected for women with malignant germ cell tumours, where the reported 5-year survival from most studies is in excess of 75%.

The only real prospect for improving survival in epithelial cancers is either detection at an early stage or development of better chemotherapy. Screening is still the subject of research, with trials involving the combination of tumour markers (such as CA125) and ultrasound. At present it seems unlikely that screening and early detection of low-risk groups is going to be a useful proposition.

Key points

- Ovarian cancer is the commonest gynaecological cancer. The incidence is increasing with around 5000 newly diagnosed cases each year in the UK. The 5-year survival is about 25%.

- Unlike cervical cancer, there is no premalignant stage and most new cases present with advanced disease (stage III or IV).

- Genetic factors have been identified (e.g. the *BRCA1* and *BRCA2* tumour suppressor genes) which identify a small proportion of women at risk. Other risk factors include low parity. Use of the oral contraceptive pill protects against ovarian cancer.

- Presentation is usually with pelvic mass, malaise and weight loss. Treatment is primarily surgical, although advances have been seen recently in chemotherapy, particularly with platinum-based drugs and the taxanes.

- Management strategies are directed towards earlier diagnosis and improved chemotherapies. Those considered to be at high risk of developing ovarian cancer should have screening with pelvic ultrasound and CA125 blood tests. Currently available tests do not fulfil the criteria for a screening programme aimed at low-risk women.

Uterine cancer

Definition

The uterus consists of both the cervix and the body (or 'corpus' of the uterus). For many reasons, however, including their causative factors and their treatment, tumours arising from the corpus and the cervix are usually regarded as originating from two separate organs. This chapter will consider cancers arising from the uterine body; cancers arising from the cervix are discussed in Chapter 29.

The majority of malignancies arising from the uterine body emanate from the endometrium. The endometrium consists of glandular and supporting (or 'stromal') elements and it is possible for either to undergo malignant change. The majority of uterine malignancies are adenocarcinomas arising from the endometrial glands (Figs 27.1 and 27.2a). Sarcomas of the muscle of the uterus, the myometrium or the stromal tissues of the endometrium are very much rarer (Fig. 27.2b).

Incidence

Endometrial cancer is the second most common gynaecological malignancy after cancer of the ovary and there are approximately 4000 new cases per year diagnosed in England and Wales. Its incidence is low in women less 40 years of age (under 2 per 100 000) but rises rapidly between the ages of 40 and 55 years, levelling off after the menopause to around 44 per 100 000.

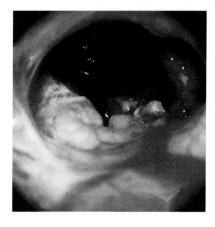

Fig. 27.1 **A hysteroscopic view of an endometrial carcinoma arising from the posterior uterine wall.** (Courtesy of Karl Storz Endoscopy (UK) Ltd.)

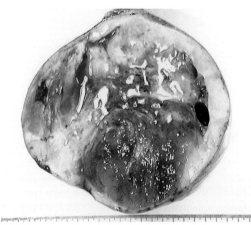

(a)

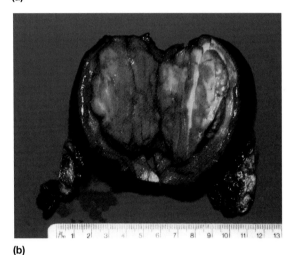

(b)

Fig. 27.2 **Macroscopic picture of (a) endometrial carcinoma and (b) endometrial sarcoma.** (Courtesy of Dr N Wilkinson, Department of Pathology, Leeds.)

Approximately 5% of endometrial carcinomas will develop in women under the age of 40 and 20–25% will be diagnosed before the menopause. There is evidence that the incidence is rising in developed countries.

Aetiology

The majority of endometrial cancers are associated with conditions in which there are relatively, rather than absolutely, high levels of oestrogen production and it is therefore postulated that oestrogen has a role in the development of the disease (Box 27.1).

High levels of oestrogen may be physiological, as with obesity (due to the aromatization in body fat of peripheral androgens to oestrogens), nulliparity (due to anovulation) and late menopause. The relationship between diabetes, hypertension and endometrial cancer

---

Box 27.1

RISK FACTORS FOR ENDOMETRIAL CARCINOMA

Increase risk

- Obesity, especially upper body obesity
- Nulliparity
- Late menopause
- Unopposed oestrogen therapy, including tamoxifen
- Oestrogen-secreting tumours (granulosa/theca cell ovarian tumours)
- Carbohydrate intolerance
- Polycystic ovary syndrome
- Personal history of breast or colon cancer
- Family history of breast, colon or endometrial cancer

Decrease risk

- The combined oral contraceptive pill
- Progestogens

---

is a result of increased incidence of obesity in these groups of women. Non-physiological causes of increased oestrogen include unopposed oestrogen hormone replacement therapy (HRT) which increases the risk fourfold. This risk is reduced to a relative risk of less than 1.0 with opposed HRT (i.e. with the addition of progestogen for at least 10 days per cycle). The levonorgestrel-releasing intrauterine system (Mirena) protects the endometrium effectively when used in conjunction with oestrogen-only HRT in postmenopausal women. Oestrogen-secreting tumours, which are rare, also increase the risk of endometrial carcinoma.

Endometrial cancer is also seen less frequently in women who have used the combined oral contraceptive pill, probably because it administers progestogens throughout the cycle. Women who smoke, and are therefore likely to reach an earlier menopause, also have a lower than expected incidence of the disease.

The more common and oestrogen-dependent type of endometrial cancer is sometimes called type I disease and is seen in women around the time of the menopause or soon after. It is generally diagnosed at an earlier stage and as a result has a better prognosis. There may be premalignant change (see 'Endometrial hyperplasia' below) and the tumour cells of type I disease usually have oestrogen and progesterone receptors. This form of the cancer has characteristic growth factor alterations which distinguish it from normal endometrium.

Type II endometrial cancer is probably not related to oestrogen production. It is seen in older women, progresses more rapidly, and is not associated with a hyperplastic or in situ phase. The chances of surviving 5 years with this type of cancer are considerably lower than for the type I form, even with early-stage disease.

Clinical features and diagnosis

Abnormal uterine bleeding is the cardinal symptom of endometrial carcinoma. The bleeding is most commonly postmenopausal, and women with this symptom should be regarded as having malignancy until proven otherwise. Around 10% of women with postmenopausal bleeding will have a primary or secondary malignancy, most commonly endometrial cancer (80%), cervical cancer, or (rarely) an ovarian tumour. As the condition can occur in premenopausal women, any irregular uterine bleeding in those over 40 years of age should also be investigated.

A less common mode of presentation in the postmenopausal group is that of vaginal discharge – either blood stained, watery or purulent. Pain is rarely associated with early disease and usually indicates late spread to involve bone or nerve roots. Endometrial carcinoma can also present with abnormal cells on a smear consistent with endometrial origin.

There are four main methods of investigation as listed below. The method chosen depends on the patient's risk factors and the local facilities.

Hysteroscopy   The inside of the uterine cavity can be visualized directly using a hysteroscope, which can be introduced with or without anaesthesia depending on the instrument and the local arrangements (Fig. 27.1). Biopsy or curettage (see below) can also be performed at the same time. Hysteroscopy with biopsy is considered to be the 'gold standard' investigation.

Dilatation and curettage   This is usually carried out under general anaesthesia. The cervix is dilated sufficiently to allow the introduction of a sharp curette, which is used to sample the endometrium. Used alone this will miss around 10% of endometrial cancers.

Endometrial biopsy   An outpatient biopsy can be obtained using one of a number of samplers, for example the Pipelle (Fig. 19.5), or the Vabra aspirator. These are both 3 mm in diameter, the Pipelle being a thin plastic tube and the Vabra a stainless steel device attached to an electrical suction pump. The Pipelle is the most convenient, best tolerated and least expensive, but samples only around 4% of the endometrial surface and will miss around a third of tumours. The Vabra samples around 40% of the endometrial surface and picks up more tumours, but is more painful and more expensive.

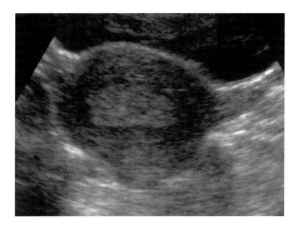

Fig. 27.3 **Ultrasound of endometrium, with thickness measuring 10 mm.** Endometrial carcinoma is very unlikely if the postmenopausal thickness is less than 4 mm. (Courtesy of Dr M Weston, Department of Radiology, St James's Hospital, Leeds.)

In view of the relatively high false negative rates, endometrial biopsy alone is appropriate only for those at relatively low risk of carcinoma.

Ultrasound   Transvaginal scanning can be used to measure the endometrial thickness in postmenopausal women (Fig. 27.3). If the thickness is less than 4 mm, endometrial cancer is very unlikely. Fluid in the endometrial cavity on ultrasound in these women is associated with malignancy in 25% of cases.

Pathology

Endometrial pathology can be divided into hyperplasia, carcinoma or sarcoma.

Endometrial hyperplasia

Endometrial hyperplasia is a potentially premalignant condition which is thought to result from persistent and prolonged oestrogenic stimulation of the endometrium. The nomenclature of this condition is confusing and the terms simple hyperplasia, glandular hyperplasia, cystic glandular hyperplasia and endometrial hyperplasia are synonymous. Complex hyperplasia (previously known as adenomatous hyperplasia) can occur with or without cytological atypia. The atypia may be severe enough to create difficulty in distinguishing the hyperplastic state from a well-differentiated carcinoma.

To diagnose hyperplasia histologically, there should be an increase in the glands-to-stromal ratio. The glands may vary in size and shape or they may branch abnormally. Cytological atypia includes a loss of polarity of cells within the glands, an increase in the nuclear–cytoplasmic ratio and nuclear irregularity with hyperchromatic changes, chromatin clumping and prominent nucleoli. This atypia is the only feature distinguishing benign endometrial lesions from those with invasive potential.

Simple hyperplasia often occurs in anovulatory teenagers and in the perimenopausal years. Atypical hyperplasia coexists with endometrial carcinoma in 25–50% of cases, and many will progress to carcinoma. This progression depends on the severity of atypia and it is thought that about 20% will develop carcinoma within 10 years.

Hyperplasia is usually discovered by endometrial biopsy as part of the investigation of abnormal uterine bleeding. There are no other symptoms or physical signs. It is common to treat hyperplasia with progestogens in young women but to consider hysterectomy, particularly if there are atypical changes, in those who have completed their family.

Endometrial carcinoma

Endometrial adenocarcinoma can have a variety of histological appearances depending upon whether it is purely glandular, or has areas of squamous differentiation (which may appear malignant or benign), or whether it demonstrates a papillary or clear cell pattern. The latter two forms are associated with a poorer prognosis.

Endometrial sarcoma

Endometrial sarcoma is very rare.

Prognostic factors

Endometrial cancer is falsely regarded as a less aggressive tumour than other gynaecological malignancies but this is simply because it more commonly presents at an earlier stage (Table 27.1). Stage for stage, endometrial cancer has a prognosis similar to that of cancer of the ovary.

There are many factors that affect the prognosis, the most obvious being the stage of disease. This is an indication of how far the cancer has spread as well as of how aggressive the tumour is. The histological type of endometrial cancer is also important. Papillary serous cancer, which is more common in older women, spreads in a manner similar to cancer of the ovary and, as noted above, is associated with a significantly poorer prognosis. Other factors which affect the prognosis are outlined in Box 27.2.

Treatment

Endometrial carcinoma is staged using the FIGO scheme (Table 27.1). This is a surgico-pathological system based on the histology results from the excised

---

Box 27.2

PROGNOSTIC FACTORS IN ENDOMETRIAL CANCER

- Histological type
- Histological differentiation
- Stage of disease
- Myometrial invasion
- Peritoneal cytology
- Lymph node metastasis
- Adnexal metastasis

---

uterus, tubes, ovaries and lymph nodes and the results of peritoneal cytology. Before operation, however, in addition to any usual preoperative investigations, the patient should have a chest X-ray and liver function tests to look for evidence of metastases.

Other possible preoperative investigations to search for metastases include ultrasound scan and magnetic resonance imaging (MRI). Ultrasound examination can determine the size of the tumour and predict the presence of myometrial invasion. It is also useful in determining the presence of advanced disease. MRI, which is becoming more commonly used, is able to assess the condition of the myometrium more specifically and also to determine the extent of myometrial invasion. More importantly, MRI may be used to determine whether the cervix has been invaded by the tumour (Fig. 27.4). If there is no cervical involvement a staging laparotomy may be carried out.

In addition to a hysterectomy and bilateral salpingo-oophorectomy, there is considerable debate as to whether the pelvic lymph nodes should be removed, sampled or left alone. Any of these strategies is acceptable and none is mandatory. Nevertheless it would seem sensible to have at least some idea if there is a risk of retroperitoneal disease, although the risk of this can be predicted from other risk factors such as tumour grade and depth of myometrial invasion. As with any tumour the more lymph nodes which are removed the more likely it is that metastases will be found. There are, however, potential complications to lymphadenectomy and the risks of surgery should be weighed against the benefits. If the tumour is of high grade, or there is deep myometrial invasion, extrapelvic spread is more likely and a surgical assessment of the para-aortic lymph nodes may be appropriate.

If the disease has spread to the cervix and no obvious disease is present elsewhere, a radical hysterectomy is

Table 27.1
FIGO staging of endometrial carcinoma

Stage	Definition	Stage at presentation	Pelvic nodes	5-year survival
I$_A$	Tumour limited to the endometrium			
I$_B$	Growth that has invaded < 50% of myometrial thickness	73%	< 20%	85%
I$_C$	Growth that has invaded > 50% of myometrial thickness			
II$_A$	Endocervical glandular involvement only	11%	20%	65%
II$_B$	Cervical stroma involved			
III$_A$	Invades sero-serosal surface of uterus, ± adnexa, ± positive washings			
III$_B$	Vaginal metastases	13%	35%	40%
III$_C$	Metastases to pelvic or para-aortic nodes			
IV$_A$	Tumour invasion of bladder and/or bowel	3%	50%	10%
IV$_B$	Distant metastases including intra-abdominal and/or inguinal lymph nodes			

Histopathology: degree of differentiation
Uterine adenocarcinoma should be grouped according to the degree of differentiation as follows:

G1 – 5% or less of a solid growth pattern
G2 – 6–50% of a solid growth pattern
G3 – More than 50% of a solid growth pattern

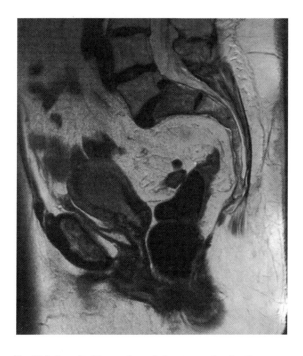

Fig. 27.4 **A sagittal image through the uterus showing the endometrial cavity distended by tumour.** The tumour extends into the endocervical canal and is invasive posteriorly at the fundus. (Courtesy of Dr S Swift, Department of Radiology, St James's Hospital, Leeds)

indicated. The difference between a radical and a simple hysterectomy is the amount of paracervical disease which is removed. A radical hysterectomy removes tissue adjacent to the cervix, the parametrium, and the proximal uterosacral and cardinal ligaments. In a simple hysterectomy the plane of excision is close to the cervix.

If, during the preoperative investigations or at the time of laparotomy, the disease is discovered to have spread beyond the uterus, treatment should be individualized. Treatment of disease in the fallopian tubes or ovaries is relatively easy to manage and for stage III disease has a relatively good prognosis. More widespread tumour, however, should be managed depending on the degree and location of spread and the condition of the patient.

The treatment of those with endometrial cancer after surgery is related to the stage of the disease (Table 27.1). Radiotherapy may be used as adjuvant (postoperative) treatment if the tumour invades the myometrium deeply, as there is a high risk of extrauterine disease. Local radiotherapy to the vault of the vagina (brachytherapy) may prevent recurrence developing in this area. Radiotherapy to the whole pelvis (teletherapy) will also prevent local disease recurring in this area, but surprisingly, does not improve overall survival.

Radiotherapy may be used for local disease if the patient is medically unfit for major surgery. Heyman's capsules are pellets containing radioactive material which are passed into the uterus through the cervix and allow local radiotherapy to be applied directly to the tumour (Fig. 27.5). For more advanced lesions, whole pelvic radiotherapy may be used.

If disease is widespread, chemotherapy may be considered. The drugs most helpful in this situation are cisplatinum and doxorubicin. Once again their influence on survival is controversial as response rates to measurable disease are only of the order of 20%.

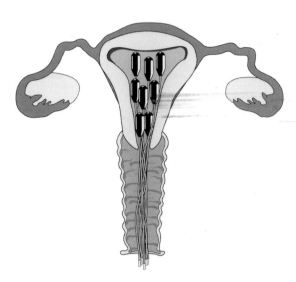

Fig. 27.5 **Heyman's capsules in the uterus.** The applicators contain an Iridium-192 source. (Courtesy of Medical Illustration at Cookridge Hospital, Leeds.)

Recurrence

Most relapses occur early (i.e. within 2 years of primary treatment). Recurrences are commonest in the lungs, bone, vagina, liver, inguinal and supraclavicular nodes. It should be remembered that 80% of those with recurrent disease will die within 2 years, and care should be taken to maximize the quality of life over this time rather than subject the patient to treatments with high morbidity and a slim chance of success.

Those with a recurrence who have not received radiotherapy should be considered for this treatment. For the remainder, the choice is between hormonal therapy and chemotherapy. The main hormonal option is high-dose progestogens which may give a response in around 30% of patients. Chemotherapy can produce tumour shrinkage in some cases but toxicity is considerable, not least because these patients are often frail and have severe coexistent medical disorders.

Summary

Endometrial cancer is often considered to be easily treatable but stage for stage its survival approximates that of ovarian cancer. It is fortunate that most women present with postmenopausal bleeding in the early stages of the disease.

To ensure the best possible outcome, women who present with bleeding 6 months or more after their last menstrual period should be referred urgently for a gynaecological opinion. From there, referral to a cancer centre specializing in the treatment of gynaecological cancer is likely to be beneficial.

> ### Key points
>
> - Endometrial cancer is the third most common gynaecological cancer after cancer of the ovary and cervix and is generally a postmenopausal disease.
>
> - The aetiology is not fully known, but exposure to unopposed oestrogens is known to increase the risk of developing the disease. Unfortunately, because the disease does not have a long premalignant phase and the sampling can be difficult, it is not suitable for a screening programme.
>
> - Endometrial cancer classically presents with postmenopausal bleeding or irregular premenopausal bleeding. Less commonly the presentation can be with vaginal discharge.
>
> - Diagnosis is made by biopsy of the endometrium. The cavity can be directly visualized with a hysteroscope, and the tissue sampled by curettage or using an outpatient sampling device. Postmenopausally, endometrial carcinoma is very unlikely if the transvaginal endometrial thickness is less than 4 mm.
>
> - Treatment is generally surgical (hysterectomy and removal of the ovaries), and in some cases lymphadenectomy may be advisable. In advanced or recurrent disease, radiotherapy is the treatment of choice.

28

Disorders of the vulva

Introduction

The vulva consists of the mons pubis, labia majora, labia minora, clitoris and the vestibule. It is covered with keratinizing squamous epithelium, unlike the vaginal mucosa which is covered with non-keratinizing squamous epithelium. The labia majora are hair-bearing and contain sweat and sebaceous glands: from an embryological viewpoint, they are analogous to the scrotum. Bartholin's glands are situated in the posterior part of the labia, one on each side of the vestibule. The lymphatics of the vulva drain to the inguinal nodes and then to the external iliac nodes. The area is richly supplied with blood vessels.

Examination of the vulva

Before direct examination of the vulva, a general dermatological examination may be useful, particularly:

- the nail beds for signs of pitting (found in psoriasis)
- the extensor surfaces (elbows and knees) also for features of psoriasis
- the flexor surfaces for lichen planus and dermatitis
- the mouth for other features of lichen planus.

The vulva may than be inspected under a good light as described on page 89. Closer inspection is possible using the colposcope.

Simple vulval conditions

Urethral caruncle

A urethral caruncle is a polypoidal outgrowth from the edge of the urethra which is most commonly seen after the menopause. The tissue is soft, red, smooth and appears as an eversion of the urethral mucosa. Most women are asymptomatic but others experience dysuria, frequency, urgency and focal tenderness. If there are any suspicious features, an excision and biopsy may be required to exclude the very rare possibility of a urethral carcinoma.

Bartholin's cysts

The greater vestibular, or Bartholin's, glands lie in the subcutaneous tissue below the lower third of the labium

271

Gynaecology

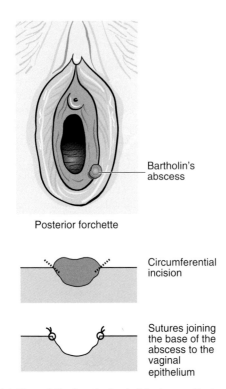

Bartholin's abscess

Posterior forchette

Circumferential incision

Sutures joining the base of the abscess to the vaginal epithelium

Fig. 28.1 **Marsupialization of a Bartholin's abscess.** The lower part of the abscess cavity granulates and heals during the subsequent weeks. (From Pitkin et al 2003.)

majorum and open via ducts to the vestibule between the hymenal orifice and the labia minora. They secrete mucus, particularly at the time of intercourse. If the duct becomes blocked a tense retention cyst forms and, if there is superadded infection, a painful abscess develops. The abscess can be incised and drained, usually under general anaesthesia, with the incision on the inner aspect of the labium so that secretions bathe the introitus rather than the outside of the vulva. To prevent the cyst reforming, the fistula is kept open by suturing its edges to the surrounding skin, a procedure known as marsupialization (Fig. 28.1). Bartholin's gland carcinoma is rare.

Small cysts

The commonest small vulval cysts are usually either inclusion cysts or sebaceous cysts. Inclusion cysts form because epithelium is trapped in the epidermis, usually following obstetric trauma or episiotomy. They are usually asymptomatic and need no treatment. Sebaceous cysts are usually multiple, mobile, non-tender, white or yellow, filled with a cottage cheese-like substance and more common in the anterior half of the vulva. Excision may be requested by the patient.

Cysts in an episiotomy scar can be tender and need excision. Infected cysts need to be excised and drained,

and recurrent infections should be treated by excision in their non-acute phase.

Moles

Vulval moles are usually asymptomatic but become more pigmented at puberty. Any other change in a vulval naevus is an indication for removal. There is a good case to be made for removing all vulval moles as approximately 10% of malignant melanomas in women arise from the vulva.

Fibroma, lipoma, hydradenoma

Fibromas and lipomas are benign, mobile tumours of fibrous tissue and fat respectively. Hidradenomas are rare tumours of sweat glands near the surface of the labia. All are benign but the diagnosis is usually only made once they have been excised.

Haematoma

The commonest cause of a vulval haematoma is vaginal delivery. It may also occur following any vulval operation, or by 'falling astride' accidents, particularly in children. The possibility of sexual assault should be borne in mind in this situation. Vulval haematomas usually present with severe pain, and evacuation under general anaesthesia is often required.

Simple atrophy

Elderly women develop vaginal, vulval and clitoral atrophy as part of the normal ageing process of skin. In severe cases the thin vulval skin, terminal urethra and fourchette cause dysuria and superficial dyspareunia. The labia minora fuse and bury the clitoris. Introital stenoses can make coitus impossible. A simple effective moisturizer rubbed into the vulva is effective, although some advocate topical oestrogen replacement. There is a small amount of systemic absorption with topical therapy and, if this route is chosen, treatment should be for no more that 2 or 3 months without either a break or a short course of progesterone to prevent endometrial stimulation.

Ulcers

These may be:

● aphthous (yellow base)
● herpetic (exquisitely painful multiple ulceration, p. 202)
● syphilitic (indurated and painless, p. 204)
● associated with Crohn's disease ('like knife cuts in skin')
● a feature of Behçet's syndrome (a chronic painful condition with aphthous genital and ocular ulceration)

- malignant (see below)
- associated with lichen planus (see below) or Stevens–Johnson syndrome
- tropical (lymphogranuloma venereum, chancroid, granuloma inguinale).

Treatment depends on the cause. The management of Behçet's syndrome is difficult, but the combined oral contraceptive or topical steroids may be tried.

Infection

Candida, vulval warts, herpes, lymphogranuloma venereum, scabies, granuloma inguinale, tinea, chancroid and syphilis are discussed in Chapter 18.

Hidradenitis suppurativa is a chronic unrelenting infection of the sweat glands. The glands become obstructed and chronic inflammation follows. Long-term antibiotics reduce further attacks but the only cure is local excision.

Dermatoses

Vulval 'dystrophy' is an abnormality of vulval epithelium. Epithelial growth may be hypoplastic, hyperplastic or abnormal in some other way.

Lichen sclerosis

This chronic and recurrent condition can present at any age, but is more common in the older patient and usually presents with pruritus. Less commonly presentation is with dyspareunia or pain. It is an auto-immune condition and there is an association with other autoimmune disorders, including pernicious anaemia, thyroid disease, diabetes mellitus, SLE, primary biliary cirrhosis and bullous pemphygoid. Histologically the epidermis appears thin, with loss of rete ridges. The superficial dermis is hyalinized and a band of chronic inflammatory cells is seen beneath it.

Clinically the skin appears white, thin and crinkly but may be thickened and keratotic if there is coexistent squamous cell hyperplasia (Fig. 28.2). There may also be clitoral or labial adhesions. Diagnosis is by biopsy. Lichen sclerosis is non-neoplastic but may coexist with vulval intraepithelial neoplasia and there is an association with subsequent development of vulval squamous cell carcinoma in 2–5% of cases. Long term 6- to 12-monthly follow-up is probably therefore warranted.

Treatment is required particularly if the condition is symptomatic, and initially is usually with a potent topical steroid cream (e.g. Dermovate b.d.), reducing gradually to a milder preparation (e.g. hydrocortisone b.d., o.d. or less) as symptoms require. Eosin paint or testosterone ointment may also be of help. Vulvectomy

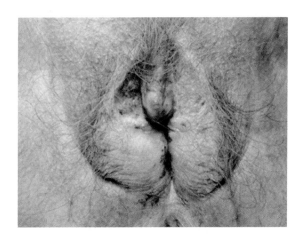

Fig. 28.2 **Lichen sclerosus.** The skin is white, with some reddened areas, and adhesions have significantly narrowed the introitus.

has no role, the recurrence rate after surgery being around 50%.

Squamous cell hyperplasia

Squamous epithelial hyperplasia is characterized by thickened hyperkeratotic skin with white, itchy plaques. Pruritus is usually severe. Diagnosis is again by biopsy, and treatment is as for 'lichen sclerosis'.

Other dermatoses
Allergic/irritant dermatosis

The vulval skin, especially the introitus, is not uncommonly affected by dermatitis. The dermatitis is either due to an irritant (non-immunological) or a true allergy (immunological aetiology). The chemicals causing hypersensitivity of the vulval skin include cosmetics, perfumes, contraceptive lubricants, sprays and douches. Detergents, dyes, softeners, bleaches, soaps and chlorine used to clean undergarments can also cause irritation. In severe cases hypersensitivity may develop to local anaesthetic creams and even steroid preparations.

Women with contact dermatitis have a red inflamed vulva with features of eczema, and patch testing may identify local irritants. Temporary relief may be obtained with vulval moisturizers (e.g. Emulsiderm in a daily bath), emollients (e.g. topical aqueous cream) and topical corticosteroids (e.g. a month's course of topical Dermovate). As before, lesions that do not respond should be biopsied to confirm the diagnosis.

Psoriasis

Psoriasis manifests as a dry red papular rash that is usually well circumscribed and extends to the thigh. The diagnosis is easier to make if bleeding occurs when

Gynaecology

the classic silvery scales are removed. Because the vulva is often moist, it is often difficult to distinguish psoriasis from candida infection or dermatitis. Candida should be excluded. The lesions may be treated topically with coal tar preparations, ultraviolet light, steroid creams or other suitable formulations.

Intertrigo with candida

Intertrigo refers to a moist inflammatory dermatitis which can occur in any body fold because of apposition and chafing of skin surfaces. Skin folds are more likely to rub together in those who are overweight and in those who use occlusive clothing.

The skin is sore, macerated and often red, inflamed and cracked. Weight loss, local hygiene, and ventilation should be encouraged, for example the use of stockings and cotton underclothes rather than tights and nylon pants. Dusting powder (e.g. talcum powder), astringents (e.g. zinc) or barrier preparations may also be helpful.

Candida often complicates intertrigo and should be treated as on page 200. Providing there is no candidal infection, steroid creams may be used to relieve inflammation.

Lichen planus

Lichen planus is a chronic papular rash with a dark blue hue, involving the vulva and flexor surfaces. It can affect other flexor surfaces and oral mucous membranes, and the diagnosis is supported by the finding of other lesions. It is usually idiopathic, but can be drug related. Treatment is with potent topical steroids or ultraviolet light, and it tends to resolve within 2 years. Surgery should be avoided.

Pruritus

Pruritus describes an intense itching with a desire to scratch. It is commoner in those aged over 40 years, and symptoms are often most severe under times of stress or depression. There are numerous aetiologies (Box. 28.1).

A biopsy may be necessary to establish the diagnosis and patch testing may be of help. If no cause is found, it may be worth considering the possibility of previous sexual abuse or psychosexual problems.

It is important to break the scratch/itch cycle and strong short-term topical steroids will reduce the local inflammation caused by scratching. Irritants and bath water additives should be avoided, soap substitutes used, the area dried gently (e.g. with a hairdryer), loose cotton clothing worn and nylon tights avoided. A strong steroid cream b.d. for 3 weeks followed by hydrocortisone cream 1% daily as maintenance is useful, as is the use of soap substitutes (e.g. Oilatum). Antihistamines may also be of help. Primary or secondary depression may also warrant treatment.

Box 28.1

CAUSES OF PRURITUS VULVAE

- Infection (candida, pediculosis, thread worms)
- Eczema
- Dermatitis (consider patch testing)
- Irritation from a vaginal discharge
- Lichen sclerosis
- Lichen planus
- Vulval intraepithelial neoplasia (VIN)
- Vulval carcinoma
- Medical problems, e.g. diabetes mellitus, uraemia or liver failure
- Psychogenic

Vulvodynia

This is chronic vulvar discomfort, especially that characterized by the complaint of burning, stinging, irritation or rawness. There may also be pruritus. No one factor can be identified as the specific cause, and indeed there appear to be no clinically definable differences between groups of patients. It may also occasionally be associated with previous sexual abuse. There may be a response to low-dose tricyclic antidepressants (e.g. amitriptyline).

Vulvar vestibulitis is a chronic clinical syndrome with erythema, severe pain on entry or to vestibular touch, and tenderness to pressure localized within the vestibule. If symptoms are of less than 3 months' duration there is often response to topical corticosteroids. If the condition is chronic, treatment is empirical and symptomatic, with vestibular resection being considered only as a last resort.

Vulval intraepithelial neoplasia (VIN)

Vulval intraepithelial neoplasia refers to the presence of neoplastic cells within the confines of the vulval epithelium. There are three types of VIN: squamous; melanoma in situ; and non-squamous.

Squamous VIN (Bowen's disease, Bowenoid papulosis)

This is classified as grade I, II or III depending on the severity, and it is considered, much like with cervical

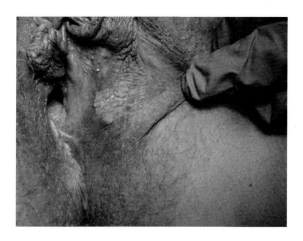

Fig. 28.3 **Squamous VIN 3 of the left labia majora.** In this case the lesion is rough surfaced, not unlike the appearance of wart virus infection, but lesions are also commonly macular with indistinct borders.

intraepithelial neoplasia (CIN), that the human papilloma virus may be important in the aetiology. Many are asymptomatic, although pruritus is present in perhaps one- to two-thirds and pain is an occasional feature. Lesions may be papular and rough surfaced, resembling warts (Fig. 28.3), or macular with indistinct borders. White lesions represent hyperkeratosis, and pigmentation is common. The lesions tend to be multifocal in women under 40 and unifocal in the postmenopausal age group.

Diagnosis is by biopsy which may be taken at vulvoscopy, using 5% acetic acid as at colposcopy, under either local or general anaesthesia. The opportunity should be taken to look at the cervix at the same time as there is an association with CIN. As the natural history is so uncertain, treatment is controversial. Regression has been observed (particularly with low-grade VIN) but progression of high-grade VIN to invasion may occur in approximately 5% of cases, and up to 15% of those with VIN III may have superficial invading vulval cancer.

Treatment of VIN may be indicated in those over the age of 45, those who are immunosuppressed and those with multifocal lower genital tract neoplasia. Such treatments include surgical excision, Nd-YAG laser therapy or imiquimod cream (Aldara).

Melanoma in situ

This is uncommon.

Non-squamous VIN (Paget's disease)

This is also uncommon. There is a poorly demarcated, often multifocal, eczematoid lesion associated in 25% with adenocarcinoma either in the pelvis or at a distant site. Treatment is by wide local excision.

Vulval carcinoma

Squamous cell carcinoma accounts for 90% of vulval cancers. Approximately 5% of vulval malignancies are malignant melanomas and the others include Bartholin's gland cancer, basal cell carcinomas and sarcomas. It is usually a disease of older women (60+ years) and, like cervical cancer, is commoner in cigarette smokers and women who are immunocompromised.

Clinical presentation

Most women will present with a history of long-standing vulval irritation or pruritus, and some will have had a previous history of lichen sclerosus. A lump or ulcer is common (Fig. 28.4). As the disease advances, the tumour grows and focal necrosis may cause discharge and pain. The diagnosis is confirmed by histological examination of a biopsy.

Pathophysiology

Squamous cell carcinoma spreads to the inguinal nodes and from there to the external iliac nodes in the pelvis (Table 28.1). Unless the lesion has only penetrated the basement membrane by < 1 mm, node involvement is common and may include both the superficial and deep inguinal lymph node systems. Clitoral lesions have extensive lymphatic drainage and cells may embolize along the inferior vesical vessels and drain directly to the internal iliac nodes.

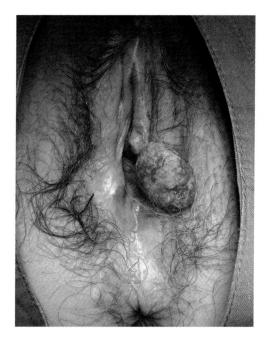

Fig. 28.4 **A stage II left-sided squamous vulval carcinoma.**

Table 28.1
FIGO staging of vulval carcinoma

Stage	Definition
I$_A$	Tumour less than 2.0 cm in dimension and less than 1 mm of stromal invasion. No lymph vascular space invasion (LVSI) and no nodal disease
I$_B$	Tumour less than 2.0 cm in dimension but with more than 1 mm of stromal invasion
II	Tumour of more than 2.0 cm dimension confined to vulva or perineum with negative nodes
III	Tumour of any size with spread to lower urethra, ± vagina, ± anus, ± unilateral groin lymph node metastases
IV$_A$	Tumour invades any of the following: upper urethra, bladder mucosa, rectal mucosa, pelvic bone ± bilateral groin nodes
IV$_B$	Any distant metastases including pelvic nodes

Surgical management

The treatment of vulval carcinoma is usually some form of surgical excision, either a wide local excision or vulvectomy. The decision about whether to undertake additional groin node exploration depends on whether there are any clinically suspicious groin nodes, the grade of tumour (more likely if poorly differentiated), and the depth of invasion on the initial specimen. It may be appropriate to only carry out a unilateral exploration if the lesion is well lateralized. Distant metastases are not a contraindication to radical vulval surgery, as death from a large fungating genital neoplasm or erosion of the femoral artery or vein by metastatic groin nodes is very unpleasant.

The groin explorations are carried out through separate incisions, and the wound should be drained for around 7–10 days under suction, as lymph fluid accumulates and breakdown is common. If there is significant groin node involvement, it may be necessary to give adjuvant pelvic node radiotherapy as well.

The commonest complication of a radical vulvectomy is breakdown of the wound, which may take weeks to heal. In addition these women are often elderly, immobile, and have had surgery on their pelvic vessels close to the femoral vein leaving them at a high risk of venous thromboembolic disease. Long-term sequelae of surgery include vulval mutilation and lymphoedema. The 5-year survival is around 80% if groin nodes are negative and 40% if positive.

Recurrence

Recurrence of the excised tumour at the primary site is unusual providing a 10-mm margin has been achieved. The epithelium is likely to be unstable, however, and new vulval tumours may arise. Treatment of recurrence is surgical, although interstitial radiotherapy may be appropriate. A check should be made at follow-up for signs of tumour spread to nodes.

Key points

- A swollen symptomatic Bartholin's gland or abscess should be marsupialized and not simply incised.
- Lichen sclerosus is associated with squamous carcinoma of the vulva in around 2–5% of women.
- VIN is analogous to CIN in the cervix. Treatment of VIN is local excision of severely dysplastic lesions with careful follow-up.
- Vulval carcinoma is usually of squamous cell type and tends to afflict the more elderly population. The treatment is excision ± unilateral or bilateral inguinal lymphadenectomy. Pelvic radiotherapy may also be indicated if there is a significant chance of nodal spread.

29

Cervical intraepithelial neoplasia and cancer

Introduction

Cervical cancer is the most common cancer among women in many developing countries, and worldwide there are over 450 000 cases each year. The overall lifetime risk is about 5% in parts of Africa, India, and Latin America, compared with 1% in Europe and North America. About 3000 cases of cervical cancer are diagnosed each year in the UK, and 1300 of these women will die from the disease.

Fortunately cervical cancer has a premalignant phase and many of the criteria for a suitable screening programme are fulfilled. The aim of this screening is to detect premalignant cervical disease by means of a 'smear test' and treat the premalignant disease before invasion occurs. Both the incidence and mortality have fallen considerably since the introduction of this screening programme.

Cervical intraepithelial and cervical cancer screening

Transformation zone

Cervical intraepithelial neoplasia (CIN) develops in the transformation zone of the cervix. Understanding the transformation zone is the key to understanding cervical cancer screening. The endocervix is lined by columnar epithelium and the ectocervix by squamous epithelium. Under the influence of oestrogen, part of the endocervix everts, thereby exposing the columnar epithelium to the chemical environment of the upper vagina (Fig. 29.1). The change in pH, along with other factors, causes the delicate columnar epithelium cells to transform into squamous epithelium through the process of metaplasia. CIN develops in this transformation zone and it is this area which is sampled cytologically.

Cells shed from the surface may be sampled by a variety of devices, so that cells from both the endocervix and ectocervix can then be examined microscopically for cytological abnormalities. Cellular abnormalities are classified into different degrees of 'dyskaryosis'. Although dyskaryosis is a *cytological* diagnosis (Fig. 29.2), the degree of dyskaryosis correlates to some degree with the degree of cervical intraepithelial neoplasia, which is a *histological* diagnosis (Figs 29.3 and 29.4). As well as examining the desquamated cervical cells, cervical smear reports may also identify infection such

Gynaecology

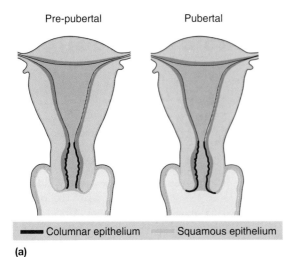

Pre-pubertal   Pubertal

━━ Columnar epithelium   Squamous epithelium

(a)

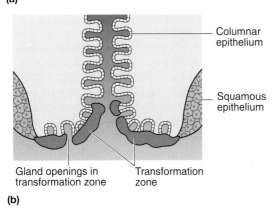

Columnar epithelium

Squamous epithelium

Gland openings in transformation zone   Transformation zone

(b)

Fig. 29.1 **The transformation zone. (a)** The cervix everts at puberty, exposing the columnar epithelium of the endocervical canal. **(b)** This epithelium, referred to as the transformation zone, gradually undergoes metaplasia to squamous epithelium.

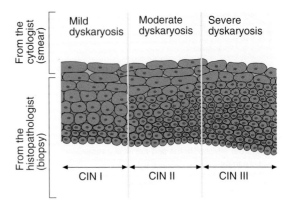

Fig. 29.3 **The CIN grading system.**

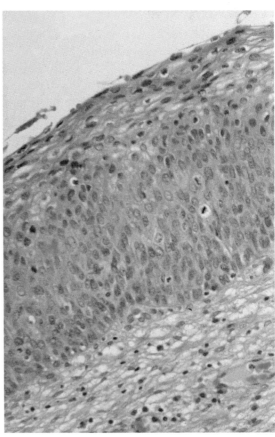

Fig. 29.4 **CIN II in a biopsy specimen.** There are abnormal cells arising from the basal layer, but not extending to the full thickness of the epithelium.

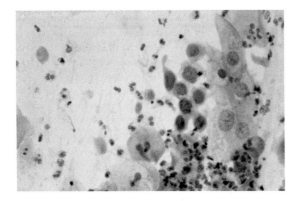

Fig. 29.2 **Slide prepared from a cervical smear.** There is moderate dysplasia with hyperchromasia, irregular nuclei and multinucleation. This slide also shows *Trichomonas vaginalis*, leucocytosis and a spermatozoon.

as candida, trichomonas or wart virus infection. Rarely they may identify cells from other parts of the genital tract such as malignant endometrial or ovarian cells.

The precise rate of progression and spontaneous resolution of the disease is unknown. Roughly one-third of lesions will progress to the next stage (CIN I to II, CIN II to III, etc.), a third will remain unchanged and a third will regress. The duration of progression to invasive carcinoma is variable but the average is perhaps around 10 years.

Screening recommendations

In the UK there is an organized systematic computerized screening programme with national recommendations to screen from the ages of 20–65 years. Different regions, however, have different protocols.

Colposcopy

Significant dyskaryosis on a cervical smear is an indication for further assessment with colposcopy. This is a procedure by which the cervix is examined in more detail using a type of binocular microscope referred to as a colposcope (Fig. 29.5). Although moderate and severe dyskaryosis are absolute indications for colposcopy, controversy exists as to whether it is required for mild dyskaryosis. Some believe it is important, while others are concerned it may lead to overtreatment of lesions which will often regress spontaneously. The indications for colposcopy are listed in Box 29.1.

The patient is placed in the lithotomy position and a bivalve speculum is then inserted to allow visualization of the cervix. It is important to identify the squamocolumnar junction (SCJ). Abnormal epithelium, such as CIN, contains an increased amount of protein and lower levels of glycogen than normal epithelium. If acetic acid is applied to the cervix, the protein coagulates and the abnormal cells appear 'aceto-white' (Fig. 29.6). There may also be a mosaic pattern with patches of aceto-white separated by areas of red vessels (Fig. 29.7).

Box 29.1

THE INDICATIONS FOR COLPOSCOPY

1. **Abnormal cervical cytology**

Smear result	Action
Severe dyskaryosis	Colposcopy
Moderate dyskaryosis	Colposcopy
Mild dyskaryosis	Repeat cytology/ colposcopy
Borderline	Repeat cytology
Glandular dyskaryosis	Colposcopy

2. **Clinical suspicion of invasive disease**

3. **Mild or borderline on two occasions 6 months apart**

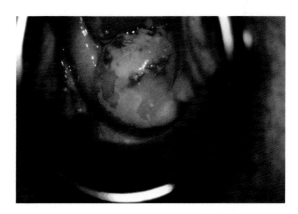

Fig. 29.6 **Acetic acid coagulates protein, and the abnormal cells, which have more protein, appear 'aceto-white'.**

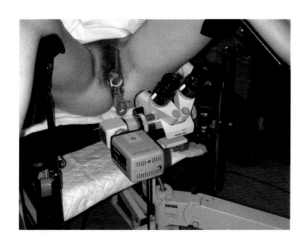

Fig. 29.5 **Colposcopy, using a high-powered microscope, allows detailed examination of the cervix.**

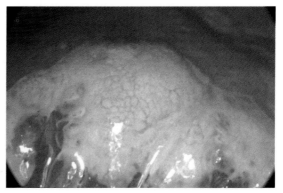

Fig. 29.7 **Patches of aceto-white may be separated by areas of blood vessels creating a mosaic pattern.**

Some of the vascular patterns may appear punctated if the vessels are viewed end on. The inter-vessel distance increases with more severe lesions, and bizarre branching with coarse punctation and atypical vessels suggests invasive disease. Lugol's iodine (Schiller's iodine) stains glycogen mahogany brown, and the abnormal cells, which have less glycogen and therefore take up less iodine, can also be viewed in this way.

Treatment of CIN

If CIN is suspected colposcopically the options are to treat immediately using an excisional method (e.g. large loop excision) or to biopsy to confirm high-grade CIN and treat thereafter. This depends on the certainty of the colposcopic findings and the likelihood that the patient will attend for the follow-up.

The cervix is infiltrated directly with local anaesthetic, and a loop diathermy excision or some other form of excision is performed (Fig. 29.8). The alternative of ablating the area has the disadvantage that the histological assessment is less complete (see Table 29.1).

Follow-up

Any woman who has had CIN, whether treated or not, continues to be at risk of developing cervical cancer due to either incomplete treatment of her CIN or the development of new disease. Follow-up is therefore important and this is usually carried out cytologically by repeating smears. Colposcopy can also be used. Protocols vary, but following successful treatment of CIN it is reasonable to arrange a follow-up smear after 6 months, and then annually for 5–10 years before

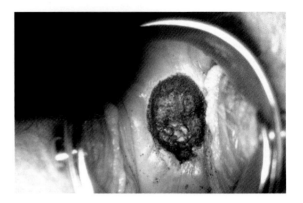

Fig. 29.8 **An area of CIN II has been excised using a loop** (Table 29.1). The cauterized area heals spontaneously.

returning to the national screening programme if the smears have been negative.

Cervical cancer

Aetiological factors

Cervical cancer arises from areas of CIN as noted above. At least 30% of patients with CIN III, if left untreated, will probably go on to develop invasive disease over a period of 5–20 years.

Sexual behaviour

Cervical cancer is usually a disease of sexually active women and has been linked mainly to human papilloma virus. Women with cervical cancer are likely to

Table 29.1
Treatment modalities for CIN

Method	Summary of method	Pros	Cons
Loop excision of the transition zone	Wire loop with high-frequency current	Easy outpatient procedure. Tissue is available for pathology	Small association with cervical incompetence and stenosis
Radical electrodiathermy	Cervical cautery using a monopolar high-frequency current	Easy outpatient procedure	No tissue available for pathology. Depth of tissue destruction not known
Cryotherapy	Freezing the cervix with a nitrogen probe	Easy outpatient procedure	No tissue available for pathology. Depth of tissue destruction not known
Laser vaporization	Destruction with CO_2 laser	Easy outpatient procedure. Known depth of tissue destruction	No tissue available for pathology
'Cold' coagulation	Heating to approx 100°C	Easy outpatient procedure	No tissue available for pathology. Depth of tissue destruction not known
Cone biopsy	Surgical excision, often under anaesthesia	Large specimen obtained. Tissue is available for pathology	Often needs general anaesthesia. Associated with cervical incompetence and stenosis

have had more sexual partners and to have started inter-course earlier, and are less likely to have used barrier methods of contraception than other women. The sexual behaviour of their partners may also be important. The disease is more frequent in parous women.

Human papilloma virus

A strong association has been observed between the human papilloma virus (HPV) serotypes 16 and 18, pre-invasive disease, and invasive cervical cancer. It may be that certain serotypes of HPV are important cofactors in the development of cervical cancer and may act by producing proteins (E6/7) which affect the action of the 'p53' gene product. The 'p53' gene is important in repairing DNA and, if damaged, may predispose to malignant change. HPV is present in around a third of all women in their 20s in the UK.

The combined oral contraceptive pill

Studies have shown that prolonged use of the oral contraceptive pill increases the risk of cervical cancer up to fourfold, but only in women who carry the human papilloma virus. It can be argued that this effect is attributable to differences in sexual behaviour rather than to the pill itself.

Smoking

Women who smoke are also at increased risk of developing cervical cancer. This may be due to alterations in immune function in the cervical epithelium or chemical carcinogenesis.

Presentation

Patients with cervical cancer may present with post-coital bleeding, intermenstrual bleeding, menorrhagia or an offensive vaginal discharge. In early cases there may be no symptoms, and the diagnosis is made only after abnormal cervical cytology is discovered. Other symptoms such as backache, referred leg pain, leg oedema, haematuria or alteration in bowel habit are usually associated with advanced-stage disease. General malaise, weight loss and anaemia are also late features.

Three categories of clinical appearance are described:

1. The most common is an exophytic lesion (Fig. 29.9). It usually arises on the ectocervix, often producing a large friable polypoid mass which bleeds easily. It can also arise from within the endocervical canal so that the canal becomes distended and 'barrel shaped'.
2. An infiltrating tumour that shows little ulceration or exophytic growth but tends to produce a hard indurated cervix.

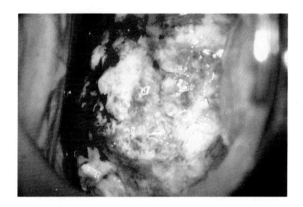

Fig. 29.9 **This squamous cell carcinoma was staged II$_A$.**

3. An ulcerative tumour which erodes a portion of the cervix and vaginal vault producing a crater with local infection and seropurulent discharge.

Pathology

The majority of cervical cancers are squamous, and may be of keratinizing (the commonest), large cell, non-keratinizing and small cell subtypes. Around 10–25% are adenocarcinomas. There may also be coexistent squamous metaplasia or neoplasia (adenosquamous carcinoma).

Spread

Cervical cancer spreads by direct extension into adjacent structures and via the draining lymphatics. Blood-borne metastases are rare. Direct invasion beyond the cervix is usually into the upper vagina, parametrium and pelvic sidewall, and this tumour may lead to ureteric obstruction. There may also be invasion of the bladder and rectum.

There is no predictable pattern of lymphatic spread, with paracervical, parametrial and both internal and external iliac nodes potentially involved. There may also be spread to the common iliac, para-aortic and left supraclavicular area.

The risk of lymph node metastases correlates with both stage and tumour volume. Around 10% of patients with stage I disease have pelvic node involvement, rising to around 35% in those with stage III disease. The incidence of para-aortic node involvement is less, at around 5% of patients with stage I disease and 25% with stage III disease.

Staging, investigation and prognostic factors

Cervical cancer is staged by clinical examination (Table 29.2), which is often carried out under anaesthetic, and the diagnosis confirmed histologically by biopsy.

Table 29.2
FIGO staging of cervical cancer

Stage	Invasion	Prognosis 5-year survival	Treatment
1_{A1}	Depth of invasion up to 3 mm and width up to 7 mm (includes early stromal invasion of up to 1 mm)	84–90% if tumour < 3 cm; 85% will have negative pelvic nodes and 95% of these patients will be 'cured'	Local excision; if margins of a cone clear (i.e. no residual tumour or CIN) then conization is adequate, with no need for pelvic lymphadenectomy
1_{A2}	Depth of invasion between 3 and 5 mm (i.e. 3.1–5 mm) and width up to 7 mm		Simple hysterectomy and pelvic lymphadenectomy
1_{B1}	Tumour confined to cervix and diameter less than 4 cm	66% if tumour > 3 cm	Radical hysterectomy or radiotherapy
1_{B2}	Tumour confined to cervix and diameter more than 4 cm		Radical hysterectomy or radiotherapy
II_A	Upper 1/3 vagina	62%	Radical hysterectomy or radiotherapy
II_B	Upper 2/3 of vagina plus parametrial disease		Radiotherapy ± chemotherapy
III_A	Lower 1/3 vagina	40%	Radiotherapy ± chemotherapy
III_B	Pelvic sidewall and/or hydronephrosis		Radiotherapy ± chemotherapy
IV_A	Bladder, rectum	15%	Radiotherapy ± chemotherapy
IV_B	Beyond pelvis		Radiotherapy ± chemotherapy

The examination should include a rectovaginal examination to assess parametrial involvement. The use of ultrasound, MRI and CT scanning has replaced the use of cystoscopy and intravenous urography (IVU) in many centres. If nodes are radiologically suspicious, for example, it may be more appropriate to avoid surgery and treat with radiotherapy.

Although in developed countries a greater proportion of cases present with stage I disease, in worldwide terms the majority (> 75%) of women with cervical cancer present with advanced stage (stage III/IV) disease. The prognosis for patients with early-stage disease is relatively good (Table 29.2) but the prognosis for patients with advanced-stage disease is poor.

Management

Treatment: stage I–II$_A$

Stage I$_{A1}$–I$_{A2}$

Stage I$_A$ can be cured by simple excision. If preservation of fertility is required a cone biopsy with close cytological follow-up may be adequate treatment; where preservation of fertility is not important simple hysterectomy is preferable. In all other cases of stage I disease more aggressive treatment with either radical radiotherapy or radical surgery is required.

Stage I$_B$–II$_A$

The choice between radical hysterectomy and radical radiotherapy is determined by the clinical condition of the patient. There is no difference in survival between the two methods but there are significant differences in morbidity.

Radical hysterectomy and pelvic lymphadenectomy involve total hysterectomy, excision of the parametria, upper third of the vagina and paracolpos, as well as dissection of the pelvic lymph nodes. Oophorectomy may be performed if appropriate but the ovaries are rarely the site of metastatic spread and can be safely conserved. The operative mortality is considerably less than 1%, although potential morbidity includes infection, thromboembolic disease, haemorrhage and vesicovaginal fistulae. There are also medium-term problems with reduced bladder sensation and voiding difficulties together with long-term problems of high residual volumes, recurrent urinary infections, stress incontinence and lymphocyst formation.

Radical radiotherapy usually consists of external beam therapy (teletherapy) to the pelvis and local vaginal therapy (brachytherapy). Teletherapy is delivered in fractions over a number of weeks to treat the pelvic lymphatics, whereas with brachytherapy a vaginal delivery system is inserted and left in situ for 12–18 hours to irradiate central disease. The radiation dose which can be given is limited by the size of the lesion and the proximity of the bladder and bowel, both of which are particularly susceptible to radiation damage. The principal morbidity results from vaginal dryness, which can lead to sexual dysfunction, radiation cystitis, proctitis and vaginal stenosis. As this morbidity often gets worse with time, surgery is considered to be more suitable for those patients who are younger. In those found to have positive pelvic nodes postoperatively, it is appropriate to offer adjuvant radiotherapy.

Treatment: stage II$_B$–IV

The treatment of advanced-stage disease usually involves radical radiotherapy and may be further improved with the additional use of platinum-based chemotherapy. Failure to cure inoperable cervical cancer may result from suboptimal treatment of the central disease or the existence of lymph node metastases. With large lesions, the sensitivity of adjacent structures to radiation may prevent use of curative radiation doses at the tumour periphery and, furthermore, some tumours may be radio-resistant.

Recurrent disease

Those patients with recurrence have a 1-year survival of around 10–15%. Most recurrences are suitable for palliative care only. If the patient has not been previously treated with radiotherapy then this may be a treatment option but the majority of patients will have already had radical radiotherapy. Patients with a central pelvic recurrence may be cured by pelvic exenteration (excision of vagina/uterus with the bladder or rectum or both). With careful selection up to 60% of these cases may survive 5 years, but the operation is associated with major morbidity.

The remaining patients may benefit from chemotherapy to palliate symptomatic recurrence or radiotherapy to palliate recurrence involving bone or nerve roots. The most active chemotherapy agents are cisplatin and ifosfamide and combinations based on these drugs cause initial tumour shrinkage in up to 70% of cases.

The main benefit from chemotherapy is the relief of disease-related symptoms, such as pelvic pain, but chemotherapy itself can cause considerable toxicity and does not improve survival in these women.

Key points

- Cervical cancer is the most common cancer among women in many developing countries and worldwide there are over 450 000 cases each year.

- The risk of cervical cancer is related to sexual behaviour. Early age of first intercourse and a high number of sexual partners are risk factors. Smoking may also increase the risk.

- An important causative agent appears to be human papilloma virus serotypes 16 and 18.

- Screening is possible because of a relatively long precancerous phase and involves a programme of regular cervical smears. Cytological abnormalities on smears (dyskaryosis) correlate to some degree with histologically abnormal cervical intraepithelial neoplasia (CIN).

- When cervical smears demonstrate dyskaryosis, colposcopy allows identification of abnormal epithelium suggestive of CIN to be localized, biopsied and treated.

- Although cervical cancers are mainly of squamous type, around 10–25% are adenocarcinomas.

- FIGO staging of cancer is from stage I–IV. Stage I can be treated by surgery or radiotherapy. More advanced cancer can be treated by radiotherapy ± chemotherapy.

30

Trophoblastic disorders

Gestational trophoblastic tumours are rare but the subject is an important one because some forms of the disease, which previously carried a high mortality, are now usually curable with appropriate therapy. The genetics and pathophysiology of the condition are fascinating and the very sensitive response to chemotherapy is both interesting and unusual.

Normal trophoblast

In the normal placenta, villi of trophoblastic cells penetrate deeply into maternal tissue to form a branching labyrinthine network. The distal branches of these villi are contained within a 'lobule' into which the maternal spiral artery flows. The trophoblastic cells of the villus are therefore in direct contact with the maternal circulation, and it is not uncommon for them to embolize into the maternal circulation. While this could be considered to be a form of metastasis, the life expectancy of these cells is limited and it is not therefore a 'malignant' process. It is the limited survival capacity of normal trophoblast, and not the nature of its invasion or secondary spread, which distinguishes it from malignant tissue. These principles apply to the behaviour of hydatidiform moles, which should be differentiated from the malignant form of trophoblastic disease, choriocarcinoma.

Normal and abnormal trophoblastic cells secrete human chorionic gonadotrophin (hCG), making it an excellent serum marker to monitor disease progress.

Trophoblastic disease (Table 30.1)

A hydatidiform mole is a tumour of trophoblastic villi with an incidence of between 0.5–2/1000 pregnancies. The name is derived from the Greek word *hydatis*, meaning a watery vesicle and the Latin *mola*, meaning a shapeless mass. There are two sorts of hydatidiform mole – 'partial' and 'complete' – and both of these can become 'invasive' moles. Despite this invasion and the potential to metastasize, however, they are still classified as benign. Choriocarcinoma is a malignant gestational trophoblastic tumour which may arise from either a normal pregnancy, an abnormal pregnancy, or a molar pregnancy.

There have been a number of reports suggesting that the incidence of molar pregnancy varies between

Table 30.1
Classification of trophoblastic disease

Classification	Pathology	Usual karyotype	Clinical features
Partial hydatidiform mole	Focal hyperplasia of villi Benign	69XXY: two paternal haploid sets and one maternal haploid set	Often an embryo. Vesicular appearance of placenta on ultrasound. Although 1% invade ('invasive mole') and a few of these develop metastases, they virtually never become choriocarcinoma
Complete hydatidiform mole	Generalized hyperplasia Benign	46XX: two haploid sets, both paternal ('androgenically diploid')	Uterine cavity filled with vesicular tissue on ultrasound. No embryo. 10% invade ('invasive mole') and the incidence of choriocarcinoma is 3%
Invasive mole	Features of invasion Benign	Virtually all are androgenically diploid	Invades the myometrium, and is therefore strictly speaking a histological diagnosis
Choriocarcinoma	Is histologically differentiated from a hydatidiform mole by the absence of villi Malignant	Contains maternal and paternal chromosomes (unlike choriocarcinoma of ovarian origin)	May arise from a hydatidiform mole or follow a live birth, stillbirth, miscarriage or ectopic pregnancy. There are often blood-borne metastases

certain racial groups. Studies suggesting a higher incidence in Africa and South America may have been biased by the population sampled, but there is some evidence that the incidence is truly higher in the Japanese population (2.5/1000) when compared to Chinese studies (0.8/1000). It has also been noted that the incidence has been falling in Japan and Korea over the past three decades, but the reason for this is unclear. There is no doubt, however, that the incidence increases with increasing maternal age such that the risk by the age of 50 years approaches 1 in 3 live births.

These risk factors also probably apply to choriocarcinoma, but history of a previous molar pregnancy is itself a significant additional risk factor. Women with type A blood group are at a greater risk than those with type O.

Partial hydatidiform mole

Trophoblastic disease is the result of an error in embryogenesis. Normal fertilization combines a 23X set of haploid chromosomes from the ovum and either a 23X or 23Y haploid set from the spermatozoa, the result being a diploid 46XX or 46XY zygote which has a mixture of maternal and paternal genes. With rare exceptions a partial mole exhibits triploidy, that is to say it has 69 chromosomes; 23 chromosomes are maternal in origin and the other 46 are paternally derived, usually from the entry of two spermatozoa into the ovum.

There is often an embryo or fetus which usually dies in the first or early second trimester. Histologically the placental tissue is characterized by focal hyperplasia and swelling of the villi. Some villi appear normal. Although 1% of partial moles become invasive moles, transformation to choriocarcinoma is rare. Only 0.5% of partial moles require chemotherapy after surgical evacuation.

Complete hydatidiform mole

The majority of complete hydatidiform moles (there are again some rare exceptions) have a 46XX karyotype but all the genetic material is paternal in origin, i.e. they are 'androgenically diploid'. There are two possible mechanisms by which this may occur:

- The maternal 23X haploid set of chromosomes in the ovum may be lost and the 23X haploid set of paternal chromosomes from the fertilizing sperm may reduplicate itself (homozygote).
- Alternatively, an 'empty' ovum may be fertilized by two separate spermatozoa (dispermy) leading to a heterozygous molar pregnancy.

In a complete molar pregnancy there is no embryo, membranes or cord. There is hyperplasia and gross vesicular swelling of all villi, and a classical complete molar pregnancy looks macroscopically like a 'bunch of small grapes'. 10% become invasive moles and the incidence of subsequent choriocarcinoma is 3%. Around 15% of complete moles will require treatment after surgical evacuation.

Invasive mole

When the villi of either a complete or partial hydatidiform mole penetrate into the myometrium and its blood vessels, the hydatidiform mole is said to be invasive. Invasion follows a complete mole much more commonly than it does a partial one. The natural history is of spontaneous regression, but metastases to the lung, vagina, liver, brain and the GI tract may occur. Emboli of molar tissue can undergo spontaneous resolution.

Choriocarcinoma

Choriocarcinoma is a malignant tumour arising from trophoblastic cells, and it lacks the villous structure of an invasive mole. The tumour cells invade aggressively and infiltrate between the maternal muscle fibres and blood vessels. The frequent invasion of blood vessels themselves explains why distant metastases are found, and these are particularly in the lung, brain, liver and kidney. Choriocarcinoma is extremely rare, arising in only approximately 1 in 50 000 pregnancies, with 50% following a molar pregnancy, 30% following a miscarriage and 20% following an apparently normal pregnancy. The exact aetiology of why choriocarcinoma develops is unknown, and cytogenetic analysis has not identified a common karyotypic change.

Clinical presentation

Partial and complete mole

Molar pregnancy becomes clinically apparent because of its pathophysiological features. Most molar pregnancies will miscarry spontaneously and the commonest clinical presentation therefore is pain and vaginal bleeding. It may also be asymptomatic and discovered at a routine early pregnancy ultrasound scan. The uterus is often large for dates. Excessive production of hCG may be one of the reasons why a molar pregnancy may present with hyperemesis gravidarum or even (very rarely) with extremely early-onset pre-eclampsia.

Invasive mole and gestational choriocarcinoma

An invasive mole is usually identified because of persistent hCG levels or ongoing bleeding after surgical evacuation of the uterus. Choriocarcinoma may present either because of the primary intrauterine lesion, in which case the pathology after surgical evacuation will confirm the diagnosis, or because of a metastasis. Metastases may be to:

- the lung, causing haemoptysis
- the brain, leading to neurological abnormalities
- the GI tract, causing chronic blood loss or melaena
- the liver, leading to jaundice
- the kidney, causing haematuria.

Management

Ultrasound of a complete mole is traditionally said to show a 'snowstorm appearance'. This describes the older B-scan pictures and on a real-time scan it more correctly looks as if the cavity is filled with relatively homogeneous solid tissue which has a vesicular appearance (Figs 30.1 and 30.2). There may also be multiple luteal cysts on the ovaries owing to ovarian stimulation from the very high hCG levels. A missed miscarriage can have similar macroscopic appearances to a hydropic placental tumour as it is often cystic and hydropic. Such a pregnancy may also have a triploid karyotype but can be differentiated from a molar pregnancy by the absence of trophoblastic hyperplasia (there is usually hypoplasia), and the fact that the hCG level is usually very much lower.

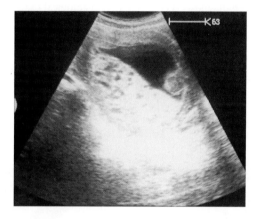

Fig. 30.1 **Ultrasound of a partial mole.**

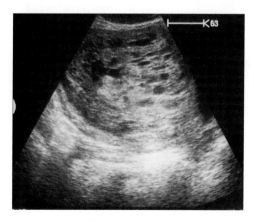

Fig. 30.2 **Ultrasound of a complete mole.**

Following an ultrasound scan suggestive of a molar pregnancy, it is important to:

- take a history and perform a physical examination
- arrange a chest X-ray
- measure the serum hCG concentration
- check the maternal and paternal blood group and rhesus status
- crossmatch maternal blood prior to theatre
- arrange for surgical evacuation of the uterus under anaesthesia.

The risks of bleeding and perforation during surgical evacuation are significant, but surgical evacuation for a complete mole is superior to both medical evacuation of the uterus (which may lead to increased risk of dissemination) and hysterectomy. Ultrasound may be used in theatre to minimize this risk. Medical evacuation may be appropriate for a partial mole, particularly if a larger fetus is present, but should be followed with a surgical evacuation of any retained products of conception (ERPOC). It is recommended that oxytocics be avoided until after the uterine evacuation, to minimize distant spread by uterine contractions.

The diagnosis is confirmed on histological examination of the intrauterine contents and supported by cytogenetic studies of the trophoblastic cells. Follow-up of molar pregnancy is discussed below. If a choriocarcinoma is identified a computerized axial tomography scan (CT scan) is also required to look for secondaries, and chemotherapy should be offered (Figs 30.3 and 30.4).

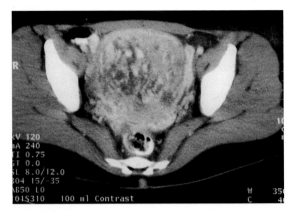

Fig. 30.4 **CT scan of pelvis in the same patient showing a large vascular mass.**

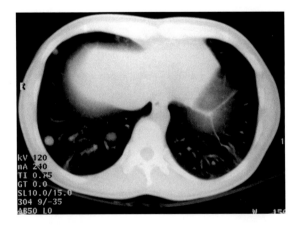

Fig. 30.3 **CT scan of pulmonary metastases with choriocarcinoma.**

Follow-up

As there is an approximately 10% chance of a complete mole becoming invasive and a 3% risk of a choriocarcinoma, it is important to monitor the postoperative hCG titres closely for 6 months in those whose hCG is normal 8 weeks post-ERPOC, and for 2 years where the hCG is still raised after 8 weeks. In Britain, follow-up of hydatidiform mole is organized through three central laboratories, London, Sheffield and Dundee. Each case of trophoblastic disease should be registered with the nearest laboratory which will then organize follow-up directly. Early detection of rising hCG titres offers the best chance of successful treatment of invasive disease. This system of well-organized centralized follow-up has been a major factor in the reduction in morbidity and mortality from choriocarcinoma.

As a subsequent normal pregnancy will also cause a rise in hCG titres, and may therefore confuse the follow-up process, women who have had a molar pregnancy should be encouraged to use contraception for at least a year. Condoms or an IUCD are appropriate but the combined oral contraceptive pill should only be taken when the hCG has returned to zero (although some advocate waiting an extra 6 months beyond this time, again to minimize recurrence risk).

Of those who have subsequent pregnancies, 85% have normal pregnancies, but the risk of a further molar pregnancy is 2% after the first mole, and 20% after the second. Follow-up with hCG monitoring must be undertaken after any subsequent pregnancy.

Chemotherapy

Chemotherapy may be required if the hCG rises progressively following the uterine evacuation, or if the serum level is > 20 000 IU/l at 4 weeks, or if the pathology is reported as choriocarcinoma. The natural history of an invasive mole is spontaneous regression but chemotherapy is offered to prevent the potential complications of uterine haemorrhage and perforation. Trophoblastic disease is exquisitely sensitive to chemotherapy, and whereas almost all women with choriocarcinoma died prior to the advent of chemotherapy, the survival with treatment is over 90%.

Regimes vary and depend on the severity of the disease, with more aggressive regimes for those with significant risk factors. These risk factors include:

- age over 39
- long interval from previous pregnancy
- high hCG level
- B or AB blood group
- tumour > 5 cm
- metastases, especially in the liver or brain
- previous chemotherapy.

Of the low-risk group, 80% respond to low-dose methotrexate and 20% will need additional chemotherapy because of methotrexate resistance. Virtually all low-risk patients are cured. High-risk patients are usually given combination chemotherapy over repeated cycles.

Key points

- Gestational trophoblastic disorders represent an abnormal proliferation of trophoblastic tissue and may be benign (hydatidiform mole) or malignant (choriocarcinoma).

- A hydatidiform mole may be complete or partial. A complete mole is diploid (but all the chromosomes are paternally derived) and there is no fetal tissue (only trophoblast). A partial mole is usually triploid (with 46 of the 69 chromosomes being paternally derived) and there may be a fetus.

- Choriocarcinoma can occur after a normal pregnancy, miscarriage or hydatidiform mole. Approximately 3% of moles develop into a malignant choriocarcinoma.

- Trophoblast secretes hCG, making it a very good tumour marker for follow-up.

- The diagnosis of a molar pregnancy is often suggested by ultrasound in which there is homogeneous solid tissue with a vesicular appearance. The diagnosis is confirmed by histopathological examination of tissue.

- Management of a mole is to carry out a surgical evacuation of the uterus, and follow-up is required to ensure that the hCG level is falling. Chemotherapy may be required if the hCG rises progressively following the uterine evacuation, or if the pathology is reported as choriocarcinoma.

- Choriocarcinomas are exquisitely sensitive to chemotherapy and the cure rate is high.

- There is an increased recurrence risk in subsequent pregnancies.

Pregnancy and the puerperium

31

The physiology of pregnancy

Introduction

Pregnancy brings huge physiological changes and, teleologically, it is assumed that these changes are in the fetal interest (see Box 31.1). The changes are proactive; in other words they are not proportional to the size of the fetus, such that by the end of the first trimester many systems are functioning at levels close to those at term. The systems are reviewed in order below.

Respiratory system

Oxygen consumption is increased by around 15–20%. This consumption is partly maternal, to supply the increased cardiac, renal and respiratory function, as well as for breast and uterine development. The remainder is for the fetoplacental unit. To supply this increased oxygen requirement the mother hyperventilates, increasing minute ventilation by about 40% above the normal 7 l/min. This increase is predominantly by increasing tidal volume rather than respiratory rate; in other words the mother breathes more deeply. Maternal serum CO_2 falls, favouring CO_2 transfer from the fetus to the mother. The change is thought to be mediated by progesterone (Fig. 31.1).

Dyspnoea is a common symptom in pregnancy. This dyspnoea is perceptual rather than a reflection of inadequate gas exchange, and is often worse at rest. In late pregnancy, the gravid uterus may restrict diaphragmatic movement, exacerbating any feelings of breathlessness. Nevertheless it is important to consider pathological causes of breathlessness, particularly pulmonary thromboembolic disease.

Box 31.1

TELEOLOGY

A 'teleological' explanation for an event is one where the explanation is sought directly from the effects. For example, if a change in P_{CO_2} favours the fetus, it is teleological to say that the reason for the change is fetal advantage. The change has arisen by natural selection, and is therefore assumed to be in the fetal interest.

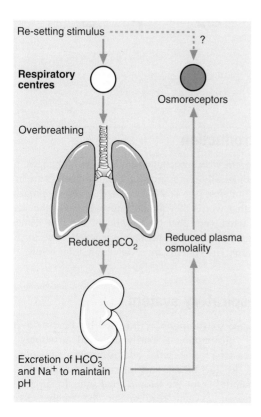

Fig. 31.1 **The postulated events leading to the resetting of the respiratory centre in pregnancy.**

Cardiovascular system

In pregnancy there is an increase in cardiac output and a decrease in peripheral vascular resistance. Cardiac output rises by about 40%, from around 3.5 to 6 l/min, from increases in both stroke volume and heart rate. These changes are complete by the start of the second trimester, but the cardiac output may rise by a further 2 l/min in established labour. The fall in peripheral vascular resistance is not quite compensated for by the increased cardiac output so the overall effect is a slight fall in blood pressure in the second trimester. The blood pressure may rise slightly again in the third trimester and it may be difficult to separate this from the pathological state of pre-eclampsia.

Late in pregnancy the mass of the uterus is liable to press on, and partially occlude, the inferior vena cava, especially when the mother lies supine. This leads to hypotension, which is worse when a mother lies flat on her back. Therefore mothers are often placed on a left lateral tilt during labour, especially if in the lithotomy position or undergoing anaesthesia.

The fetus benefits because this high blood flow maximizes P_{O_2} on the maternal side of the placenta (also see below). The plasma volume expansion and increased cardiac output may also help heat loss by increasing blood flow through the skin, thus compensating for the increased metabolic rate of pregnancy. Peripheral vasodilatation causes a feeling of warmth and a tolerance to cold, and may be a factor in the palmar erythema and spider naevi of pregnancy.

Blood, plasma, and extracellular fluid volume

On average the total red cell mass increases by 25% from 1300 ml to 1700 ml but the circulating plasma volume increases by 40% from 2600 ml to 3700 ml. There is thus a dilutional drop in the haemoglobin (Hb) concentration and in the haematocrit.

Plasma colloid osmotic pressure falls in pregnancy and, as a result, fluid shifts into the extravascular compartment causing oedema. Not only do almost all pregnant women have some dependent oedema, but so also do non-pregnant women in the post-ovulatory (high progesterone) phase of the cycle.

Blood constituents and anaemia

The typical changes in the full blood count in pregnancy are shown in Table 31.1.

Iron requirements are increased (Table 31.2) and the serum ferritin level falls. It has been found that the haemoglobin drop mentioned above can be minimized by giving iron supplements, and some authors have concluded that there must therefore be a pathological iron deficiency. Despite this, trials of supplementation have not demonstrated a reduction in any important adverse pregnancy outcome, and observational data indicate that maternal and perinatal mortality do not rise with low Hb concentrations until levels fall below 7 g/dl. Despite these reservations, it is likely that

Table 31.1
Blood changes in pregnancy

	Non-pregnant	Pregnant
Haemoglobin (g/dl)	12–14	10–12
Red cell count ($\times 10^{12}$/l)	4.2	3.7
Haematocrit (venous)	40%	34%
MCV (fl)	75–99	80–103
MCH (pg)	27–31	No change
MCHC (g/dl)	32–36	No change
White cell count ($\times 10^9$/l)	4–11	9–15
Platelets ($\times 10^9$/l)	140–440	100–440
ESR (mm/h)	< 10	30–100

ESR, erythrocyte sedimentation rate; MCH, mean corpuscular haemoglobin: MCHC, mean corpuscular haemoglobin concentration; MCV, mean corpuscular volume

Table 31.2
The requirements of elemental iron during pregnancy

Fetus and placenta	500 mg
Red cell increment	500 mg
Postpartum blood loss and 6 months' lactation	360 mg
Total	1360 mg
Saving from amenorrhoea approximately	360 mg
Net increased demand approximately	**1 gram**

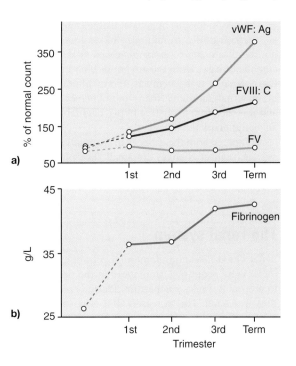

Fig. 31.2 **The levels of the procoagulants (a) factor VIII, von Willebrand factor and (b) fibrinogen rise in pregnancy.** FV, factor V.

iron deficiency does occasionally occur, particularly if iron stores are low before pregnancy. The WHO have suggested iron supplementation at haemoglobin levels below 10.5 g/dl.

Folate metabolism

The daily folate requirement rises from 50 µg to 400 µg, and folate deficiency may also occur. It is usually possible to meet this increased requirement through a normal diet, although intake in those with a poor diet is likely to be inadequate.

Haemostasis in pregnancy

Pregnancy is a hypercoagulable state with an increase in procoagulants (fibrinogen, platelets, factor VIII, von Willebrand factor) and a reduction in naturally occurring anticoagulants (for example antithrombin III). Fibrinolysis is also increased so that there is an increased net turnover of coagulation factors (Figs 31.2 and 31.3).

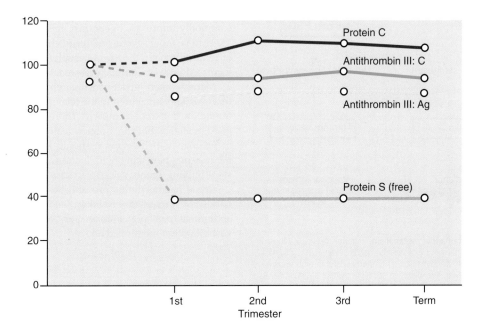

Fig. 31.3 **The levels of the anticoagulants antithrombin III and protein S fall in pregnancy.**

The reason for this hypercoagulable state is presumably, teleologically, to minimize blood loss at delivery but the disadvantage is the increased risk of thromboembolic disease. Until the advent of blood transfusion, haemorrhage was a much more important cause of maternal mortality than thromboembolic disease, and it is therefore likely that hypercoagulability offered an evolutionary advantage.

Compared with the changes in coagulation and fibrinolysis, platelet changes are small. The platelet count falls only slightly but there is an increased aggregability, probably in relation to prostaglandin changes (Fig. 31.4).

The renal system

Renal blood flow and glomerular filtration rate (GFR) increase by about 60% from early in the first trimester to around 4 weeks postpartum. Plasma creatinine and urea levels fall. The increased GFR is not matched by increased tubular reabsorption and there would therefore be a tendency to lose sodium were it not for a compensatory increase in aldosterone levels. Glycosuria is common because the filtered load of glucose is greater than the tubular reabsorption capacity. Although glycosuria is therefore often normal in pregnancy, it may still be pathological.

Dilatation of the renal pelvis and ureters is caused by both a progesterone and local pressure effect. It occurs from early in the first trimester and results in urinary stasis, which increases the chance of urinary tract infection. The chance of infection may be exacerbated by the presence of glycosuria.

Gastrointestinal system

There is a general reduction in gut motility and slowing of transit times. This may benefit the fetus by increasing the absorption of certain nutrients. Delayed gastric emptying is a feature of pregnancy, and is particularly marked in labour. It becomes clinically important if the woman requires a general anaesthetic because of the risk of aspiration pneumonia (Mendelson's syndrome).

Nausea and vomiting are common in early pregnancy. It is not clear whether they are caused by rising human chorionic gonadotrophin (hCG) or oestrogen or some other factor, but management is discussed further on page 319. Most pregnant women report increased appetite and thirst, and many have cravings for, or aversions to, certain foods. Perhaps the most common aversions are to tea and coffee. Pica, a craving for non-food substances such as coal, chalk or soap, is rare but well known. The cause is unknown.

Gastric acid secretion is reduced in pregnancy, which is presumably the reason that peptic ulcer disease commonly improves. In contrast, reflux oesophagitis is likely to be more severe, and results from a combination of reduced tone in the lower oesophageal sphincter and increased intra-abdominal pressure.

Many women report constipation in pregnancy and this is usually attributed to the relaxing effect of progesterone on gut smooth muscle. There is, however, little good evidence that constipation really is more common in pregnancy. If it occurs it should be managed, as in the non-pregnant state, with increased dietary fibre and stool-bulking agents.

Rectal haemorrhoids probably result from a combination of increased straining, and increased intra-abdominal pressure, and as part of the generalized vasodilatation mentioned above.

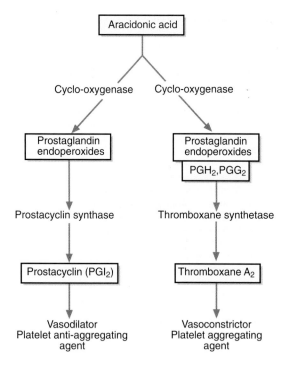

Fig. 31.4 **Prostaglandin metabolism.** In normal pregnancy there is increased biosynthesis of eicosanoids – particularly prostacyclin (PGI_2), a vasodilator with platelet inhibitory properties, and thromboxane A_2, a vasoconstrictor with a tendency to stimulate platelet aggregation. As both usually increase in proportion to each other, there is a net neutralization and homeostasis is maintained. This homeostasis is disrupted in pre-eclampsia because of a relative deficiency in prostacyclin owing to either a decrease in its synthesis and/or an increase in the production of thromboxane A_2. This imbalance leads to vasoconstriction, hypertension, and platelet stimulation.

Liver and bile ducts

Normal pregnancy is a mildly 'cholestatic' state. Biochemical tests of liver function lie within the normal range. Alkaline phosphatase levels are almost doubled, but most of this increase comes from placental secretion of this enzyme. Pathological cholestasis is discussed on page 334.

Oestrogen increases the serum cholesterol and this is translated into bile salt production, which supersaturates the bile. Since progesterone also reduces gall bladder emptying the stage is set for gallstone formation.

Skin and appendages

The skin participates in the generalized increase in blood flow in pregnancy. Increased pigmentation is also seen in the nipples and in the midline of the abdomen (linea nigra). Striae gravidarum, or stretch marks, occur in the presence of high oestrogen levels, in skin subject to stretching, such as that over the breasts and abdomen. Initially reddish/purple they fade after delivery to a faint silvery colour. There is no effective prevention or treatment despite the efforts of the cosmetic industry.

The cycle of hair growth is altered in pregnancy with a greater proportion (95% vs 85%) of hairs in the actively growing phase. As a result there are many over-aged hairs at the end of pregnancy, which fall out and lead to the common symptom of hair coming out 'in handfuls' postnatally. It recovers.

Metabolic changes

Extra energy is required not only for the developing fetus but also to fuel the increase in maternal physio-logical parameters. The resting metabolic rate is increased by around 20% and weight increases on average by around 12 kg (Fig. 31.5). Initially there is an increased sensitivity to insulin which leads to increased glycogen synthesis, increased fat deposition and an increase in amino acid transfer into cells. After mid-pregnancy there is a degree of insulin resistance. The serum glucose level at this stage may therefore rise, a change presumably in the fetal interest as fetal glucose levels will also rise. The insulin resistance also leads to increased levels of serum lipids which can be used by the mother as an alternative energy source to glucose. Although maternal amino acid levels fall, there is increased transport across the placenta.

Pregnancy is a diabetogenic state. Cortisol, progesterone, oestrogen and human placental lactogen (HPL) are all insulin antagonists, and tend to increase the glucose level. If the pancreatic islet β-cells are unable to produce sufficient insulin to balance this increase, or if there is maternal insulin resistance, the maternal glucose level may rise pathologically (Fig. 31.6). This is discussed further on page 327.

Thyroid function

In pregnancy there is increased iodine uptake activity and the total serum levels of T_3 and T_4 are also raised. Only the unbound portion of thyroxine is metabolically active, however, and as oestrogens also induce synthesis of thyroid-binding globulin, the levels of free T_3 and T_4 remain within the normal range or may even fall slightly. Clinically, it may be difficult to separate the

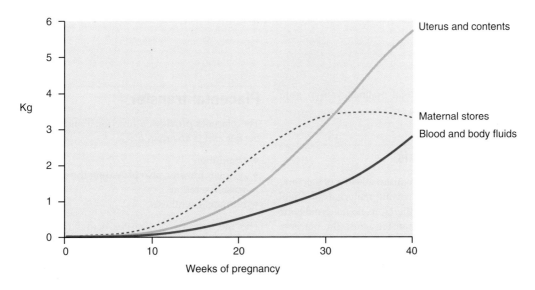

Fig. 31.5 **Components of weight gained in normal pregnancy.**

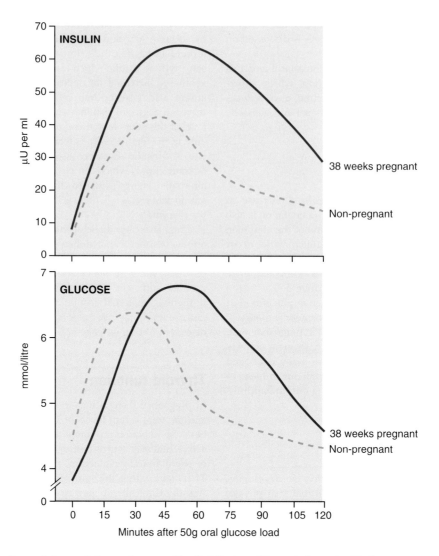

Fig. 31.6 **The patterns of change of plasma glucose and insulin following a 50 g oral glucose load in the non-pregnant woman compared to late pregnancy.**

hypermetabolic state of normal pregnancy from mild hyperthyroidism.

Calcium homeostasis

Fetal skeletal development requires 20–30 g of calcium, and this need is met by increasing maternal intestinal absorption. There is usually, therefore, no maternal bone demineralization. Calcium transfer across the placenta is an active process occurring against a concentration gradient and it is therefore not surprising that maternal free calcium levels are not significantly changed. Serum protein and albumin fall as part of the plasma dilution of pregnancy so that total calcium is reduced.

Placental transfer

The placenta provides a functional and immunological barrier and is an organ of:

● respiration
● nutrient transfer, also providing the mechanism for waste excretion
● hormonal synthesis.

The mechanisms of transfer across the placenta are outlined in Table 31.3. The nuclei and other intracellular organelles in the syncytiotrophoblast come to lie in groups to form areas of thick metabolically active tissue which are probably the sites of active diffusion. Between them are other areas with only a very fine layer separ-

Table 31.3
Some examples of the mechanism of placental transfer

Mechanism	Substance
Passive diffusion	CO_2, O_2, water
Facilitated diffusion (by a carrier molecule)	Glucose
Active transport by enzymatic action	Amino acids, Ca, Fe, vitamins B and C, free fatty acids
Organelle transport by pinocytosis	IgG

Box 31.2

MATERNO-FETAL OXYGEN EQUILIBRIUM

Consider the hypothetical situation of the fetomaternal circulation at oxygen equilibrium with a P_{O_2} of 4 kPa (30 mmHg), maternal Hb 11 g/dl and fetal Hb 17 g/dl. Maternal haemoglobin will be 60% saturated and fetal 80% saturated. Each gram of fully saturated haemoglobin carries 1.38 ml of oxygen. Maternal oxygen carriage (saturation × haemoglobin concentration × 1.38) is thus $0.6 \times 11 \times 1.38 = 0.91$ ml/dl, while fetal oxygen carriage is $0.8 \times 17 \times 1.38 = 1.88$ ml/dl. The oxygen molecules would therefore equilibrate in a ratio of 2 : 1 in favour of the fetal circulation. In practice, although equilibrium may be reached locally on either side of the vasculosyncytial membrane, it is not achieved overall. Firstly there is functional shunting in both circulations, and secondly the fetal P_{O_2} remains well below maternal levels because of local oxygen consumption by the placenta. This is to the fetal advantage since a high P_{O_2} would stimulate premature closure of the ductus arteriosus.

The final result of all this is that even though the P_{O_2} is much lower in the fetus, the O_2 content of fetal blood is higher than in the mother's blood. Fetal umbilical venous blood (Hb 17 g/dl) at a P_{O_2} of 4 kPa (30 mmHg) will be 75% saturated and carry $17 \times 0.75 \times 1.38 = 17.5$ ml/dl of oxygen. Maternal uterine venous blood (Hb 11 g/dl), even at a higher P_{O_2} of 5.3 kPa (40 mmHg), will be only 70% saturated and carry $11 \times 0.7 \times 1.38 = 10.6$ ml/dl.

ating maternal and fetal blood, the vasculosyncytial membrane, and these are where most passive gas transfer occurs.

Respiration

The following changes maintain the diffusion gradient:

1. The high O_2 affinity of fetal haemoglobin. The dissociation curve of fetal haemoglobin is shifted to the right so that at a given P_{O_2} the percentage saturation is higher than for adult haemoglobin (Box 31.2). More importantly for the fetal interest, at a given level of oxygen transfer the P_{O_2} will be lower (see Fig. 31.7).

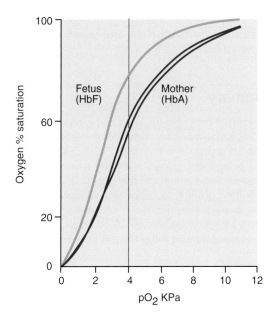

Fig. 31.7 **Fetal haemoglobin has a higher affinity for O_2 than maternal haemoglobin.** The dissociation curve of fetal haemoglobin is shifted to the right so that at a given P_{O_2} the percentage saturation is higher than for adult haemoglobin. More importantly for the fetal interest, at a given level of oxygen transfer the P_{O_2} will be lower.

2. The high fetal Hb (normal 14–20 g/dl) also results in a lower P_{O_2} for a given saturation.
3. Finally, the passage of CO_2 from fetus to mother helps increase maternal oxygen dissociation and fetal association. This shift of the oxygen dissociation curve to the right caused by CO_2 accumulation is called the Bohr effect.

The CO_2 dissociation curves are similar in fetal and maternal blood. Although most CO_2 is carried as bicarbonate, bicarbonate is a charged molecule and cannot cross the placenta. Only dissolved CO_2 can cross the placenta, and this is again by diffusion. This transfer is facilitated by maternal hyperventilation, which lowers maternal P_{CO_2}, and lower fetal concentrations of carbonic anhydrase, which slows the establishment of equilibrium between CO_2 and HCO_3^-. Furthermore as maternal Hb gives up oxygen, its CO_2 affinity increases (the Haldane effect), and the opposite (reverse Haldane effect) decreases CO_2 affinity of fetal haemoglobin as it in turn takes up oxygen.

Table 31.4
Roles of selected placental hormones

Hormone	Role
Human chorionic gonadotrophin (hCG)	Initially maintains the corpus luteum's secretion of progesterone and oestrogen; later it may have a role in regulating placental oestrogen secretion and in modulating the maternal immune response
Oestrogen	Over 90% is in the form of oestriol; it is involved in uterine growth, cervical changes, and breast development
Progesterone	Smooth muscle relaxation, acting on the uterus, GI tract and ureters. Also has a role in regulating maternal physiological changes
Human placental lactogen (HPL)	Mobilizes maternal free fatty acids, improving glucose availability for the fetus

Nutrition

The developing fetus requires energy, largely provided by glucose, amino acids and fatty acids. These are mostly transported across the placental membrane by active processes as outlined in Table 31.3. In later pregnancy, excessive glucose is converted into glycogen and fat such that by term, 15% of the body weight is fat. In preterm babies and those with in-utero growth restriction these energy stores are lower.

Hormone synthesis

The placenta produces a large number of hormones. Although the function of many of these is not understood, the roles of the main ones are outlined in Table 31.4.

Immunology

Most human cells have a gene on chromosome 6 that codes for a particular protein called the human leucocyte antigen or 'HLA'. Each of us has a unique HLA gene and the protein synthesized from this gene coats the surface of all the cells in our body, allowing our immune cells to recognize 'self' cells. If leucocytes identify a 'non-self' code, they initiate a process of cell destruction. The fetus is genetically unique and will have a different HLA complement from that of either parent. If a skin graft is taken from a child and grafted onto its mother, the graft will be rejected. Yet while the fetus is 'grafted' onto the lining of the maternal uterus, it is not rejected. There must therefore be some protective mechanism, or mechanisms, to prevent immunological fetal rejection.

HLA has different subtypes. The classical genes, *HLA-A*, *-B* and *-C*, provide the highly individual molecules coding for 'self,' and these molecules are absent on many of the placental cells. This would render these placental cells less susceptible to maternal leucocyte recognition and therefore less liable to destruction. Some immunological reaction, however, may be important to prevent placental over-invasion, and some placental cells do express the classical genes, particularly *HLA-C*. Further modulation of this uneasy fetomaternal immune relationship may be modified by another HLA molecule, HLA-G, specific only to placental tissue. Much more work is required before these mechanisms are understood more clearly, particularly as it is becoming apparent that immunological disparity may lie behind recurrent miscarriage, fetal growth restriction, and pre-eclampsia.

Summary

Women who are pregnant overbreathe, retain fluid and calories, and increase the perfusion of most organs. This makes pregnancy uncomfortable. In the process many blood parameters change, and there may be anaemia, glycosuria, constipation and cholestasis. This sometimes makes their doctors uncomfortable. Nevertheless most of the changes are, directly or indirectly, in the fetal interest. Minor symptoms, and blood values outside the normal non-pregnant range, do not necessarily require treatment.

Key points

- Pregnancy exerts profound physiological changes on a mother's body in virtually every organ system.

- The ventilation rate increases by 40%. The alveolar ventilation rate increases, and there is a fall in the physiological dead space. These profound changes in respiratory function provide the developing fetoplacental unit with the 250–290 ml/min rise in oxygen consumption needed for pregnancy to progress and develop.

- Cardiac output increases during pregnancy by approximately 40% from increases in both stroke volume and heart rate. Blood pressure falls in early pregnancy but by late pregnancy it returns to normal again or may even be slightly raised.

- The red cell mass increases by 25% but a 40% increase in circulating plasma volume leads to a dilutional fall in haemoglobin concentration and the haematocrit. A policy of routine iron supplementation for healthy women with singleton pregnancies is not appropriate, but supplementation is useful in the presence of iron-deficiency anaemia.

- Progesterone concentrations rise in pregnancy and have effects in many parts of the body. They can cause constipation, delayed gastric emptying, reflux oesophagitis, urinary frequency and urinary stasis, and have the effect of exacerbating varicose veins.

- Some women may develop impaired glucose tolerance in pregnancy.

Maternal mortality

In the UK about 90 women die each year as a direct or indirect result of pregnancy – a small number compared with the annual total of over 600 000 deliveries. In most parts of the world, however – particularly developing countries – pregnancy is much more risky than it is in Britain. Worldwide over half a million women die every year due to pregnancy – one every minute of every day (Fig. 32.1). This global tragedy is largely preventable.

Definitions

Maternal deaths are clearly defined to allow comparisons over time and between countries.

Maternal death   Death of a woman while pregnant or within 42 days of termination of pregnancy, from any cause related to or aggravated by the pregnancy or its management, but not from accidental or incidental causes.

Direct death   Death resulting from obstetric complications of the pregnant state (pregnancy, labour and puerperium), from interventions, omissions, incorrect treatment or from a chain of events resulting from any of the above.

Indirect death   Death resulting from previous existing disease, or disease that developed during pregnancy and was not due to direct obstetric causes, but which was aggravated by the physiological effects of pregnancy.

Late death   Death occurring between 42 days and 1 year after abortion, miscarriage or delivery, due to direct or indirect maternal causes.

Coincidental death   Death from an unrelated cause which happens to occur in pregnancy or the puerperium. The word 'coincidental' has replaced the term 'fortuitous'.

The maternal mortality rate is usually expressed as the number of deaths per 100 000 maternities. A 'maternity' is a clinical pregnancy ending in live birth, stillbirth, miscarriage or abortion.

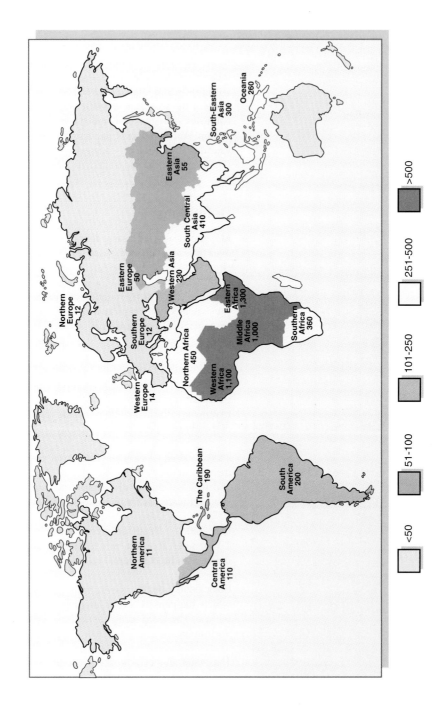

Fig. 32.1 **Maternal mortality by sub-region, 1995 (deaths per 100 000 live births)**. (Source: WHO/UNICEF/UNFPA.)

Historical aspects

Safe pregnancy is a relatively recent development in Britain. Between 1847 and 1936 the maternal mortality rate remained virtually unchanged at around 400 (1 death in 250 births) but after 1936 it fell sharply (Fig. 32.2). This remarkable reduction is often dismissed as part of a general improvement in public health, but other indicators, such as infant mortality, fell slowly and steadily during the 20th century. The fastest fall in maternal mortality, by contrast, was during the Second World War, when social conditions could hardly be said to be improving. This timing suggests that the fall was due to other factors.

Before 1936

Most deliveries used to take place at home and the maternal mortality rate may have been kept high by general practitioner obstetricians, some of whom used forceps under chloroform anaesthesia in up to 70% of deliveries. In the 1920s public concern about maternal mortality grew. Training of midwives was improved (Midwives Acts were passed in 1902 and 1936), and the British (later Royal) College of Obstetricians and Gynaecologists was founded in 1929.

After 1936

The first breakthrough was the introduction of sulphonamides in 1936, followed by penicillin and other antibiotics. Puerperal sepsis had been the leading cause of maternal mortality, and deaths from this cause fell quickly. Other factors were:

- safe blood transfusion
- ergometrine, for the treatment and prevention of postpartum haemorrhage
- better treatment of pre-eclampsia and prevention of eclampsia
- better contraception leading to reduced family size
- the Abortion Act of 1967 (Fig. 32.3)
- confidential enquiries into maternal deaths.

Confidential Enquiries into Maternal Deaths (CEMD)

A national system of enquiries was set up in England and Wales in 1951 and has continued to the present day, making it probably the longest-running professional self-audit in the world. Enquiries are conducted by clinicians – doctors and, nowadays, midwives. Confidentiality is maintained to encourage those involved with the case to be as frank as possible.

Full information is sought about every death during pregnancy or within a year after delivery. A form is filled in by all staff involved – general practitioner, midwife, obstetrician, anaesthetist and others – and sent for comment to regional assessors in obstetrics, pathology and other specialties if appropriate. It is then sent to the Department of Health and anonymized before being seen by national assessors.

Similar systems exist in Scotland, Wales and Northern Ireland. Every 3 years a UK-wide report is published which lists the causes of death, draws attention to areas of substandard care and makes recommendations for improving practice. As the data from the UK are so thorough, this chapter will focus on the trends in the UK to illustrate the potential for change.

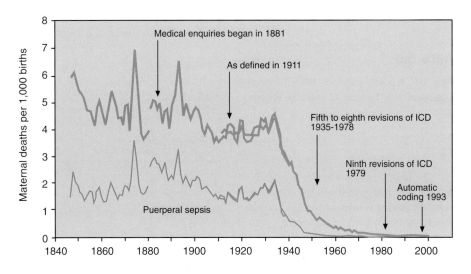

Fig. 32.2 **Maternal mortality rate in England and Wales, 1847–2000.**

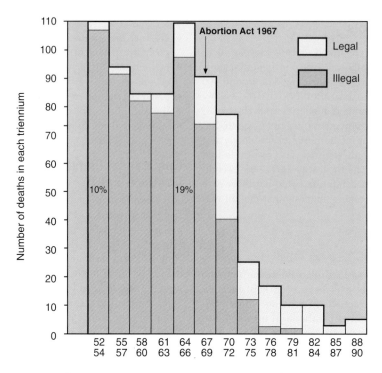

Percentages within columns indicate that of all direct maternal deaths in that triennium, 10% and 19% were caused by abortion

Fig. 32.3 **Maternal deaths from abortion, 1952–1989.** (From *Maternal and Child Health*, 1994, 19:348, with permission.)

Recent trends

From 1937 to 1984 in Britain the maternal mortality rate halved every decade. Since 1985, however, the overall rate has remained constant at around 10/100 000 maternities. It has not, however, reached an irreducible minimum. Standards keep improving and there has been little if any fall in the proportion of cases with substandard care.

Why mothers die

The most recent UK reports, entitled 'Why Mothers Die', identify general risk factors as well as specific causes of death.

Risk factors

Age and parity   The highly parous woman (the 'grand multipara') has long been recognized as a high-risk case, and still is. In 1997–99 among women of parity 4 or more the maternal mortality rate was 35 while among primigravidae it was 6.2 (Fig. 32.4).

Age and high parity used to go together but as high parity is becoming less common the importance of maternal age is becoming clearer. Between 1985 and 1999 the maternal mortality rate among women aged over 40 was 35.5 while among women aged 20–24 it was 7.2 (Fig. 32.5). This is important as more women are now choosing to delay childbearing.

Social class   The 1997–99 report identified for the first time the high risk among the lowest social class in Britain (Table 32.1). The maternal mortality rate in this group, which includes itinerant and unemployed people, is similar to that of a Third-World country.

Table 32.1
Risk factors for maternal death in relation to social class

Social class	Direct and Indirect deaths	Maternal mortality rate/ 100 000 maternities
1	5	2.94
2	25	4.19
3	31	15.21
4	33	5.32
5	26	8.31
6	12	11.35
7	7	23.81
8	5	38.96
9	97	135.46

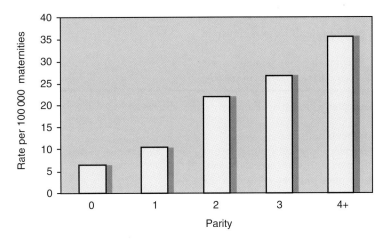

Fig. 32.4 **Maternal mortality rate and parity, 1997–99.**

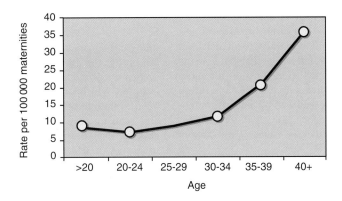

Fig. 32.5 **Maternal mortality rate and maternal age, 1985–1999.**

40% of the maternal deaths in the UK occur in social class 9. This wretched state of affairs is illustrated in the 1997–99 report by brief case-histories – for example, a homeless teenager who was discharged from hospital and froze to death in a front garden.

Ethnicity   Several countries including the USA, France and The Netherlands have reported higher maternal mortality rates among black women. Recent reports from the UK have confirmed that the maternal mortality rate is two to three times higher among black and Asian women than among whites. The reasons for this are unclear.

Other risk factors include infertility and multiple pregnancy. This is relevant to couples undergoing assisted conception.

Causes of death

Table 32.2 shows the number of maternal deaths notified to the CEMD during the 1990s.

Since 1988 there has been a steady fall in Direct deaths and a rise in Indirect deaths, which now outnumber Direct deaths. Coincidental deaths have remained fairly constant but Late deaths have risen, probably because of increasing awareness that such cases should be reported to the CEMD. The maternal mortality rate, which includes only Direct and Indirect deaths, rose from 9.9 in 1988–90 to 12.1 in 1994–96, and fell slightly to 11.4 in 1997–99.

Table 32.2
Deaths notified to the UK CEMD

	1988–90	1991–93	1994–96	1997–99
Direct	145	129	134	106
Indirect	93	100	134	136
Coincidental	39	46	36	29
Late	48	46	72	107
Total	325	321	376	378

Direct deaths

In 1997–99 the causes of Direct death were as shown in Table 32.3.

'Substandard care' may involve only a minor aspect of the treatment and does not necessarily mean that the death could have been avoided. Standards are rising all the time and are particularly high in anaesthesia.

Thrombosis and thromboembolism

At the beginning of pregnancy levels of clotting factors change, and later in pregnancy pressure on pelvic veins causes venous stasis, as does immobility during the puerperium (for example, after caesarean section). All these factors increase the risk of thrombosis.

The 31 deaths from pulmonary embolism in 1997–99 were almost equally divided between antepartum and postpartum deaths. (In addition there were four deaths from cerebral embolism.) Eight of the 31 deaths occurred before 12 weeks of pregnancy.

Ten women died after vaginal delivery, almost all of whom had risk factors. Four women collapsed and died after caesarean section, a marked reduction from the 15 cases in 1994–96. This fall was probably due to the publication in 1995 of RCOG guidelines on thrombo-prophylaxis after caesarean section (Fig. 32.6). In future a similar reduction may be achieved by better thrombo-prophylaxis during pregnancy and after vaginal de-livery for all women with risk factors. Risk factors include:

- obesity
- bed rest
- past history or family history of thromboembolism
- long-haul air travel
- age over 35.

Most deaths from thromboembolism are preceded by symptoms of chest pain, cough or leg pain. Deaths may be prevented by prompt investigation, especially in high-risk women.

Table 32.3
Causes of Direct death, 1997–99

	Cases	No. (%) with substandard care
1. Thrombosis and thromboembolism	35	20 (57%)
2. Early pregnancy deaths	17	11 (65%)
3. Hypertensive disorders of pregnancy	15	12 (80%)
4. Genital tract sepsis	14	7 (50%)
5. Amniotic fluid embolism	8	2 (25%)
6. Haemorrhage	7	5 (71%)
7. Anaesthesia	3	3 (100%)
8. Other Direct deaths	7	4 (57%)

Early pregnancy deaths

Deaths before 20 weeks' gestation include, apart from thromboembolism, those due to ectopic pregnancy, spontaneous miscarriage and termination of pregnancy.

Ectopic pregnancy is notoriously deceptive. With modern pregnancy tests, diagnosing pregnancy is easy, but only if the doctor thinks of the possibility. Ectopic pregnancy sometimes causes bowel symptoms, for example, which can be misleading. GPs and casualty officers should perform a urinary pregnancy test on any woman of reproductive age with unexplained abdominal pain. In 1997–99 13 women died of ectopic pregnancy, 10 of whom had had substandard care.

Spontaneous miscarriage caused two deaths in 1997–99. One was a woman with alcohol dependence and the other was the very young teenager, mentioned above, who had run away from home and was abusing drugs.

Termination of pregnancy Before the Abortion Act of 1967, illegal abortion caused about 30 deaths a year in Britain (Fig. 32.3). For the last 20 years there have been no deaths from criminal abortion, but there are a small

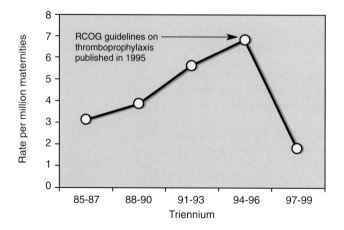

Fig. 32.6 **Deaths from pulmonary embolism after caesarean section (rate per million maternities), UK 1985–1999.**

number of deaths from legal abortion. In 1997–99 there were two such deaths, the exact causes being unclear.

Hypertensive disorders of pregnancy

In 1952–54 there were 246 deaths from hypertensive disease in England and Wales. In 1997–99 in the UK there were 15. This dramatic fall has occurred because of better care, not because the condition has become less common. Treatment can still be improved, however. Almost 50% of the 20 deaths in 1994–96 were due to pulmonary or cerebral oedema, i.e. to fluid balance problems during treatment. In 1997–99, none of the 15 deaths was due to oedema but seven were due to intracranial haemorrhage, i.e. to failure of hypotensive therapy. Of these 15 women, 12 had had substandard care, usually in the form of inadequate monitoring, delay in treatment, or lack of multidisciplinary care. The recommendations in the 1997–99 report include:

- investigation of symptoms such as headache or abdominal pain
- clear guidelines for hospital treatment
- the use of magnesium sulphate as the anticonvulsant of choice
- early collaboration with intensive care specialists.

Genital tract sepsis

Until 1936, streptococcal puerperal sepsis accounted for over 1000 deaths a year in Britain. With the introduction of antibiotics the numbers fell rapidly until the 1982–84 Report was able to state 'No deaths could be directly attributed to puerperal sepsis'. This brief sentence recorded one of the greatest triumphs of 20th century medicine. Since then, puerperal sepsis has reappeared. There were 10 deaths from this cause in 1994–96 and four (including two Late deaths) in 1997–99. The condition may occur after the woman leaves hospital and as it is now so rare it can be difficult for GPs and midwives to recognize the very early signs of rapidly progressive infection.

Controlled trials have shown that prophylactic antibiotics should routinely be given for caesarean section. In 1997–99 sepsis caused one death after caesarean section but also caused 13 antenatal deaths. When infection develops, urgent and repeated bacteriological specimens should be taken and a microbiologist's advice should be sought. In severe cases parenteral antibiotics should be given before the diagnosis is confirmed.

Amniotic fluid embolism (AFE)

In this condition amniotic fluid enters the maternal circulation, causing an intense vascular reaction. At autopsy fetal squames are usually found in the mother's lungs. Sudden collapse occurs during labour, or rarely before labour or during caesarean section. In 1997–99 AFE caused eight deaths, all but one being in women aged 25 or over. In five of the cases labour had been

induced or augmented, and of the other three, one was a twin pregnancy and another had had a previous caesarean section. AFE is rare when there has been no obstetric intervention whatsoever. It carries a high mortality but if death does not occur quickly, the woman may be saved by prompt transfer to intensive care. A register of surviving cases is being maintained to see if lessons for treatment can be learned.

Haemorrhage

In 1952–54 in England and Wales there were 188 deaths from obstetric haemorrhage. In 1997–99 in the UK there were seven. The number fell to single figures in 1982–84 but rose again as lessons were forgotten. Of the seven deaths in 1997–99, three were from placenta praevia, three from placental abruption and one from postpartum haemorrhage.

Placenta praevia carries particular dangers when the placenta is implanted over a uterine scar. Caesarean section for placenta praevia must be carried out by a very experienced operator, preferably a consultant.

Abruptio placentae is usually complicated by coagulo-athy, and although nowadays this can usually be treated successfully, serious problems can develop quickly. The three women who died in 1997–99 were lost despite satisfactory or even exemplary care.

Postpartum haemorrhage played a role in six deaths in 1997–99, though only one death was solely due to this cause. Life-threatening haemorrhage occurs after at least one in 1000 deliveries, so several hundred cases are treated successfully every year in the UK.

Nevertheless, as severe obstetric haemorrhage becomes less frequent, teams become less experienced in treating these life-threatening emergencies. A multi-disciplinary massive haemorrhage protocol should be available in all units and updated and rehearsed regularly in conjunction with the blood bank. Women at known higher risk of haemorrhage should be delivered in a consultant unit with an on-site blood bank.

Guidelines have also been produced for the management of haemorrhage in women who refuse blood transfusion for religious reasons. Hysterectomy may be life-saving in such cases, and consultant involvement in their management is important.

Anaesthesia

The safety of obstetric anaesthesia has improved dramatically over the last 20 years, with the risk of anaesthetic death falling from over 10 per million maternities in the 1970s to around 1 per million in the 1990s, despite a marked increase in the number of anaesthetics given. Reasons for this improvement include greater use of epidural rather than general anaesthesia, and the exclusion of the most junior training grades from obstetric anaesthesia.

In 1997–99 there were three deaths due directly to anaesthesia. Substandard care was judged to be present in all three cases but some of the cases were difficult and, as mentioned above, standards in anaesthesia are high.

Other Direct deaths

Four deaths in 1997–99 were due to acute fatty liver of pregnancy, and one to spontaneous rupture of the caecum. Two were due to genital tract trauma – one after a vaginal tear during an unattended spontaneous delivery at home and the other after uterine rupture in a woman with a previous caesarean section, delivered by vacuum extraction.

Indirect deaths

The causes of Indirect deaths in 1997–99 are shown in Table 32.4.

The proportion of cases with substandard care is lower among Indirect deaths than among Direct deaths, but there is nevertheless potential for improvement, particularly with psychiatric cases and some specific medical conditions.

Cardiac disease

In Britain, cardiac disease now includes a wide spectrum of conditions. Formerly the major problem was rheumatic heart disease, as it still is in many developing countries. The cardiovascular changes of pregnancy put a strain on the heart. In 1997–99, cardiac disease was the indirect cause of 35 deaths (the same number as thromboembolism, the leading cause of Direct death). The causes are shown in Table 32.5. Substandard care was present in only three of the 35 cases.

Women with pulmonary vascular disease have a high risk of dying in pregnancy (the risk is around 30% for those with Eisenmenger's syndrome) and should be strongly advised against getting pregnant, though they should not be alienated from seeking care if pregnancy occurs. Women with known heart disease should be managed by a cardiologist in cooperation with an

Table 32.4
Causes of Indirect deaths, 1997–99

	Cases	No. (%) with substandard care
Cardiac disease	35	3 (9%)
Psychiatric	43*	17 (39%)
Other indirect	75	13 (25%)

*This total of psychiatric deaths includes Late deaths, mainly from suicide.

Table 32.5
Causes of death from cardiac disease

Cardiac disease	Deaths
Congenital heart disease	10
Cardiomyopathy	12
Ruptured aortic aneurysm	5
Myocardial infarction	5
Endocarditis/heart failure	3

obstetrician. The possibility of endocarditis should be considered in a pregnant woman with an obscure febrile illness.

Psychiatric deaths

The importance of psychiatric illness as a cause of maternal death has only recently been recognized. Mental illness, new or recurrent, is commonly associated with childbirth: 10% of new mothers suffer from a depressive illness, which is severe in up to half of cases; 2% see a psychiatrist within 1 year of delivery and 2 per 1000 suffer from puerperal psychosis.

In 1997–99 13 women committed suicide within 6 weeks of delivery. Another 15 suicides after 6 weeks were classified as late Indirect deaths. When other causes of death such as drug overdose were examined, 42 cases were identified in which psychiatric disorder caused or contributed to the woman's death. In addition, a study by the Office of National Statistics, linking birth certificates and death certificates, found another 40 deaths from suicide or violent causes, eight more in which the coroner had recorded an open verdict and another 11 cases of accidental drug overdose. Although details of all cases were not available, it is now clear that suicide is the leading cause of maternal death in the UK.

Suicide in this group of women is often violent, such as jumping from a height, or by hanging. All social classes are equally affected. Women with a past history of severe mental illness complicating pregnancy have a 33–55% chance of this recurring in future pregnancies, and this cannot be prevented by hormonal treatment.

The booking history should include sensitive enquiry about such a past history and, when appropriate, psychiatric assessment should be arranged during pregnancy. Each unit should have a protocol for management of women at high risk, and every region should have a mother and baby unit to which women may be admitted. The vague term 'postnatal depression' or 'PND' should be avoided as it may fail to identify the seriousness of an episode of mental illness.

Other Indirect deaths

This category includes a wide variety of diseases, the commonest single condition being intracranial haemorrhage (including subarachnoid and intracerebral haemorrhage). The most important preventable cause is epilepsy, which led to 19 deaths in 1994–96 and nine in 1997–99. Women with epilepsy need specific specialist advice in pregnancy, if possible from a combined clinic run by an obstetrician, a physician and a specialist nurse or midwife. Another recurring lesson from analysis of Indirect deaths is that pregnancy is not a reason for withholding plain X-rays of the chest or abdomen, some computed tomography films or magnetic resonance imaging from sick women.

Coincidental deaths

Formerly known as 'fortuitous' deaths, this group includes road traffic accidents and murder, each of which accounted for eight deaths in 1997–99. All eight murder victims were killed by their male partner or a member of their close family. Domestic violence may begin or worsen during pregnancy and units are being encouraged to develop programmes to identify and offer help to women experiencing violence from men they know.

International comparisons

Safe childbirth is limited to Western Europe, North America, Australasia, Singapore and Japan. In many countries maternal mortality rates are as high as they were in Britain before 1937, and in some countries even higher, reaching 1000 per 100 000 deliveries in parts of sub-Saharan Africa. The World Health Organization estimates that at least 600 000 maternal deaths occur every year, from the causes shown in Table 32.6.

International agencies including the World Health Organization and the World Bank are promoting initiatives to try to reduce these appalling figures. The World Bank points out that as well as the individual human tragedies, there are also major economic consequences of losing women who are productive members of society. Some countries have introduced confidential enquiries based on the UK model. The leading causes of death differ from country to country, but include:

- lack of access to contraception
- unsafe abortion
- lack of primary care or transport facilities
- inadequate equipment and staffing in district hospitals.

Comparison of different states in India shows that high rates of female literacy correlate with high rates of contraceptive use and low maternal mortality rates. Better education of women is important but in the meantime safer care could be provided for pregnant women if there is the will to do so.

Key points

- Maternal death is the death of a woman while pregnant or 42 days after the end of pregnancy. *Direct* deaths result from obstetric complications and *Indirect* deaths from disease aggravated by pregnancy but not directly due to pregnancy.

- In developed countries the maternal mortality rate is around 10 per 100 000 maternities. In many developing countries it is still around 400 per 100 000. Across the globe over 600 000 women die during pregnancy every year, mainly in developing countries.

- The fall in maternal mortality in Britain after 1936 is attributable to antibiotics, safe blood transfusion, ergometrine for the prevention of postpartum haemorrhage, better training of midwives and obstetricians and, later, the Abortion Act of 1967.

- The commonest direct causes in the UK are thromboembolism, hypertensive disease and ectopic pregnancy. The commonest indirect cause is cardiac disease.

- Risk factors include age, parity, low social class and being an ethnic minority.

- Taking into account Late deaths and those not reported to the Confidential Enquiry, psychiatric disease is now the leading cause of maternal death in the UK.

- Many of the deaths are preventable, both in Britain and worldwide.

Table 32.6
WHO estimates of maternal deaths

Causes of maternal death	Estimated number of deaths worldwide per year	
Haemorrhage	150 000	(25%)
Indirect (including HIV/AIDS)	120 000	(20%)
Sepsis	90 000	(15%)
Unsafe abortion	78 000	(13%)
Eclampsia	72 000	(12%)
Obstructed labour	48 000	(8%)
Other direct causes	48 000	(8%)

33

Antenatal care

Introduction

Most pregnancies are uneventful and uncomplicated and would progress normally without medical intervention. One of the purposes of antenatal care is to provide appropriate surveillance for all pregnancies in the hope of identifying the small number that do develop complications, with the aim of ensuring an optimum outcome for both the mother and her baby.

Ideally this should be achieved with as little interference as possible and tailored to a given woman's risk factors. Care, however, is usually based on a traditional arrangement of antenatal visits. The schedule varies, with the initial, or 'booking', visit somewhere between 10 and 18 weeks with subsequent visits often 4-weekly until 30 weeks, 2-weekly until 32 weeks and then weekly thereafter. While there is ongoing debate about rearranging this care according to evidence-based practice, the incentive for change from parents and care providers is weak.

In western societies antenatal care is provided by some combination of midwives, obstetricians and family doctors, depending on local preferences and resources. Care may be shared, and may include some hospital visits and some more local visits to other practitioners, allowing the hospital to focus on those who need more intensive input.

In the developing world many mothers have little or no antenatal care. This may have serious consequences. Haemorrhage, for example, remains the single most important cause of maternal death in less affluent countries and the risk of death is exacerbated by the underlying anaemia recognized to be present in two-thirds of women at booking. As the anaemia results from a combination of chronic undernutrition and malaria, these women would receive major benefits from antimalarial prophylaxis and iron supplementation. Access to healthcare is limited by poverty, lack of facilities, lack of education and cultural resistance. These issues have been discussed in Chapter 1.

The booking visit

The purpose of the antenatal booking visit is to detect any risk factors that may require extra surveillance above that provided to low-risk women. It is also an opportunity to identify any social difficulties and to discuss the parents' own wishes for the pregnancy and delivery.

Past obstetric history

A detailed account should be documented of the previous pregnancies and labours including gestation at delivery and whether the labour was induced or of spontaneous onset. The duration of labour, mode of delivery, birth weight, sex, neonatal outcome and any postnatal complications should also be noted.

Women who have experienced obstetrical difficulties in a previous pregnancy are often anxious to talk these through and consider the likelihood of recurrence. This is frequently a listening exercise so that anxieties and occasionally anger can be expressed, especially in cases of previous fetal or neonatal loss. An explanation followed by discussion of possible recurrence risks and a plan for the next pregnancy is useful. It is also an opportunity to identify those with abnormal grief reactions who might benefit from further counselling.

Medical and surgical history

This history should include details of previous operations, particularly gynaecological procedures such as a previous cone biopsy that may predispose to cervical incompetence, and must include a history of whether blood transfusions have been given. Questions should be asked about relevant medical disorders such as hypertension, diabetes, heart disease, renal disease, epilepsy, asthma or thyroid dysfunction.

Family history

The family history should cover potential congenital problems such as thalassaemia, cystic fibrosis, sickle cell anaemia, chromosomal disorders and previous congenital structural abnormalities.

History of present pregnancy

The date of the first day of the last menstrual period and details of the menstrual cycle prior to conception should be noted. If there has been a regular 28-day cycle the estimated date of delivery may be calculated by Naegele's rule: 9 months and 7 days are added to the date of the last period. For example, if the last menstrual period was on 1.1.03, then the estimated date of delivery would be 8.10.03. If the cycle is longer, then these extra days are also added on.

Drug history

It is essential to note all drugs and medications taken by the mother during the pregnancy as some preparations may be teratogenic.

Examination

A general examination is performed to include measurement of pulse rate, blood pressure and baseline weight. Auscultation of the heart may identify previously unrecognized structural problems. Abdominal examination gives an indication of the uterine size, and excludes abnormal masses and other abnormalities. There is no indication to carry out a routine vaginal examination although it remains sensible to check a cervical smear if one is due.

Ultrasound scan

This very useful investigation establishes fetal viability and gestational age, and excludes multiple pregnancy. It may also be an opportunity to measure the nuchal translucency (see p. 340).

Urine analysis

The urine is checked for the presence of protein and glucose.

Booking blood samples

- Full blood count to exclude maternal anaemia and thrombocytopenia (p. 316).
- Blood group to determine the ABO and rhesus status of the mother and to detect the presence of any irregular antibodies (p. 387).
- Rubella status to identify those mothers who are not immune to rubella and are therefore at risk of a primary rubella infection during pregnancy. Such women are offered rubella vaccination after delivery (p. 350).
- Haemoglobin electrophoresis may be offered to all women, or restricted to those of certain ethnic origin, particularly those of Asian, Afro-Caribbean or Mediterranean origin, and will identify those mothers who may be carriers of sickle-cell anaemia or thalassaemia.
- Hepatitis B status allows for neonatal vaccination if the result is positive (see p. 348).
- Serological testing for syphilis. Those with positive tests should receive penicillin.
- HIV (see p. 204).

Screening discussion

It is essential to use the booking visit to discuss screening options for chromosomal and structural abnormalities. This is an emotive area and parents should be aware of the implications of any tests they decide to take (p. 337).

Antenatal planning

Mothers at the extremes of reproductive age are at increased risk of obstetric complications, particularly hypertensive disorders, and they also carry an increased risk of perinatal mortality. Pre-eclampsia tends to improve with subsequent pregnancies, with the possible exception of severe preterm disease. The incidence of proteinuric pre-eclampsia in a second pregnancy is 10–15 times greater if there was pre-eclampsia in the first pregnancy, compared to those with a normal first pregnancy. It has been suggested that low-dose aspirin taken from early pregnancy (< 17 weeks and probably from the first trimester) may reduce the incidence of fetal growth restriction or perinatal mortality in those with previous severe disease. Studies in this area have provided conflicting evidence.

Those who have had a previous difficult instrumental delivery usually have a much more straightforward delivery next time around, but may occasionally request an elective caesarean section. This is controversial, and careful consideration of the advantages and disadvantages is required. In general, those with a previous caesarean section for a non-recurrent indication, e.g. breech, fetal distress or relative cephalopelvic disproportion secondary to fetal malposition, should be offered a trial of labour, although repeat elective caesarean section may be considered in certain circumstances.

In situations where there has been previous fetal growth restriction or an intrauterine death, subsequent management depends on the cause and the estimated likelihood of recurrence. More intensive antenatal monitoring is usually offered and the outcome is usually good, particularly when the loss was 'unexplained'.

Smoking is associated with low-birth-weight babies, probably related to fetal hypoxaemia and ischaemia from both carbon monoxide and nicotine. Although there is no evidence to support an association with fetal abnormality, long-term follow-up has demonstrated intellectual and emotional impairment. Smoking is also associated with an increased risk of abruption, preterm labour, intrauterine fetal demise and sudden infant death syndrome. Alcohol and drug misuse also carry significant fetal risks and, in the ideal world, all of these substances should be avoided in pregnancy.

Those whose work environment exposes them to radiation, hazardous gases or specific chemicals should be appropriately counselled. There is no evidence that VDUs are harmful, or indeed that work itself is harmful to the mother or fetus. The mother should be advised that she can continue working providing she is not unduly tired. Moderate exercise is likely to be of benefit and should be encouraged, but should probably be avoided if there are significant complications such as hypertension, cardiorespiratory compromise, antepartum haemorrhage or threatened preterm labour.

Antenatal surveillance

Subsequent visits are then used to identify obstetric complications.

Gestational hypertension and pre-eclampsia

The blood pressure and a urinalysis should be checked at every visit, and there should be a low threshold for acting on any abnormalities (see Ch. 39).

Fetal growth restriction (FGR) and small for gestational age (SGA) (see also Ch. 38)

'Small for gestational age' describes the baby whose birth weight is below the centile for a specified gestation, the most commonly used threshold being the 10th centile. The term 'fetal growth restriction' describes 'a fetus which fails to reach its genetic growth potential'. In practice it may be difficult to differentiate the two antenatally, but it is clear that fetal growth restriction carries a significant risk of chronic hypoxia, intrapartum asphyxia, neonatal hypoglycaemia, long-term neurological impairment and perinatal death. It is therefore important to try to identify these babies at an early stage to enable more intensive monitoring or delivery.

Screening for small babies can be by clinical palpation, with or without a tape measure, and is recognized to identify 40–50% of the babies that are truly small. Ultrasound studies have been shown to identify 25–90% of small babies depending on the criteria used, but there are currently no studies to support routine ultrasound growth measurements in low-risk pregnancies.

Impaired glucose tolerance and diabetes

Some centres offer a glucose tolerance test to women who fulfil certain criteria. Other centres screen all women by checking random blood sugar measurements, and others offer a glucose tolerance test to all women. The choice in part depends on the prevalence of the condition in the immediate population, and the significance is discussed further on page 327.

Haemolytic disease

Maternal IgG antibodies to fetal red cell antigens cross the placenta and may lead to fetal haemolysis, anaemia and hydrops fetalis. Initial sensitization usually occurs at delivery, but may also occur with vaginal bleeding at any stage, amniocentesis, external cephalic version or at some unrecognized event. The most significant antibody is to the rhesus antigen, which rhesus negative mothers may develop against rhesus positive fetal cells. All women should be screened for all antibodies at booking and again in the third trimester. Those with antibodies require further investigation (p. 387).

Breech presentation

The incidence of breech presentation is 40% at 20 weeks, 25% at 32 weeks and 3% at term, with the chance of spontaneous version after 38 weeks less than 4%. It is associated with multiple pregnancy, bicornuate uterus, fibroids, placenta praevia, polyhydramnios and oligohydramnios. Planned caesarean section at term is associated with less perinatal mortality and less serious neonatal morbidity than is planned vaginal birth, making it important for breech presentation to be identified prior to the onset of labour. This allows the option of external cephalic version, and a more planned delivery.

Breech presentation can be suspected following clinical palpation and confirmed by ultrasound scan. For further management, see page 432.

Anaemia

As there is a physiological fall in haemoglobin (Hb) as pregnancy advances, there is controversy about the treatment of mild anaemia (e.g. Hb 8–10 g/dl). Iron supplements may lead to gastrointestinal side-effects and have no proven benefits. Artificially raising the haemoglobin levels carries theoretical worries about increasing the risks of 'sludging' within the placenta.

On the other hand, iron supplements have no proven harmful effects and may lead to improvements in mitochondrial function and generalized well-being. Most practitioners will prescribe oral $FeSO_4$ if the Hb is < 10 g/dl or if the mean corpuscular volume (MCV) is low (e.g. < 80 fl), but it may be worth checking folate, vitamin B_{12} and ferritin before deciding on therapy. Oral iron is very well absorbed and the only indication for parenteral iron is when there are compliance worries or prohibitive side-effects with the oral route. Parenteral iron should never be given in thalassaemia.

Polyhydramnios

In the second and third trimester liquor is produced by fetal kidneys and is swallowed by the fetus. Excess liquor, polyhydramnios, may be defined as more than 2–3 litres of amniotic fluid. In the past, polyhydramnios was diagnosed by clinical examination – the uterus felt tight and fetal parts were difficult to palpate – but nowadays the amount of liquor is assessed by ultrasound. For practical purposes it may be considered as:

- a single pool > 8 cm in depth, or
- an amniotic fluid index > 90th centile. This is a measurement of the maximum depth of liquor in the four quadrants of the uterus (Fig. 33.1).

Polyhydramnios occurs in 0.5–2% of all pregnancies and is associated with maternal diabetes (~ 20%) and congenital fetal anomaly (~ 5%) (Table 33.1).

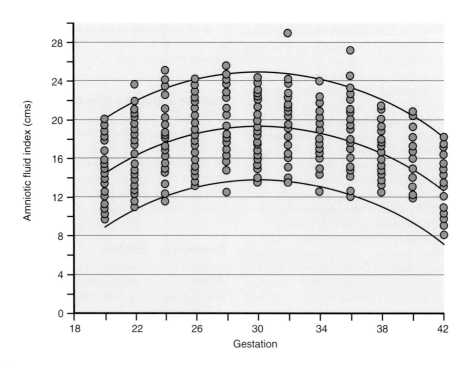

Fig. 33.1 **Amniotic fluid index (sum of the ultrasound depth of liquor in cm measured in the four quadrants of the uterus) according to gestation.**

Antenatal care   33

Table 33.1
Polyhydramnios

Cause of polyhydramnios	Pathology
Increased production from high urine output	Macrosomia, diabetes, recipient of twin–twin transfusion, hydrops fetalis
GI obstruction	Oesophageal atresia, duodenal atresia, bowel obstruction or Hirschsprung's disease
Poor swallowing because of neuromuscular problems or mechanical obstruction	Anencephaly, myotonic dystrophy, maternal myasthenia, facial tumour, macroglossia or micrognathia

Even in the absence of an identifiable cause (> 60%), polyhydramnios is associated with an increased rate of:

- placental abruption
- malpresentation
- cord prolapse
- carrying a large for gestational age infant
- requiring a caesarean section
- perinatal death.

It is important to arrange a growth and detailed ultrasound scan, glucose tolerance test, and fetal well-being assessment. Antibody titres should be checked to exclude alloimmune haemolytic disease (p. 387). Only rarely does it become necessary to aspirate liquor for maternal comfort or to decrease the chance of preterm labour. If it is aspirated, it quickly reaccumulates. Increased antenatal fetal surveillance is important, as is an increased awareness of the risks of intrapartum complications. A paediatrician should be present for delivery to check the baby for congenital anomalies.

Investigations may suggest that the baby is large for dates. It should be remembered that clinical examination and ultrasound measurements are relatively poor predictors of birth weight, and it is rarely justifiable to use these assessments alone to plan an elective caesarean section.

Prolonged pregnancy (> 42 weeks)

This is defined as pregnancy beyond 42 weeks' gestation. It occurs in 10% of pregnancies and is associated with a very slight increase in perinatal mortality due to unexplained intrauterine death, intrapartum hypoxia and meconium aspiration syndrome.

Monitoring of postdates pregnancy

Monitoring pregnancies over 40 weeks with ultrasound or cardiotocography (CTG) confers no demonstrable benefit.

Sweeping the membranes

This involves performing a vaginal examination and inserting a finger through the internal os to separate the membranes from the uterine wall, thus releasing endogenous prostaglandins. It may be uncomfortable for the mother. If a sweep is carried out once after 40 weeks' gestation, it increases the incidence of spontaneous labour before 42 weeks over controls, especially in those with a low Bishop's score. The risk of infection is considered to be minimal.

Induction of labour

Induction of labour after 41 weeks reduces the incidence of fetal distress and meconium staining compared with pregnancies managed conservatively with monitoring. There is also a reduction in the caesarean section rate and no increase in the incidence of uterine hypertonus. Despite this, no demonstrable effect on perinatal mortality has been observed, and it has been estimated that 500 inductions may be required to prevent one perinatal death.

Antenatal assessment of fetal well-being

Many hospitals have 'Day Unit' facilities for mothers who require additional assessment after their routine antenatal screening has identified some problem, most commonly possible pre-eclampsia or fetal growth restriction. Fetal monitoring may be by fetal movement charts, fetal cardiotocography, biophysical scoring and Doppler blood flow studies.

Fetal movement monitoring

This is used as a screening test for further investigations (Fig. 33.2). The woman is asked to choose a starting time (usually 9 a.m.) and record how long it takes to feel 10 separate movements. If there have been < 10 movements by say 5 p.m. she is asked to contact the hospital for further tests. There is great variation in what may be considered as normal and 'a change in the usual movements' may be more important than absolute numbers. The true value of movement counting, however, is unclear and a number of studies have failed to demonstrate any benefit.

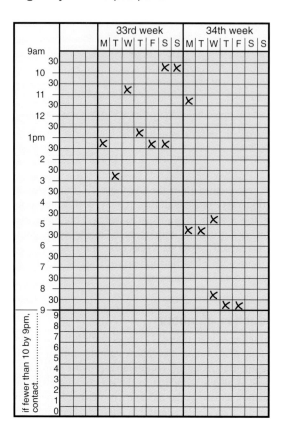

Fig. 33.2 **The 'count to ten' chart.** The mother is asked to start recording fetal movements at 9.00 a.m. and to contact the hospital for further tests if she has not recorded a total of 10 movements by 5.00 p.m.

Fetal cardiotocography (CTG)

The interpretation of CTGs is discussed on page 407. The CTG gives an indication of fetal well-being at a particular moment but has little longer-term predictive value. The routine use of antenatal cardiotocography does not seem to be associated with an improved perinatal outcome.

Fetal biophysical score

In the standard biophysical score five parameters are assessed, each scored out of 2, and the total out of 10 is used to give an indication of fetal well-being (Table 33.2). The CTG may be considered separately and the score therefore given out of 8. Of all the parameters, liquor volume is probably the most predictive of fetal well-being. As most babies with an abnormal biophysical score also have abnormal umbilical artery Doppler flow, it seems more appropriate to use Doppler studies. Furthermore, Doppler abnormalities also probably precede abnormalities in the biophysical profile.

Table 33.2
Parameters of the biophysical profile

CTG	More than two accelerations of 15 b.p.m. lasting longer than 15 seconds in 20 minutes
Fetal breathing	Lasting more than 30 seconds in 30 minutes
Fetal movements	More than three limb or trunk movements in 30 minutes
Fetal tone	One return to flexion (of neck) after extension, or one hand opening and closing
Liquor	More than 3 cm depth in two planes

Doppler blood flow studies

Doppler ultrasound examination of the umbilical arteries is used as an assessment of placental vascular resistance further downstream. It assesses blood flow, and reduced blood flow correlates with fetal compromise. In severe compromise it may stop altogether during diastole, or may even reverse. Reduction or loss of end-diastolic flow identifies a fetus at high risk of hypoxia, and indeed this hypoxia probably precedes Doppler abnormalities. A normal Doppler study, therefore, does not exclude hypoxia and tests of fetal well-being (e.g. CTG and amniotic fluid volume) must also be employed for complete assessment. There is probably no useful screening role for routine Doppler studies in low-risk pregnancies.

The test is useful in pregnancies considered at risk of hypoxia due to impaired placental function. In particular, a normal waveform would suggest that a small for gestational age fetus was constitutionally small rather than growth restricted due to impaired placental function. Abnormal waveforms are associated with an increased risk of structural and chromosomal abnormalities, and detailed sonography is indicated to avoid inappropriate iatrogenic morbidity.

Common antenatal problems
Backache

This occurs as ligaments relax, and a support brace, a firm mattress, and flat shoes are of help. Symptoms of nerve involvement warrant thorough clinical examination.

Carpal tunnel syndrome

The median nerve passes under the flexor retinaculum and supplies sensation on the radial half of the hand. Oedema may result in compression, which leads to paraesthesia of the thumb, index finger and lateral aspect of the middle finger. Holding the wrist hyperflexed for 2 minutes reproduces the symptoms. Treatment is by resting with the arm elevated, the use of splints, a local hydrocortisone injection or, in severe cases, surgical division of the retinaculum.

Constipation

Constipation is a common complaint in pregnancy and can be exacerbated by iron therapy. Usually dietary advice with recommendation of adequate intake of fibre and fresh fruit and vegetables is all that is required. Laxatives may be used, although bowel stimulants should be avoided.

Haemorrhoids

The weight of the gravid uterus reduces venous return and this, in addition to bearing down during labour, predisposes to haemorrhoids. Treatment is by avoiding constipation and local application of proprietary creams. Rarely, thrombosed prolapsed haemorrhoids require surgical treatment.

Heartburn

Relaxation of smooth muscle by high circulating levels of pregnancy hormones (particularly progesterone) causes relaxation at the oesophageal–gastric junction and reduces lower oesophageal sphincter pressure. This can result in the passage of acidic gastric juice into the lower oesophagus. It is helpful to avoid large meals, spicy meals, fatty foods, alcohol and cigarette smoking. Sleeping in a more upright posture can also help. Aluminium- and magnesium-based antacids appear to be safe during pregnancy and there has been no reported teratogenicity with the H_2 antagonist ranitidine.

Itching

This may be localized to the perineum or may be generalized. Localized itching may be due to infection (particularly candidiasis but less commonly pediculosis pubis or *Trichomonas vaginalis*). Generalized itching may occur with eczema, urticaria or scabies. If there is a systemic rash, consider one of the four pregnancy-associated dermatoses (see Table 33.3). Itching may also be due to intrahepatic cholestasis of pregnancy, particularly if on the palms of the hands (see p. 334).

Leg cramps

This affects a third of women in pregnancy and will be severe in 5%. Elevating the end of the bed 20 cm or so may help. Salt supplements are of unproven benefit and quinine should not be used.

Nausea and vomiting

This commonly starts at approximately 6 weeks' gestational age and, while it usually settles between 12–16 weeks, it sometimes continues throughout the pregnancy. It is sometimes referred to as morning sickness but often persists throughout the day. The sickness often takes the form of retching, rather than true vomiting, and rarely affects the mother's health. The cause of vomiting is unknown, but the onset and resolution of symptoms mirror the rise and fall of human chorionic gonadotrophin (hCG) in maternal serum. Furthermore, conditions associated with high levels of hCG, for example multiple pregnancies or molar pregnancies, are often associated with more severe symptoms.

Those admitted to hospital for excessive vomiting are said to have 'hyperemesis gravidarum'. Inability

Table 33.3
Dermatoses of pregnancy

	Incidence	Features	Usual timing of onset	Fetal problems	Treatment
Polymorphic eruption of pregnancy	1 : 240	Abdominal urticaria and vesicles (with no bullae), rarely occurring in the periumbilical area, sometimes extending to the proximal limbs	32 weeks' gestation to term	None	Antihistamines and topical steroids
Prurigo of pregnancy	1 : 300	Excoriated pustules on extensor surfaces	25–30 weeks' gestation	None	Antihistamines and topical steroids
Pruritic folliculitis		Acneiform rash	16–40 weeks' gestation	None	Topical steroids
Pemphigoid gestationis	1 : 10 000	Pruritic erythematous papules, plaques and wheals spreading from the periumbilical area to the breasts, thighs and palms. Diagnosed by the presence of immunofluorescence on biopsy	9 weeks' gestation to 7 weeks' postpartum	FGR and increased incidence of fetal abnormality	Antihistamines, topical steroids, systemic steroids and rarely plasmapheresis

to keep down fluids or solids leads to weight loss, dehydration and electrolyte disturbances, and may very rarely lead to vitamin B deficiency (and polyneuropathy). Liver failure, renal failure and fetal or maternal death are rare. On admission the urine should be tested for ketones, and blood sent for urea, electrolytes and haematocrit (urea and haematocrit may be elevated in dehydration). Liver function tests may also be deranged in severe hyperemesis, with reduced albumin and increased transaminase levels. It is also worth checking an ultrasound scan to exclude multiple pregnancy or a hydatidiform mole.

Treatment with i.v. fluids is usually sufficient in itself to reduce nausea and should be the only initial management. Anti-emetics may be used but only if the vomiting is not settling. No anti-emetics are licensed for use in pregnancy, but the risk of teratogenesis is probably very low with metoclopramide, cyclizine or prochlorperazine. Only extremely rarely are B-vitamin supplementation, enteral feeding or parenteral feeding required.

Vaginal discharge

'Normal' vaginal discharge may be heavier during pregnancy, but pathological causes should be excluded. Cándidiasis (thrush) is common and is typically a thick white or cream discharge with a cottage-cheese-like appearance. It may cause vulval itching. When a heavy vaginal discharge is noted, appropriate swabs should be taken to confirm the presence of infection and to suggest appropriate treatment.

Varicose veins

Varicose veins and ankle oedema are common, as the weight of the gravid uterus impairs venous return. They seldom improve until after delivery. Symptomatic relief in pregnancy may be gained from rest, elevation of the legs at rest, and the use of support stockings or tights.

Patient education (parentcraft)

This very important function is most often undertaken by a nominated midwife but may also have input from delivery suite staff, obstetricians and anaesthetists. Many women request guidance and information about normal and abnormal antenatal events and what to expect during the antenatal period, in labour and after delivery. The knowledge gained and the opportunity to discuss her pregnancy with an interested midwife can make a significant difference to the mother's perception of the pregnancy.

Parentcraft provides education for primigravidae, who have had no previous experience of pregnancy and labour, and advice is given about diet, dental care, stopping smoking and reducing alcohol intake. Multigravidae may request 'refresher' classes. Labour, normal and abnormal, can be explained. Visits to the delivery ward are offered, allowing women to become familiar with the delivery rooms, and provide the first contact with the staff of the delivery suite. Information about analgesia in labour can also be given so that women may make an informed decision as to their preference, although they should be encouraged to keep an open mind.

Parentcraft classes targeting a particular group are becoming popular, e.g. multiple pregnancy or teenage classes where women can meet others in similar circumstances to themselves. In this way, particular difficulties experienced by a group can be discussed and addressed.

Drug misuse

The prevalence of drug misuse is on the increase, particularly in women of childbearing age. Serious problem misuse (especially i.v.) and poly-drug misuse is associated with socio-economic deprivation and an increase in obstetric complications including miscarriage, antepartum haemorrhage, fetal growth restriction, intrauterine death and preterm labour. Care must usually be directed firmly towards social factors before any impact on obstetric problems can be achieved. Pregnancy may provide a window of opportunity to provide real help, breaking a cycle of poor parenting which might in turn lead to further problems in the next generation (Fig. 33.3).

The history should cover:

- type of drug (Table 33.4)
  - street drugs, e.g. heroin, amfetamines
  - pharmacological preparations (usually illicit and/or prescribed), e.g. benzodiazepines, buprenorphine and analgesics, particularly DF118 and other codeine compounds
  - prescribed preparations, usually methadone
- pattern of use, dose, route, frequency and method of financing supply
- social support, the other children, partner, family, friends, social work involvement, clothing, food, shelter and transport
- impending legal problems
- risks of infection including HIV, hepatitis B/C counselling with or without testing
- domestic abuse, which is a common occurrence with all groups of pregnant women, and all women should be asked about this (surprisingly, it is not any more common in association with socio-economic deprivation): among women, drug misuse is often a consequence, rather than a cause, of violence.

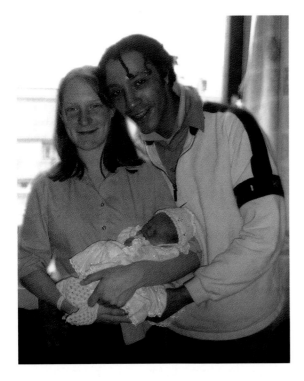

Fig. 33.3 **This mother, who was taking methadone, required induction of labour as for fetal growth restriction. (reproduced with permission)**

There may be poor self-esteem following a lack of trusting relationships, lack of positive body image and concerns about the woman's abilities to be a parent.

Management

Social factors   Illegal drugs are expensive and addicts are often forced into theft (and therefore problems with the police and courts) or prostitution (with its risks of violence and sexually transmitted diseases including HIV). In addition, lifestyle may be erratic and pregnancy outcome is compounded by various additional nutritional and social factors. Attendance for antenatal care may often compete with more immediate problems (e.g. seeing the social worker or lawyer, or getting money/drugs etc.) but if such care can be delivered locally with truly flexible access and be combined with confidentiality, non-judgemental consistency, access to social workers and legal aid, then fuller and more holistic care can be achieved.

Users of opiates/opioids   For opiate/opioid users it is worth considering transfer to methadone (which is metabolized more slowly, and therefore has more stable levels, and less risk of fetal distress and preterm labour associated with sudden withdrawals or fluctuations in serum opiate levels). Those stabilized on methadone alone probably have a lower neonatal mortality than those still taking heroin. There may also be improved prenatal attendance.

Detoxification   There are theoretical fetal risks from very rapid opiate/opioid detoxification but in practice the true fetal risks from even 'cold turkey' detoxification are relatively small. Despite this, patients undergoing

Table 33.4
Fetal effects of drugs

Alcohol	There is no clear dose relationship. Fetal alcohol syndrome is rare (fetal growth restriction, microcephaly, craniofacial abnormalities and mental retardation). Consumption of even small amounts of alcohol has been associated with a reduction in birth weight and intellectual impairment
Amfetamines	There is no good evidence of fetal abnormality. Fetal thrombocytopenia is very rare
Benzodiazepines	Neonatal withdrawal occurs at levels associated with abuse, even after quite brief use. 'Floppy infant syndrome' may occur if high doses have been given to a non-abusing mother in the 15 hours prior to delivery
Ecstasy	No increased risk has been demonstrated
Cannabis (hash, marihuana)	There have been no demonstrable teratogenic effects, but there is almost certainly fetal growth restriction
Opiates/opioids (e.g. heroin, methadone, DF118, buprenorphine)	Methadone and heroin are also associated with fetal growth restriction, and heroin is also associated with amenorrhoea (± anovulation) and preterm labour. Buprenorphine and DF118 probably have similar associations to those of heroin, but with DF118 there is increased severity of withdrawal
Cocaine and 'crack'	There is an increased risk of abruption, premature rupture of membranes and possibly fetal growth restriction and sudden infant death syndrome
Nicotine	There is an association with fetal growth restriction, preterm labour, perinatal death and delayed development. Tobacco use, if heavy, may lead to neonatal withdrawal symptoms
LSD	No increased risk has been demonstrated

rapid detoxification should ideally be managed on an obstetric unit, or at least under the close supervision of an obstetrician. It has been suggested that the risks of detoxification (whether rapid or gradual) may be higher in the first and third trimesters, but practical experience does not bear this out. The goal should be to reduce drug use to a level compatible with stability (e.g. with methadone), not necessarily aiming for abstinence. It may be more acceptable for a mother taking a moderate dose of methadone to top up with very small amounts of a similar non-injected substance (e.g. smoking heroin) than increasing methadone doses to very high levels in a futile attempt to achieve total abstinence from illicit drugs. If, however, women attempt unrealistic reductions in methadone and top up with other drugs, the dose of methadone should be increased. Topping up with benzodiazepines is particularly inadvisable.

Neonatal complications

There is an increased incidence of low birth weight due to fetal growth restriction, preterm delivery and sudden infant death syndrome. Neonatal withdrawal problems are particularly associated with opiates/opioids and benzodiazepines, and are worse if they have been used together. Severity is dose related and timing depends on the rate of drug metabolism, e.g. heroin and morphine are metabolized rapidly and signs usually develop within 1 day, whereas methadone is metabolized more slowly, and signs usually occur between 3 and 5 days. Classically, babies are hungry but feed ineffectually. There is CNS hyperexcitability (increased reflexes and tremor), GI dysfunction (finger sucking, regurgitation, diarrhoea) and respiratory distress. Treatment options include replacement for those who have been taking opiates/opioids, but it is not appropriate for benzodiazepine withdrawals. The severity of withdrawal symptoms is reduced by breast-feeding.

Key points

- Pregnancy is a physiological event, not an illness, and medical interference should be limited to those women who are truly likely to benefit. Nonetheless, complications can arise.

- Antenatal care is a multifaceted screening programme aimed at identifying problems at an early stage to minimize the risks to mothers and their babies. How best to deliver this care remains a subject for debate, but uncertainties about this should not give way to neglectful complacency.

34

Postnatal care

The puerperium is defined as being from delivery of the placenta to the end of the sixth postnatal week. This arbitrary definition, however, has no true physiological basis as some pregnancy changes revert to the pre-pregnancy state within a few minutes while others never revert at all.

The uterus contracts within just a few minutes from a cavity capable of containing 4 or 5 litres to a space barely able to contain an adult's fingers. It involutes over the next 4 weeks from 1000 g to just 50–100 g in size, with the lochial discharge changing from red to brownish pink and finally yellowish/white. Maternal weight reduces, plasma volume, red cell mass and haemostasis revert back to normal, and the other systemic, endocrine and metabolic adaptations return to the pre-pregnancy state. Lactation, instigated by the falling progesterone levels and maintained by oxytocin, inhibits the return of menstruation and fertility until weaning.

Routine postnatal assessment is useful to help provide the mother with support as she cares for her baby, and to identify any puerperal complications at an early stage.

Normal puerperium

For those delivering in hospital, the postnatal stay should be tailored to each individual mother. The length of this stay depends largely on maternal wishes and on her clinical condition, and may be anything from an immediate discharge to several days or longer. Problems with breast-feeding, difficulties with bonding, the development of medical problems, poor social circumstances or lack of home support may all warrant more inpatient support.

If the woman is rhesus negative, a Kleihauer test should be sent and the baby's blood group checked to determine whether anti-D prophylaxis is required. The mother should also be offered rubella vaccination if she is known to be non-immune.

Early postnatal checks

In the UK, the midwife sees the woman each day after delivery and checks on:

- general emotional and physical well-being
- infant feeding and care – breast-feeding should be encouraged if possible

- urinary and bowel function (see below)
- lochia – this may continue for up to 4–8 weeks
- contraceptive plans.

On examination, the following should be checked as a matter of routine:

- Pulse, blood pressure and temperature, looking for signs of haemorrhage, anaemia or sepsis.
- Abdominal examination to ensure that the uterus is involuting. On the first day after delivery the uterine fundus should be palpable at the umbilicus and it gradually reduces in size until, by the 10th–14th day, it is no longer palpable above the symphysis pubis.
- The perineum, looking particularly for evidence of wound breakdown in those who have had sutures. Ice or cold packs may be applied, simple analgesia prescribed and local anaesthetic gels or sprays may sometimes be of help.

Late postnatal check

This usually takes place around 6 weeks after delivery and should be a chance to review the delivery, answer any doubts or questions, and place these in context for future deliveries. It is important to assess the baby and how well the mother is coping, looking particularly for tiredness or depression.

The maternal haemoglobin should be checked and a cervical smear taken if appropriate. Contraception can again be discussed and enquiries made about whether intercourse has been resumed and whether there were any specific problems.

Postnatal problems

Anaemia

The incidence of postnatal anaemia is 25–30%. It is reasonable simply to treat non-symptomatic anaemia with oral iron, reserving transfusion for those with significant symptoms.

Bowel problems

Constipation may in part be due to narcotic analgesia in labour and is reported by up to 20% of postnatal women. Haemorrhoids also affect around 20% of women and these often persist for some time after delivery. They are more common in primiparous women and after instrumental delivery.

Breast problems

Two-thirds of women will have some problem, including nipple pain, engorgement, cracks and bleeding. These can largely be prevented by proper advice regarding positioning of the baby's mouth and supportive counselling. Mastitis, if it occurs, is usually the result of a blocked duct although it can occur secondary to infection (e.g. with *Staphylococcus aureus*).

Episiotomy breakdown

This is not uncommon, but long-term problems are rare. If the wound is clean, resuturing should be considered. If there is any suggestion of infection, however, it is probably better to allow healing by secondary intention.

Incontinence

In the first year after delivery, 3–5% of women experience urinary tract infection and about 5% report urinary frequency for the first time. Low-grade urinary tract infection is possible especially after catheterization.

At least 20% of women suffer from stress incontinence if assessed 3 months after delivery. This is mostly from neuropraxia and commonly resolves spontaneously. A few will still be incontinent a year later. Postnatal exercises are of help.

Inability to control flatus or faeces occurs in around 5% of women after delivery, but as it is often embarrassing, women frequently fail to report it. According to ultrasound studies, 35% of primiparae have demonstrable damage to the anal sphincter although many of these women do not have symptoms (Fig. 34.1). Both direct perineal trauma and nerve damage following spontaneous or instrumental delivery contribute to the problem. Investigation and treatment of symptoms is warranted.

Psychiatric problems in the puerperium

These range from 'the blues', which can be so common as to be normal, to the much more serious puerperal psychosis, which is rare, but can have fatal consequences.

'The postnatal blues'

This occurs in over 50% of women, usually beginning on days 2–4, peaking at days 4–6 and lasting for 2–7 days. It is a mood disturbance rather than a mood illness, which may have a hormonal basis, and it is unrelated to obstetric or cultural factors. There is emotional lability, tearfulness, sadness, sleep disturbance, poor concentration, restlessness and headaches. The mother may feel vulnerable and/or rejected, and may show undue concern for the baby. Treatment is with reassurance and support. Antenatal preparation may be of help.

Postnatal depression

The incidence of postnatal depression is between 10–25% of women in the first postnatal year, with the peak onset around weeks 3–4. In two-thirds, the illness

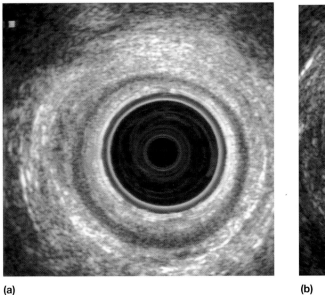 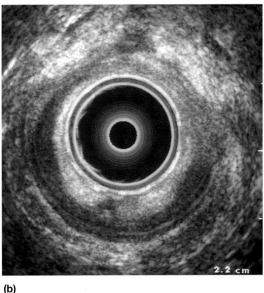

(a) (b)

Fig. 34.1 **Anal sphincter damage on endoanal ultrasound. (a)** Normal anal sphincter scan. **(b)** Anterior anal sphincter defect between the 10 o'clock and 3 o'clock position.

is self-limiting; in one-third it may be sustained or severe. There are the usual features of depression, but particularly increased irritability, tiredness, decreased libido, guilt at not loving or caring enough for the baby, inability to cope with the baby or undue anxieties over the baby's health and feeding. It is more likely in those who have had adverse life events shortly before or during pregnancy, those in marital conflict and those ambivalent to motherhood. It is not related to obstetric factors, but may be associated with a past history of depression. Treatment depends on severity, circumstances and patient preferences, but includes brief psychotherapy, supportive psychotherapy, counselling and antidepressants. The outcome is generally good.

Puerperal psychosis

This has an incidence of 1:500–800 deliveries, beginning around days 3–7 and peaking at 2 weeks. There may be serious risks to both the mother and child. One study has suggested that 5% of patients commit suicide and 4% kill their baby. There are variable psychotic symptoms, sometimes superimposed upon postnatal blues. The clinical picture is a shifting one, often ushered in by one or two nights' insomnia. Mood abnormality is common and the mother may be suspicious, sometimes denying the pregnancy and baby. There may be delusions, hallucinations, confusion and cognitive impairment. The condition is associated with a past history of psychosis (especially manic depression), with being unmarried, having a caesarean section, developing an

infection or suffering a perinatal death. Mother and baby should be admitted to hospital, ideally to a specialized mother and baby unit. The prognosis is good for the incident episode, particularly if the family is supportive, but 20% of those who become pregnant again will develop a further puerperal psychosis. 50% will have another psychotic episode at some time in their life.

Puerperal pyrexia

This is defined as a temperature of > 38°C on any occasion in the first 14 days after delivery or miscarriage (a slight fever is not uncommon in the first 24 hours). Pyrexia is usually due to urinary or genital infections (including endometritis) but may also be related to infection in the chest or breast. Deep venous thrombosis and pulmonary thromboembolism must not be forgotten. After a full clinical examination (including breasts, legs, perineum, chest, and abdominal palpation of the uterus) a midstream specimen of urine should be sent, as well as endocervical and wounds swabs as appropriate. If there is any suggestion of a chest infection sputum should also be sent for culture. Blood cultures need only be taken if the patient is systemically unwell.

In general, if the mother is well and the temperature only mildly elevated, conservative treatment may be warranted. If she is unwell and the source of infection is not clear, treatment should be started with either co-amoxiclav or with a combination of amoxicillin and metronidazole. Breast infections should be treated with flucloxacillin and breast-feeding continued if possible.

Secondary postpartum haemorrhage

See page 358.

Superficial thrombophlebitis

This affects about 1% of women. There is a painful, erythematous and tender (usually varicose) vein. Treatment is with support stockings and anti-inflammatory drugs.

Key points

- The puerperium is a time of major physiological change, and a time of major emotional and personal upheaval.

- Postnatal checks are useful to assess both the mother and baby. The major maternal complications are sepsis, haemorrhage, thromboembolic disease and depression.

35   Medical disorders in pregnancy

Medical disorders are relatively common in pregnancy and often have no implications for the mother or her baby. The alteration in maternal physiology which occurs in pregnancy, however, may affect the medical condition, or the medical condition itself may affect the pregnancy and the baby. Treatment options for the mother may be limited by concerns for fetal welfare and there is therefore the potential for difficult ethical dilemmas.

The following conditions will be considered, but see also hypertension (p. 367), and infection in pregnancy (p. 347):

- diabetes mellitus
- venous thromboembolic disease
- cardiac disease
- connective tissue disease
- epilepsy
- hepatic disorders
- renal disorders
- respiratory disorders
- thrombocytopenia
- thyroid disorders.

Diabetes mellitus

Diabetes mellitus may be known to be present before pregnancy or may be discovered for the first time during pregnancy. Discovery during pregnancy is rare for type I (insulin-dependent) diabetes, but not uncommon in type II. In addition to these, however, a transient self-limiting state of hyperglycaemia may occur in pregnancy as a result of maternal endocrine changes.

Glucose homeostasis is maintained by the balance between insulin, which reduces glucose levels by increasing cellular uptake, and other hormones such as glucagon and cortisol, which increase glucose production. In pregnancy the placenta produces additional cortisol as well as other insulin antagonists such as human placental lactogen, progesterone and human chorionic gonadotrophin, all of which tend to increase the glucose level. If the pancreatic β islet cells are unable to produce sufficient insulin to balance this increase, or if there is maternal insulin resistance, the mother may develop a state of hyperglycaemia referred to as 'gestational diabetes'. A lesser rise in glucose levels that does not reach the criteria required for a diagnosis of gestational diabetes is termed 'impaired glucose tolerance of pregnancy'.

Women with pre-existing diabetes mellitus may have high glucose levels in the first trimester at the time of organogenesis, and there is an increase in the rate of congenital abnormality in these pregnancies. The abnormalities are mainly cardiac defects, neural tube defects and renal anomalies and are more likely to occur if the diabetic control has been poor. Although the mechanism of this teratogenesis is unclear, there is very good evidence that improved pre-pregnancy and early pregnancy control reduces this congenital abnormality risk.

Fetal glucose levels closely follow those of the mother, with glucose crossing the placenta through facilitated diffusion. Maternal insulin does not cross the placenta and the fetus produces its own insulin from around 10 weeks' gestation. This insulin is recognized to have a significant role in promoting fetal growth. As maternal levels of glucose are higher in mothers with diabetes, fetal levels are also increased and, in turn, there is increased insulin production from the fetal β islet cells. This excess insulin leads to macrosomia (large babies) and organomegaly as well as increased erythropoiesis and neonatal polycythaemia.

In addition to the risk of congenital abnormality there is also a risk of unexplained intrauterine fetal death, possibly because fetal hyperinsulinaemia leads to chronic hypoxia and lactic acidaemia. A macrosomic fetus may be more at risk of these complications because of its increased oxygen demands.

Although fetal growth restriction occurs, in that a neonate may weigh 4 kg rather than 5 kg, only 15% of babies of diabetic mothers weigh less than the normal 50th centile, and to be less than the 5th centile is very uncommon. Labour and delivery may therefore be complicated by dystocia and in particular shoulder dystocia. Neonates may have hypoglycaemia, hypocalcaemia, hypomagnesaemia and polycythaemia. There is also an increased incidence of respiratory distress syndrome.

Effects of pregnancy on diabetes

Insulin requirements may be static or decrease during the first trimester. They increase during the second and third trimesters and may reduce slightly towards 40 weeks. Pregnancy, and tighter glucose control, exacerbate diabetic retinopathy, and the eyes should be assessed for signs of proliferative retinopathy, with laser treatment if required.

Effects of diabetes on pregnancy

The incidence of pre-eclampsia is increased. There is also an increased incidence of maternal infection, particularly of the urinary tract, which may account in part for the increased incidence of pre-term labour. Poly-hydramnios, which probably results from increased fetal polyuria, may result in unstable lie, malpresentation and preterm labour.

Screening for impaired glucose tolerance and gestational diabetes

This is an extremely controversial subject. Some centres offer a glucose tolerance test (GTT) to women who fulfil certain criteria, for example those with significant glycosuria, or with a family history of diabetes, or previous babies above the 90th centile, or those with a history of previous gestational diabetes. Other centres screen all women by checking random blood sugar measurements and offering a glucose tolerance test to those with abnormal levels (e.g. those with a blood sugar level ≥ 6 mmol/l 2 hours after food or ≥ 7 mmol/l at any time). Others offer a glucose tolerance test to all women. The choice in part depends of the prevalence of the condition in the local population.

The normal fasting plasma glucose is < 5.5 mmol/l. For an oral GTT patients should fast overnight. Venous blood is taken for fasting blood glucose and a 75-g glucose drink is given. Further venous blood samples are taken after 1 hour and 2 hours. The WHO non-pregnant diagnostic criteria are:

- diabetes: fasting glucose > 7.8 mmol/l and/or 2-hour level > 11.2 mmol/l
- impaired glucose tolerance: fasting glucose ≤ 7.8 mmol/l and the 2-hour level ≤ 11.2 mmol/l but ≥ 8 mmol/l.

When these criteria are applied to a European population in the third trimester of pregnancy, 10% will have impaired glucose tolerance.

Management of impaired glucose tolerance and gestational diabetes

The management is controversial. There is no evidence that treatment is beneficial unless the criteria for diabetes are actually reached. It is reasonable to treat with diet in the first instance (unless the preprandial glucose is greater than 8 mmol/l) and to consider insulin if the glucose level remains above 6 mmol/l or the postprandial level is greater than 8 mmol/l on dietary treatment. Insulin treatment should aim to keep the preprandial glucose less than 6 mmol/l.

One-third of women with impaired glucose tolerance in pregnancy go on to develop diabetes mellitus in the subsequent 25 years.

Antenatal management of established diabetes

At pre-pregnancy counselling, advice should be given about good diabetic control, diet, smoking and folate supplements. If possible, pregnancy management should be in a combined obstetric/diabetic clinic with frequent visits planned as required. Blood glucose should be measured several times a day at home, aiming for tight control (e.g. with preprandial levels < 5 mmol/l and 1- to 2-hour postprandial levels of < 7.5 mmol/l). Glycosylated haemoglobin (HbA_{1c}) should be checked monthly, aiming for levels below about 8% depending on the laboratory reference range.

Insulin is commonly given in a soluble form three times a day (before meals), with an intermediate insulin overnight. Ketoacidosis should be avoided as it is associated with significant perinatal mortality.

Maternal renal function and optic fundi should be checked in early pregnancy, and a detailed anomaly scan offered at 18–20 weeks to look for congenital abnormalities. The abdomen should be examined for polyhydramnios, macrosomia or fetal growth restriction, and serial growth scans may also be useful.

In the third trimester regular assessments of fetal well-being (cardiography (CTG) or biophysical profile) may be carried out. While reduced liquor volume is associated with fetal compromise, polyhydramnios in diabetes may also be a sign of chronic fetal compromise.

With regard to delivery each case should be considered individually. There is no need for intervention before 38 weeks if there is no evidence of complications, and there is no indication for elective caesarean section on the basis of diabetes alone. If preterm labour occurs, steroids may be given as for the non-diabetic patient, but may lead to marked deterioration in diabetic control.

Delivery

There are numerous different regimens of intravenous dextrose and insulin, but the aim of all is to maintain tight intrapartum control whether during labour or for caesarean section. In the immediate postpartum period insulin requirements rapidly return to pre-pregnancy levels and the previous subcutaneous regimen can be re-established.

In view of the probability of diabetes in later life, it is appropriate to consider some form of subsequent screening in any mother known to have had gestational diabetes.

Venous thromboembolic disease

Antenatal

In pregnancy the balance of the clotting system is altered towards clot formation. There are increased levels of fibrinogen, prothrombin and other clotting factors, together with reduced thrombin inhibitor action. This tendency to clot formation is only in part offset by an increase in fibrinolysis. In addition to the clotting system changes, the gravid uterus causes some mechanical obstruction to the venous system and leads to peripheral venous stasis in the lower limbs.

Venous thromboembolic disease appears to be very rare in Africa and the Far East but is the commonest direct cause of maternal mortality in the UK. The reason for such wide racial difference may be that the factor V Leiden mutation and prothrombin gene variants are rare in African and Asian populations. In the UK just over 40% of maternal deaths from thromboembolism occur antenatally, often in the first trimester. Over 80% of deep venous thromboses (DVTs) in pregnancy are left-sided, in contrast to only 55% in non-pregnant woman. The underlying explanation is not established, but it may reflect compression of the left common iliac vein by the right common iliac artery and the ovarian artery, which cross the vein on the left side only. Furthermore, more than 70% of DVTs in pregnancy are iliofemoral compared to the non-pregnant rate of around 9%, and are therefore more likely than lower calf vein thromboses to give rise to pulmonary embolism.

Risk factors for thromboembolic disease include:

- obesity
- age > 35 years
- family history
- high parity
- previous thromboembolism
- immobility
- pre-eclampsia
- varicose veins
- congenital or acquired thrombophilia
- intercurrent infection
- caesarean section (particularly emergency caesarean section).

Thromboembolism may be asymptomatic but usually presents with the traditional symptoms and signs such as calf tenderness, cough and chest pain. It may also present with lower abdominal pain. It is essential to make a definitive diagnosis if at all possible, not just for management of the current pregnancy but because there are major implications for subsequent pregnancies as well.

Blood testing may be helpful and a normal D-dimer implies a low risk of venous thromboembolic disease. Radiological investigations are often required. Duplex Doppler ultrasound is particularly useful for identifying femoral vein thromboses although iliac veins are less easily seen (Fig. 35.1). It is safe and should be the first-line investigation. Venography is more specific, but has the disadvantage of radiation exposure. It may be used if Doppler studies give equivocal results or are not available. It is also essential to fully investigate a suspected pulmonary embolism. Pregnancy is not a contraindication to carrying out a ventilation–perfusion ($\dot{V}/\dot{Q}$) scan – any risks are far outweighed by the

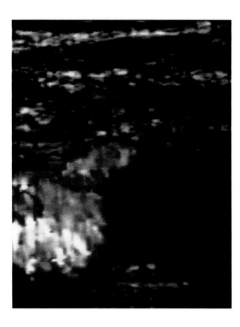

Fig. 35.1 **Normal Doppler flow in the femoral artery (red, left) with no flow through the occluded femoral vein (black, right).**

benefits of accurate diagnosis (Fig. 35.2). A normal scan virtually excludes the diagnosis of pulmonary embolism. A computerized tomography (CT) scan of the pulmonary artery may also be appropriate if a large pulmonary embolism is suspected.

Treatment of DVT or pulmonary embolism in pregnancy is with intravenous (i.v.) or subcutaneous (s.c.) heparin, continued into labour. Low-molecular-weight heparin is appropriate in most instances although i.v. unfractionated heparin is still appropriate for those with a major pulmonary embolus. Low-molecular-weight heparin probably carries a lower risk of thrombocytopenia and possibly also of osteoporosis. After delivery the woman may choose to continue with s.c. heparin

or start warfarin, continuing anticoagulation for 6–12 weeks as decided by timing of onset and clinical severity of the thrombosis. Once anticoagulants are stopped, women should be screened for thrombophilia (Box 35.1).

Management of those with a previous history of thromboembolism carries more uncertainties. Women who have had a single episode of DVT/PTE should be screened for thrombophilia. If the screen is negative, and the event occurred outside pregnancy and was not severe, thromboprophylaxis may not be required. If positive, or there are other risk factors, antenatal and postnatal prophylaxis can be considered. Heparin treatment may induce thrombocytopenia and may also rarely lead to osteoporotic fractures.

Postnatal risk assessment

The risks of thromboembolism should be assessed in all patients who undergo caesarean section (see Box 35.2). It is also essential to consider prophylaxis in women who have vaginal delivery, whether instrumental or not, who may be at increased risk.

Cardiac disease

Heart disease of variable types complicates less than 1% of all pregnancies but accounts for around 10% of UK maternal deaths. Rheumatic heart disease remains a significant problem in the developing world but in western countries there are increasing numbers of fertile women who have had surgery as children for congenital heart disease. Maternal mortality is highest in conditions where pulmonary blood flow cannot be increased to compensate for the increased demand during pregnancy, particularly Eisenmenger's syndrome where maternal mortality rates reach 40–50%.

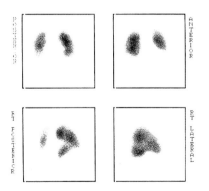

Fig. 35.2 **Positive Q̇ scan.** Note the lack of perfusion in the right lower lobe. The ventilation scan was normal. (From Pitkin et al 2003.)

valve prolapse) the prognosis is good and there may be no need for cardiac follow-up. If there are potential haemodynamic problems, pregnancy termination is often advisable (e.g. with Eisenmenger's syndrome, primary pulmonary hypertension and pulmonary veno-occlusive disease). With atrial fibrillation, anticoagulation is required to prevent atrial clot forming and subsequent embolic problems. If the maternal P_{O_2} is decreased, the fetus is at risk from hypoxia and fetal growth restriction, and should be monitored closely.

Severe cardiac disease can cause problems at delivery, particularly in those with prosthetic valves, aortic stenosis, severe mitral stenosis and again those with pulmonary hypertension (Box 35.3).

Myocardial infarction is very rare in pregnancy but carries a high mortality, especially in the puerperium (25–50%). Puerperal cardiomyopathy is also rare (< 1 : 5000), carries a 25–50% mortality, and is associated with hypertension in pregnancy, multiple pregnancy, high multiparity and increased maternal age. It presents with sudden onset of heart failure and on echocardiography there is a grossly dilated heart (Fig. 35.3).

Connective tissue disease

These diseases are not uncommon and, as they often affect women during their childbearing years, they are not infrequently found in association with pregnancy. See also the antiphospholipid syndrome page 166.

Unfortunately, many of the symptoms and signs of heart disease occur commonly in normal pregnancy, making a clinical diagnosis difficult. Breathlessness and syncopal episodes are present in 90% of normal pregnancies, atrial ectopic beats are common and up to 96% of normal women may have an audible ejection systolic murmur. Further investigation should be considered if the murmur is > 2/6, if a thrill is present, or if there are any other suspicious features.

If problems are discovered a cardiologist should be involved in the antenatal care. If there is no haemodynamic compromise (e.g. as with congenital mitral

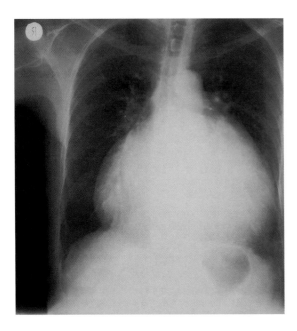

Fig. 35.3 **Postpartum cardiomyopathy after twin delivery in a mother aged 42 years.** There is massive cardiomegaly. The patient very nearly required cardiac transplantation, but improved spontaneously.

Systemic lupus erythematosus (SLE)

Pregnancy does not affect the long-term prognosis of SLE. There is probably an increased chance of flare-ups occurring in pregnancy, and particularly in the postnatal period (Fig. 35.4). Women should be discouraged from becoming pregnant during disease flare-ups to minimize fetal problems. Active SLE nephritis during pregnancy is associated with a significant maternal and perinatal mortality and in particular with a risk of pre-eclampsia.

SLE is associated with increased fetal loss rates from spontaneous miscarriages and preterm delivery. This is particularly so in those with raised anticardiolipin antibodies. There is an increased incidence of pre-eclampsia and this may be difficult to differentiate from a disease flare-up, as both are associated with hypertension and proteinuria. There is no increase in the rate of fetal abnormalities, although there is a risk of fetal congenital heart block associated with the presence of anti-Ro and anti-La antibodies (Fig. 35.5). Neonatal lupus may rarely occur and is characterized by haemolytic anaemia, leucopenia, thrombocytopenia, discoid skin lesions, pericarditis and congenital heart block.

If lupus anticoagulant or anticardiolipin antibodies are present, low-dose aspirin should be given and, in women with a previous history of thromboembolic disease, low-dose heparin may also be required. Careful monitoring of renal function is appropriate. Flare-ups should be managed where possible with oral prednisolone (if the woman is not already on oral prednisolone) and there should be regular growth scans looking for fetal growth restriction, as well as regular fetal monitoring with CTG and biophysical profiles in the third trimester.

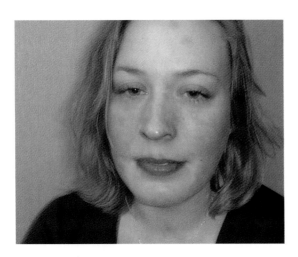

Fig. 35.4 **Facial rash of a severe second trimester flare-up of systemic lupus erythematosus** (with permission).

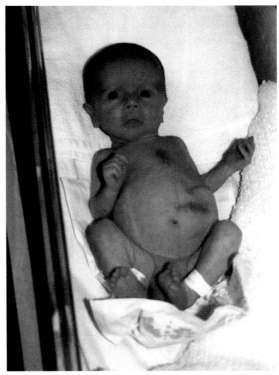

Fig. 35.5 **Pacemaker in baby with congenital heart block in association with anti-Ro antibodies** (with permission).

Epilepsy

A seizure in pregnancy should be assumed to be eclampsia until proven otherwise. Around a third of pregnant women with epilepsy have an increase in seizure frequency independent of the effects of medication, particularly those with secondary generalized or complex partial seizures. For epileptic women on treatment, the fall in anticonvulsant levels due to dilution, reduced absorption, reduced compliance and increased drug metabolism is partially compensated for by reduced protein binding (and therefore an increase in the level of free drug). There is an increased incidence of fetal anomalies in association with epilepsy irrespective of the effects of drugs (3–4% vs 2% in the general population) possibly due to a combination of hypoxic and genetic factors (Fig. 35.6). For those on anticonvulsants, the incidence of anomalies is ≈ 6%. Single-drug regimens are less teratogenic than multidrug therapy (Table 35.1).

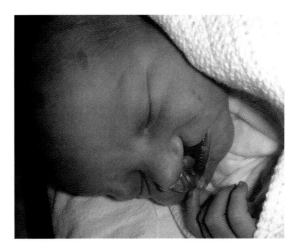

Fig. 35.6 **Anticonvulsants are associated with neural tube defects, cardiac and craniofacial defects** (with permission).

Hepatic disorders

There are a large number of potential causes of liver dysfunction in pregnancy (Tables 35.2 and 35.3). A history of a prodromal illness, overseas travel or high-risk group for blood-borne illness may suggest viral hepatitis. Itch is suggestive of cholestasis. Abdominal pain is associated with gallstones, HELLP syndrome (p. 372) or acute fatty liver. Clinical signs are often unhelpful in diagnosis. Urea and electrolytes (U&Es), urate, liver function tests (LFTs), blood glucose, platelets and coagulation screen should be checked and blood sent for hepatitis serology. Abdominal ultrasound of the liver may show obstruction or fat infiltration. It is usual for the alkaline phosphatase level to increase in pregnancy (1.5–2 times normal).

Renal disorders

In pregnancy, there is an increase in the size of both kidneys as well as dilatation of the ureter and renal pelvis (Fig. 35.7). This dilatation is greater on the right than the left because of the dextrorotation of the uterus. There is also an increase in creatinine clearance owing to the increased glomerular filtration rate (maximal in the second trimester). In pregnancy the normal serum urea should be < 4.5 mmol/l and creatinine < 75 μmol/l.

Table 35.1
Management of epilepsy in pregnancy

Pre-pregnancy counselling	Monotherapy ideal. Folate supplementation should be continued until at least 12 weeks
Anticonvulsant dosage	Anticonvulsant doses adjusted on clinical grounds. There are fetal risks from the anticonvulsant medication as well as from not taking the drugs (from increased fit frequency)
	Checking plasma levels is usually not necessary, but can occasionally be useful to check compliance and exclude toxicity ('free' drug levels rather than 'total' drug levels are ideal)
Detailed ultrasound scan at 18–22 weeks	Neural tube, cardiac and craniofacial abnormalities as well as diaphragmatic herniae are more common
Vitamin K for women on enzyme-inducing anticonvulsants	Oral vitamin K should be given daily from 36 weeks (anticonvulsants are vitamin K antagonists and increase the risk of haemorrhagic disease of the newborn). The baby should be given intramuscular vitamin K stat at birth and the paediatrician alerted to the possibilities of anticonvulsant drug withdrawal
Fits	Most fits in pregnancy will be self-limiting but if prolonged, rectal or intravenous diazepam p.r./i.v. with or without ventilation may be required
Postnatal	The mother may breast-feed safely (drugs pass into the milk but are of no clinical significance). Advice should be given about safe and suitable settings for feeding, bathing, etc. Carbamazepine, phenytoin, primidone and phenobarbital induce liver enzymes, reducing the effectiveness of the standard-dose combined oral contraceptives, and a higher-dose oestrogen preparation is therefore required

Table 35.2
Liver disorders specific to pregnancy

Hyperemesis gravidarum	This may occasionally be associated with abnormal LFTs
Obstetric cholestasis	Usually presents after 30 weeks' gestation possibly due to a genetic predisposition to the cholestatic effect of oestrogens. Pruritus affects the limbs and trunk, and it is often severe. There may be a positive family history in up to 50% of cases
	Serum total bile acid concentration is increased early in the disease and is the optimum marker for the condition. Transaminases may be increased (less than threefold). Bilirubin is usually < 100 µmol/l, and there may be pale stools and dark urine
	There are no serious long-term maternal risks but there is a risk of preterm labour, fetal distress and intrauterine fetal death. The fetus must be monitored closely and there is growing evidence that delivery at 37–38 weeks is appropriate. The combined oral contraceptive pill is contraindicated
HELLP syndrome	See page 372
Acute fatty liver of pregnancy	This is very rare, carries a high maternal and fetal mortality and may progress rapidly to hepatic failure. It usually presents with vomiting in the third trimester associated with malaise and abdominal pain followed by jaundice, thirst and alteration in consciousness level. LFTs are elevated, urate is very high and there is often profound hypoglycaemia. There may be hypertension and proteinuria. Coagulopathy, hypoglycaemia and fluid imbalance should be corrected and the fetus monitored or delivered, usually by caesarean section. Following delivery there is a risk of postpartum haemorrhage (PPH), and liver dysfunction may be prolonged. Hepatic encephalopathy may develop and liver transplant is occasionally necessary. If the patient recovers, there is no long-term liver impairment

Table 35.3
Liver disorders coincidental with pregnancy

Viral hepatitis	This is the commonest cause of abnormal LFTs in pregnancy. Titres should be checked for hepatitis A, B and C as well as for cytomegalovirus (CMV) and toxoplasmosis
Gallstones	Asymptomatic gallstones do not require treatment. Cholecystitis should be managed conservatively if possible
Cirrhosis	In severe cirrhosis there is usually amenorrhoea. If pregnancy occurs, and the disease is well compensated, there is usually no long-term effect on hepatic function. The main risk is bleeding from oesophageal varices
Chronic active hepatitis	This is usually associated with amenorrhoea. Pregnancy does not usually have any long-term effect on liver function. Obstetric complications are common and fetal loss rate is high. Immunosuppressant therapy with prednisolone and azathioprine should be continued in those with autoimmune disease
Primary biliary cirrhosis	This is variable in severity. The prognosis for mother and fetus is good in mild disease. It may present during pregnancy for the first time in a similar way to intrahepatic cholestasis of pregnancy

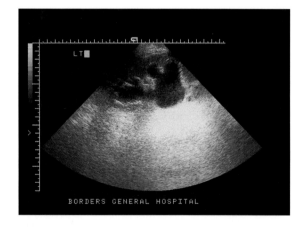

Fig. 35.7 **Ultrasound of left kidney with ureteric obstruction and calyceal clubbing.** There was a calculus in the lower third of the ureter.

Infection

Urinary tract infections occur in 3–7% of pregnancies and, if untreated, may lead to septicaemia and premature labour. Asymptomatic bacteriuria should be treated in all pregnant women, as there is a 30–40% risk of developing a symptomatic urinary tract infection (UTI). Pyelonephritis should be treated aggressively.

Obstruction

Acute hydronephrosis is characterized by loin pain, ureteric colic, sterile urine and a renal ultrasound scan showing dilatation of the renal tract greater than normal for pregnancy. If the symptoms are not settling and the ultrasound scan does not demonstrate the cause of the obstruction, a limited intravenous urogram should be considered. Treatment is with ureteric stenting or nephrostomy. There may be no obvious cause of obstruction and complete resolution may occur following delivery. Renal tract calculi are associated with an increased incidence of UTIs but otherwise do not usually affect pregnancy (unless obstruction is severe).

Chronic renal impairment

With chronic renal disease in pregnancy the fetal prognosis is best if maternal renal function and blood pressure (BP) are optimized. If the plasma creatinine is < 125 µmol/l the maternal and perinatal outcome is usually good. If > 250 µmol/l there is usually amenorrhoea, and if pregnancy occurs there may be a risk of renal deterioration. Between these levels women should be advised that pregnancy may cause their renal function to deteriorate and that there are also risks to the fetus (mainly fetal growth restriction). Some renal diseases carry a worse prognosis than others and specialist advice is required.

Ideally patients should receive pre-pregnancy counselling. The patient should be seen frequently antenatally, particularly in the third trimester. Raised BP should be treated aggressively, U&Es, plasma protein, urinalysis and midstream urine (MSU) samples checked at each visit, and a 24-hour urine collection sent each month for quantitative protein and creatinine clearance. Close fetal monitoring is important in the third trimester. It is difficult to distinguish pre-eclampsia from increasing renal compromise as both may present with hypertension and proteinuria.

Pregnancy should be discouraged in patients on dialysis as the fetal prognosis is poor. Pregnancy in women who have had a renal transplant is possible.

Respiratory disorders

Breathlessness due to the physiological increase in ventilation is a common symptom in pregnancy and is maximal around 28–31 weeks. Although there is an increased tidal volume from early pregnancy, the exact cause of the feeling of breathlessness is unclear. Investigation should be considered only if there is excess breathlessness, or if there are clinical signs. It should be remembered that breathlessness can also be a feature of pulmonary thromboembolic disease.

Asthma is a common condition. In most patients the disease is unchanged in pregnancy, but it may improve or, less commonly, deteriorate. Treatment is similar to that in the non-pregnant patient and patients already established on treatment should continue. Inhaled beta-sympathomimetics and inhaled steroids are considered safe. Oral steroids should be given if clinically indicated.

Thrombocytopenia

Maternal thrombocytopenia in pregnancy

In the second half of 8% of normal pregnancies there is a mild thrombocytopenia (platelet count 100–150 × 10^9/l) which is not associated with any risk to the mother or fetus. Platelets may also be reduced in pre-eclampsia.

Autoimmune thrombocytopenic purpura is the commonest cause of thrombocytopenia in early pregnancy (but can also arise in later pregnancy) and may be acute or chronic. Antiplatelet antibodies may be detected. These may cross the placenta and cause fetal thrombocytopenia, although this is rarely associated with long-term morbidity (cf. alloimmune thrombocytopenia below). No treatment is required in the absence of bleeding, providing the platelet count remains above 50 × 10^9/l. If the platelet count falls below this level, steroids and immunoglobulin can be given.

Fetal (alloimmune) thrombocytopenia

This is a rare disorder in which there are maternal antibodies to fetal platelets. This has similarities to rhesus disease in which there are maternal antibodies to the fetal red cells. The maternal platelet level is normal but there may be profound fetal thrombocytopenia and antenatal or intrapartum intracranial bleeds. The diagnosis should be suspected when a previous child has had neonatal thrombocytopenia and maternal antiplatelet antibodies have been identified (often to the HPA-1a antigen). Treatment is usually with antenatal immunoglobulin and elective caesarean section.

Thyroid disorders

1% of pregnant women in the western world are affected by thyroid disease, with hypothyroidism being commoner than hyperthyroidism. The fetal thyroid gland secretes thyroid hormones from the 12th week and is independent of maternal control.

Hypothyroidism

This may present with fatigue, hair loss, dry skin, abnormal weight gain, poor appetite, cold intolerance, bradycardia and delayed tendon reflexes. If untreated there is double the rate of spontaneous miscarriages and stillbirths compared to the normal population, as well as a risk of fetal neurological impairment. There is minimal fetal risk if the mother is treated and is euthyroid. Thyroid function should be regularly monitored, aiming to keep TSH within the normal range and free T_4 at the upper end of the normal range. If the woman is already on treatment and euthyroid at booking, the dose probably need not be increased. Fetal hypothyroidism may occur when the mother carries antithyroid antibodies or is receiving antithyroid drugs.

Hyperthyroidism

Thyrotoxicosis presents with weight loss, exophthalmos, tachycardia and restlessness. It is usually due to Graves' disease but may occur secondary to a toxic thyroid adenoma or multinodular goitre. Untreated thyrotoxicosis is associated with a high fetal mortality and a risk of maternal thyroid crisis at delivery. Well-controlled hyperthyroidism is not associated with an increase in fetal anomalies but there is a tendency for babies to be small for gestational age. Graves' disease usually improves during pregnancy. Carbimazole and propylthiouracil cross the placenta and can potentially cause fetal thyroid suppression but in low doses this is rarely significant. Radioactive iodine is absolutely contraindicated and surgery is indicated only for those with a very large goitre or poor compliance with oral therapy.

Postpartum thyroiditis

This occurs following 5–10% of all pregnancies, with initial hyperthyroidism followed by hypothyroidism and then recovery. As the hypothyroidism occurs around 1–3 months the condition may be confused with puerperal depression. Symptoms of hyperthyroidism may be treated with propranolol (antithyroid drugs accelerate the appearance of hypothyroidism). Hypothyroidism should be treated with thyroxine as above, withdrawing around 6 months after delivery. A small proportion may require long-term treatment or may develop hypothyroidism later in life.

Key points

- Diabetes carries risks of congenital abnormality and intrauterine death for the fetus.
- Pregnancy-related venous thromboembolic disease is the commonest direct cause of maternal mortality in many western countries. Any symptoms should be investigated fully, even if this requires X-rays or isotope scanning. Prophylaxis is important in both obstetrics and gynaecological practice.
- Structural heart disease in pregnancy has potentially serious implications for both mother and fetus.
- The fewer anticonvulsants, the less the risk of fetal abnormality.
- Abnormal liver function tests may be related to the pregnancy, but are commonly coincidental.
- Asymptomatic UTIs should be treated.
- Well-controlled thyroid disease poses little serious risk to mother or fetus.

36

Prenatal diagnosis

Introduction

The finding of some 'abnormality' in pregnancy transforms what was previously an exciting and joyous event into an extremely worrying and distressing time. Tact, understanding and reassurance (if appropriate) are paramount. The very greatest of care should be taken in explaining any findings to parents. The advice given to parents is of such importance that it will frequently be necessary to involve senior members of the obstetric team as well as members of other specialties, particularly paediatricians, and clinical geneticists and radiologists.

The aims of prenatal diagnosis are fourfold:

- the identification at an early gestation of abnormalities incompatible with survival, or likely to result in severe handicap, in order to prepare parents and offer the option of termination of pregnancy (TOP)
- the identification of conditions which may influence the timing, site or mode of delivery
- the identification of fetuses who would benefit from early paediatric intervention
- the identification of fetuses who may benefit from in-utero treatment (rare).

It should not be assumed that all parents are going to request TOP even in the presence of lethal abnormality. Many couples have opted to continue pregnancies in the face of severe defects that have resulted in either intrauterine or early neonatal death, and have expressed the view that they found it easier to cope with their grief having held their child. Others say that they were glad of the opportunity to terminate the pregnancy at an early stage and that they could not have coped with going on. More controversial still are the problems of chronic diseases with long-term handicap and long-term suffering for both the child and its parents. The parents themselves must decide what action they wish to take – it is they who will have to live with the decisions we place in front of them. It is our role to advise, guide and respect their final wishes, irrespective of our own personal views (see also Ethics, p. 19).

Non-directive counselling

When parents are found to have an abnormal baby they often know little or nothing about the abnormality, about termination or about recurrence risks. They need information, and it is the role of obstetricians and genetic counsellors to inform accurately and in language that is clear to understand. Often parents ask the doctor what he or she would do, but it remains important to encourage the couple towards their own decision.

Non-directive counselling has to be truly non-directive. The sentence 'the risk of handicap is 5%' sounds worse than 'the baby has a 95% chance of being normal'. Expressions like 'high risk' or 'severe handicap' imply a value judgement and should be avoided if possible. 'Common' may be interpreted as anything from 1% to 99% depending on the context and the listener.

It is sometimes helpful to give information in writing, as well as verbally. Parents may need time to take in information, and it is often important that they take time to consider any decisions carefully. It can be extremely useful to arrange a review a day or two after the initial appointment.

The spectrum of congenital abnormality

Although most congenital abnormalities are individually rare, together they cause an enormous burden of suffering. Approximately 2% of newborn babies have a serious abnormality detectable at, or soon after, birth. The main ones are listed in Box 36.1.

Assessing the risk

In general, the risks for most couples are very small, although the risk of Down's syndrome increases with increasing maternal age. In some instances, however, there may be a family history of an inherited condition, for example Duchenne muscular dystrophy, cystic fibrosis, sickle cell disease or myotonic dystrophy. Consanguinity increases the risk of genetic problems, particularly in relation to autosomal recessive conditions. Structural abnormalities are also usually slightly more likely to occur in those with a family history, for example a woman who has had a child with spina bifida has an approximately 2% risk of a recurrence compared to the background risk of ≈ 0.2%.

In addition, it is important to consider medical conditions. Those with diabetes have an increased risk of cardiac and neural tube defects, and those with epilepsy are also at increased risk of structural problems, particularly if taking potentially teratogenic anticonvulsants. The majority of structural and chromosomal problems, however, occur in those who have no predisposing history or recognized risk factors, and screening tests may be offered even to those apparently at low risk.

Box 36.1

SELECTED CONGENITAL ABNORMALITIES

Genetic disorders
- Down's syndrome (trisomy 21)
- Edward's syndrome (trisomy 18)
- Patau's syndrome (trisomy 13)
- Triploidy
- Sex chromosome abnormalities
- XO (Turner's syndrome)
- XXY (Klinefelter's syndrome)
- XYY
- XXX
- Apparently balanced rearrangements (translocations or inversions)
- Unbalanced chromosomal structural abnormalities
- Gene disorders (e.g. fragile X syndrome, Huntington's chorea, Tay–Sachs disease)

Structural disorders
- Congenital heart disease
- Neural tube defects (e.g. anencephaly, encephalocele, spina bifida)
- Abdominal wall defects (e.g. exomphalos, gastroschisis)
- Genitourinary abnormalities (e.g. renal dysplasia, polycystic kidney disease, pyelectasis, posterior urethral valves, Potter's syndrome)
- Lung disorders (e.g. pulmonary hypoplasia, diaphragmatic herniae, cystic fibrosis)

Congenital infection
- Toxoplasmosis
- Rubella
- Cytomegalovirus
- Herpes simplex virus
- Chickenpox
- Parvovirus B19
- Hepatitis
- *Listeria monocytogenes*
- Syphilis
- β-haemolytic streptococci – group B

Screening for fetal abnormalities

The decision to screen for abnormality rests with each individual couple. Some wish no screening tests at all, others may be keen to consider all of the options below. A number of screening strategies are available (Table 36.1).

Ultrasound scanning

Structural anomalies are best seen on ultrasound scan and many clinicians advocate that all mothers should be offered at least one detailed ultrasound at around 18–20 weeks' gestation. This has the advantage that those with major or lethal anomalies (e.g. spina bifida or renal agenesis) can be offered termination, and it also allows planned deliveries of those conditions which may require early neonatal intervention (e.g. gastroschisis or transposition of the great arteries).

Scanning has the disadvantage, however, that many defects are not identified. It is likely, for example, that less than 50% of cardiac defects are recognized and the false reassurance provided by a scan may become a source of parental resentment. Furthermore, a 'soft marker' may be uncovered, the significance of which is often unclear. These soft markers are structural features found on ultrasound scan which in themselves are not a problem, but which may point to other problems, particularly chromosomal abnormalities. They are found in approximately 5% of all pregnancies at a second trimester scan and cause of a lot of parental anxiety. Such markers include choroid plexus cysts (Fig. 36.1), mild renal pelvic dilatation, echogenic foci (Fig. 36.2), and mild cerebral ventricular dilatation. If the soft marker is isolated, the risk of chromosomal problems is low, but if more than one is found, or if there are

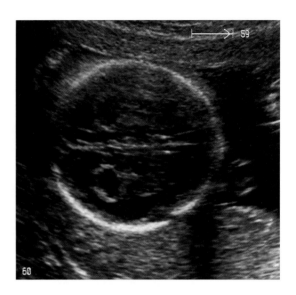

Fig. 36.1 **Although there are bilateral choroid plexus cysts, the baby was karyotypically normal.**

any other structural defects, the risk of a chromosomal problem is very much higher.

Unlike structural abnormalities, chromosomal abnormalities can be much more difficult to identify on ultrasound scan. Around two-thirds of fetuses with Down's syndrome (trisomy 21) will look normal at 18 weeks, and the remaining third may demonstrate only minor defects not necessarily pathognomonic of a chromosomal problem. Most babies with the less common trisomies, e.g. Edward's syndrome (trisomy 18) or Patau's syndrome (trisomy 13), do show some abnormality, although the abnormality is often neither specific nor diagnostic. As Edward's and Patau's syndromes are usually lethal in the perinatal period, there are fewer

Table 36.1
Overview of potential screening programmes for chromosomal and structural abnormalities

Programme	Advantages	Disadvantages
NT alone at 11–14 weeks	Good detection of Down's syndrome at early gestation (11–14 weeks)	Use of CVS may increase miscarriage rate Minimal detection of structural abnormalities
NT at 11–14 weeks and FDS at 18 weeks	Good detection of Down's syndrome at early gestation (11–14 weeks)	Use of CVS may increase miscarriage rate Good detection of structural abnormalities
FDS at 18 weeks	Good detection of structural abnormalities	Minimal detection of Down's syndrome
Serum screening alone at 16 weeks	Good detection of Down's syndrome Amniocentesis may be safer than CVS	Reasonable detection of open lesions, particularly neural tube defects Minimal detection of other structural abnormalities
Serum screening at 16 weeks with FDS at 18 weeks	Good detection of Down's syndrome Amniocentesis may be safer than CVS	Good detection of structural abnormalities Down's syndrome not identified until relatively late (17–18 weeks)

CVS, chorionic villus sampling; FDS, fetal detailed scan; NT, nuchal translucency

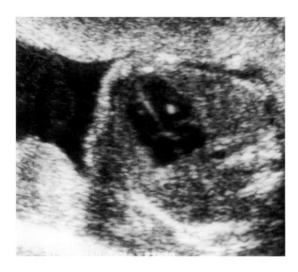

Fig. 36.2 **Echogenic focus in the left ventricle of a four-chamber cardiac view.**

lifelong implications than for Down's syndrome. Much of the screening work has therefore been directed at Down's, in particular measuring specific markers in the maternal blood (serological screening), or measuring the thickness of nuchal fluid behind the fetal neck (nuchal translucency assessment).

Serological screening

This is used almost exclusively to detect two abnormalities, spina bifida and Down's syndrome. Alpha-fetoprotein (αFP) is an alpha-globulin of similar molecular weight to albumin which is synthesized by the fetal liver. If there is a break in the fetal skin (for example with spina bifida), αFP escapes into the maternal circulation and the maternal serum level becomes elevated on testing.

Normal serum αFP levels rise with advancing gestation and most laboratories report results as multiples of the median (MoMs) for unaffected pregnancies at the gestation of sampling. A level of 1.0 is normal, and for screening purposes levels raised to more than 2.0–2.5 MoM indicate the need for detailed scanning to look for neural tube defects, twins, gastroschisis, or intrauterine death. As there is a large overlap between normal and affected pregnancies, a raised level of maternal serum αFP is therefore only a screening test and not a diagnostic test. The scan provides the diagnosis.

It has also been observed that the level of maternal serum αFP is lower than expected when the fetus has Down's syndrome. The reason for this remains unclear but the result can be combined with maternal age to give an estimated risk of the fetus being affected. This risk can be further modified by measuring human chorionic gonadotrophin (hCG; raised in Down's) and unconjugated oestriol (low in Down's) – the so-called 'triple test.' Again there is considerable overlap between the levels in unaffected and affected pregnancies so any test which uses these markers can only give an estimation of risk, not a definite diagnosis. Unfortunately as we have seen there is no simple ultrasound test for Down's syndrome and the parents have to weigh up the risks of the more invasive tests of amniocentesis or chorionic villus sampling (CVS).

Nuchal translucency

Screening for Down's syndrome is also possible by measuring the fetal nuchal thickness on first trimester ultrasound scanning (Fig. 36.3). Chorionic villus sampling may then be used to establish an earlier diagnosis than with amniocentesis (see below), thereby allowing an early surgical termination of pregnancy rather than a late medical termination. There is, however, evidence to suggest that parental psychological morbidity is independent of whether a diagnosis is made in the first or second trimester, and indeed medical termination may carry less psychological morbidity than surgical (even if medical complications are higher). In very experienced hands, chorionic villus sampling may carry the same complication rate as an amniocentesis, but for most practitioners chorionic villus sampling probably carries a higher risk of miscarriage (2–3%).

Increased nuchal translucency is also a marker for structural defects, particularly cardiac, renal and abdominal wall as well as diaphragmatic herniae. The overall survival for those with a nuchal thickness > 5 mm is ≈ 50%.

Diagnosis of chromosomal abnormalities

Diagnostic tests are offered if screening tests suggest that the mother is above a certain risk level of carrying a baby with a chromosomal abnormality.

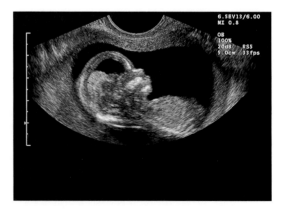

Fig. 36.3 **This is the view required to measure the nuchal translucency.** (Reproduced with permission from Seimens)

Amniocentesis

Diagnostic amniocentesis may be performed after 15 weeks' gestation. A 22 gauge needle is inserted into the amniotic cavity under ultrasound control and 10–15 ml of amniotic fluid are drawn off (Fig. 36.4). Rhesus negative women are given anti-D immunoglobulin to prevent immunization. The risk of miscarriage is around 0.5%.

Karyotype results are usually available within 3 weeks, but rapid FISH (fluorescence in-situ hybridization) or PCR (polymerase chain reaction) techniques may be used to exclude the commoner aneuploidies (Figs 36.5 and 36.6).

Chorionic villus sampling

CVS or placental biopsy may be performed any time after 10 weeks' gestation. Either a flexible cannula is

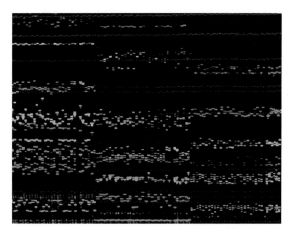

Fig. 36.6 **PCR.**

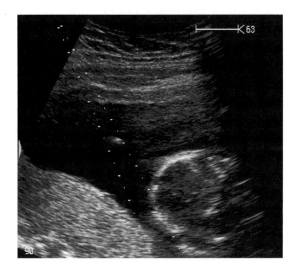

Fig. 36.4 **Amniocentesis is carried out under direct ultrasound guidance.** The tip of the needle can be seen between the dotted guidelines 2 cm above the fetal head.

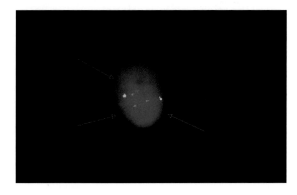

Fig. 36.5 **FISH.** Probes to chromosome 21 appear red in this cell, demonstrating trisomy 21.

passed through the cervix, or a needle is passed trans-abdominally – both under ultrasound control. Results are usually available within 48 hours.

Structural and chromosomal abnormalities

Down's syndrome (trisomy 21)

The overall incidence is 1 : 650 live births, but the incidence increases with increasing maternal age:

20 years	1 : 2000
30 years	1 : 900
35 years	1 : 350
36 years	1 : 240
38 years	1 : 180
40 years	1 : 100
44 years	1 : 40

Most Down's syndrome children, however, are born to younger mothers, as there are overall many more younger mothers than older ones. Although walking, language and self-care skills are usually attained, independence is rare. There is mental retardation (with a mean IQ around 50) and an association with congenital heart disease. Gastrointestinal atresia is common, and there is early dementia with similarities to Alzheimer's disease. 20% die before the age of 1 year and 45% by the age of 60 years.

95% of cases are due to non-dysjunction, with translocation 14 : 21 accounting for 2%, other translocations 2% and mosaicism 1%. Half of the translocations occur de novo. The recurrence risk for non-dysjunction is ≈ 1 : 100 if the mother is less than 35 years old and approximately four times the baseline risk if she is more than 35 years old. If there is a 14 : 21 translocation in the mother, the recurrence risk is 1 : 10, and if in the father, 1 : 50.

Edward's syndrome (trisomy 18)

The incidence is around 1 : 2500 live births and most are due to non-dysjunction. The baby has fetal growth restriction (FGR), a small elongated head (strawberry shaped on ultrasound), severe mental retardation, rocker bottom feet and an increased incidence of gastro-intestinal and renal anomalies. Virtually all have congenital heart disease, often a ventriculoseptal defect. 50% die before the age of 2 months and 90% before the end of the first year.

Patau's syndrome (trisomy 13)

This is rare, at around 1 : 5000 live births. There is FGR, severe mental retardation and an increased incidence of cleft palate, gastrointestinal atresias and holoprosencephaly. Again, most have congenital heart disease. The majority of children die before the age of 3 months, and survival is rare after the age of 1 year.

Triploidy

These children rarely survive to birth and there is no survival beyond the neonatal period.

Turner's syndrome (XO)

This occurs in around 1: 3000 live births: 60% are pure XO; just over 15% are mosaics (usually XO/XX); and the rest are deletions, rings or isochromosomes of Xq or Xp. The incidence is increased with increasing paternal age and decreased with increasing maternal age. Antenatally there may be a cystic hygroma ± generalized oedema and cardiac defects (Fig. 36.7). The child may

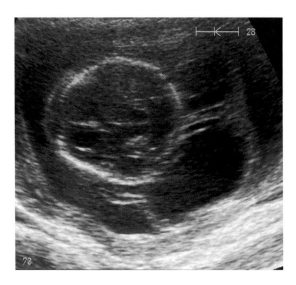

Fig. 36.7 **Cystic hygroma.** There is a massive loculated cystic swelling behind the fetal neck.

have short stature, cubitus valgus, coarctation of the aorta, a bicuspid aortic valve, streak gonads and only occasionally a lowered IQ. A small proportion may have fertility (particularly mosaics and deletions), although the incidence of premature ovarian failure is high.

XXX

The incidence of 1 : 1000 live births is doubled or tripled when the maternal age is more than 40 years. The phenotype and fertility are normal and the abnormality frequently goes unnoticed. There is, however, an increased risk of sex chromosome abnormalities ($\approx 4\%$) and premature menopause in the offspring. XXX+ (i.e. more than three X chromosomes) is rare. Dysmorphism and mental retardation in this group are common, as is menstrual dysfunction. The individual may be fertile.

Klinefelter's syndrome (XXY)

This is uncommon, at around 1 : 700–2000 live births. The individual is phenotypically a tall male, with occasionally a reduced IQ, sparse facial hair and gynaecomastia. It is the commonest single cause of male hypogonadism and is usually diagnosed in the investigation of male infertility. There is an association with hypothyroidism, diabetes and asthma. Azoospermia is the rule.

XYY

Again this is uncommon at around 1 : 700 live births, and there is no association with maternal age. The IQ and fertility are usually normal and the suggestion of increased impulsive behaviour may be biased by the population sampled. Individuals are usually tall. The risk of sex chromosome abnormalities in offspring is $\approx 4\%$.

Apparently balanced rearrangements (translocations or inversions)

If apparently balanced rearrangements are found at amniocentesis it is essential to check the karyotype of both parents. If one parent has the translocation and is phenotypically normal, it is likely that the fetus will be phenotypically normal as well. There is a chance that other offspring (or offspring of the fetus) will have an unbalanced translocation, and counselling ± karyotyping should be offered. In general the smaller the section of chromosome involved, the greater the likelihood of a fetus surviving to term with an unbalanced translocation. Offspring may, of course, also have normal karyotypes without the translocation. If the translocation has occurred de novo, the overall risk of phenotypic abnormality is in the order of 10%, but as some chromosomal rearrangements are normal population variants, genetic advice should always be sought.

Unbalanced chromosomal structural abnormalities

Many chromosomal structural abnormalities are well characterized, but it is often difficult to be specific. Parental karyotyping is required and genetic advice should be sought. Mental impairment is common, and physical abnormality is possible.

Congenital heart disease

This is the commonest congenital malformation in children and affects about 5–8 : 1000 live births. Of defects diagnosed antenatally, about 15% are associated with aneuploidy, most commonly trisomies 18 and 21.

The four-chamber view of the heart can be used as a screening test (Fig. 36.2) and will identify 25–40% of all major abnormalities, particularly ventriculoseptal defect, ventricular hypoplasia (Fig. 36.8), valvular incompetence and arrhythmias. Moving above the four-chamber view allows the aorta and pulmonary artery to be visualized (Fig. 36.9). This increases the sensitivity to identify over 60% of cardiac defects by screening for Fallot's tetralogy and transposition of the great arteries. At 18 weeks most of these major connections can be seen, but high-risk pregnancies (e.g. those with diabetes, or women taking anticonvulsants, or who have a personal or family history of congenital heart disease) should be re-scanned at 22–26 weeks for more minor defects.

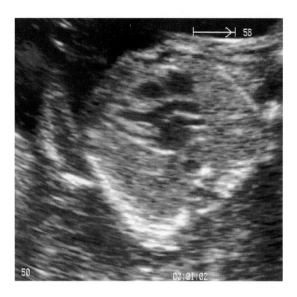

Fig. 36.9 **Aorta.** The aorta in this normal heart is seen to be arising exclusively from the left ventricle, excluding the diagnosis of Fallot's tetralogy.

Neural tube defects

The neural tube is formed from the closing of the neural folds, with both anterior and posterior neuropores closed by 6 weeks' gestation (Fig. 36.10). Failure of closure of the anterior neuropore results in anencephaly or an encephalocele, and failure of posterior closure results in spina bifida.

Spina bifida and anencephaly make up more than 95% of neural tube defects. There is wide geographical variation, with a higher incidence in Scotland and Ireland (3 : 1000), and a lower incidence in England (2 : 1000), USA, Canada, Japan and Africa (< 1 : 1000).

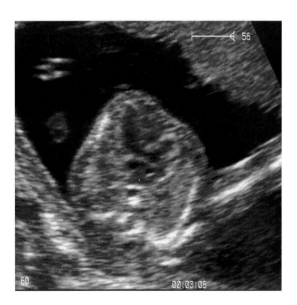

Fig. 36.8 **Hypoplastic right heart.** The baby died in the early neonatal period.

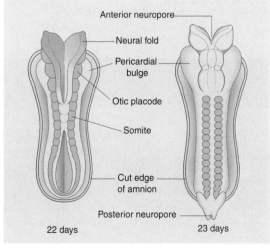

Fig. 36.10 **Dorsal view of embryo on days 22 and 23, demonstrating neural tube closure.**

Pregnancy and the puerperium

There is good evidence that the overall incidence has fallen over the past 15 years, independent of any screening programmes.

Anencephaly The skull vault and cerebral cortex are absent. The infant is either stillborn or, if live born, will usually die shortly after birth (although some may survive for several days).

Encephalocele There is a bony defect in the cranial vault through which a dura mater sac (± brain tissue) protrudes (Fig. 36.11). This may be occipital or frontal. Small isolated encephaloceles carry a good prognosis, whereas those with microcephaly secondary to brain herniation carry a very poor prognosis.

Spina bifida (Figs 36.12 and 36.13) This may take the form of a meningocele or a myelomeningocele. In a meningocele the meninges of the neural tissue bulge

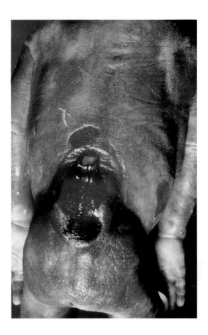

Fig. 36.13 **Spina bifida.**

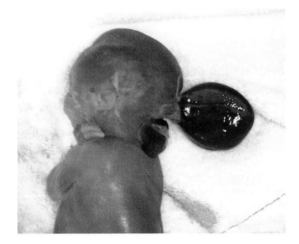

Fig. 36.11 **Encephalocele.** There is a defect in the posterior aspect of the skull, allowing brain tissue to herniate into the sac.

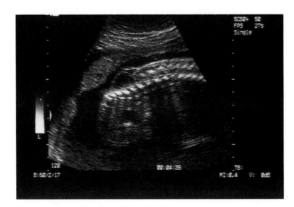

Fig. 36.12 **Spina bifida.** There is a large lumbosacral defect, with the sac of the myelomeningocele clearly visible.

through a posterior spinal wall defect, whereas in a myelomeningocele the central canal of the cord is also exposed. Those with spinal meningoceles usually have normal lower limb neurology and 20% have hydrocephalus. Those with myelomeningoceles usually have abnormal lower limb neurology and many have hydrocephalus. In addition to immobility and mental retardation there may be problems with urinary tract infection, bladder dysfunction, bowel dysfunction, social and sexual isolation.

Daily folic acid taken from before conception reduces the recurrence risk of neural tube defects in those who have had a previously affected child. A preconceptual prophylactic dose for all pregnant women probably also offers some protection. There are, at present, no known teratogenic effects from folate.

Abdominal wall defects

Exomphalos (Fig. 36.14a,b)

This occurs following failure of the gut to return to the abdominal cavity at 8 weeks' gestation and results in a defect through which the peritoneal sac protrudes. The sac may contain both intestines and liver. There are chromosomal abnormalities in 30% (especially trisomy 18) and 10–50% have other lesions, particularly cardiac and renal. There is also an association with ectopia vesicae and ectopia cardia (midline bladder and cardiac herniae). If the exomphalos is isolated (i.e. no other structural abnormalities), the chromosomes are normal and there is no bowel atresia or infarction, the prognosis

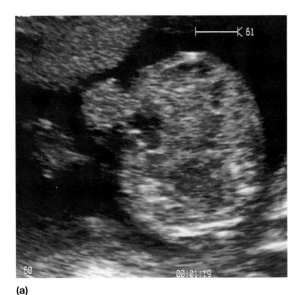

(a)

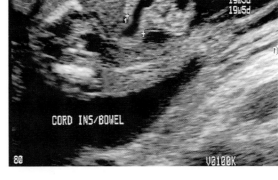

Fig. 36.15 **Gastroschisis, with Doppler flow to highlight the cord.** (Reproduced with permission from Seimens)

(b)

Fig. 36.14 **Small exomphalos in a baby terminated for multiple abnormalities.**

is good (> 80% long-term survival). The sac rarely ruptures at vaginal delivery.

Gastroschisis (Fig. 36.15)

There is an abdominal wall defect usually to the right and below the insertion of the umbilical cord. Small bowel (without a peritoneal covering) protrudes and floats free in the peritoneal fluid. Gut atresias and cardiac lesions occur in 20% but the association with chromosomal abnormality is very small (probably < 1%). The prognosis is good if the bowel is viable, although 10% end in stillbirth despite apparently normal growth. Gut dilatation may be associated with bowel obstruction or ischaemia but is not directly linked to prognosis.

These babies are usually small for dates and require very close surveillance. The recurrence risk is less than 1%.

Genitourinary abnormalities

Renal dysplasia (Fig. 36.16a,b)

Multicystic dysplastic kidneys   The kidneys have large discrete non-communicating cysts with a central, more solid core and are thought to follow early developmental failure. The inheritance is sporadic. If the cysts affect only one kidney, the other is normal, and there is adequate liquor, the prognosis is good. If the cysts are bilateral and the liquor is reduced, the prognosis is poor.

Polycystic kidney disease

Adult polycystic kidney disease has an autosomal dominant inheritance and is relatively benign, often not producing symptoms until the fifth decade of life. Many individuals have ultrasonically normal kidneys at birth.

Infantile polycystic kidney disease has an autosomal recessive inheritance. There is a wide range of expression with the size of cysts ranging from microscopic to several millimetres across. Both kidneys are affected, and there may also be cysts present in the liver and pancreas. Ultrasound features of oligohydramnios, empty bladder and large symmetrical bright kidneys (Fig. 36.17) may not develop until later in pregnancy. If there is survival beyond the neonatal period, there may be later problems with raised blood pressure and progressive renal failure. Long-term survival is rare.

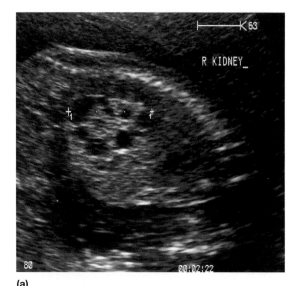

(a)

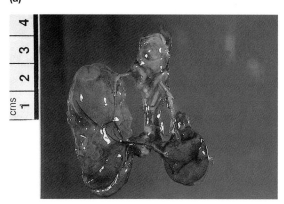

(b)

Fig. 36.16 **Dysplastic renal scan.** Note the enlarged kidney containing fluid-filled cysts: **(a)** ultrasound; **(b)** post-mortem specimen.

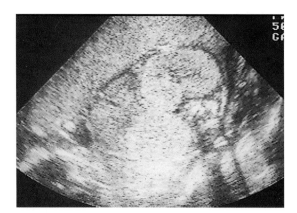

Fig. 36.17 **Infantile renal cystic scan.** Note anhydramnios and bright renal echoes from the microscopically small cysts.

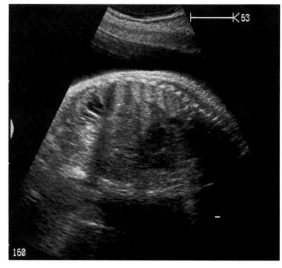

Fig. 36.18 **Pyelectasis.** The renal pelvis is markedly dilated, although the renal cortex looks well preserved.

Pyelectasis (Fig. 36.18)

Renal pelvic dilatation may be unilateral (79–90%) or bilateral. It is probably caused by a neuromuscular defect at the junction of the ureter and the renal pelvis, and presents with increasing pelvic dilatation in the presence of a normal ureter. As there is an association with postnatal urinary tract infections and reflux nephropathy, it is reasonable to start all affected neonates on prophylactic antibiotics and arrange postnatal radiological follow-up. Even in those with mild dilatation (≥ 5 mm and < 10 mm) there is vesicoureteric reflux in 10–20%, although only a small proportion require surgery.

Posterior urethral valves

In this condition, folds of mucosa at the bladder neck prevent urine leaving the bladder. The fetus is usually male, there is often oligohydramnios and on ultrasound there are varying degrees of renal dysplasia. There is a chromosomal abnormality in 7% of isolated defects, and in one-third of those with other abnormalities. It may be possible to insert a 'pigtail' shunt between the bladder and amniotic cavity to relieve the obstruction, but the long-term prognosis is still poor as the renal damage may not be reversible.

Potter's syndrome

Bilateral renal agenesis (Potter's syndrome) is associated with extreme oligohydramnios which leads to the Potter's sequence of pulmonary hypoplasia (see below) and limb deformity (due to fetal compression). The condition is lethal. The recurrence risk is approximately 3% although autosomal dominant forms with variable penetrance have been described.

Lung disorders

Pulmonary hypoplasia

Liquor is important for alveolar maturation, particularly in the second trimester. Without liquor there will be pulmonary hypoplasia. Severe oligohydramnios occurs if there is very preterm pre-labour membrane rupture or Potter's syndrome (see above). Pulmonary hypoplasia also occurs with diaphragmatic herniae as there is no room for lung expansion.

Diaphragmatic hernia

Stomach, colon and even spleen can enter the chest through a defect in the diaphragm, usually on the left. The heart is pushed to the right and the lungs become hypoplastic. The incidence of aneuploidy is 15–30% and there is an association with neural tube defects, congenital heart disease and renal and skeletal abnormalities. The overall survival of those diagnosed antenatally is ~ 20% with a better prognosis for isolated left-sided herniae. Polyhydramnios, mediastinal shift and left ventricular compression are poor antenatal prognostic factors. Babies who survive postnatally undergo surgery to reduce the hernia and close the diaphragmatic defect.

Other disorders

Cystic fibrosis

The UK gene frequency for cystic fibrosis is 1 : 20 (i.e. heterozygote frequency) and the estimated overall couple risk for a live birth is around 1 : 2500 (there is probably an increased miscarriage rate in homozygotes). Clinically there is respiratory, gastrointestinal, liver and pancreatic dysfunction and azoospermia is the rule. The prognosis is very variable and although death around the age of 20–30 still occurs, the prognosis is improving and many affected individuals now live considerably longer. The health of an affected sibling is not a prognostic guide to the health of other siblings. Four mutant alleles account for 85% of the gene defects in the UK (the commonest being ΔF508), and antenatal screening for these is possible using saliva specimens, with CVS being performed if both parents are gene carriers.

Cystic hygroma (see Fig. 36.7)

Cystic hygromas are fluid-filled swellings at the back of the fetal neck which probably develop because of a defect in the formation of lymphatic vessels. It is likely that the lymphatic and venous systems fail to connect and lymph fluid accumulates in the jugular lymph sacs. Larger hygromas are frequently divided by septae and may be associated with skin oedema, ascites, pleural and pericardial effusions, cardiac and renal abnormalities. There is also an association with aneuploidy (particularly Turner's, Down's, Edward's) and it is appropriate to offer karyotyping. If generalized fetal hydrops is present the prognosis is bleak. Isolated hygromas may be surgically corrected postnatally and have a good prognosis. Only rarely are they so large as to result in problems with labour.

Fragile X syndrome

This is the commonest cause of moderate mental retardation after Down's syndrome and the commonest form of inherited mental handicap. It is X-linked. Males are usually more severely affected than females. Speech delay is common and there is an associated behavioural phenotype with gaze aversion. The condition is caused by the expansion of a CGG triplet repeat on the X chromosome. Normal individuals have an average of 29 repeats but for an unexplained reason this may increase to a pre-mutation of 50–200 repeats. Those with a pre-mutation are phenotypically normal but the pre-mutation is unstable during female meiosis and can expand to a full mutation of more than 200 repeats. There is an approximately 10% chance of this occurring (in the absence of a full mutation in that generation already). This causes the fragile X phenotype in 99% of males and around 30–50% of females. Parental screening is possible and CVS may be used to identify the degree of amplification of the CGG repeats in potential offspring.

Huntington's chorea

The onset of this autosomal dominant condition is usually after the age of 30, although it may present as early as 10–15 years of age. There is dementia, mood change (usually depression) and choreoathetosis progressing to death in approximately 15 years. There is a CAG trinucleotide expansion on chromosome 4p allowing accurate carrier and prenatal testing.

Tay–Sachs disease

The gene frequency is 1 : 30 in Ashkenazi Jews, but is rare in other groups. There is a build-up of gangliosides within the CNS leading to mental retardation, paralysis and blindness. By the age of 4 years, the child is usually dead or in a vegetative state. Carriers may be screened by measuring the level of hexosaminidase A in leucocytes.

Prenatal congenital infection

Infections in pregnancy are important because of potential risks to the fetus. A number of agents are known to be teratogenic, particularly in the first and early second trimesters. Others carry the risk of miscarriage,

Table 36.2
Foods that carry potential infection risks in pregnancy

Soft cheeses	Unpasteurized milk and its products may contain listeria. Those made from pasteurized milk are safe
Raw eggs	Must be avoided as there is a risk of salmonella (including puddings)
Meat or pâté	Undercooked meat may transmit toxoplasma or rarely listeria
Fruit	This should always be washed before eating as it may be contaminated with salmonella, toxoplasma or one of several intestinal parasites

premature labour, severe neonatal sepsis or long-term carrier states.

Risk factors

Farm workers are at risk of chlamydial infection (which causes abortion in sheep) and listerial infection, both of which can cause abortion in humans. Care is required particularly at lambing time. Toxoplasma may also be acquired from cows, sheep and domestic cats. Certain foods have also been implicated in congenital infection (Table 36.2).

Specific infections (see also Table 36.3)

Infections in general raise the maternal levels of immunoglobulins of both the IgG and IgM variety.

Maternal IgG crosses the placenta while IgM, a much larger molecule, does not. The fetus does not make IgM until beyond 20 weeks' gestation and its presence in fetal or early neonatal blood implies infection. Infection does not necessarily mean that the infection has caused a problem, and absence of fetal or neonatal IgM at sampling does not completely exclude infection.

Chickenpox at term (see Table 36.3 for early pregnancy)

Severe and even fatal cases of chickenpox can occur in neonates whose mothers develop chickenpox just before delivery, as the baby is born before maternal IgG production has increased sufficiently to allow passive transplacental protection. If maternal infection occurs 1–4 weeks before delivery, up to 50% of babies are infected and approximately a quarter of these develop clinical varicella. Severe infection is most likely to occur if the infant is born within 7 days of onset of the mother's rash when cord blood IgG is low.

If delivery occurs within 5 days of maternal infection, or if the mother develops chickenpox within 2 days of giving birth, the neonate should be given passive varicella zoster immunoglobulin and the infant should be monitored for around 2 weeks. If neonatal infection occurs, it should be treated with aciclovir.

Hepatitis

Hepatitis A has not been associated with significant complications in pregnancy. All mothers should be screened antenatally for hepatitis B virus. The initial

Table 36.3
Infections in pregnancy

Agent	Epidemiology	Maternal features	Fetal features	Risk	Treatment
Rubella	Person to person. UK immunity now 97% and congenital infection is rare	Asymptomatic or mild maculopapular rash	FGR, ↓ platelets, hepatosplenomegaly, jaundice, deafness, congenital heart disease, mental retardation, cataracts, microphthalmia, abortion, microcephaly and cerebral palsy	Risk of affected fetus: < 4 weeks 50% 5–8 weeks 25% 9–12 weeks 10% > 13 weeks 1%	Consider TOP if < 12 weeks. Postnatal vaccination if not immune
Toxoplasmosis (protozoan – *Toxoplasma gondii*)	From cats, uncooked meats and unwashed fruits	May have fever, rash and lymphadenopathy, but most are asymptomatic	Hydrocephalus, chorioretinitis, intracranial calcification, ↓ platelets	< 12 weeks: transmission is 10–25%, of which 75% will be severely affected 12–28 weeks: transmission is 54% of which 25% will be severely affected > 28 weeks: transmission is 65%–90% of which << 10% will be severely affected	Consider TOP only if primary infection < 20 weeks

Table 36.3 (cont.)

Agent	Epidemiology	Maternal features	Fetal features	Risk	Treatment
CMV (herpesvirus)	Person to person	Nearly always asymptomatic	Hepatosplenomegaly, ↓ platelets, FGR, microcephaly, sensorineural deafness, cerebral palsy, chorioretinitis, hydrops fetalis, exomphalos	40% fetuses infected. Risk is unaffected by gestation. Of these, 90% are normal at birth, although 20% develop late sequelae. Of the 10% who are symptomatic, 33% die and the rest have long-term problems	Even primary infection carries only a 10–25% risk of severe abnormality
Parvovirus B19	Respiratory transmission. Seroprevalence 50%	Erythema infectiosum (slapped cheek disease). May be asymptomatic	Aplastic anaemia, hydrops fetalis (Fig. 36.19) and myocarditis ± fetal loss (if < 20 weeks). Transmission < 20 weeks ≈ 10% of which ≈ 10% are lost. If > 20 weeks, transmission 60%, but no adverse effects been demonstrated	If < 20 weeks and fetus survives the infection (≈ 90%), it is likely to result in a healthy live birth	Intrauterine transfusion may be possible
Chickenpox (varicella zoster virus)	Person to person	Papules and pustules	Limb hypoplasia, skin scarring, FGR, eye abnormalities, neurological abnormalities and hydrops fetalis	25% transmission. Probably < 1–2% have problems if < 20 weeks. No structural problems > 20 weeks. See also 'Chickenpox at term' (p. 348)	Give ZIG (zoster immuno-globulin) if < 10 days from contact or < 4 days from onset of rash, although the benefits are not proven

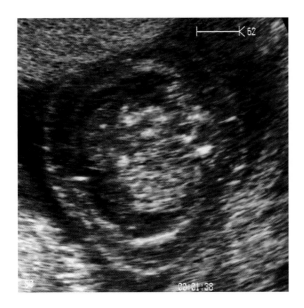

Fig. 36.19 **Hydrops fetalis caused by infection with human parvovirus B19.** There is ascites and marked skin oedema. The baby survived with problems.

serological response to infection is with HBsAg, followed by HBeAg, a marker of high infectivity. Vertical transmission to the fetus is most likely to occur with acute infection (especially third trimester) or in the presence of HBeAg and may lead to neonatal infection or long-term carriage. The baby should be given passive hepatitis B immunoglobulin at birth as well as an active hepatitis B immunization.

With hepatitis C, vertical transmission is related to viral load but is unlikely in the absence of detectable RNA. There is no evidence that treatment during pregnancy reduces the chance of transmission and ribavirin is probably teratogenic. Hepatitis E infection in pregnancy, whilst uncommon, carries a 30% maternal mortality rate and possible risk of fetal loss.

Herpes simplex virus

An acute attack of primary herpes shortly before delivery may lead to a localized or systemic neonatal infection, including encephalitis. The risk of infection is greatest with a primary infection, but can occur with recurrence, although this risk decreases with time from the first attack. Screening is of no proven value, but caesarean section may be indicated in the presence of a primary infection.

Rubella

Rubella infection is discussed in Table 36.3 but its importance lies in the potential for prevention through vaccination. Immunity from natural infection is lifelong. Seroconversion and lifelong immunity occur in about 95% of vaccinated individuals and, as the benefits of herd immunity have been clearly demonstrated, many countries now immunize all pre-school children. Rubella antibodies are commonly checked at booking, and postnatal vaccination is offered to those with low titres.

Listeria monocytogenes

This is a rare bacterial infection transmitted by food, usually soft ripe cheeses, pâté, cooked–chilled meals and ready-to-eat foods that have not been thoroughly cooked. Following an initial gastroenteritis, which may be fleeting, bacteraemia results in bacilli crossing the placenta and causing amnionitis, preterm labour (which may result in stillbirth) or spontaneous miscarriage. There may be meconium, neonatal jaundice, conjunctivitis or meningoencephalitis. Diagnosis is made by blood culture or by culture of liquor or placenta. Treatment is with high-dose amoxicillin or erythromycin.

β-haemolytic streptococci – group B

Between 5 and 20% of women carry this organism in the vagina. It is associated with preterm rupture of the membranes. About 50% of babies become colonized at delivery but only about 1% of these develop infection. The neonatal mortality from infection may be as high as 80%, with 50% of those surviving meningitis having subsequent neurological impairment. Antenatal screening is not indicated in the UK (initial screen positives may become negative and vice versa) but those with known infection should receive intrapartum antibiotics

(e.g. amoxicillin or erythromycin). There is no evidence to support antenatal treatment of asymptomatic carriers, as carriage is rapidly re-established following treatment.

Syphilis

Congenital syphilis is rare, and those identified antenatally with positive serology should be treated with penicillin.

Termination for abnormality

Prenatal diagnoses are often made relatively late in pregnancy and termination has to be performed by inducing labour, rather than by surgical means. This needs to be handled sensitively. Parents may initially be reluctant to see the baby, but should be offered the opportunity. Many mothers are later grateful that they underwent a delivery and saw and named the baby. Photographs of the baby can also be taken for the parents.

Post-mortem examination should be encouraged, and if parents decline, they may accept post-mortem investigation with X-rays, clinical photographs and specimens for karyotype studies instead. Follow-up to discuss the results and their implications for subsequent pregnancy is important.

Key points

- Approximately 2% of newborn babies have a serious abnormality detectable at, or soon after, birth. The main ones are listed in Box 36.1. Many of these can be diagnosed antenatally.

- There are a number of different strategies for prenatal screening programmes. These are summarized in Table 36.1.

37

Obstetric haemorrhage

Antepartum haemorrhage

Introduction

Obstetric haemorrhage is one of the leading causes of maternal mortality worldwide and, even in the more affluent societies with ready access to resuscitation, oxytocics, blood transfusion and surgery, deaths still occur. Haemorrhage may be rapid. It is important to recognize its severity promptly, institute effective therapy and keep ahead of the loss.

A vaginal examination should never be performed in the presence of vaginal bleeding without first excluding placenta praevia – 'No PV until no PP'.

Definitions

Vaginal bleeding associated with intrauterine pregnancy is divided into the following categories:

- threatened miscarriage – up to 24 weeks' gestation
- antepartum haemorrhage – from 24 weeks' gestation until the onset of labour
- intrapartum haemorrhage – from the onset of labour until the end of the second stage
- postpartum haemorrhage – from the third stage of labour until the end of the puerperium.

Causes

Antepartum haemorrhage is further classified according to the source of the bleeding.

Local

There may be local bleeding from the vulva, vagina or cervix. Bleeding from the cervix is not uncommon in pregnancy and may be provoked by sexual intercourse. A cervical ectropion is often found, and only very rarely is there a carcinoma. Later in pregnancy a 'show' of mucus along with a small amount of blood may simply herald the onset of labour as the cervix becomes effaced or 'takes up'.

Placental

Placenta praevia

This is defined as a placenta encroaching on the lower segment with the lower segment arbitrarily defined on ultrasound scanning as extending 5 cm from the internal os. Placenta praevia is commoner in older mothers and those with a previous caesarean section. It is classified either as major or minor, or graded I–IV (Table 37.1, Fig. 37.1).

It is not possible to avoid haemorrhage in labour with a major placenta praevia, but it may be possible to deliver successfully with a minor degree of praevia. In the assessment of suitability for such a delivery, engagement of the presenting part is probably more important than the actual distance of the placenta from the internal os on ultrasound scan (Fig. 37.2). Those who do not have an at least partially engaged head should be delivered by caesarean section. These sections should be personally supervised or performed by a senior obstetrician and a large blood loss should be anticipated.

A low-lying placenta may be identified in an asymptomatic woman at the time of an ultrasound scan early in pregnancy. As the uterus grows from the lower segment upwards, the placenta appears to move upwards with advancing gestation. 2% of those with a low-lying placenta before 24 weeks, 5% of those at 24–29 weeks and 23% of those at 30+ weeks will still have a placenta praevia at term. This is not a reflection of placental migration, but simply a feature of uterine growth. When a low-lying placenta is detected on ultrasound scanning early in pregnancy, it is reasonable to repeat the scan early in the third trimester and then review the management if the placenta is still low.

The risk of placenta praevia is of a sudden, unpredictable, major haemorrhage and some clinicians advocate hospital admission from 30–32 weeks onwards so that facilities for resuscitation and delivery are immediately available. This can be socially difficult for the woman, particularly if she has existing children at home, and immobility in hospital may predispose to thromboembolic disease. There is therefore a trend towards outpatient management, particularly for those who have had no bleeding, or just light bleeding, and who live close to the hospital. Those who have had heavy bleeds, or who live further away, are often advised to stay in hospital. Elective delivery is usually planned for 38–39 weeks, but may be earlier if there is a major haemorrhage.

If the placenta invades the myometrium it is termed 'placenta accreta', and this markedly increases the chance of severe haemorrhage (p. 444).

Placental abruption

Placental abruption is defined as retroplacental haemorrhage and usually involves some degree of placental separation. Its management depends on the amount of bleeding, the maturity of the baby and the fetal condition. It is essential to remember, however, that with placental abruption the amount of 'revealed' bleeding from the vagina may not reflect the degree of internal retroplacental bleeding and indeed a woman may have considerable internal bleeding without any external loss at all – a 'concealed abruption' (Fig. 37.3).

Light bleeding from the edge of a normally situated placenta does not normally compromise the fetus and can be treated by a short spell of rest with subsequent close supervision of fetal growth and placental function until normal labour.

Major revealed haemorrhage is obvious, and urgent delivery is usually required. A major concealed abruption is inferred from the degree of pain, uterine tenderness and evidence of shock, and again urgent delivery may be required. The decision between vaginal delivery and caesarean section can be difficult, but depends on the severity of bleeding and the fetal condition.

If there is no fetal heartbeat, vaginal delivery is indicated as the mother should not be subjected to an unnecessary caesarean section if the baby is dead. However, it is very likely that there will have been a major degree of blood loss. Hypovolaemic shock may develop and may progress to multisystem failure if not corrected. In addition, release of thromboplastins from the damaged placenta may lead to disseminated intravascular coagulation with depletion of platelets, fibrinogen and other clotting factors. Waiting for vaginal delivery therefore carries risks, and caesarean section may occasionally be indicated to minimize these systemic risks. The decision is further complicated by the risks of carrying out an operation in the presence of disseminated intravascular coagulation.

Unknown cause

A specific explanation for the bleeding is often not found, even after the pregnancy is over, and it is then presumed to have come from a normally situated placenta.

Clinical presentation

Bleeding can be light, moderate or severe and can occur with or without pain. Admission to hospital is advised, as even light bleeding may be a sign of premature labour, or a warning of further haemorrhage to come.

Table 37.1
Classification of placenta praevia

Minor	I	Encroaches on lower segment
	II	Reaches internal os (marginal)
Major	III	Covers part of os (partial)
	IV	Completely covers the os (complete)

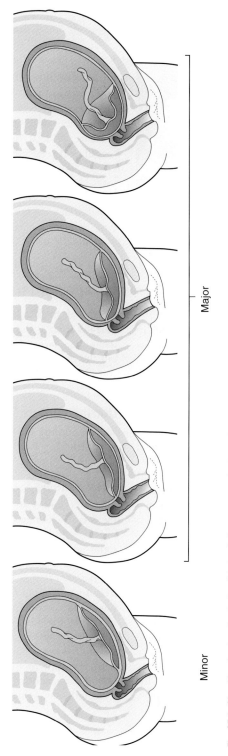

Minor

Major

Fig. 37.1 **Classification into 'major' and 'minor' placenta praevia depends on the distance of the placenta from the internal os.** It is also important to note whether the placenta is anterior or posterior, as caesarean section is more difficult through an anterior placenta.

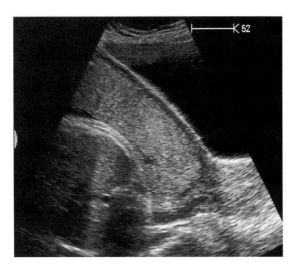

Fig. 37.2 **An anterior placenta praevia extending to just beyond the internal os.**

An attempt should be made to determine the cause of the bleeding. In practice, history and initial examination are carried out simultaneously. It is relevant to ask when the bleeding started, how much blood has been lost and when the baby was last felt to move. Observation will tell if the mother is in pain, which suggests abruption or labour, and there may be visible blood on the bed or legs or floor. If she is pale, with low blood pressure and rapid pulse, there is probably hypovolaemic shock. With an abruption the uterus is hard and tender and there may be no discernible fetal heartbeat. When the bleeding has been from a placenta praevia, the uterus is usually soft, the presenting part will be free and the fetal heartbeat is usually present.

Subsequent management depends on the estimated severity of haemorrhage.

Light bleeding, with a soft uterus and normal cardiotocography

An ultrasound scan should be arranged to check the placental site and, providing the placenta is not low-lying, a speculum examination should be performed to look for cervical effacement or dilatation, an ectropion or a carcinoma. If all is normal it is common practice to admit the woman until the bleeding settles. Many clinicians, however, will not admit the patient if the bleeding is light and seen to be coming from an ectropion.

Women who are rhesus negative should be given prophylactic anti-D.

If there is a placenta praevia and the patient is at more than 37–38 weeks' gestation, it is reasonable to arrange for delivery. If less than this gestation, a conservative approach is probably appropriate as above.

Light bleeding, but with a hard tender uterus

The diagnosis is probably a concealed abruption, and management is undertaken as above. The route of delivery will depend on a number of factors including evidence of fetal distress and the presence of any coagulopathy. Resuscitation will be required.

Heavy bleeding

Whether the diagnosis is placenta praevia or an abruption, delivery is likely to be required irrespective of gestation. Resuscitation will again be required.

Intrapartum haemorrhage

Abnormal bleeding during labour must be distinguished from a 'show' that may occur during cervical dilatation. Placental abruption can occur during labour but the possibility of uterine rupture also needs to be considered.

Uterine rupture

Uterine rupture is relatively rare, and is discussed on page 449.

Vasa praevia

This is very rare, and occurs when cord vessels run in the fetal membranes and cross the internal os. These vessels may rupture in early labour and this leads to rapid fetal exsanguination. It may be that the cord is inserted into the membranes rather than directly into the placenta (Fig. 37.4), or that the vessels are running from the placenta to a separate succenturiate placental lobe. The condition presents as severe fetal distress following a relatively small intrapartum haemorrhage. A Kleihauer test on a sample of the blood may distinguish fetal from maternal red cells but in practice the baby is usually delivered immediately because of the fetal distress and the diagnosis is made retrospectively by examination of the placenta and membranes.

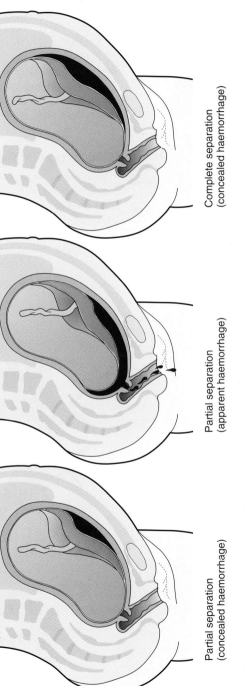

Complete separation
(concealed haemorrhage)

Partial separation
(apparent haemorrhage)

Partial separation
(concealed haemorrhage)

Fig. 37.3 **Classification of placental abruption.**

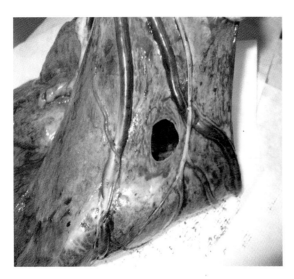

Fig. 37.4 **Cord vessels running through the membranes.** If these vessels overlie the internal os, they are termed 'vasa praevia'.

Postpartum haemorrhage

Introduction

It is impossible to predict with certainty which patients will have a postpartum haemorrhage, and it is important to appreciate that a major haemorrhage can very rapidly lead to maternal death.

Definitions

There is always some bleeding during the third stage of a normal delivery, usually around 200–300 ml.

- A primary postpartum haemorrhage is defined as a blood loss of 500 ml or more within 24 hours of the delivery of the baby.
- A secondary postpartum haemorrhage is any significant loss between 24 hours and 6 weeks after the birth.

Primary postpartum haemorrhage

This occurs in around 5% of all deliveries. It is commoner in grand multiparity, multiple pregnancy, those with fibroids and placenta praevia, and in those who have had a long labour. It may also follow an antepartum haemorrhage and is more likely in women with a past history of postpartum haemorrhage.

Causes

- *Atony* (90%). Normally, contraction of the uterus in the third stage of labour causes compression of intramyometrial blood vessels, and bleeding usually settles (Fig. 37.5). If there is uterine atony this compression does not occur. Atony is more likely if the placenta is retained, as its physical presence prevents contraction occurring.
- *Trauma* (7%). Bleeding may come from an episiotomy, a vaginal or cervical laceration (Fig. 37.6), or a rupture in the uterine wall. Lacerations are more common after an instrumental delivery than after a spontaneous one.
- *Coagulation problems* – usually disseminated intravascular coagulation (DIC) (3%) – DIC may be present from a number of different causes.
- *Multiple causes* may be present

Clinical presentation

The bleeding is usually obvious but occasionally an atonic uterus can fill up without obvious external loss and the first real sign can be cardiovascular collapse. Another problem is a prolonged undrammatic 'trickle', the significance of which may not be appreciated. With blood-soaked pads and bedding it is easy to

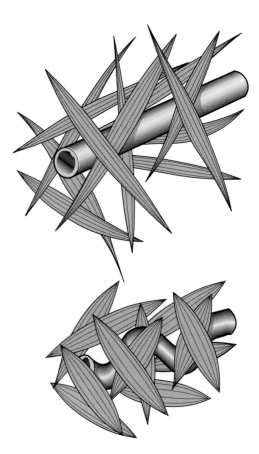

Fig. 37.5 **Postpartum haemostasis is achieved largely because the contracting myometrial fibres constrict the vessels within the uterine wall.**

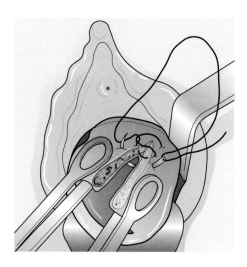

Fig. 37.6 **Cervical lacerations often bleed profusely.** They are best repaired under general anaesthesia.

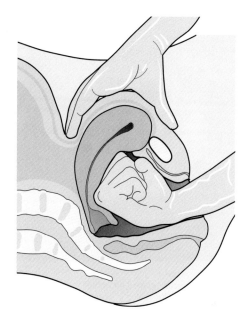

Fig. 37.7 **Some clinicians advocate bimanual compression in postpartum haemorrhage to aid uterine contraction.**

underestimate the real loss. The most critical factors are the signs of shock, pallor, rising pulse and falling blood pressure.

The key questions are:

1. Has the placenta been delivered and is it complete?
2. Is the uterus firmly contracted?
3. If so, is the bleeding due to trauma?

Management

A controlled reassuring presence is important.

Assessment
- Make a rough but realistic estimate of the loss.
- Check the pulse and blood pressure.
- Feel the abdomen to assess the size and tone of the uterus.

Treatment
- If the uterus is atonic, a contraction can be 'rubbed up' by abdominal massage. Bimanual compression may also be tried (Fig. 37.7).
- Intravenous access should be established with *two* wide-bore cannulae and blood taken for haemoglobin, haematocrit, platelets, clotting and a red cell crossmatch (the number of units depends on volume lost).
- Syntocinon 10 IU stat i.v. should be given to further contract the uterus, followed by a Syntocinon infusion.
- Crystalloid and/or colloid should be rapidly infused to maintain the circulating volume.

- If the placenta has not been delivered, a gentle attempt at controlled cord traction should be tried. If still retained, a regional block or general anaesthetic will be required for a manual removal. If the placenta is pathologically adherent (placenta accreta) in the presence of haemorrhage a hysterectomy is likely to be required.
- Further oxytocics may be given, e.g. Syntocinon i.v., ergometrine i.m., or carboprost i.m. or intramyometrially.
- If there is ongoing loss, a general anaesthetic will allow assessment for vaginal or cervical lacerations

  If the haemorrhage continues:

- A CVP line should be considered and a blood transfusion commenced. Group specific un-crossmatched blood or even O negative blood may be used in extreme emergency.
- The coagulation defects of DIC should be corrected with fresh frozen plasma or cryoprecipitate depending on specialist advice.
- Hysterectomy (or subtotal hysterectomy) may be indicated, especially if there is a non-lower-segment uterine rupture or placenta accreta. Internal iliac artery ligation is only likely to be suitable for atony, is of less use with placenta accreta and is of no use for uterine lacerations. Uterine packing is an option for atony, but may in itself prevent an adequate uterine contraction and therefore haemostasis.
- Radiologically directed arterial embolization is also an option for uncontrolled haemorrhage (Fig. 37.8).

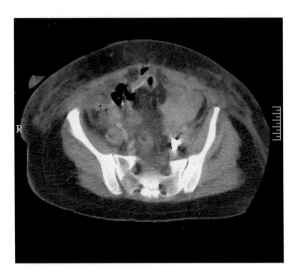

Fig. 37.8 **Radiologically guided internal iliac artery embolization can be life-saving in severe postpartum haemorrhage.** The embolizing 'coils' are visible as a bright area anterior to the left side of the sacrum, just behind a large intra-abdominal haematoma.

In practice, the decision is usually between conservative management with antibiotics, or arranging for an evacuation of retained products with antibiotic cover under anaesthesia. In the first week the evacuation can often be carried out digitally without the need to instrument the uterus and risk perforation. Clinical judgement is important, perhaps giving antibiotics in the first instance if the bleeding is not severe, and arranging an evacuation if it does not settle. Ultrasound scans can be unhelpful as many normal women have asymptomatic retained products after entirely normal deliveries and the temptation may be to carry out an unnecessary and potentially hazardous uterine evacuation.

Secondary postpartum haemorrhage

This is defined as bleeding between 24 hours and 6 weeks postnatally. It is usually due to infection or retained products of conception, rarely to a vulval haematoma, very rarely to caesarean scar dehiscence and only exceptionally to trophoblastic disease. Checks should be made of pulse, blood pressure and temperature, the uterus palpated for tenderness, and an endocervical swab sent for culture.

> ### Key points
>
> - Obstetric haemorrhage is one of the leading causes of maternal mortality worldwide.
>
> - It can be rapidly fatal, and it is extremely important to establish adequate i.v. access, resuscitate and identify the cause of the bleeding.
>
> - A mother who has experienced an obstetric haemorrhage is often apprehensive about a subsequent pregnancy, particularly if the bleeding has been severe. The chance of recurrence is relatively small.

38

Small for gestational age and fetal growth restriction

Introduction

Babies are born with a wide range of birth weights. While those born prematurely are more likely to be of low birth weight, this chapter is not specifically concerned with preterm delivery problems. The focus is on those babies who are small for their gestation. These babies may simply be small, in other words they are normal babies who just happen to be at the smaller end of a normal range, and these are termed 'small for gestational age'. A few babies, however, are small for some pathological reason and are referred to as having 'fetal growth restriction'.

The key issues are how to screen a low-risk population in order to identify these small babies and, once identified, how best to identify those that are risk of developing problems.

Accuracy of dating

It is impossible to diagnose small for gestational age or fetal growth restriction without accurate knowledge of gestation. Menstrual dating has significant inherent inaccuracies. The dates may be inaccurately recalled, the cycle may be irregular, and bleeding in early pregnancy may be mistaken for menses. Gestation is most accurately determined by an ultrasound scan undertaken before 20 weeks' gestation, as it is a reasonable approximation to assume that all fetuses are of similar size up until this point. The natural variation in size after this stage makes accurate dating very difficult and an estimate is required from menstrual dates. The most reliable measurements are based on the crown–rump length between the 8th and 10th weeks, and the biparietal diameter between the 16th and 20th weeks.

The estimated date of delivery is taken as 40 weeks after the date of the start of the last menstrual period (LMP) providing the cycle length is 28 days. A correction may be made for those with regular longer or shorter cycles; for example if the cycle is 35 days long then 7 days should be added to the date of the LMP. The date of the first positive pregnancy test can also be of some help. A pregnancy test usually becomes positive on the day when the next period would have been due and therefore the gestation must be at least 4 weeks on that date. Abdominal palpation is a relatively inaccurate way of establishing dates, as is the date that fetal movements were first noted. Fetal movements are usually noted around 20 weeks' gestation but the range either side of this figure is wide.

The rest of this chapter will assume that the dates are correct and that the gestation is known.

Definitions

Low birth weight (LBW)

This is defined as any baby born with a weight under 2.5 kg. It is recognized to be associated with significant neonatal and post-neonatal mortality. Over 25 million babies a year worldwide are born below this cut-off, and overall 90% of these are born in developing countries where perinatal and infant mortality is already high. As LBW is uncorrected for gestation, however, it does not differentiate between those babies born prematurely and those born small for gestational age.

Small for gestational age (SGA)

Small for gestational age describes the baby whose birth weight is below a specified centile for its gestation at birth. The chosen centile may be the 10th, 5th or 3rd depending on different policies, and this choice reflects a trade-off between sensitivity and specificity. If the 10th centile is chosen it will correctly identify most babies liable to be at risk on account of their small size but will also include many other babies who are not at risk. If the 3rd centile is chosen then specificity will be good, in other words a greater proportion of identified babies will be at risk, but more 'at-risk' babies might be missed. The most commonly used threshold is the 10th centile.

Fetal growth restriction (FGR)

The term fetal growth restriction (which is the same as intrauterine growth restriction or IUGR) was first used in the 1950s to describe babies born after term with meconium staining of the liquor who were wasted and had evidence of peripartum asphyxia. These findings were attributed to placental failure and were in part responsible for some obstetricians adopting a policy of inducing labour at term (a policy that was later abandoned).

A more appropriate definition of fetal growth restriction is that of 'a fetus which fails to reach its genetic growth potential'. (The previous term 'fetal growth retardation' should no longer be used as the word 'retarded' has connotations of cerebral impairment.) Fetal growth restriction presents as a fetus whose growth on ultrasound scanning is noted to be falling away from its initial centile. A fetus whose measurements are found to be on the 50th centile having originally been on the 90th centile, strictly speaking has FGR, whereas a baby growing continuously on the 5th centile, while small for

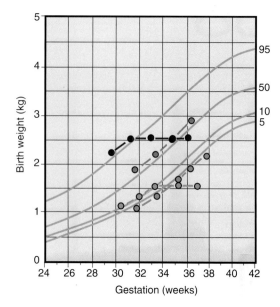

Fig. 38.1 **Fetal growth charts.** ◒ The baby is growing along the 50th centile. ◒ The baby is small for dates but does not have fetal growth restriction. ◒ The baby is laterally small for dates and has fetal growth restriction. ● The baby has fetal growth restriction but is not small for dates.

gestational age, does not have FGR. SGA and FGR are therefore not synonymous, with SGA babies growing parallel to the centiles and FGR babies falling away from their original centiles. The two cannot be differentiated without at least two measurements taken more than 2 weeks apart. The incidence of SGA is 10% (if the 10th centile is chosen) whereas the incidence of FGR is perhaps only 3%. In practice therefore most babies with FGR are SGA, while most babies who are SGA do not have FGR (Fig. 38.1).

Postnatally, babies with FGR appear thin as measured by the ponderal index (the ratio of body weight to length). The skin-fold thickness is reduced and there is often catch-up growth in the following months. This is, of course, of little value to an obstetrician who needs to make the diagnosis prior to birth.

Aetiology

Fetal growth is determined by the baby's intrinsic genetic drive, which is then modified by various fetal, maternal and placental factors (Box 38.1).

Fetal factors affecting fetal growth

The genetic make-up of the fetus is the main determinant of the intrinsic drive and is related to a number of factors including ethnicity. Asian mothers, for example, have smaller babies than their European counterparts.

seen with chromosomal abnormalities, for instance trisomies 18, 13, 21 and triploidy. Small babies are also found in association with structural abnormalities of all the major organ systems as well as with fetal infection. These infections include toxoplasmosis, cytomegalovirus and rubella but worldwide the main association is with malaria. There is good evidence that routine use of antenatal malarial prophylaxis in endemic areas increases the average birth weight.

The role of endocrine factors in fetal growth has been studied through various congenital diseases. Most hormones appear to have little effect on growth rates. Insulin, on the other hand, does appear to be important, and babies born with hypoinsulinism, as a result of the very rare condition of congenital diabetes, are small. Conversely those with hyperinsulinism secondary to maternal diabetes tend to be obese.

Maternal factors affecting fetal growth

Small variations in diet do not have a measurable effect on fetal growth but extreme starvation does cause significant growth impairment. This was seen in the Dutch winter famine of 1944 and during the Siege of Leningrad from 1941 to 1944. There is no evidence, however, that food supplementation above a normal diet can improve growth in utero.

Oxygen supply is important. Babies born at high altitude are small, presumably as a result of the decreased oxygen content found in the rarefied atmosphere. This is also true of babies born to mothers with chronic hypoxia secondary to congenital heart disease. The fetus is able to partly compensate through placental hypertrophy, but this compensation is incomplete.

Drugs such as tobacco, heroin, cocaine and alcohol may decrease fetal growth velocity. It has been estimated that smoking, for example, will decrease neonatal weight by an average of approximately 150 grams. Maternal chronic disease also has an adverse effect on fetal growth, particularly if there is renal impairment.

Placental factors affecting fetal growth

Adequate placental function depends on adequate trophoblastic invasion. In the first trimester trophoblast cells invade the maternal spiral arteries in the decidua. In the second trimester a secondary wave of trophoblast extends this invasion along the spiral arteries and into the myometrium. This results in the conversion of thick-walled muscular vessels with a relatively high vascular resistance to flaccid thin-walled vessels with a low resistance to flow. In certain conditions, such as proteinuric hypertension, it would appear that there has been failure of this secondary trophoblastic invasion, the consequences being subsequent placental ischaemia, atheromatous changes and secondary placental insufficiency. Why this failure should occur is unclear, but

The smallest babies are born to the Lumi tribe of Papua New Guinea with a mean birth weight of 2.4 kg. The largest, with a mean birth weight of 3.9 kg, are to the North American Cheyenne.

This intrinsic genetic drive is more related to the maternal genome than the genome of the father, and involves 'genomic imprinting'. It is well recognized that while large women often have correspondingly large babies, the correlation between large men and the size of their baby is poor. The importance of this maternal contribution is demonstrated by the experience of mating Shire horses, which are large, with Shetland ponies, which are small. When the stallion is a Shire and the mare a Shetland the result is a small foal, but conversely when the Shetland is the stallion and the Shire the mare the foal is large. Further experiments with mouse eggs suggest that the maternal genome may be responsible for imprinting an appropriate fetal growth trajectory and the paternal genome for regulating placental development.

There is also evidence that uniparental disomy, the process by which both chromosomes of a homologous pair are inherited from the same parent rather than one chromosome from each, may also lead to FGR. Whether this is due to fetal or placental problems is unclear.

Many abnormal fetuses are small, presumably as a result of a decreased intrinsic drive. This is particularly

Table 38.1
Factors controlling local uterine blood flow

Thromboxane	Prostacyclin
Vasoconstrictor	Vasodilator
Platelet aggregation	Inhibits platelet aggregation

may be related to the immunological interface between the fetal and maternal cells.

In pre-eclampsia there may be additional impaired placental flow from vasoconstriction. Local placental blood flow is under the control of prostacyclin and thromboxane A_2, with thromboxane causing vasoconstriction, and prostacyclin vasodilatation (Table 38.1). There is a relative deficiency of prostacyclin in pre-eclampsia and an increase in the production of thromboxane A_2, the net result being placental vessel vasoconstriction. Release of thromboxane, which is produced and stored within platelets, can be suppressed by low-dose aspirin therapy and this offers the possibility of some useful intervention.

Another cause of poor placental function may be confined placental mosaicism. It is recognized that placental mosaicism can occur even when the fetal karyotype is normal, the most commonly recognized abnormality being placental trisomy 16. The mechanism of this impaired function remains unclear.

The overall effect of uteroplacental insufficiency, whatever the cause, is a decrease in the nutrient supply to the fetus. It is not surprising therefore that these fetuses are often found to be hypoxic, hypoglycaemic, and sometimes acidotic. To compensate for this hypoxia the fetus increases erythropoiesis in order to increase its oxygen-carrying capacity, and redistributes blood away from the peripheral circulation, gut and liver towards the brain, heart and adrenal glands.

The result is a baby with normal axial growth and brain development, but who is thin and has little or no subcutaneous fat. Glycogen stores are minimal. As these babies have relatively large heads compared to their bodies their growth is referred to as 'asymmetrical'.

Screening and diagnosis

A history may give some pointers towards the possibility of a small baby, particularly if there has been a previous small baby, an antepartum haemorrhage or decreased fetal movements. The diagnosis should also be considered in any mother with signs of pre-eclampsia. Usually, however, small babies are identified following routine clinical or ultrasound examination.

Clinical examination

Estimation of fetal weight from clinical examination is notoriously difficult. The fundus reaches the umbilicus by around 20–24 weeks and the xiphisternum by approximately 36 weeks. Some clinicians try to gain an impression of the fetal weight from bimanual abdominal palpation, while others prefer using a tape measure. After 20 weeks' gestation the height of the uterus, measured from the uterine fundus to the symphysis pubis in centimetres, is approximately equal to the gestation in weeks. This provides a simple and cheap screening test that can be expected to identify 30–80% of all SGA babies.

Ultrasound examination

Ultrasound is a more accurate method of assessing the fetal size. Measurements can be made of the fetal head (circumference or biparietal diameter), the abdominal circumference and the femur length, and various equations have been used to estimate fetal weight. For practical purposes it is reasonable to consider the abdominal circumference alone, as measurements below the 10th centile have an approximately 80% sensitivity in the prediction of SGA neonates in high-risk pregnancies. The use of customized ultrasound charts adjusted for variables such as maternal weight, maternal height, ethnic group and parity has a better sensitivity than standard population charts. There is no evidence that routine ultrasound screening is of value in low-risk women.

SGA or FGR?

This is the key question and one which it is not always possible to answer. As noted above, those babies less than the 10th centile include those who are simply constitutionally small (perhaps around 70%) and those who have FGR (perhaps 30%). The increased risks of stillbirth, birth hypoxia, neonatal complications and impaired neurodevelopment are likely to be in the FGR group only, and it would be of great value to differentiate these two groups.

Those fetuses which have been measured serially and whose growth is falling away from the original centiles are, by definition, in the FGR group. Ultrasound measurements, however, have a significant inherent inaccuracy that sometimes makes this distinction difficult. As also noted above, attempts have been made to classify small fetuses into those with a reduced abdominal circumference and normal head size (asymmetrical) and those with both small head and small abdominal circumference (symmetrical). Those with asymmetrical measurements are more likely to have FGR as the baby is demonstrating redistribution of blood flow towards the brain, but again the concept may be difficult to apply in practice because of the inaccuracy in ultrasound measurements.

A detailed scan is warranted to look for any evidence of structural or chromosomal abnormality which makes FGR much more likely than SGA. A normal structural scan, however, does not prove the absence of FGR, and it is then necessary to check other parameters of fetal well-being. These parameters are considered below. In practice, most fetuses less than the 10th centile require close observation and whether they have FGR or are SGA only becomes apparent in retrospect.

Management

The main principle is to monitor the fetus and deliver at the appropriate time (Box 38.2). No in-utero treatment is of any proven benefit. Although smoking cessation programmes can be effective in increasing birth weight, there are no data to suggest this improves perinatal outcome.

As discussed on page 317, the options for fetal monitoring include fetal movement charts, fetal cardiotocography, biophysical scoring and Doppler blood flow studies. Of these, Doppler flow studies are likely to be the most valuable.

Fetal movement monitoring

A starved fetus will attempt to conserve energy by becoming less active and it may be useful to ask the mother about fetal movements. Most women experience a decrease in fetal movements as they approach term but any sudden change in the pattern of movements may be of significance. The true value of movement counting, however, is unclear and a number of studies have failed to demonstrate any benefit from using this technique.

Fetal cardiotocography

The interpretation of cardiotocographs (CTGs) is discussed on page 407. The CTG gives an indication of fetal well-being at a particular moment but has little longer-term value. The routine use of antenatal cardiotocography does not seem to be associated with an improved perinatal outcome.

Biophysical profile

This is discussed in detail on page 318 but the predictive value in FGR is low. The test takes a long time to carry out, sometimes up to an hour. As most babies with an abnormal biophysical score also have abnormal umbilical artery Doppler flow, it seems more appropriate to rely on Doppler studies. Furthermore, Doppler abnormalities probably precede abnormalities in the biophysical profile.

Doppler ultrasound

Doppler ultrasound of the umbilical artery is used as an assessment of placental vascular resistance further 'downstream' (p. 318). A normal waveform indicates that a SGA fetus is constitutionally small rather than growth restricted because of impaired placental function. Reduction or loss of end-diastolic flow identifies a fetus at high risk of hypoxia, and absent end-diastolic flow has been shown to be a useful discriminator between those FGR babies at high risk of perinatal death and those at a lower risk. Other studies have shown that use of umbilical artery studies to monitor high-risk fetuses reduces perinatal morbidity and mortality.

Doppler studies of the fetal cerebral circulation can also provide additional useful information (Fig. 38.2). As the growth-restricted fetus redistributes its blood flow away from the less vital organs towards the brain in response to hypoxia it is reasonable to expect an increased cerebral flow. This is indeed observed to happen, with Doppler studies showing a decreased resistance of the middle cerebral artery (Fig. 38.3). As the hypoxia becomes more severe this resistance increases again, possibly secondary to cerebral oedema.

Overall strategy

Figure 38.4 illustrates the probable sequence of events in fetal decompensation. As umbilical Doppler abnormalities are the first to appear, it is logical to use Doppler as the main screening tool. Thereafter, the optimal surveillance strategy in fetuses with absent or reduced end-diastolic flow is unclear but some form of frequent

---

Box 38.2

CLINICAL MANAGEMENT OF FGR

- Screening by palpation
- Ultrasound confirmation that the baby is small
- Exclude fetal structural (± chromosomal) abnormality
- Consider whether the fetus is SGA or whether it has FGR. Use Doppler studies ± biophysical scoring and CTGs
- Monitor, again with Doppler studies, biophysical scoring and CTGs as appropriate
- Consider steroids if preterm
- Deliver if problems, depending on gestation

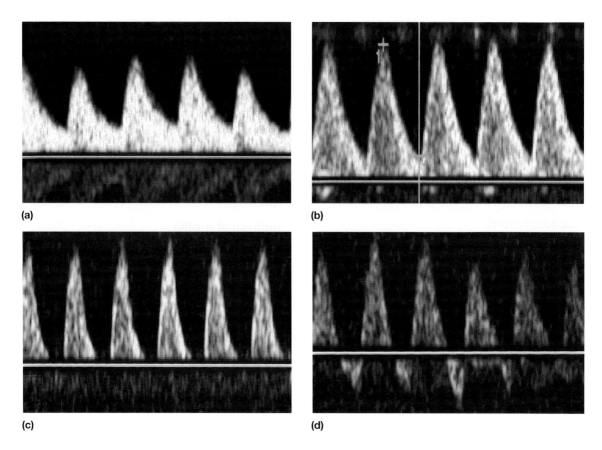

(a)

(b)

(c)

(d)

Fig. 38.2 **Doppler ultrasound of the umbilical cord demonstrating (a) normal, (b) reduced, (c) absent and (d) reversed end-diastolic flow.** Absent and reversed end-diastolic flow are associated with fetal compromise of placental origin.

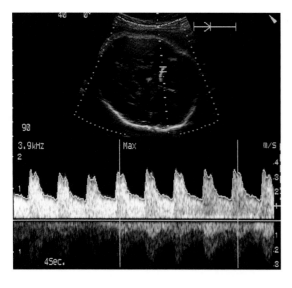

Fig. 38.3 **In fetal growth restriction there is an increased flow in the middle cerebral artery.**

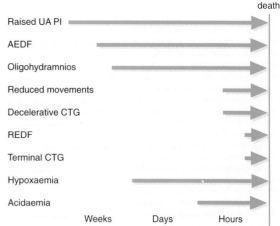

Fig. 38.4 **The 'decompensation cascade' of fetal growth restriction.** Absent end-diastolic flow (AEDF) is a relatively early sign of hypoxaemia, with reduced fetal movements, cardiotocographic abnormalities and reversed end-diastolic flow (REDF) late features. UA PI, urinary artery pulsatility index.

(e.g. daily) monitoring with CTGs, biophysical profile and further Doppler studies seems appropriate. The timing of the delivery will be decided by weighing up the risks of leaving the baby in utero against the risks of prematurity, but delivery is likely to be appropriate when the CTG becomes pathological (decelerations or reduced variability), the biophysical profile becomes abnormal (e.g. < 4) or there is reversal of end-diastolic flow. If FGR is suspected before 34–36 weeks, it is appropriate to consider giving steroids to the mother to enhance fetal lung maturation (p. 377).

The actual mode of delivery depends on the individual circumstances, but it must be remembered that the placental reserve of some of these fetuses may be extremely low and careful monitoring in labour is required. Early recourse to caesarean section is appropriate if the monitoring shows signs of fetal compromise. Pre-labour caesarean section may be appropriate if there are significant pre-labour concerns about fetal well-being.

Long-term implications of FGR

Babies with FGR are at increased risk of perinatal mortality and have a significant risk of stillbirth (Box 38.3). Antenatal hypoxia may lead to long-term neurological handicap, as may more acute intrapartum hypoxia. Even if there is no overt evidence of handicap, studies of long-term development suggest that growth-restricted fetuses may be more clumsy and that their IQ may be 5–10 points lower than a normally grown sibling.

There is also increasing evidence to suggest that FGR predisposes babies to problems much later in life, particularly non-insulin-dependent diabetes and coronary heart disease. It may be that the fetus alters its metabolism to cope with poor nutrition in utero and is subsequently less able to cope with normal carbohydrate levels in later postnatal life. It is also possible that there are vascular compensatory changes with FGR which predispose to later arterial disease. Critics of this 'fetal origins' hypothesis suggest that the genes responsible for FGR may be the same genes responsible for non-insulin-dependent diabetes and coronary heart disease. Either way, this very interesting hypothesis has only limited practical application at present but serves to highlight the importance of the uterine environment to fetal development. Research in this area is continuing.

Box 38.3

CLINICAL SIGNIFICANCE OF FGR

Increased risk of:

- fetal anomaly
- perinatal asphyxia
- operative delivery
- perinatal death
- neonatal hypoglycaemia and hypocalcaemia
- necrotizing enterocolitis
- long-term handicap
- increased incidence of non-insulin-dependent diabetes and coronary heart disease in later life

---

Key points

- An accurate estimation of gestation is a prerequisite of accurate diagnosis of fetal growth abnormality.

- Small for gestational age (SGA) refers to those fetuses whose weight is < 10th centile for their gestational age. They are simply inherently small, but may be growing along their centile with a normal growth velocity.

- Fetal growth restriction (FGR) refers to any fetus failing to achieve its growth potential. Not all small-for-gestational-age fetuses are growth restricted and not all growth-restricted fetuses are SGA. FGR carries an increased risk of intrapartum asphyxia, neonatal hypoglycaemia and possible long-term neurological impairment. There is also an increased risk of perinatal mortality.

- Most screening tests attempt to diagnose small-for gestational-age fetuses rather than growth-restricted fetuses. Diagnosis of FGR requires at least two ultrasound scans, at least 2 weeks apart.

- Management involves appropriate monitoring with delivery if required.

Pregnancy-induced hypertension

Introduction

The term 'pregnancy-induced hypertension' (PIH) suggests a disorder of blood pressure arising because of the presence of pregnancy. Such a simplistic view detracts from the fundamental pathological process underlying this condition – it is a multisystem disorder which can affect every organ system in the body, particularly the liver, lungs, kidney, brain and cardiovascular system. It appears to be caused by some placental factor, the exact nature of which is unclear, and the pathophysiology involves endothelial dysfunction.

Pregnancy-induced hypertension is unpredictable in onset and progression, incurable except by ending the pregnancy and potentially dangerous for both the mother and the fetus.

It is a very heterogeneous condition such that in some instances the most prominent feature may be liver damage, in others it may be kidney dysfunction and in still others it may be, as the name suggests, the blood pressure itself.

Definitions

Although multisystem in nature, the condition is classified into four main groups depending on the cardiovascular, renal, cerebral and hepatic manifestations:

- gestational hypertension – hypertension only
- pre-eclampsia – hypertension and proteinuria
- eclampsia – generalized convulsion
- HELLP syndrome – hepatic and haematological dysfunction.

Together they account for the second highest cause of direct maternal deaths in the UK (1997–1999) and for around 75 000 maternal deaths worldwide every year.

Hypertension

In normal pregnancy the blood pressure falls slightly during the first trimester reaching a nadir in the second trimester and rising a little again during the third. It should be measured in the sitting position with an appropriate size of cuff (Fig. 39.1). Although controversial, it is suggested that the phase IV Korotkoff sound (i.e. 'muffling' rather than 'disappearance') should be taken when reading the diastolic pressure. Hypertension in pregnancy may be coincidental (usually background

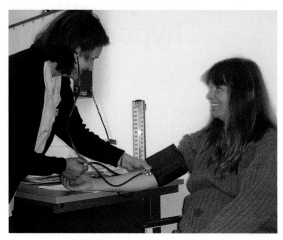

(a)

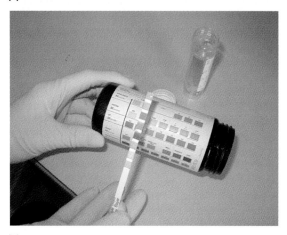

(b)

Fig. 39.1 **Early detection of pre-eclampsia is paramount.**
(a) Measurement of blood pressure (reproduced with permission).
(b) Testing for urinary protein.

essential hypertension), or related to pregnancy (gestational hypertension or pre-eclampsia).

- Hypertension in pregnancy is defined as a diastolic blood pressure > 110 mmHg on any one occasion or > 90 mmHg on two occasions more than 4 hours apart.
- Severe hypertension is a single diastolic blood pressure > 120 mmHg on any one occasion or > 110 mmHg on two occasions more than 4 hours apart.

Some authorities also consider a diastolic pressure 30 mmHg above the booking diastolic pressure to be a useful definition.

Raised blood pressure at booking (e.g. before 16 weeks) is usually due to chronic hypertension, most commonly essential hypertension rather than the rarer problems of renal disease or phaeochromocytoma. Gestational hypertension (hypertension only) and pre-

eclampsia (hypertension and proteinuria) only very rarely occur before 20 weeks, unless associated with trophoblastic disease.

Proteinuria

This is defined as a persistent urinary protein of more than 300 mg/24 hours, which approximates to '+' or more on urine dipstick testing.

Essential hypertension

Essential hypertension is commoner in older women and the prognosis for pregnancy is overall good. The main risk is from superimposed pre-eclampsia, which is more common in those who have pre-existing hypertension. Essential hypertension itself is rarely of significance although there may be a slightly increased risk of placental abruption. Those women who are already taking antihypertensive drugs, and who have mild to moderate hypertension (140/90–170/110), may be able to discontinue the medication in pregnancy. Those with more severe hypertension should continue. Appropriate preparations include methyldopa, beta-blockers (e.g. labetalol) or nifedipine. Diuretics and ACE inhibitors can cause fetal compromise and are contraindicated.

Gestational hypertension, pre-eclampsia and eclampsia

Pathophysiology

The incidence of the hypertensive disorders in pregnancy is 8–10% and the recognized predisposing factors are shown in Box 39.1. Despite extensive research, the exact aetiology and pathophysiology of the condition remain unclear. It is likely, however, that inadequate placental perfusion resulting from inadequate placental invasion precipitates the release of some form of chemical trigger which, in susceptible mothers, leads to endothelial damage, metabolic changes and a form of inflammatory response. This process is discussed below.

Placental invasion

In normal pregnancy trophoblastic invasion of the maternal spiral arteries causes the diameter of these arteries to increase around fivefold, converting the supply from a high-resistance low-flow system to one with a low resistance and high flow. In pre-eclampsia adequate invasion does not seem to occur, or is limited to the decidual portions of the vessels, and the result is inadequate placental blood flow. Inadequate placental invasion is also associated with fetal growth restriction (FGR), but not all those with this form of growth restriction develop pre-eclampsia.

As the degree of trophoblastic invasion is regulated by the maternal decidual barrier, probably by the action of a specific form of leucocyte, it is has been suggested that the primary aetiological factor in pre-eclampsia may be immunological in origin. The predominance of pre-eclampsia in first pregnancies, and the protective effect of parity, further support an immunological mechanism but the exact nature of this has yet to be elucidated. Nonetheless, inadequate placental invasion certainly occurs and may be the trigger to release some factor, or alter the level of some factor, which brings about a response in a susceptible mother.

Maternal susceptibility

As noted above, placentally mediated growth restriction can occur in isolation, but is also common with pre-eclampsia. It is therefore reasonable to assume that, while inadequate invasion occurs in both, only mothers who develop pre-eclampsia have a susceptibility to the placental stimulus. This susceptibility may be genotypic or phenotypic.

The evidence for genotypic susceptibility is strong. It has long been recognized that there is a familial pattern to pre-eclampsia and studies of pregnant women who have developed eclamptic seizures show that these women are more likely to have had sisters, mothers or grandmothers who have suffered from the same problem. Analysis suggests a single gene inheritance, either recessive with high penetrance, or dominant with incomplete penetrance. A number of genes on a variety of chromosomes have been found to be associated with pre-eclampsia, as has an angiotensin gene variant on chromosome 4. A genetic predisposition

is also observed in those with certain congenital thrombophilias.

Certain phenotypes are also more susceptible. Those with insulin resistance and central obesity are at increased risk of pre-eclampsia, possibly on account of an exaggerated metabolic response. Those with systemic lupus erythematosus are also at increased risk, possibly because of an exaggerated immune response, and it has already been noted that those with a congenital thrombophilia are more likely to develop problems, possibly because of an increased coagulation response. These associations suggest that the pathophysiology involves a significant interrelation between metabolic processes, an immunological response and coagulation problems, possibly mediated through endothelial damage. These maternal responses are now considered.

Metabolic changes, inflammatory response and endothelial damage

In normal pregnancy there is increased biosynthesis of eicosanoids – particularly prostacyclin (PGI_2), a vasodilator with platelet-inhibitory properties, and thromboxane A_2, a vasoconstrictor with a tendency to stimulate platelet aggregation. As both usually increase in proportion to each other, there is a net neutralization and homeostasis is maintained. This homeostasis is disrupted in pre-eclampsia because of a relative deficiency in prostacyclin because of a decrease in its synthesis and/or an increase in the production of thromboxane A_2. This imbalance leads to vasoconstriction, hypertension, and platelet stimulation. These observations form the theoretical basis behind the use of low-dose aspirin, a prostaglandin inhibitor, in preventing pre-eclampsia. The dose of aspirin required to inhibit thromboxane synthesis is less than that required for prostacyclin inhibition and it should, in theory, therefore reduce the vascular and thrombotic effects.

Normal pregnancy is also associated with an increase in angiotensin II, a potent vasoconstrictor, yet despite this it is usual in pregnancy for the peripheral vascular resistance to fall. This appears to be because of a resistance to the effects of angiotensin II in normal pregnancy, a phenomenon which seems to be lost in women who are destined to develop pregnancy-induced hypertension. This suggests that abnormalities in the renin–angiotensin–aldosterone system may play a role in the pathogenesis of the condition. Most agree that it seems unlikely, however, that derangements in this system are the primary cause of the pre-eclampsia.

In addition to these changes, there also appears to be some form of inflammatory process. There is an increase in the pro-inflammatory cytokines, evidence of neutrophil activation, and an increase in substances capable of causing inflammatory damage, particularly proteases and oxygen radicals. These are also recognized to damage vessel walls. Other systemic metabolic

Table 39.1
Potential secondary effects of the metabolic, inflammatory endothelial alterations in pre-eclampsia

CVS	Increased peripheral resistance leading to hypertension Increased vascular permeability and reduced maternal plasma volume
Lungs	Laryngeal and pulmonary oedema
Renal	Glomerular damage leading to proteinuria, hypoproteinaemia and reduced oncotic pressure which further exacerbates the hypovolaemia. May develop acute renal failure ± cortical necrosis
Clotting	Hypercoagulability, with increased fibrin formation and increased fibrinolysis, i.e. disseminated intravascular coagulation
Liver	HELLP syndrome Hepatic rupture
CNS	Thrombosis and fibrinoid necrosis of the cerebral arterioles Eclampsia (convulsions), cerebral haemorrhage and cerebral oedema
Fetus	Impaired uteroplacental circulation, potentially leading to FGR, hypoxaemia and intrauterine death

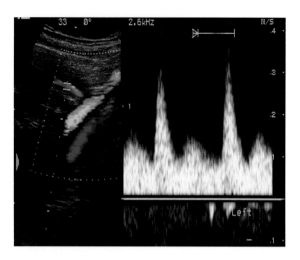

Fig. 39.2 **Uterine artery Doppler notching at 24 weeks is predictive of pre-eclampsia and intrauterine growth restriction in high-risk mothers.**

changes include hypertriglyceridaemia and a significant increase in free fatty acids, both associated with acute atherosis.

Some of these metabolic changes may cause endothelial damage, which in turn promotes platelet adhesion, stimulates clotting activity and disturbs the normal physiological modulation of vascular tone, further amplifying the response. The resulting secondary damage to other organs, as outlined in Table 39.1, gives rise to the clinical features of gestational hypertension, pre-eclampsia, eclampsia and the HELLP syndrome.

Screening and detection

Pre-eclampsia is an extremely variable and unpredictable condition and progression is often more rapid the earlier in pregnancy it occurs. Some mothers have minimal symptoms and then have fits, other look worryingly unwell and are fine. The purpose of antenatal screening is to prevent both the maternal and fetal complications by timely delivery of the baby.

Mothers are screened for hypertension and proteinuria in antenatal clinics (Fig. 39.1). A number of additional screening tests for predicting pre-eclampsia have been suggested but are of limited clinical use. In those with risk factors, however, Doppler ultrasound may reveal bilateral uterine artery Doppler notching at 24 weeks which does identify a group at increased risk of later hypertensive problems (Fig. 39.2).

Treatment of the mother with antihypertensive drugs masks the sign of hypertension but does not alter the course of the disease. It may allow prolongation of the pregnancy and thereby improve fetal outcome. The only true 'cure' is delivery of the placenta.

Clinical management of gestational hypertension without proteinuria

The following may be used as guidelines:

- If the blood pressure is found to be elevated at an antenatal clinic, it should be re-checked after 10–20 minutes. If it settles, no further action is required.
- If the blood pressure is elevated on two readings more than 4 hours apart, fetal size should be appraised clinically and enquiry made about maternal well-being. Serum urate (which rises with pre-eclampsia), urea and electrolytes (U&Es), and platelets (which fall with pre-eclampsia) should be checked twice weekly along with blood pressure and urinalysis for protein. Advice should be given to present if unwell, or if there is frontal headache or epigastric pain.
- If there are abnormal blood results or the diastolic pressure is more than 100 mmHg or there is clinical suspicion of FGR, poor fetal well-being or maternal compromise, arrangements should be made for cardiotocography, and ultrasound assessment of fetal size and liquor volume (Fig. 39.3). Blood pressure recordings and urinalysis three times per week, with at least weekly measurement of serum urate, U&Es, FBC and platelets, are also appropriate (Table 39.2). If fetal monitoring is suspicious or pre-eclampsia develops, further action may be required.

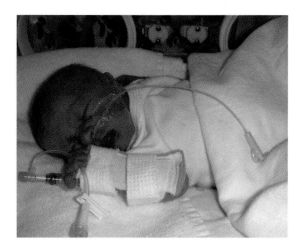

Fig. 39.3 **This baby, born at 36 weeks to a mother with severe pre-eclampsia, weighed 1.6 kg.** (Usual weight at 36 weeks: 2.2–3.3 kg.)

Table 39.2
Possible investigations

Investigation	Finding in pre-eclampsia
FBC	Reduced platelets, haemolysis on blood film
Renal function	Reduced urine output Increased urate, increased urea Reduced glomerular filtration rate Proteinuria and low serum albumin
Coagulation system	Abnormal APTT and INR
Hepatic system	Elevated alkaline phosphatase and aspartate transaminase

APTT, activated partial thromboplastin time; FBC, full blood count; INR, International Normalized Ratio

Clinical management of pre-eclampsia

With pre-eclampsia, it is important to consider the overall picture rather than make decisions on the basis of a single parameter. It is appropriate to admit the mother for more intensive monitoring if there are symptoms, or if she has significant proteinuria or severe hypertension. Antihypertensives may need to be considered as well as plans made for delivery.

The decision to deliver and the method of delivery are dependent on many of the above factors. There are usually fetal advantages to conservative management before 34 weeks if the blood pressure, laboratory values and fetal parameters are stable.

The aim is to:

- Reduce the diastolic blood pressure to < 100 mmHg with methyldopa, labetalol, hydralazine or nifedipine (Table 39.3).
- Consider delivery, the time of which depends on maternal well-being, gestation and fetal well-being.
- Assess the fluid balance. There is increased vascular permeability and a reduced intravascular compartment – giving too little fluid risks renal failure and too much risks pulmonary oedema. Urine output should be monitored. The SaO_2 should also be monitored if the pre-eclampsia is severe. U&Es, liver function tests (LFTs), albumin, urate, haemoglobin, haematocrit, platelets and clotting should also be monitored. Central venous pressure monitoring may be helpful in oliguria to differentiate intravascular depletion from renal impairment.

The use of magnesium sulphate in severe pre-eclampsia halves the risk of subsequent eclampsia, and may reduce the risk of maternal death. Magnesium sulphate, given to those who have had an eclamptic seizure, also prevents further seizures.

Table 39.3
Drug treatment for hypertension of PIH

Drug	Action	Side-effects	Comments
Methyldopa (orally)	Central acting; decreases sympathetic outflow from the brain	Initial drowsiness	Safe; oral drug of choice
Labetalol (orally/i.v.)	Alpha- and beta-blocker	Postural hypotension, tiredness, headaches	i.v. – widely used in hypertensive crisis
Hydralazine (orally/i.m./i.v.)	Direct-acting vasodilator	May mimic impending eclampsia	i.v. – widely used in hypertensive crisis
Nifedipine (orally/s.l.)	Calcium-channel blocker and vasodilator	Flushing, headache, ankle swelling	

> ### Box 39.2
>
> *SYMPTOMS AND SIGNS OF IMPENDING ECLAMPSIA*
>
> 1. Unusual headaches
> 2. Visual disturbances
> 3. Restlessness or agitation
> 4. Epigastric pain, nausea and vomiting
> 5. Sudden severe hypertension and proteinuria
> 6. Fluid retention with reduced urine output
> 7. Hyperreflexia or ankle clonus
> 8. Retinal oedema, haemorrhages or papilloedema

> ### Box 39.3
>
> *TREATMENT OF ECLAMPSIA*
>
> - The patient should be turned onto her side to avoid aortocaval compression. An airway should be inserted and high-flow O_2 should be given.
>
> - $MgSO_4$ i.v. stat should be given to terminate the convulsion and then by intravenous infusion to reduce the chance of further convulsions. $MgSO_4$ can depress neuromuscular transmission, so the respiratory rate and patellar reflexes should be monitored (reduced patellar reflexes usually precede respiratory depression). If there is significant respiratory depression, calcium gluconate can be used to reverse the effects and consideration given to ventilation.
>
> - Urgent delivery should be considered if the fit has occurred antenatally.
>
> - Paralysis and ventilation should also be considered if the fits are prolonged or recurrent.

Management of eclampsia

Eclampsia occurs when there has been a convulsion (the word 'eclampsia' originally meant bolt of lightning). The UK national incidence is 4.9/10 000 maternities, with 38% of these occurring antepartum, 18% intrapartum and 44% postpartum. Of these, over a third occurred before proteinuria and hypertension had been documented. The maternal mortality is 1.8% with a neonatal death rate of 34/1000. In less-developed countries incidences of 20–80/10 000 maternities have been quoted, with maternal death occurring in around 10%.

In the presence of PIH, certain non-specific symptoms and signs become important indicators of widespread involvement of various maternal organs and may herald eclampsia (Box 39.2). These include visual symptoms (blurring of vision, diplopia, scotomas or flashes of light), headache, epigastric or upper quadrant abdominal pain, oliguria or anuria and pulmonary oedema or cyanosis. Treatment is outlined in Box 39.3.

Prevention of PIH

Various preventive strategies have been applied to women thought to be at risk of developing pre-eclampsia. The estimated value of these interventions is shown in Box 39.4.

It has been suggested that low-dose aspirin taken from early pregnancy (< 17 weeks and probably from the first trimester) may reduce the incidence of FGR or perinatal mortality in those with previous disease. Theoretically it can favourably alter the imbalance between prostacyclin and thromboxane A_2 seen in pre-eclampsia (see above), and overall clinical studies in this area are supportive. Strategies using fish supplements are showing promise. Restriction of salt and limiting weight gain is not useful.

> ### Box 39.4
>
> *PREVENTION OF PREGNANCY-INDUCED HYPERTENSION*
>
> **Possibly of value**
> - Low-dose aspirin
> - Fish oil supplements, or high fish diet
> - Calcium supplementation
>
> **Unlikely to be of value**
> - Diet with high protein content
> - Restriction of salt in diet
> - Restriction of weight gain

HELLP syndrome

HELLP is an acronym from *h*aemolysis, *e*levated *l*iver enzymes (particularly transaminases) and *l*ow *p*latelets. It is probably a variant of pre-eclampsia, and affects 4–12% of those with pre-eclampsia/eclampsia, being commoner in multigravidae. Presentation may be with epigastric pain, nausea, vomiting, and right upper quadrant tenderness. Aspartate transaminase rises first, then lactic dehydrogenase. A blood film may show burr cells and polychromasia consistent with haemolysis, although frank anaemia is uncommon. Platelet transfusion is only rarely required. There may also be acute renal failure and disseminated intravascular coagulation (DIC), and there is an increased incidence of abruption. The management of HELLP syndrome is to stabilize coagulation, assess fetal well-being and consider the need for delivery. It is generally considered that delivery is appropriate for moderate or severe cases, but management may be more conservative (with close monitoring) if the condition is mild. Postpartum vigilance is required for at least 48 hours as deterioration may occur. The incidence of recurrence in subsequent pregnancies is about 20%.

Key points

- Pre-eclampsia is a multisystem disorder, and a major cause of fetal and maternal morbidity and mortality.

- Medication, including antihypertensive agents, does not alter the progress of the condition; the only cure is delivery.

- HELLP syndrome is a variant of pre-eclampsia and is an acronym from *haemolysis, elevated liver enzymes* (particularly transaminases) and *low platelets*.

40

Prematurity

Introduction

Prematurity is defined as delivery between 24 and 37 weeks' gestation. It occurs in 6–10% of pregnancies. Although preterm labour is more common in association with multiple pregnancy, antepartum haemorrhage, fetal growth restriction, cervical incompetence, amnionitis, congenital uterine anomaly, polyhydramnios and systemic infection, there is often no apparent predisposing cause. Almost one-third of cases in the UK are iatrogenic following deliberate medical intervention when it has been felt that the risks of continuing the pregnancy for either the mother or the fetus outweigh the risk of prematurity.

To be born prematurely is a very serious hazard. Morbidity and mortality rates are directly related to the maturity of organ systems such as the lungs, brain and gastrointestinal tract, and it is exceptional to survive if delivered before 24 weeks' gestation. In western countries up to 85% of neonatal deaths are attributed to prematurity and, of those who survive, 10% will suffer some form of long-term handicap.

Research into the exact mechanisms involved in preterm delivery and methods of preventing it has been relatively unsuccessful so that prematurity is currently one of the most challenging problems facing both obstetricians and paediatricians.

Definitions

Preterm   A gestation of less than 37 completed weeks.

Very preterm   A gestation of less than 32 completed weeks.

Preterm labour   Regular uterine contractions accompanied by effacement and dilatation of the cervix after 20 weeks and before 37 completed weeks.

Preterm pre-labour rupture of the membranes (PPROM)   Rupture of the fetal membranes before 37 completed weeks and before the onset of labour.

Low birth weight (LBW)   Birth weight of less than 2501 g. It is important to note that low-birth-weight infants may be either preterm, growth restricted or both.

Table 40.1
Aetiology of preterm delivery

Spontaneous labour, cause unknown	35%
Elective delivery (iatrogenic)	30%
Maternal and fetal conditions	25%
Multiple pregnancy	10%

Very low birth weight (VLBW)   Birth weight of less than 1501 g.

Extremely low birth weight (ELBW)   Birth weight of less than 1000 g.

Perinatal mortality rates   See Chapter 51.

Aetiology and predisposing factors

As noted above, the incidence of preterm labour (before 37 weeks) is between 6–10% (Table 40.1). Only 1.5% will deliver before 32 weeks. Although only 0.5% deliver before 28 weeks, this group accounts for two-thirds of the neonatal deaths.

The exact aetiological factors that trigger spontaneous preterm labour are unknown, but the trigger may be mediated through prostaglandins. It may also, in some instances, be related directly to uterine size or to other hormonal factors. Infection has been implicated in preterm delivery and it may be that bacterial toxins initiate an inflammatory process in the chorioamniotic membranes, which in turn release prostaglandins. Bacteria may damage membranes by direct protease action, or by stimulating production of immune mediators like 5-hydroxytryptamine which stimulate smooth muscle cells. None of these postulated mechanisms entirely explains every case of preterm labour and the aetiology is therefore considered to be multifactorial.

Risk factors associated with preterm delivery include previous preterm delivery or pregnancy loss, low socio-economic status, low body mass index before pregnancy, teenage pregnancy, smoking, previous genital infection, urinary tract infection and heavy physical activity (Box 40.1).

Diagnosis of preterm labour

The definition of preterm labour is the same as in the diagnosis of labour at term; in other words regular painful contractions associated with progressive cervical dilatation. Diagnosis may be difficult in early stages as, in at least 50% of cases, regular painful contractions may not progress to established labour. Labour may also be insidious, or heralded by a 'show', bleeding or abruption.

Box 40.1

CONDITIONS DURING PREGNANCY ASSOCIATED WITH PRETERM DELIVERY

Fetal and placental
- Congenital uterine anomaly
- Bleeding in the first or second trimester
- Antepartum haemorrhage
- Placenta praevia
- Intrauterine infection
- Pre-labour rupture of the membranes
- Fetal growth restriction
- Congenital fetal anomaly
- Multiple pregnancy
- Polyhydramnios

Maternal
- Severe maternal disease
- Pre-eclampsia
- Urinary tract infection including asymptomatic bacteriuria
- Other infections and fevers including malaria
- Bacterial vaginosis
- Psychological stress

Screening for preterm labour

There have been a number of techniques proposed to screen for preterm labour. They include risk scoring, cervical assessment, measurement of fibronectin and bacteriological vaginal assessment.

The 'risk scoring' is based on the risk factors listed in Box 40.1. Unfortunately, the performance of these scoring systems has been poor, with sensitivities quoted as less than 40%, but the system at least serves to highlight the potentially avoidable factors such as urinary tract infections, vaginal infections, smoking, drugs and lifestyle.

Clinical assessment of the cervix has also been proposed, with those who have high Bishop's scores (p. 416) judged to be at increased risk. This again has performed poorly as a test and interest has focused on transvaginal measurement of the cervix. A normal cervical length is somewhere between 34 and 40 mm and there should be no funnelling at the internal os (Fig. 40.1). A cervical length < 15 mm at 23 weeks occurs in 2% of the

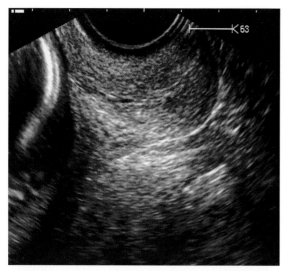

(a)

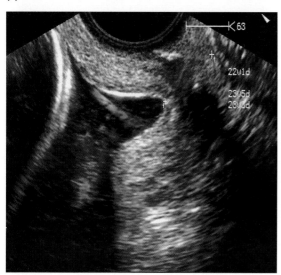

(b)

Fig. 40.1 **Cervical length as measured by transvaginal scan.**
(a) Normal. **(b)** There is shortening of the cervix and funnelling at the internal os. Note the transvaginal cervical suture in situ.

of the extracellular matrix. The presence of fetal fibronectin measured at 23 weeks predicts 60% of spontaneous preterm births at < 28 weeks in an unselected population, although with a positive predictive value of only 25%. In those suspected to be in preterm labour, a positive test has a positive predictive value of 80%, and < 3% with a negative test will deliver in the subsequent 3 weeks.

Screening for infection has also been considered, but again no benefits have been demonstrated. Bacterial vaginosis, which is present in 10–20% of pregnant women, has been associated with a doubling of the relative risk of delivery. There is no evidence, however, that treating bacterial vaginosis in low-risk groups carries any benefit. It is reasonable to treat bacterial vaginosis in those considered to have other risk factors.

Management

First ask 'is this preterm labour?', and if so 'why?' Cervical assessment, either clinically or with ultrasound, will be extremely helpful and it may also be helpful to look for fibronectin. If there is evidence of preterm membrane rupture it is inappropriate to carry out a digital vaginal examination as infection may be introduced.

Next it is important to assess maternal well-being, looking particularly for evidence of infection or haemorrhage. The white cell count may be raised in infection, as may the C-reactive protein. Vaginal swabs and urine should be sent for culture.

The fetus can be assessed with cardiotocography, and then ideally with ultrasound, looking for growth, liquor volume, presentation, Doppler flow anomalies and any evidence of fetal abnormality. If preterm delivery is likely the paediatricians should be alerted and arrangements made for in-utero transfer if local facilities are not optimal.

Steroids should be given if delivery before 34 weeks is considered likely. They cross the placenta and increase the production and release of pulmonary surfactant by a complex receptor-mediated gene transcription mechanism. Betamethasone or dexamethasone 24 mg i.m. is given in divided doses over 24 hours and their use reduces the incidence of respiratory distress syndrome by ≈ 50%. The incidence of necrotizing enterocolitis and periventricular haemorrhage is also reduced. No adverse neurological or cognitive effects following steroid treatment have been demonstrated, even with 12-year follow-up, but the possibility of unrecognized long-term effects has not been excluded. There is no identifiable increase in the incidence of maternal or fetal infection, but steroids are contraindicated if there is active maternal septicaemia. It is unknown whether it is appropriate to prescribe repeat doses (e.g. 12 mg every 10 days) if delivery does not occur and the risk

population but accounts for 90% of those who will deliver before 28 weeks. The risk of severe preterm labour with a cervical length greater than 15 mm is 4%, rising to 78% if the length is less than 5 mm. Those at high risk of preterm labour may benefit from a cervical suture (see below and Fig. 40.1b), and the opportunity also arises to give prophylactic steroids (see below).

Fetal fibronectin is a protein thought to be an adhesion molecule involved in maintaining the integrity of the choriodecidual extracellular matrix. It is usually not detectable after 20 weeks until membrane rupture, but if it is found to be present the risk of preterm labour is markedly increased. This may imply some disruption

of preterm delivery continues, but research is under way in this field. Steroids should be used with great caution in those with insulin-dependent diabetes, as they may precipitate ketoacidosis.

There is no indication for routine antibiotic prescription in spontaneous preterm labour in the absence of clinical infection.

Inhibition of preterm labour

In view of the high morbidity and mortality associated with prematurity an attempt may be made to stop preterm labour, particularly at gestations less than 33 weeks. The use of drugs to suppress uterine activity, 'tocolytics', will allow usually only a short delay at best but it may be sufficient to allow steroid administration or time to arrange an appropriate in-utero transfer. On the other hand, if there has been an abruption or there is intrauterine infection, the risk of fetal compromise may be increased. Contraindications to tocolytic therapy are listed in Box 40.2.

A wide variety of drugs have been used for tocolysis including beta-sympathomimetics, an oxytocin antagonist, cyclo-oxygenase inhibitors, calcium-channel blockers and magnesium sulphate.

Beta-sympathomimetics

Ritodrine and salbutamol, which are chemically related to adrenaline (epinephrine) and noradrenaline (norepinephrine), cause stimulation of $beta_2$-adrenergic receptors on myometrial cell membranes. This leads to a reduction in intracellular calcium concentrations and inhibition of the actin–myosin interaction necessary for smooth muscle contraction. An intravenous infusion of ritodrine has been shown to reduce the proportion of deliveries within the first 48 hours and, although this delay has not been conclusively shown to improve fetal morbidity or mortality, it may provide a useful window for steroid administration.

Beta-sympathomimetics stimulate the sympathetic nervous system, and side-effects include maternal (and fetal) tachycardia, visual disturbances, skin flushing, nausea, vomiting, hyperkalaemia and hyperglycaemia. Pulmonary oedema, severe maternal bradycardia, hypotension and arrhythmias may occur, and maternal deaths have been reported. At a minimum there must be a calibrated infusion pump and good facilities for maternal monitoring. In view of these potentially serious maternal side-effects the use of beta-sympathomimetics should be restricted to those less than 34 weeks' gestation with good evidence of preterm labour.

Oxytocin antagonist

Atosiban is a synthetic competitive inhibitor of oxytocin which binds to myometrial oxytocin receptors and leads to an inhibition of intracellular calcium release. It has been shown to be as effective as ritodrine, but has minimal maternal or fetal side-effects. Nausea and vomiting have occasionally been reported.

Cyclo-oxygenase inhibitors

Most experience in this group of drugs is with indometacin. It inhibits cyclo-oxygenase, the enzyme which converts fatty acids into prostaglandin endoperoxidases, and it thereby reduces prostaglandin production. Trials have shown that indometacin reduces the frequency of delivery within 48 hours and within 7–10 days from the beginning of treatment.

It may lead to maternal gastrointestinal irritation, peptic ulceration, thrombocytopenia, allergic reactions, headaches and dizziness but, in contrast to the beta-sympathomimetics, the main risks are to the fetus. The patency of the ductus arteriosus is prostaglandin-dependent and ductal constriction has been demonstrated in human fetuses from as early as 27 weeks' gestation in response to these drugs. There is also evidence that indometacin reduces fetal urine output, probably as a result of changes in proximal tubular reabsorption and in the effect on fetal ADH. Despite these two potential problems, significant adverse neonatal effects have not been convincingly demonstrated, but caution is nonetheless advised, particularly in those with pre-existing oligohydramnios.

Calcium-channel blockers

There has been considerable research with nifedipine, a type 2 calcium-channel blocker, which inhibits inward

---

Box 40.2

CONTRAINDICATIONS TO TOCOLYSIS

Relative contraindications
- Significant vaginal bleeding
- Pre-eclampsia
- Fetal growth restriction

Absolute contraindications
- Fetal death
- Lethal congenital anomaly
- Chorioamnionitis
- Significant fetal distress
- Maternal condition requiring immediate delivery

calcium flow across cell membranes. In vitro, nifedipine reduces myometrial contractility, but data on clinical benefit are uncertain. The side-effects of dizziness, flushing and headache are all related to peripheral dilatation, but serious adverse problems are rare. There seem to be no obvious adverse fetal effects.

Magnesium sulphate

Magnesium sulphate is the treatment of choice for pre-eclampsia but its use in preterm labour is not well established. Its mechanism of action is not fully understood but probably involves calcium uptake in smooth muscle cells. There is in-vitro evidence of smooth muscle inhibition but also clinical evidence to suggest that it may in fact increase perinatal mortality. Its use for tocolysis is therefore not recommended, although it has wide usage in the USA.

Although there is also research on glyceryl trinitrate and COX-2 inhibitors, the drugs listed above remain the primary available tocolytics. Indometacin appears to be the superior tocolytic (Table 40.2), but concerns remain about its adverse fetal side-effects. Atosiban combines effectiveness with a low side-effect profile and, although it is relatively new, may attain more widespread usage.

Delivery

If labour is allowed to continue or tocolysis is unsuccessful, then close monitoring is important as a preterm fetus is probably more susceptible to acidosis than a fetus at term. Complications such as abnormal lie, cord prolapse, abruption and intrauterine infection are also more common.

The route of delivery needs to be considered. While caesarean section may be indicated for an apparently compromised fetus, there is no evidence to support liberal use of caesarean section in the majority of instances, and indeed, preterm delivery by caesarean section may lead to significant fetal trauma. The vaginal route is preferred for those with cephalic presentation and, contrary to some texts, there is no evidence to

Table 40.2
Effectiveness of tocolytics

	Odds ratio of delivery	
	Less than 48 hours	Less than 7 days
Ritodrine	0.56	0.65
Atosiban	0.67	0.59
Indometacin	0.12	0.07
Nifedipine	0.48	
Magnesium sulphate	0.52	1.54

support routine epidurals, forceps or episiotomy. There is more controversy about route of delivery, however, in those presenting by the breech, with little good evidence to support either route. In current clinical practice most preterm breeches before 26 weeks are delivered vaginally and many of those above this gestation are delivered by caesarean section.

Prevention of preterm labour

As noted above, there is no indication for routine antibiotic treatment in uncomplicated spontaneous preterm labour. There is some evidence that elective cervical cerclage is of benefit in those with a history of cervical incompetence, particularly those with a history of more than two deliveries before 37 weeks. A Mersilene suture is inserted transvaginally around the cervix under anaesthesia and removed electively after 38 weeks' gestation or as an emergency if labour establishes before that time (see Fig. 40.1b). Transabdominal cervico-isthmic cerclage is a specialist procedure reserved for failed transcervical cerclage.

'Rescue' cerclage refers to the emergency use of a suture in early preterm labour thought to be due to cervical incompetence, and may be used following the reduction of prolapsed membranes.

Preterm pre-labour rupture of the membranes

This occurs in 2–3% of all pregnancies but in 40–60% of all spontaneous preterm deliveries and is more likely with polyhydramnios, twins, and vaginal infection. If the mother does not establish in labour, the problem is one of balancing the risks of chorioamnionitis (which accounts for approximately 20% of the neonatal deaths) against the risks of prematurity.

The outcome becomes more guarded the earlier membrane rupture occurs, on account of secondary pulmonary hypoplasia and severe skeletal deformities resulting from the absence of amniotic fluid (see Box 40.3). The amniotic fluid normally allows fetal movement and it circulates into the fetal lungs. Pulmonary hypoplasia occurs in 50% of cases with spontaneous membrane rupture before 20 weeks and in 3% after 24 weeks. It remains very difficult to predict which fetuses will be affected.

Investigation

The diagnosis of membrane rupture is established by observing liquor either draining at the introitus or pooled at the posterior fornix on speculum examination. The liquor may be flecked with vernix. Liquor has a higher pH than vaginal secretion and will turn nitrazine

> ## Box 40.3
>
> ### RISKS TO THE INFANT OF PRETERM RUPTURE OF THE MEMBRANES
>
> - Cord prolapse
> - Premature delivery
> - Ascending intrauterine infection
> - Pulmonary hypoplasia and deformities associated with oligohydramnios

sticks black (they are usually orange) but false positives are common, particularly with vaginal discharge, semen, blood, water and urine. An ultrasound scan will often show severe oligohydramnios, and the biophysical profile will therefore be more difficult to interpret.

Chorioamnionitis is potentially extremely serious for both mother and baby as both may develop rapid and overwhelming fatal septicaemia. Infection supervenes after the membranes have ruptured in between 0.5% and 25% of cases depending on criteria employed for diagnosis, and is more likely if vaginal examinations have been performed. Vaginal examinations are therefore contraindicated unless there is strong evidence of labour. It may be considered appropriate to carry out a sterile speculum examination to confirm the diagnosis, exclude cord prolapse and take a high vaginal swab (HVS), but an HVS is not a predictor of subsequent infection and the procedure may actually introduce infection.

The diagnosis of chorioamnionitis is suggested by maternal pyrexia, abdominal pain, uterine tenderness and a raised white cell count. It is also more likely if there has been a proven vaginal or urinary infection. It is therefore important to check the maternal temperature and white cell count, and send urine for microscopy. It should be noted that the white cell count rises after maternal steroid administration (see below), and C-reactive protein measurements are therefore preferred by some as a better predictor of infection.

Management

Most mothers will establish in labour, with around 75% of those at 28 weeks' gestation delivering within 7 days. There is no research evidence that tocolysis is beneficial. For those who do not establish in labour, regular fetal monitoring is essential. It is considered acceptable practice to manage these patients on an outpatient basis following an initial inpatient stay and the patient may take her own temperature at home four times a day. It is also common practice to deliver if beyond 36 or 37 weeks.

As there is such a high risk of delivery, dexamethasone or betamethasone should be given if PPROM occurs at less than 34 weeks (see above). Prophylactic oral erythromycin has been shown to be associated with improved neonatal outcome when compared to placebo. The use of co-amoxiclav in this circumstance has been associated with an increased incidence of necrotizing enterocolitis after delivery.

> ### Key points
>
> - Preterm labour occurs in 6–10% of pregnancies.
> - Predicting preterm labour is difficult, but there are encouraging results from transvaginal cervical assessment and measurement of fibronectin.
> - The choice of tocolytic is difficult. Indomethacin appears to be the most effective, but atosiban has a lower side-effect profile.
> - Antenatal steroids are effective in reducing respiratory distress syndrome in the neonate.

41

Multiple pregnancy

The incidence of twinning ranges from 54/1000 in Nigeria to 4/1000 in Japan. This difference is almost entirely due to variations in the rate of non-identical twins, while the incidence of identical twins remains remarkably constant at around 3/1000. In the UK, the incidence of twins is around 12/1000 pregnancies. Overall the perinatal mortality in twin pregnancies is four or five times higher than for singleton pregnancies, largely because of preterm delivery (40% deliver before 37 weeks compared to 6% of singletons), fetal growth restriction, feto-fetal transfusion sequence (FFTS), malpresentation and a slightly increased incidence of congenital malformations.

The incidence of multiple pregnancy is higher after ovulation induction, whether with clomifene (10%) or gonadotrophins (30%). Around 50–60% of triplet pregnancies, 75% of quadruplet pregnancies and most quintuplet pregnancies are associated with assisted reproductive techniques.

The process of twinning

'Zygosity' refers to whether the twins have come from the same ovum or from different ova – in other words whether they are identical or non-identical. 'Chorionicity' refers to the number of placentae (Fig. 41.1).

Dizygotic twinning (non-identical)

This process occurs when two ova are fertilized and implant separately into the decidua. Each developing fetus will have its own separate placenta and membranes, and both placentae have their own separate circulation. The placental unit is, therefore, dichorionic and diamniotic (Table 41.1).

Monozygotic twinning (identical)

Monozygotic twins are derived from the splitting of a single embryo, and the exact configuration of placentation depends on the age of the embryo when the split occurs. A split that occurs at or before the eight-cell stage (3 days post-fertilization) will result in two separate embryos and implantation sites. The placenta would therefore be diamniotic and dichorionic. Embryo-splitting at the blastocyst stage (4–7 days post-fertilization) will result in a monochorionic, diamniotic placenta with almost inevitable anastomoses devel-

Table 41.1
Chorionicity in monozygous twins

Timing of embryonic separation after fertilization	Number of chorions (placentae)	Number of amniotic sacs	Percentage of monozygous twins
< 4 days	Dichorionic	Diamniotic	30%
4–7 days	Monochorionic	Diamniotic	66%
7–14 days	Monochorionic	Monoamniotic	3%
> 14 days	Conjoined		< 1%

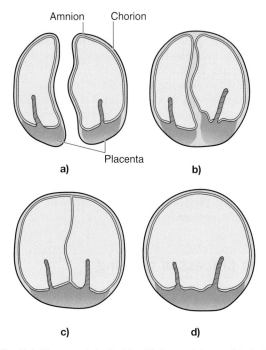

a) b)

c) d)

Fig. 41.1 **Diagram of chorionicity.** All dizygous twins are dichorionic (a,b). Monozygotic pregnancies may form any of the following combinations: **(a)** dichorionic diamniotic; **(b)** dichorionic diamniotic (placentae beside each other); **(c)** monochorionic diamniotic; **(d)** monochorionic monoamniotic.

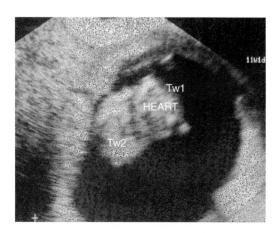

Fig. 41.2 **Conjoined twins.** Diagnosed at 12 weeks' gestation. This is a cross-sectional view through the thoraces of both of the twins. In view of the shared cardiac structures, termination was offered.

oping between the two fetal circulations. This is the more common form of monozygotic twinning. Between 7–14 days, the amnion will be shared. Splitting beyond 14 days following fertilization is extremely rare and may give rise to conjoined twins (Fig. 41.2).

Chorionicity

This refers to the number of placentae. All dizygous pregnancies are dichorionic, and therefore have separate chorions and amnions. The placental tissue may appear to be continuous but there are no significant vascular communications between the fetuses. Most monochorionic placentae have inter-fetal vascular connections.

Chorionicity determination is essential to allow risk stratification (Table 41.2), and has key implications for prenatal diagnosis and antenatal monitoring. It is most easily determined in the first or early second trimester by ultrasound:

- Widely separated first trimester sacs or separate placentae are dichorionic.
- Those with a 'lambda' or twin-peak' sign at the membrane insertion are dichorionic (Figs 41.3, 41.4 and 41.5).
- Those with a dividing membrane thicker than 2 mm are often dichorionic.
- Different sex fetuses are always dichorionic (and dizygous!).

Table 41.2
Fetal loss by chorionicity

	Dichorionic	Monochorionic
Fetal loss before 24 weeks	1.8%	12.2%
Fetal loss after 24 weeks	1.6%	2.8%
Delivery before 32 weeks	5.5%	9.2%

The high early fetal mortality in monochorionic pregnancy before 24 weeks is probably due largely to severe early-onset feto-fetal transfusion sequence (see below).

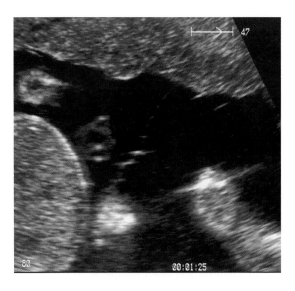

Fig. 41.3 **Monochorionic twins – no lambda sign.**

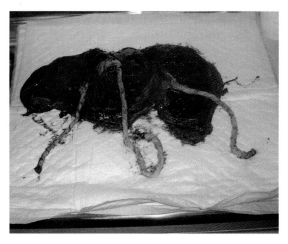

Fig. 41.5 **Trichorionic placenta following delivery at 36 weeks.**

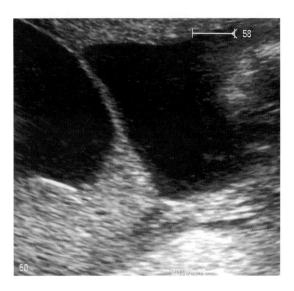

Fig. 41.4 **Dichorionic twins – lambda sign.**

Maternal complications

The incidence of maternal complications is only slightly increased.

Anaemia

There is a slight increase in the incidence of anaemia associated with multiple pregnancy which is not completely explained by a haemodilutional effect of the increased plasma volume. The extra iron and folate requirement may justify routine supplementation.

Antepartum haemorrhage

Placenta praevia seems to be commoner with multiple gestation as a result of a larger placental surface. The management of this condition with multiple pregnancy is similar to that of a singleton pregnancy.

Pre-eclampsia

The incidence of pre-eclampsia in twin pregnancy is three or four times greater than that of singleton pregnancies. It tends to develop earlier and may be more severe.

Fetal abnormality

Fetal abnormality may be considered in terms of structural and chromosomal problems.

Structural defects

The incidence of structural fetal abnormality is no different per fetus in a dichorionic pregnancy compared to a singleton pregnancy, but it is greater with mono-chorionicity. Characteristic abnormalities include hydrocephalus, gastrointestinal atresia and cardiac defects, and it is therefore reasonable to offer all those with multiple pregnancies a detailed mid-trimester ultrasound scan. The abnormalities are usually confined to one twin (i.e. non-concordant); for example if there is a neural tube defect in one twin, the other twin is normal in 85–90% of cases. Selective termination with intracardiac KCl is possible in dichorionic pregnancies only, and is most safely carried out before 16–20 weeks. The procedure, however, carries a small risk of miscarriage of both twins.

Chromosomal abnormalities

These are usually discordant in dizygotic twins and almost always concordant in monozygotic twins. For Down's screening in multiple pregnancies, nuchal translucency measurement is probably more appropriate than serum screening, although the nuchal measurement may be slightly increased in normal monochorionic gestations. Two amniocenteses are required in dichorionic pregnancies, and very great care must be taken to document which sample has come from which amniotic sac. Chorionic villous sampling is not appropriate for twin pregnancies as it is difficult to be sure that both placentae have been sampled, particularly if they are lying close together.

Management of pregnancy

Initial visit

As many as 50% of twin pregnancies diagnosed in the first trimester will proceed only as singleton pregnancies despite the absence of vaginal bleeding, and parents should be made aware of this if the diagnosis is made in the first trimester. It is important to ensure that chorionicity has been established at the first scan, as it becomes increasingly difficult to do so with advancing gestation. It may also be worth considering starting iron and folate at this stage.

The parents are often quite excited, and often shocked, so initial counselling should be brief and focus mostly on the positive aspects.

More details should be discussed at a subsequent visit at least a couple of days later, emphasizing particularly the increased risk of preterm labour and the importance of presenting if suspicious symptoms or signs occur. The parents should consider whether they want antenatal screening and should particularly consider the potential problems of finding one normal and one abnormal twin. Finally it should be explained that more frequent antenatal visits will be required and that ultrasound will be used to monitor growth.

Following the initial visit, follow-up with scans may be arranged at:

- 18 weeks for growth discrepancy, with or without fetal abnormality screening if the patient wishes
- 24 weeks for growth (average weight for twins is 10% lighter than singletons)
- every 2–4 weeks thereafter depending on chorionicity for growth measurements, and more frequently if there is a significant size discordance.

Doppler, cardiotocographic and biophysical profile studies may be arranged if appropriate.

Antenatal problems specific to multiple pregnancies

Feto-fetal transfusion sequence (FFTS) (or twin–twin transfusion syndrome)

This complicates 4–35% of monochorionic multiple pregnancies and accounts for around 15% of perinatal mortality in twins. It does not occur in dichorionic twins.

In this condition there is a net blood flow from one twin to the other through the shared placental vasculature of the monochorionic placentae, probably as the result of a relative deficiency of arteriovenous connections in one direction. The circulation of the recipient becomes hyperdynamic, with the risk of high-output cardiac failure, polyhydramnios and raised amniotic pressure. Conversely, the donor develops oliguria and oligohydramnios and often suffers growth restriction (Fig. 41.6).

The ultrasound finding of amniotic fluid discordancy in the absence of demonstrable fetal abnormality is the key to establishing an antenatal diagnosis. Although FFTS is also often associated with discordant growth measurements, their inherent inaccuracy makes them less useful diagnostic criteria. The features of amniotic fluid discrepancy have largely superseded the previous postnatal criteria of differing weights and haemoglobin levels.

Treatment is often indicated. Most centres advise serial amnioreductions if the amniotic fluid index exceeds a certain limit or if the uterus becomes tense. This involves removing liquor by amniocentesis, often > 1000 ml at a time. Other centres prefer laser division of placental vessels, which, although technically more difficult, may have some advantages.

Twins with one fetal death

First trimester intrauterine death in a twin has not been shown to have adverse consequences for the survivor. This probably also holds true for the early second trimester, but loss in the late second or third trimester commonly precipitates labour such that 90% will have delivered both twins within 3 weeks of the loss. Prognosis for a surviving dichorionic fetus is then influenced primarily by its gestation. When a monochorionic twin dies in utero, however, there are additional risks of death (approximately 20%) or cerebral damage (approximately 25%) in the co-twin. As these are probably related to acute hypotension in the co-twin at the time of the other's death, it is unlikely that early delivery will affect the risk of cerebral injury or death in the survivor.

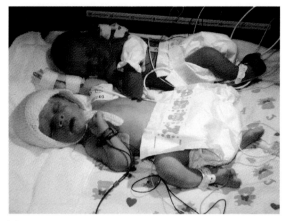

(a)

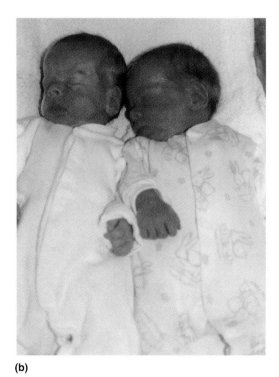

(b)

Fig. 41.6 **Twin–twin transfusion sequence.** These monochorionic twins were born at 37 weeks' gestation. Although their weights were almost identical, there was significant oligohydramnios around the recipient. **(a)** Pre-transfusion. **(b)** Post-transfusion. (with permission)

Twin reversed arterial perfusion sequence (acardia)

If the heart of one monochorionic twin stops, it may continue to be partially perfused through vascular connections from the surviving twin. The condition is very rare and there is a high incidence of mortality in the donor twin due to intrauterine cardiac failure and prematurity. Cord ligation has been used with success in isolated cases.

Management of twin delivery

Presentations at term may be:

- cephalic/cephalic (40%)
- cephalic/breech (40%)
- breech/cephalic (10%)
- other, e.g. transverse (10%).

It is common practice at 38–40 weeks to induce labour in those who are suitable for vaginal delivery, and to carry out a caesarean section at 38 weeks in those who are not. In general with twins, providing the presentation of the first twin is cephalic, evidence would suggest that a trial of labour is appropriate. Significant growth discordance, particularly if twin II is the smaller, may be a reason to consider caesarean section. If the labour is preterm (< 34 weeks), many clinicians would also consider delivery by caesarean section. Triplets and higher-order multiples are probably also best delivered by caesarean section.

An epidural may be very useful in assisting the delivery of a second twin. The first stage of labour is managed as for singleton pregnancies and care should be taken to ensure that both twins are being monitored with cardiotocography (CTG), rather than one twin twice. Although some feel this is best achieved by monitoring twin I with a fetal scalp electrode and twin II abdominally it is probably more useful to scan in early labour, confirm the lie of each twin and note the position of each heart to enable reliable abdominal monitoring of both.

An experienced obstetrician, an anaesthetist, two paediatricians and two midwives should be present for delivery, and a Syntocinon infusion should be ready in case uterine activity falls away after delivery of the first twin. After delivery of the first twin it is often helpful to have someone 'stabilize' the second twin by abdominal palpation while a vaginal examination is performed to assess the station of the presenting part. If a second bag of membranes is present, it should not be broken until the presenting part has descended into the pelvis. If twin II lies transversely after the delivery of twin I, external cephalic or breech version is appropriate. If the lie is still transverse (particularly likely if the back is towards the fundus), the choice is between breech extraction (gentle continuous traction on one or both feet through intact membranes) or caesarean section. Twin delivery carries an increased incidence of postpartum haemorrhage (PPH).

Triplets and higher multiples

In these cases, the perinatal mortality is high, mostly because of the very high risk of premature labour, and it may be appropriate to discuss reducing the number of fetuses to twins at 12–14 weeks' gestation. With quadruplets or higher-order pregnancies, there is likely to be a greater chance of a least one or two survivors if fetal reduction is carried out, despite the miscarriage risk associated with the procedure itself. For triplets, the situation is much less clear. The emotional and ethical problems associated with these decisions are very great.

High-order multiple pregnancies require very intensive antenatal care. Most clinicians would deliver by caesarean section because of problems with mal-presentation and difficulties with intrapartum fetal monitoring.

Key points

- It is essential to establish chorionicity early to help advise about prenatal diagnosis and stratify subsequent care. Prenatal screening should only be undertaken after careful discussion of its implications.

- Monochorionic pregnancies have the additional risks of feto-fetal transfusion sequence, loss of co-twin problems, and twin reversed arterial perfusion sequence.

Fetal haemolytic disease

Introduction

Haemolytic disease is likely to occur when maternal antibodies develop against fetal red blood cells. Red cells not infrequently cross from the fetus to the mother either antenatally or at some intrapartum event and, if they are antigenically different from the mother's red cells, there may be a maternal immune response with antibody production. IgG antibodies may cross in the opposite direction, back to the fetus, leading to haemolysis, anaemia, high-output cardiac failure and fetal death. There are numerous known red cell antigens but the rhesus antigen accounts for more than 95% of haemolytic disease.

Maternal rhesus isoimmunization exemplifies the achievements of systematic scientific and clinical research. In just 40 years it has been possible to unravel the pathophysiology, devise useful treatments and introduce an effective means to prevent a condition which had previously caused extensive fetal morbidity and mortality. Among those with access to an anti-D prophylaxis programme, the fully developed clinical condition of haemolytic disease of the newborn is rare.

The blood group system

Blood groups are determined by antigens on the erythrocyte cell wall. In the ABO system the letter 'O' is used to refer to those who lack both the 'A' and 'B' antigen. If the mother is group 'O' and the fetus has paternally inherited the 'A' or 'B' antigens the mother may, if exposed, develop antibodies to these fetal cells. In practice these antibodies rarely cause significant haemolytic disease and no antenatal investigations are warranted.

The next most important system is the rhesus system which comprises at least 40 antigens, the most important of which are C, D and E. 'C' and 'E' have immunologically distinct isoforms which are designated 'c' and 'e,' but it seems unlikely that a 'd' isoform exists. If there is a 'd' antigen, it seems to have little if any immunogenic potential and the notation 'd' is used to indicate the absence of 'D'. A parent contributes one or other antigen (e.g. C or c) to the offspring from each of these three alphabetically designated pairs. An individual can therefore be homozygous or heterozygous for any of the six (e.g. Cde/cDE, cde/cdE). Those who carry the D antigen, which is inherited as an autosomal dominant, are referred to as rhesus D positive whether in the homozygous or heterozygous form.

Any of the rhesus antigens are capable of stimulating antibody formation but the 'D' antigen is by far the most immunogenic, followed by c and E. If a rhesus negative mother has a rhesus positive baby and is at some stage sensitized to the baby's red cells, there is a chance of anti-D antibodies developing against the fetal cells. These antibodies may cross back to the fetus and lead to fetal haemolytic anaemia.

There are other significant antigens in addition to the ABO and rhesus systems. Many of these (e.g. Ce, Fy^a, Jk^a, C^w) are poorly developed on the red cell surface and usually stimulate only low levels of antibody production, often of the IgM category (which does not cross the placenta). Some, however, will cause significant haemolytic disease. The one notable exception is the anti-Kell antibody which seems to cause marrow aplasia rather than haemolytic disease and is therefore much more complex to manage.

Incidence

This varies widely. Before the availability of anti-D prophylaxis, rhesus haemolytic disease was common in populations where there was a high prevalence of Rh (D) negative individuals and where high parity caused an accumulation of isoimmunized women. In the UK 17% of the population is Rh (D) negative and, assuming random mating without intervention, around two-thirds of Rh (D) negative mothers would be expected to carry a rhesus positive fetus. Approximately 10% of pregnant women are therefore at risk of developing anti-D antibodies.

Since the effective use of prophylactic anti-D, the perinatal mortality from haemolytic disease has fallen from around 46/100 000 to 1.9/100 000. Newly sensitized cases are detected at a rate of approximately 1/1000 maternities.

Aetiology and predisposing factors

Transfer of fetal erythrocytes to the maternal circulation during pregnancy (fetomaternal haemorrhage) may occur without any obvious predisposing event and about 75% of women may be found to have fetal red cells circulating at some stage during the pregnancy or delivery. Fetomaternal haemorrhage is more likely, however, with disruption of the placental bed and this may occur with:

- miscarriage and ectopic pregnancy
- invasive intrauterine procedures, e.g. amniocentesis
- external cephalic version
- abdominal trauma
- antepartum haemorrhage

- labour and delivery, particularly with delivery of the placenta.

An immune response may, but does not inevitably, follow fetomaternal haemorrhage. The response depends in part on the volume of blood, its antigenic potential and on the maternal responsiveness. ABO incompatibility between mother and fetus may paradoxically offer some protection as the transfused cells are likely to be haemolysed by circulating maternal antibodies, reducing the risk of immunization. This observation illustrates the mechanism for the use of prophylactic anti-D immunoglobulin in that exogenous anti-D is used to bind and lyse any rhesus positive fetal red cells that reach the maternal circulation.

Pathophysiology of haemolytic disease

Initial exposure leads to a small antigen-specific antibody response largely of IgM (which does not cross the placenta). On subsequent exposure, for example in a second pregnancy, the already primed B cells produce a much larger response, this time with IgG, which does cross the placenta. In the fetal circulation it forms an antibody–antigen complex on the red cell membrane which provokes phagocytosis of the cell by the reticuloendothelial system and results in a reduction in fetal red cells numbers. This will lead to anaemia unless there is sufficient compensatory haemopoiesis from the marrow, spleen and liver.

Increasing anaemia causes progressive fetal hypoxia and acidosis leading to hepatic and cardiac dysfunction. Generalized oedema of skin develops as well as ascites, a pericardial effusion and pleural effusions. This syndrome is known as immune hydrops fetalis and it may be fatal.

With haemolysis there is also an increased production of bilirubin, most of which passes across the placenta to the mother and is cleared by the maternal system. The fetus therefore does not become jaundiced antenatally but after delivery its own liver is unable to metabolize bilirubin sufficiently quickly and the neonatal bilirubin level rises (Fig. 42.1). If untreated, the bilirubin can rise to levels which endanger the nervous system. Bilirubin deposition in the basal ganglia leads to a condition called 'kernicterus'.

Although most fetal bilirubin is readily cleared, some also passes into the fetal urine and then into the amniotic fluid. The level of amniotic bilirubin is therefore an indicator of the severity of the haemolysis.

Prevention of haemolytic disease
Anti-D prophylaxis

The most effective preventive measure is the use of intramuscular anti-D to provide passive immunization

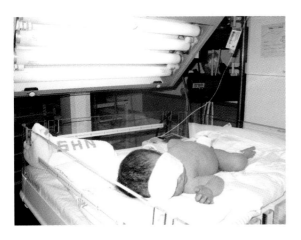

Fig. 42.1 **Baby delivered at 37 weeks because of high anti-D levels.** The bilirubin level rose steeply in the first 24 hours but, with phototherapy, exchange transfusion was avoided.

of unsensitized women around the time of exposure. A Rh (D) negative mother who has a potentially sensitizing event (see Box 42.1) before 20 weeks' gestation should be given 250 IU of anti-D as soon as possible after the event, and certainly within 72 hours if possible. At more than 20 weeks the dose is 500 IU. At de-

livery a sample of fetal cord blood should be rhesus grouped and, if positive, a film made of the mother's blood for Kleihauer testing. The Kleihauer test estimates the volume of fetomaternal transfer and allows an appropriate dose of anti-D to be calculated.

As immunization can occur without a recognized predisposing event, prophylaxis is likely to be more effective if anti-D is given to all rhesus negative mothers routinely in the third trimester (either 500 IU at 28 and 34 weeks, or a single larger dose early in the third trimester). This is already standard practice in some areas.

Surprisingly, there is some evidence of benefit from anti-D prophylaxis even for women already mildly sensitized, in that subsequent children appear less severely affected by haemolytic disease than would otherwise have been expected.

Clinical presentation of haemolytic disease

Clinical symptoms and signs of fetal haemolytic anaemia occur late, are easily missed and are of little help in management. In advanced disease, fetal movements may become feeble or even absent and there may be fetal growth restriction. Polyhydramnios, which is associated with fetal hydrops, may also be detected. In reality, however, detection is based on routine antenatal screening.

Routine maternal screening

All pregnant women at their first visit have serum sent for ABO and Rh (D) grouping with screening for irregular antibodies. The maternal serum level of any antibody discovered (usually anti-D) is used as an initial screening test for further action. There are regional variations, but an example of when to check for antibody levels is shown in Table 42.1.

Fetal assessment

If screening demonstrates the presence of an alloimmune antibody, further assessment is required to determine its significance. This depends in part on the clinical details and on the likely antigen status of the fetus. Additional investigation may be warranted with amniocentesis or fetal blood sampling, either of which may indicate a need for treatment by intrauterine transfusion. An important principle is that invasive investigations carry significant acute fetal risks and also increase the chance of fetomaternal haemorrhage which may exacerbate the alloimmune condition itself.

Box 42.1

INDICATIONS FOR ANTI-D IMMUNOPROPHYLAXIS

First trimester
- Ectopic pregnancy
- Surgical or medical termination of pregnancy
- Miscarriage with heavy loss or requiring surgical evacuation of products

Second trimester
- Amniocentesis
- Chorionic villous sampling
- Threatened miscarriage or antepartum haemorrhage

Third trimester
- Routine prophylaxis
- Antepartum haemorrhage
- External cephalic version
- Delivery

Table 42.1
Possible screening programme for antibodies in haemolytic disease of the newborn

All pregnant women (whether D +ve or D –ve)	ABO + Rh D group and antibody screen Rh D group and antibody screen	At 10–16 weeks At 28–36 weeks
Patients identified with autoantibodies Anti-D, c or Kell related	Antibody screen ± titre	At least monthly to 28 weeks then 2-weekly to term
Other antibodies	Antibody screen ± titre	At 28–36 weeks, thereafter depending on the titre

Clinical significance of the antibody

As noted above, red cell antigens vary in their likelihood of stimulating an immune response, with the D antigen being the most immunogenic. Most of the other antigens are less likely to lead to significant clinical problems and are not discussed further in this section. The D antibody titre in maternal serum can be measured and the level is recognized to correlate well with disease severity. Severe disease is rare if the maternal antibody level is < 4 IU/ml, and additional specific intervention is probably not required. The risk of significant problems is only moderate between 4 and 15 IU/ml but above 15 IU/ml there is a risk of severe anaemia in 50% of fetuses. These higher levels call for invasive investigation and the management of these relatively uncommon cases should be centralized within specialized units. A sudden rise in levels, rather than a particular absolute level, is also likely to be significant.

The next stage is to assess the likely rhesus status of the baby by establishing the genotype of the putative father and remembering that the D antigen is inherited as an autosomal dominant. If the father is found to be d/d it is likely that anti-D antibodies in a rhesus negative woman have developed from exposure to some other source of incompatible red cells, for example a previous blood transfusion or the fetus of a previous partner. Assuming confident paternity, the fetus will be unaffected and further specific action is unnecessary. Where the father is believed to be D/d, half of his offspring will be rhesus positive, and direct testing of fetal blood would be required to establish the risk. If the father is homozygous for the D antigen, it follows that the fetus will also be rhesus D positive and will be at risk of haemolytic disease.

Non-invasive testing

Non-invasive testing largely involves the use of ultrasound, which, as well as measuring growth and liquor volume, can be used to look for evidence of hydrops fetalis. This presents with signs of ascites, a pericardial effusion, pleural effusions, and oedema of the skin. These signs are unfortunately present only in advanced disease, and fetal Doppler blood flow studies, particu-

larly of the middle cerebral artery, are very helpful in identifying problems at an earlier stage. A hyperkinetic circulation implies anaemia and it appears to occur prior to the onset of hydrops itself.

Cardiotocography is also used and may reveal an unreactive pattern or even decelerations, but again only in advanced disease. A sinusoidal fetal heart pattern is thought to be fairly specific for severe anaemia. Between assessments, maternal counting of fetal movements may be of some use as they are usually reduced in severe fetal anaemia.

If ultrasound assessment is normal and the antibody level relatively low, a conservative approach with delivery at term is appropriate. If there are abnormal parameters, or a high antibody level, invasive testing by amniocentesis or fetal blood sampling may be indicated. Both are carried out under continuous ultrasound monitoring.

Invasive testing

Amniocentesis will allow the clinician to establish the fetal rhesus genotype by PCR amplification of the appropriate gene locus on amniocytes. It also allows the spectrophotometric estimation of amniotic fluid bilirubin, which is optimally measured at a wavelength of 450 nm. This can be plotted on one of a number of different charts, most of which are modified from the original data by AW Liley (1961), whose chart is commonly known as the Liley chart. Based upon this and other associated observations a decision can be made between continued monitoring, intrauterine fetal blood transfusion or premature delivery. Amniocentesis has advantages over fetal blood sampling in that there is less immediate risk to the fetus and the chance of fetomaternal haemorrhage is smaller.

Although fetal blood sampling carries more immediate fetal risk it enables an immediate haemoglobin estimation to be made and provides a mechanism by which blood may be infused in utero. Group O rhesus negative blood is crossmatched to the mother's own serum prior to the procedure and, if the haemoglobin (or in some centres the haematocrit) is low, a calculated volume may be infused during the same sampling procedure. Fetal blood sampling carries the risk of cord haematomata, fetal bradycardia, intrauterine death and further sensitization of the mother to fetal red cell antigens. It may need to be repeated on a number of occasions depending on severity.

If an intravascular transfusion is too technically difficult it is possible to inject the red cells directly into the peritoneal cavity from which they are subsequently absorbed by the fetal lymphatic system.

Additional measures

In severe early cases, when hydropic change occurs before fetal transfusion is technically possible, repeated maternal plasma exchange may reduce the levels of maternal antibody. The technique requires special equipment to separate red cells from plasma and is both time-consuming and expensive. Maternal immunosuppression has also been tried in very severe cases.

Delivery

All babies with haemolytic disease should be delivered in a specialist unit with full neonatal intensive care facilities. If premature delivery is anticipated, maternal corticosteroid therapy is warranted. Induction of labour with a view to vaginal delivery may be appropriate in mild cases although it is of note that an anaemic fetus is particularly vulnerable to hypoxic insult. Delivery should ideally be as atraumatic as possible and caesarean section may be preferred for more severely affected cases. Experienced paediatric attendance at delivery is essential and cord blood must be collected for assessment of haemoglobin, platelets, blood grouping, bilirubin and direct Coombs' testing. The neonate may require intensive support with measures to control anaemia, hyperbilirubinaemia and any associated cardiorespiratory problems.

Prognosis

For mildly to moderately affected fetuses in whom intrauterine therapy is unnecessary the outlook, in experienced units, is excellent. Perinatal mortality is increased where there is a past history of stillbirth, and especially if fetal transfusion is necessary. Reported survival rates in these circumstances vary widely from 30–80%.

Long-term sequelae

Early reports suggested serious neurological impairments including cerebral palsy, abnormal development and hearing problems, especially in those children who were transfused in utero. Recent experience is very much more reassuring and suggests there are few, if any, additional risks beyond the well-recognized hazards of prematurity.

Key points

- Isoimmunization occurs when maternal antibodies develop against fetal red blood cells. These antibodies cross to the fetus and may lead to haemolysis, anaemia, high-output cardiac failure and fetal death. There are numerous known red cell antigens but the rhesus D antigen accounts for more than 95% of haemolytic disease.

- Entry of fetal cells to the maternal circulation is particularly likely with disruption of the placental bed, for example with antepartum haemorrhage. Passive immunization with anti-D IgG prevents sensitization in most cases.

- Appropriately regular serological screening of all pregnant women for irregular antibodies is essential to ensure timely detection of isoimmune fetal haemolytic disease.

- Treatment of severe disease is highly specialized and requires referral to appropriately experienced units. Assessment may involve the use of ultrasound, and invasive testing by amniocentesis or fetal blood sampling. Intrauterine fetal transfusion is possible.

43

Labour

Introduction

Human labour is surprisingly hazardous. Evolution ought to favour those mothers who deliver without problems and yet, for those without access to good medical care, the lifetime risk of dying from labour may be 10% or more. Why has natural selection not selected out those who labour poorly, favouring those who labour safely and go on to reproduce again?

Apes are able to give birth with little problem. Their pelvises are relatively large, the fetal head is relatively small and the fetus is born facing anteriorly. When the Australopithecines adopted an upright posture around 4 million years ago, the pelvic shape became narrower in the anteroposterior plane to allow more efficient weight transfer from the trunk to the femurs. As the fetal head was still relatively small, the Australopithecines were also able to deliver without much problem, although the head was this time in the transverse position.

With further evolution 1.5 million years ago to *Homo erectus* and then *Homo sapiens* the volume of the brain increased from around 500 ml to between 1000–2000 ml. This increased the chance of the head being bigger than the pelvis (cephalopelvic disproportion) and to deliver successfully it became necessary for the head to rotate during delivery. The head entered the pelvic brim in the transverse position, as the inlet is widest in the transverse plane, but rotated at the pelvic floor to the anteroposterior plane, which is the widest diameter of the pelvic outlet.

This process requires efficient uterine activity and is aided by 'moulding' of the fetal head. Moulding is possible because the individual skull bones are unfused and can therefore move or even override each other to form the most efficient shape for delivery. The pelvic ligaments, particularly the cartilaginous joint of the symphysis pubis, relax antenatally under the influence of a hormone called relaxin to maximize the pelvic diameters. Successful delivery also requires the fetus to enter the pelvis in the appropriate position. When these criteria are not met, problems may occur and these are discussed further in Chapter 48. The difficulty with human delivery, then, is related to the balance between our need to run (and therefore have a narrow pelvis) and our need to think (and therefore have a big head).

Table 43.1
The difference between a normal primigravid and multigravid labour

Primigravida	Multigravida
Unique psychological experience	
Inefficient uterine action common, therefore labour often longer	Uterine action efficient and genital tract stretches more easily, therefore labour usually shorter
The functional capacity of the pelvis is not known – cephalopelvic disproportion is a possibility	Cephalopelvic disproportion is rare. If it does occur, it is usually secondary to some serious problem
Serious injury to the child relatively more common. The incidence of instrumental delivery is higher	Serious injury to the child rare. Furthermore, the risk of birth injury is less when the baby is born by propulsion rather than traction
Uterus virtually immune to rupture	There is a small risk of uterine rupture, particularly if there is a pre-existing caesarean section scar

Primigravid vs multigravid labour

It is fundamentally important to appreciate that there is an overwhelming difference between the labour of a primigravida (a mother having her first labour) and that of a parous woman who has had a previous vaginal delivery (Table 43.1). A first labour is one of the most profound emotional experiences any individual will experience. A successful well-managed vaginal delivery first time around usually leads to subsequent deliveries being relatively uneventful. Conversely, a poorly managed first labour can add to subsequent obstetric problems, and have emotional ramifications far beyond any obstetrical complications that may have occurred.

The uterus during pregnancy

The uterus is a thick-walled hollow organ normally located entirely, in the non-pregnant state, within the lesser pelvis. The smooth muscle fibres interdigitate to form a single functional muscle which increases markedly during pregnancy mainly by hypertrophy (an increase in size of cells) and to a lesser extent hyperplasia (an increase in the number of smooth muscle cells).

From early pregnancy onwards the uterus contracts intermittently, and the frequency and amplitude of these contractions increase as labour approaches. These 'Braxton Hicks' contractions are irregular, low frequency and high amplitude in character and are only occasionally painful. They normally begin at a pacemaker point close to the junction of the uterus and the fallopian tube and spread from this point downwards. Intensity is maximal at the fundus (where the muscle is thickest), intermediate at the mid-zone and least at the lower segment.

The initiation of labour

The mechanisms controlling the onset of labour are different for different mammals. In some mammals, it is the changing levels of oestrogen and progesterone which regulate the timing of onset. In other animals, for example sheep, there is some evidence that the fetal adrenal secretion of corticosteroids is the responsible trigger. In humans, however, there is no evidence of any sudden hormonal changes prior to the onset of labour and the precise trigger mechanism remains unclear. Any proposed mechanism must therefore be considered to be a hypothesis.

It seems that there is a balance between pro-pregnancy factors and pro-labour factors (Box 43.1), the pro-pregnancy factors promoting pregnancy continuation and the pro-labour factors stimulating the onset of labour. Labour may be triggered when the pro-pregnancy factors become overwhelmed by increasing

Box 43.1

PRO-PREGNANCY FACTORS AND PRO-LABOUR FACTORS

Pro-pregnancy factors
- Progesterone
- Nitric oxide
- Catecholamines
- Relaxin

Pro-labour factors
- Oestrogens
- Oxytocin
- Prostaglandins
- Prostaglandin dehydrogenase
- Inflammatory mediators

levels of the pro-labour factors, although why this should occur at one particular point remains uncertain. There is some limited evidence that the human fetus may play a role in regulating this balance, but the mother also has a role.

Pro-pregnancy factors

Progesterone is derived from the corpus luteum for the first 8 weeks or so of pregnancy and thereafter from the placenta. It has the direct effect of decreasing uterine oxytocin receptor sensitivity and therefore promotes uterine smooth muscle relaxation. That it plays a significant pro-pregnancy role is illustrated by the fact that the progesterone antagonist mifepristone increases myometrial contractility, and has been successfully used to induce labour. Nitric oxide, a highly reactive free radical, is also a possible pro-pregnancy factor. Some studies have observed a fall in uterine nitric oxide synthetase activity as pregnancy advances, but these findings are not confirmed in other studies. Catecholamines act directly on the myometrial cell membrane to alter contractility and beta-sympathomimetics are used as tocolytics to prevent preterm labour. The role for these catecholamines in physiological terms, however, and the role of the hormone relaxin, are unclear.

Pro-labour factors

Oxytocin, a nonapeptide from the posterior pituitary, is a potent stimulator of uterine contractility. Circulating levels, however, do not change as term approaches. Oestrogen levels do increase, and oestrogens increase oxytocin receptor expression within the uterus. This gradual rise may be mediated in part by fetal adrenocorticotrophic hormone (ACTH). Prostaglandin levels also increase prior to the onset of labour. These are synthesized from arachidonic acid by cyclo-oxygenase (COX), and COX-2 enzyme expression in the fetal membranes has been observed to double by the time labour begins. Prostaglandins promote cervical ripening and stimulate uterine contractility both directly and by up-regulation of oxytocin receptors, and there is some evidence that the increased levels may be mediated by maternal corticotrophin-releasing hormone (CRH) secretion.

Hypothesis

The proposed hypothesis for the onset of labour is that the uterus is under strong initial progesterone repression but the rising oestrogen and CRH concentrations activate cell surface receptors and COX-2 activity. The increased myometrial activity is further promoted by an inflammatory reaction in both the myometrium and the cervix, a process which also promotes cervical ripening. The actual timing of onset may therefore be determined by the oestrogen or CRH concentration reaching a sufficient level to overcome the pro-pregnancy suppression, but to what extent this is under maternal or fetal control is unclear.

The mechanism of normal labour

(See also pelvic anatomy, Ch. 7.)

The mechanism of labour involves effacement and then dilatation of the cervix followed by expulsion of the fetus by uterine contraction. The lower part of the uterus is anchored to the pelvis by the transverse cervical (or cardinal) ligaments as well as by the uterosacral ligaments, allowing the shortening uterine muscle to drive the fetus downwards (Box 43.2).

The cervix is composed of a network of collagen fibres embedded in proteoglycans and it needs to soften and efface before delivery can occur. Prostaglandins increase cervical ripening by inhibiting collagen synthesis and stimulating collagenase activity to break down the collagen. This collagenase activity comes in part from fibroblast cells but also from an influx of inflammatory cells, supporting the theory that labour is in part like an inflammatory process. Within the cervix the result is an overall reduction in the firm collagen fibres, leaving it softer and ready to dilate.

The fetus then needs to traverse the pelvis. The widest two points of the fetus are the head in the antero-posterior plane (Fig. 43.1) and the shoulders, laterally from one shoulder tip to the other. As noted above, the

---

Box 43.2

SUMMARY OF THE MECHANISM OF THE LABOUR

- Head at pelvic brim in left or right occipitolateral position
- Neck flexes so that the presenting diameter is suboccipitobregmatic
- Head descends and engages
- Head reaches the pelvic floor and occiput rotates to occipitoanterior
- Head delivers by extension
- Descent continues and shoulders rotate into the anteroposterior diameter of the pelvis
- Head restitutes (comes into line with the shoulders)
- Anterior shoulder delivered by lateral flexion from downward pressure on the baby's head; posterior shoulder delivered by lateral flexion upwards

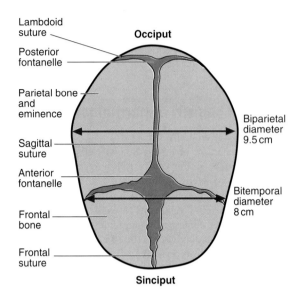

Fig. 43.1 **The fetal skull.** The widest diameter is anteroposterior.

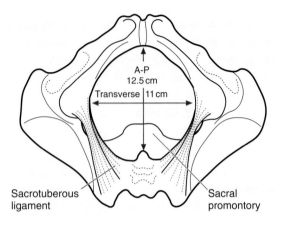

Fig. 43.3 **The maternal pelvic outlet.** The widest diameter is anteroposterior.

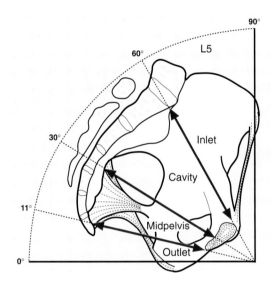

Fig. 43.4 **Lateral view of the pelvis.**

head rotates from a lateral position at the pelvic brim to the anteroposterior position at the outlet (Figs 43.2, 43.3 and 43.4). This rotation has the advantage that by the time the head is delivering through the outlet, the shoulders will be entering the inlet in the transverse position, maximizing the chance of successful delivery.

The position of the head as it traverses the canal is described according to the position of the occiput. The head usually enters the pelvic brim in either the right or the left occipitotransverse position (Fig. 43.5a). The contracting uterus above causes the head to flex, so that the minimum head diameter is presented for delivery.

As the head descends it reaches the V-shaped pelvic floor at the level of the ischial spines (Fig. 43.5b,c,d). It is the fact that this V-shaped pelvic floor has its gutter

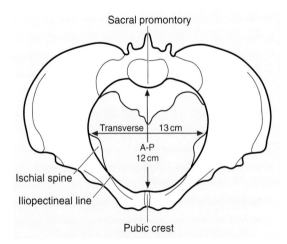

Fig. 43.2 **The maternal pelvic inlet.** The widest diameter is from one side laterally to the other.

running anteroposteriorly that encourages the fundamentally important head rotation. Figure 43.6 illustrates the tendency for the longest part of the head to fit into the lowest part of the V-shaped gutter, achievable only by a 90° rotation to either the occipitoanterior or occipitoposterior position. In most cases the head rotates anteriorly. The consequences of posterior rotation are discussed on page 436. The head, now occipitoanterior, descends beyond the ischial spines and extends, distending the vulva until it is eventually delivered (Fig. 43.5e,f).

Meanwhile back at the pelvic inlet, the shoulders are now presenting in the transverse position. They too descend to the pelvic floor and rotate to the antero-posterior position in the V of the pelvic floor (Fig. 43.5g). By this time the head has been completely delivered and it is free to rotate back to the transverse position along

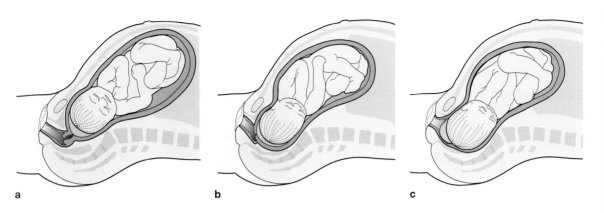

a   b   c

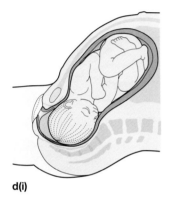

d(i)

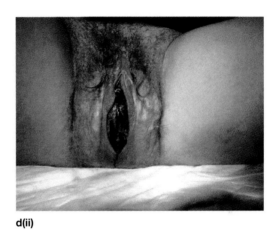

d(ii)

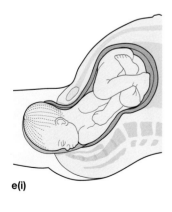

e(i)

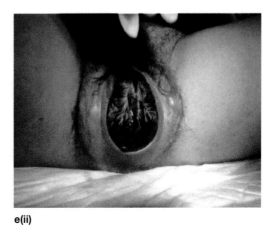

e(ii)

Fig. 43.5 **Normal labour. (a–h(i))** See text for details.

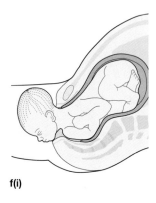

f(i)

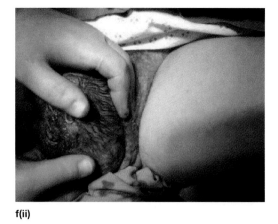

f(ii)

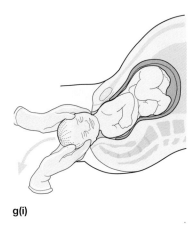

g(i)

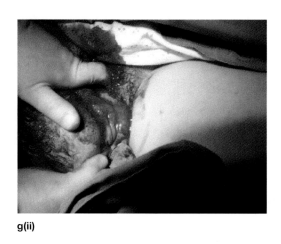

g(ii)

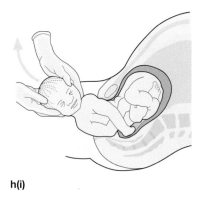

h(i)

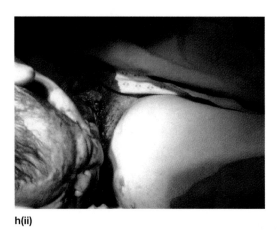

h(ii)

Fig. 43.5 **Normal labour. (d–h(ii))** See text for details.

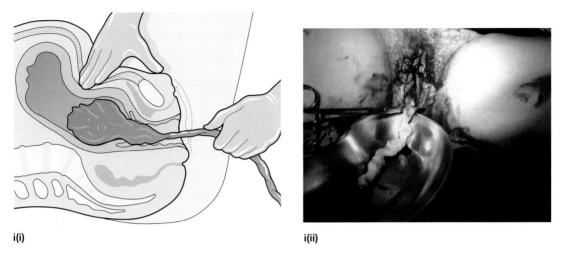

i(i)   i(ii)

Fig. 43.5 **Normal labour. (i(i)–i(ii))** See text for details.

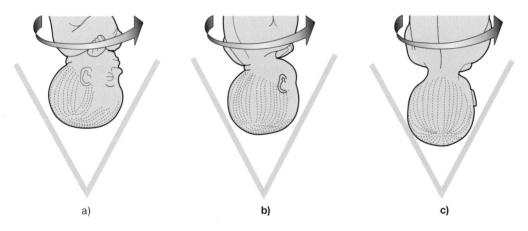

a)   b)   c)

Fig. 43.6 **The head descends onto the pelvic floor.** This runs in a V shape, and it is this V shape which encourages rotation of the fetal head.

with the shoulders. The anterior shoulder can then be delivered by downward traction of the head, so that the lateral traction on the fetal trunk allows the shoulder to be freed (Fig. 43.5g). The posterior shoulder is delivered with upward lateral traction and the rest of the baby usually follows without difficulty (Fig. 43.5h).

The third stage is from delivery of the baby until delivery of the placenta. The uterus contracts, shearing the placenta from the uterine wall, and this separation is often indicated by a small rush of dark blood and a 'lengthening' of cord. The placenta can then be delivered by gentle cord traction (Fig. 43.5i) but caution is required to avoid uterine inversion.

Diagnosis of labour

The diagnosis of 'labour' is pivotal to management. Accurate diagnosis of labour is vital and a wrong diagnosis is likely to lead to wrong management. The diagnosis is easy in retrospect, but of course a prospective diagnosis is required. The presence of palpable contractions does not necessarily mean that a woman is in labour, as Braxton Hicks contractions are common antenatally. There need to be contractions together with effacement and dilatation of the cervix.

Effacement has occurred when the entire length of the cervical canal has been taken up into the lower segment of the uterus, a process which begins at the

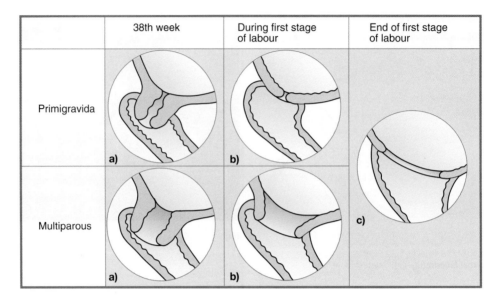

	38th week	During first stage of labour	End of first stage of labour
Primigravida	a)	b)	c)
Multiparous	a)	b)	

Fig. 43.7 **Cervical dilatation – primigravida vs multigravida.** Note that in a multigravida, the cervix may dilate before effacement is complete.

internal os and proceeds downwards to the external os. This is analogous to pulling a polo-necked sweater over your head. It is of note that 'dilatation' refers only to the dilatation of the external os. Again, there is an important difference between primigravid and multigravid labours as dilatation will not begin in a primigravida until effacement has occurred, whereas both may occur simultaneously in a parous woman (Fig. 43.7).

If there are regular contractions and a fully effaced cervix, the woman can be said to be in labour. If, however, there are contractions with an only partially effaced cervix, further objective evidence must be sought in the form of either a 'show' or spontaneous membrane rupture. A 'show', or blood-stained mucous discharge, has occurred in approximately two-thirds of women by the time of presentation and supports the diagnosis *in those with regular contractions*. Spontaneous membrane rupture *in the presence of regular contractions* also confirms the diagnosis.

Pre-labour rupture of the membranes

In around 6–12% of cases the membranes will rupture prior to the onset of uterine contractions or cervical dilatation. The mother will usually describe the feeling of 'water' leaking vaginally and, if a speculum examination is carried out, a pool of liquor can be seen in the posterior fornix. A digital vaginal examination is not indicated as this increases the risk of introducing infec-tion. If managed conservatively 70% of mothers will establish in labour spontaneously by 24 hours and 90% by 48 hours. This conservative management, however, carries a small risk of ascending infection, which may lead to chorioamnionitis. Rarely, chorioamnionitis may progress to a rapid overwhelming fetal and maternal sepsis.

Nonetheless, in view of the high chance of sponta-neous labour over the first 48 hours a conservative approach may be appropriate. This is providing that the mother is apyrexial, the baby is in cephalic presentation, the liquor is clear and the fetal monitoring is normal. On the other hand, there is also evidence that induction of labour on admission may reduce the incidence of neo-natal infection with no increase in the rate of caesarean delivery. Women with pre-labour rupture of membranes should be counselled about their options and they and their partners should be involved in the decision-making process. In those managed conservatively, if there is a clinical suspicion of chorioamnionitis with pyrexia or passage of meconium (see below) delivery must be undertaken at once, ideally by caesarean section unless labour is well established. Pain and discharge are late features of infection.

Clinical progress in labour

Labour is divided into three stages of unequal length (Table 43.2).

There is no 'normal' time for the length of labour. The mean duration of primigravid labours is 10 hours

Table 43.2
The three stages of labour

Stage	Duration	Phases
First stage	From the onset of labour until the cervix is fully dilated, further subdivided into two phases:	(a) Latent – onset of contractions until the cervix is fully effaced (b) Active – cervical dilatation
Second stage	From full cervical dilatation until the head has delivered. It also has two phases:	(a) Propulsive – from full dilatation until head has descended onto the pelvic floor (b) Expulsive – from time the mother has an irresistible desire to bear down and push until the baby is delivered
Third stage	From delivery of the baby until expulsion of the placenta and membranes	

and for second labours is 5.5 hours but the range of normality on either side of these means is wide. Even after a labour of 40 hours the chance of a vaginal delivery is still around 50%. Fetal distress is only partly related to the length of labour. The highest incidence of caesarean section for distress is in the first hour of labour, probably related to babies already compromised antenatally with some pre-existing problem. Even after 24 hours, however, the chance of fetal distress remains low. It is recognized that markedly prolonged labour is associated with subsequent pelvic floor dysfunction and fistulae. There is therefore no 'optimal' length of labour and each mother should be assessed on an individual basis. It seems likely that the rising caesarean section rates in some countries are related more to maternal choice, obstetric preference and concerns about the pelvic floor than to strict medical indications.

First stage

Progress in the first stage is measured in terms of dilatation of the cervix and descent of the fetal head. Information about the labour is plotted on a partogram, which should be commenced when a woman is admitted to the delivery suite in labour (Fig. 43.8). It forms a graphic record of clinical findings and any relevant events. The purpose is to aid continuity of care and help early recognition of abnormal labour.

Vaginal examinations should be performed every 2–4 hours depending on progress and, ideally, successive examinations should be carried out by the same person to minimize the subjective element in interpretation (Table 43.3). The average rate of cervical dilatation in primigravidae is around 1 cm per hour.

Descent of the fetal head is measured in labour by abdominal examination, when the amount of the fetal head palpable above the pelvic brim (in fifths) is documented on the partogram. If only 2/5, 1/5, or 0/5 of the fetal head is palpable abdominally, then the head is engaged (Fig. 43.9).

On vaginal examination, the 'station' of the fetal head with respect to the ischial spines is recorded. Care should be taken not to confuse increasing caput succedaneum with descent of the head itself. By notation the ischial spines are designated station zero. When the head is above the spines, it is said to be at –1, –2, –3,

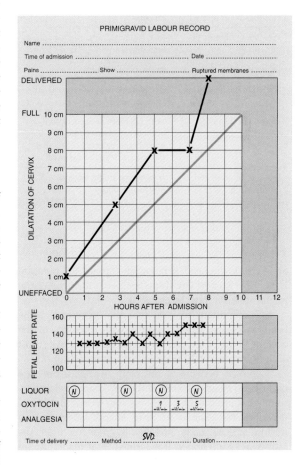

Fig. 43.8 **Partogram suitable for recording a primigravid labour.**

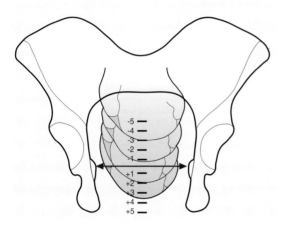

Fig. 43.9 **Descent of the head is described relative to the ischial spines.**

Table 43.3
Vaginal examinations

Findings on examination	Details
Presence or absence of meconium	Meconium staining might suggest fetal distress
Dilatation of the cervix	In cm, from 0–10 cm
Station of the presenting part	In cm above or below the ischial spines
Position of the head	With reference to the occiput if cephalic, or sacrum if breech. A note should be made of whether the head is flexed or deflexed
Presence of caput and/ or moulding	If excessive, might suggest obstructed labour

or −4 cm. If the head is below the spines the notation is +1, +2, +3, or +4 cm. If the head is at the level of the ischial spines it must be engaged.

It is important to note that the 'position' of the head on vaginal examination is with reference to the occiput – for example, occipitoanterior (OA), right occipitotransverse (ROT) or left occipitoposterior (LOT).

'Caput' is oedema of the scalp owing to pressure of the head against the rim of the cervix and is classified somewhat arbitrarily as '+', '++' or '+++'. 'Moulding' describes the change in head shape, which occurs during labour, made possible by movement of the individual scalp bones. It is termed '+' if the bones are closer together, '++' if they are opposed and '+++' if they are overlapping.

Second stage

This begins when the cervix is fully dilated. Progress is measured in terms of descent and rotation of the fetal head on vaginal examination. There are two distinct phases:

1. *The propulsive/passive phase.* This is from full dilatation until the head reaches the pelvic floor. During this time the head is relatively high in the pelvis, the position is occipitotransverse, the lower vagina is not stretched and the mother has no urge to push. In many respects it is a natural extension of the first stage of labour.
2. *The expulsive/active phase.* This begins when the fetal head reaches the pelvic floor and the mother usually has a strong desire to push.

With active pushing, the head usually delivers. Normally it does so in the occipitoanterior position. After delivery it restitutes, returning to an occipitolateral position by rotating with the shoulders as they descend into the pelvis. The birth attendant then applies lateral traction to the head, moving it in the direction of the mother's back to allow the birth of the anterior fetal shoulder (see above). At this point Syntometrine (a combination of 5 units Syntocinon and 0.5 mg ergometrine) is injected intramuscularly into the mother's thigh to encourage a tonic uterine contraction and minimize the chance of postpartum haemorrhage. The head is then lifted anteriorly to allow delivery of the posterior shoulder, after which the rest of the baby is delivered with lateral flexion of the fetal body. The umbilical cord is clamped and cut. If the baby does not require resuscitation, he or she may be placed on the mother's abdomen or wrapped in a warm towel and handed to the parents.

Third stage

The third stage of labour should be actively managed to minimize the risk of postpartum haemorrhage. This involves the use of Syntometrine (as above) and gentle controlled cord traction using the 'Brandt–Andrews' method (Fig. 43.5i). The operator exerts traction on the cord while the other hand maintains pressure upwards on the fundus. Placental separation is recognized by lengthening of the cord and a gush of dark blood per vaginam. The main risk of cord traction is uterine inversion and the fundus is continually 'guarded' to prevent this (see p. 449). Once the placenta passes the vulva it may be gently twisted to allow the membranes to peel off completely and the uterine fundus is rubbed up to ensure that the uterus is well contracted. The labia, vagina and perineum are inspected for tears and sutured if bleeding. Finally, the placenta is examined to ensure it is complete.

The normal blood loss at delivery is about 300 ml. The routine use of Syntometrine following delivery of the anterior shoulder reduces the risk of postpartum haemorrhage (PPH) by about 60%.

Episiotomies and perineal tears

It was previously felt that the use of episiotomy reduced the incidence of anal sphincter tears. There is, however, little good evidence to support this and there is certainly no evidence to support routine episiotomy in all deliveries as a preventive measure against third- or fourth-degree tears. Midline episiotomy in particular does not protect the perineum or sphincters during childbirth and may impair anal continence. If an episiotomy is to be performed at all, a right (or less commonly left) posterolateral episiotomy is preferred (Fig. 43.10).

The rate of episiotomy has wide geographic variations from 8% in The Netherlands, to 20% in England and Wales, 50% in the USA and 99% in some Eastern European countries. It is also high in many developing countries. Defining a 'good' episiotomy rate is therefore difficult. Restricting the use of episiotomy to specific fetal and maternal indications leads to lower rates of posterior perineal trauma, less need for suturing and fewer long-term complications. A tear may be less painful than an episiotomy and may also heal better.

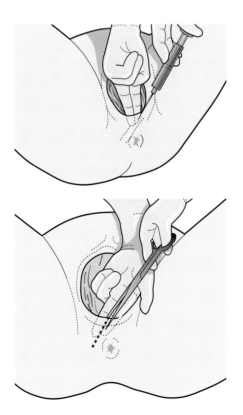

Fig. 43.10 **If required, an episiotomy is usually carried out after infiltration of the perineum with local anaesthetic.**

Table 43.4
Classification of spontaneous perineal tears

	Tear involves
First degree	Injury to the vaginal epithelium and vulval skin only
Second degree	Injury to the perineal muscles, but not the anal sphincter
Third degree	Injury to the perineum involving the anal sphincter complex
Fourth degree	Injury to the perineum involving the anal sphincter complex and rectal mucosa

Possible indications for an episiotomy are as follows:

- a rigid perineum which is preventing delivery
- if it is felt that a large tear is imminent
- most instrumental deliveries (forceps or ventouse)
- shoulder dystocia
- breech delivery.

Prior to an episiotomy, lidocaine (lignocaine) is injected into the subcutaneous tissues of the perineum and vagina. A right mediolateral cut is then made and pressure on the fetal head is maintained so that the delivery is slow and the head remains flexed, minimizing the possibility of the incision extending.

Spontaneous tears are categorized into four degrees (Table 43.4).

Some people prefer to classify perineal tears into only three degrees but the system described in Table 43.4 allows a differentiation between injuries to the anal sphincter and those involving the anal mucosa.

Anterior perineal trauma is classified as any injury to the labia, anterior vagina, urethra or clitoris and is associated with less morbidity than posterior trauma.

Repair of episiotomies and perineal tears

Repair should be with an absorbable synthetic material (Dexon or Vicryl), using a continuous subcuticular (possibly non-locking) technique to minimize short- and long-term problems (Fig. 43.11). These newer materials result in less short-term pain and less analgesic requirements than older materials such as catgut and non-absorbable sutures. Good perineal hygiene after delivery is likely to aid healing, and the use of ice packs and analgesia may be useful to control symptoms.

Repair of episiotomy and first- or second-degree tears

The perineum is infiltrated with 1% lidocaine (lignocaine) (Fig. 43.11a) (unless an epidural is in situ or there has been a pudendal block or perineal infiltration prior

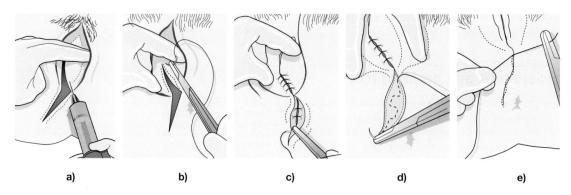

a)   b)   c)   d)   e)

Fig. 43.11 **Repair of a perineal tear or episiotomy. (a–e)** See text for details.

to delivery). The apex of the vaginal incision or tear is identified and the first suture placed above this level (Fig. 43.11b) (care is needed because the rectum is just posterior to the vaginal wall).

A continuous locking suture is used to close the vaginal wall until the hymeneal edges are opposed. The suture can then be tied, or more simply locked, and the needle threaded between the opposed vaginal edges a few centimetres back, ready to close the perineal body (Fig. 43.11c). The perineal body sutures should be interrupted. A continuous finer suture is then used for the skin (Fig. 43.11d,e). It is possible that not closing the skin (i.e. leaving the skin edges approximately 5 mm apart) reduces postnatal pain.

Repair of third- or fourth-degree tears

This should ideally be by an experienced clinician, in theatre, with good analgesia, good light and the appropriate instruments. The anal mucosa should be repaired using interrupted dissolving sutures, with the knot of each suture in the lumen of the bowel. The internal sphincter is then identified and its ends approximated and sutured with a monofilament suture such as polydioxanone (PDS). Next, the ends of the external anal sphincter are identified and either approximated or overlapped, again with the monofilament suture. The rest is as described above for first- and second-degree tears. Antibiotics, laxatives and fibre are important to allow healing. If secondary breakdown occurs, it may be necessary to perform a defunctioning colostomy before re-repairing.

> ### Key points
>
> - Diagnosis of 'labour' is pivotal to management
>
> - Labour is considered in three stages: the first from the onset of labour until the cervix is fully dilated, the second from then until delivery of the baby, and the third from that point until delivery of the placenta.
>
> - Compared to a multigravida, the labour of a primigravida is likely to be longer and more likely to result in both instrumental delivery and neonatal injury. Uterine rupture, though rare in a multigravida, virtually never occurs in a primigravida.

Monitoring of the fetus in labour

Introduction

The purpose of monitoring the fetus is to try to identify those which might be of risk of hypoxic injury so that delivery can then be expedited and potential problems prevented. This process of monitoring usually involves some form of fetal heart rate assessment either with intermittent auscultation or by continuous electronic measurement (cardiotocography). Although electronic monitoring is probably of value in 'high-risk' labours, research has yet to conclusively prove that it is useful in the 'low-risk' situation. There is a high false-positive rate in the 'low-risk' group and many fetuses labelled as 'distressed' are actually not hypoxic. As a consequence the rate of obstetric intervention may be increased in this group in return for no true neonatal benefit.

Fetal physiology

Fetal oxygenation depends on a number of factors.

Maternal blood supply to the placenta

During a contraction, the intramural vessels supplying the placenta are constricted by the smooth muscle fibres of the uterus. Providing the contractions are not too long or too frequent, the placental blood supply has time to recover before the next contraction begins. In hyperstimulation, when the uterus is contracting too frequently, placental oxygenation may be impaired. In other circumstances there may be placental hypoperfusion, for example following the distal sympathetic blockade and associated hypotension which can occur with spinal or epidural anaesthesia.

Functional capacity of the placenta

A small poorly formed placenta is less capable of adequate oxygen transfer than a larger placenta. In this condition, the fetus may already be growth restricted prior to the onset of labour and therefore more susceptible to a hypoxic stress. In abruptio placentae it is obvious that the resulting partial placental separation leaves a reduced surface area for vascular communication, and is therefore less efficient at oxygen exchange.

Fetal blood supply

This is dependent on adequate fetal cardiac output. The fetus responds to hypoxic stress with peripheral vasoconstriction and redistribution of the blood to the heart and the brain. Prolonged vasoconstriction may lead to damage in other organs, particularly the gastrointestinal tract (necrotizing enterocolitis), the lungs (respiratory distress) and kidneys (acute renal failure).

Hypoxia also leads to anaerobic metabolism and acidosis. Acidosis is therefore a reflection of the degree of oxygenation and this forms the basis of intrapartum fetal blood sampling.

Risk assessment

Some form of monitoring is appropriate for all labours, but whether this should be continuous or intermittent is unclear. As noted above, the use of continuous electronic monitoring in 'low-risk' labours may increase the rate of intervention for no demonstrable neonatal benefit. It is therefore important to consider which babies are 'high risk' and which are 'low risk'. Some of these factors are outlined in Box 44.1. It is important to take these background factors into consideration before interpreting a heart rate problem.

Box 44.1

BABIES AT 'HIGH RISK' OF DISTRESS IN LABOUR

Fetal factors

- Fetal growth restriction or any baby whose weight is estimated to be less than the 10th centile

Placental factors

- Hypertension
- Antepartum haemorrhage

Obstetric factors

- Precipitate labour
- Premature labour
- Prolonged labour
- Induced labours or those augmented with Syntocinon
- Mothers with epidurals, a previous caesarean section or significant medical problems
- Those with meconium (fetal stool) stained liquor (see below)

Meconium staining of the liquor

Meconium (fetal stool) staining of the liquor is present in 15% of all deliveries at term and in about 40% at 42 weeks. The mechanism may be stimulation of the vagus (parasympathetic) nerves in utero causing the fetal gut to contract and the anal sphincter to relax. This often happens for no particular reason but it also may occur as a response to fetal distress. While therefore often not of clinical significance, the presence of meconium staining increases the chance that there is underlying fetal compromise. A normal cardiotocograph (CTG) provides reassurance, but an abnormal CTG becomes even more significant in the presence of meconium and should lower the threshold for investigation or intervention.

As well as being a sign of fetal distress, meconium is found below the vocal cords postnatally in about one-third of cases in which it is present and may give rise to the meconium aspiration syndrome. This is a form of neonatal pneumonitis. Clinical features range from mild neonatal tachypnoea to severe respiratory compromise. The incidence is probably unrelated to fetal distress (and indeed the majority of babies with meconium aspiration syndrome are not acidotic at delivery) but the syndrome is more likely to be severe if there is associated acidosis. It is also more severe when the meconium is thick. There is no evidence to support early delivery in the absence of fetal distress as it is likely that the aspiration occurs in utero rather that at delivery itself.

Meconium can be graded as follows:

Grade 1: good volume of liquor stained lightly with meconium
Grade 2: reasonable volume of liquor with heavy suspension of meconium
Grade 3: thick undiluted meconium of 'pea-soup' consistency.

The higher the grade the more likely it is to be associated with metabolic acidosis and the meconium aspiration syndrome. As noted above, it is reasonable to consider continuous electronic fetal heart rate recording if meconium is found to be present. Some would recommend fetal blood sampling if Grade 3 meconium is present.

Fetal heart rate recording

Intermittent monitoring

Assessment of the fetal heart rate can be used to provide some information about fetal well-being. In 'low-risk' labours, providing an admission CTG is normal, it is probably reasonable to auscultate the fetal heart every 15 minutes before and after a contraction during the first stage of labour, and every 5 or 10 minutes between contractions in the second stage of labour. A baseline tachycardia or bradycardia, or the presence of decelerations are indications for further evaluation with continuous CTG monitoring. The heart can be auscultated using either a manual Pinard stethoscope or an electronic Doppler detector.

Continuous monitoring (cardiotocography)

A cardiotocograph (CTG) provides a continuous printed record of the fetal heart rate and uterine contractions. The contractions are registered by a pressure monitor supported on the mother's abdomen by an elastic belt, and the fetal heart rate is measured using either:

- an abdominal ultrasonic transmitter–receiver Doppler probe which detects fetal cardiac movements and hence the heart rate, or
- a clip, known as a fetal scalp electrode (FSE), which is attached to the baby's scalp and detects the R–R wave of the fetal ECG. It is usually used if the external abdominal monitoring is unsatisfactory.

The important features of a cardiotocograph are given in Table 44.1.

Normally the baseline fetal heart rate is between 110 and 150 beats per minute (b.p.m.). This rate represents a balance between the sympathetic and parasympathetic systems. Sustained tachycardia is associated with prematurity, and the rate slows physiologically with advancing gestation. It may also be associated with fetal acidosis (probably as a response to increased sympathetic stimulation), maternal pyrexia, and the use of exogenous beta-sympathomimetics. Baseline bradycardia is associated with severe fetal acidosis (e.g. abruption or uterine rupture) but is more commonly found with hypotension and maternal sedation. Congenital heart block is rare, but can occur especially in association with maternal systemic lupus erythematosus. Cardiac dysrhythmias are also rare but can cause extremes of heart rate, either fast or slow, with tachycardia usually being the more sinister.

Baseline variability is the variation in the fetal heart rate from one beat to the next (the beat-to-beat variation) and is again due to the balance between the parasympathetic and the sympathetic nervous systems. Since the nervous system of the baby develops as pregnancy advances, the beat-to-beat variability is reduced at earlier gestations. Baseline variability is described as normal, reduced or absent, and it gives a relatively good indication of well-being. The normal is 10–25 b.p.m. The commonest reason for loss of baseline variability is the 'sleep' or 'quiet' phase of the fetal behavioural cycle, which may last up to 40 minutes. Loss of variability is also associated with prematurity, acidosis and drugs (e.g. opiates or benzodiazepines). Fetal acidosis is much more likely if there is reduced variability in the presence of late decelerations.

Accelerations of the fetal heart rate with contractions are a sign of a healthy fetus but their absence in advanced labour is not unusual. Antenatally there should be at least two accelerations per 15 minutes, each with an amplitude greater than 15 b.p.m. and lasting for at least 15 seconds.

Decelerations are of at least 15 b.p.m. and last for more than 15 seconds. Early decelerations occur with contractions. If decelerations occur more than 15 seconds after the contraction they are termed 'late'. 'Variable' decelerations vary in both timing and shape.

- Early decelerations reflect increased vagal tone (intracranial pressure rises during a contraction) and are probably physiological.
- Variable decelerations may represent cord compression (particularly in oligohydramnios) or acidosis. A small acceleration at the beginning and end of a deceleration (shouldering) suggests that the fetus is coping well with the stress of the intermittent compressions. Variable decelerations may resolve if the mother's position is changed.
- Late decelerations suggest acidosis. Shallow late decelerations may be particularly ominous.

Table 44.1
Features of a cardiotocograph

Normal heart rate	110–150 b.p.m.	Reassuring
Baseline variability	10–25 b.p.m.	Reassuring
Accelerations		Reassuring
Decelerations	Early (type 1)	These occur at the time of the contraction and are rarely of more than 40 b.p.m. They are probably related to parasympathetic stimulation associated with head compression, and are unlikely to be of clinical significance
	Variable	These are variable in their timing in relation to the timing of the contraction. They are associated with cord compression and may indicate fetal hypoxia
	Late (type 2)	These occur after the contraction, may be of low amplitude and are suggestive of fetal hypoxia

A true sinusoidal trace is rare. This is a smooth undulating sine-wave-like baseline with no variability. It may represent fetal anaemia but can be a feature of fetal physiological behaviour. It should be considered to be serious until proven otherwise.

Fetal blood sampling (FBS)

This is the same as fetal scalp sampling (FSS). As mentioned above, CTGs are used as a screening test to detect babies who may be developing 'distress' as measured by metabolic acidosis. CTGs are highly sensitive (good at detecting *true* positives) but very poorly specific (there are many *false* positives). In other words, when the CTG is normal the baby is very likely to be well, but the majority of abnormal CTGs occur in babies who are not distressed. CTGs used on their own lead to an approximately fourfold increase in caesarean section rates for presumed fetal distress, a figure much reduced if fetal blood sampling is used to identify a normal pH in the false positives.

FBS is a diagnostic test for fetal acidosis. Using an amnioscope, a tiny amount of blood is removed from the scalp (see below) and both pH and base excess are measured. Normal maternal pH is 7.38 but the normal range of fetal pH is broader, extending to as low as 7.20. In the presence of hypoxia the fetus compensates by anaerobic glycolysis. This leads to an accumulation of lactic acid and a fall in the pH. FBS carries a very small risk of fetal scalp haemorrhage and infection.

Indications for fetal blood sampling

1. Persistent late or variable decelerations on CTG
2. Persistent fetal tachycardia
3. Prolonged and persistent early decelerations
4. Significant meconium-stained liquor (Grade 2 or 3) along with any CTG abnormality
5. Prolonged loss of baseline variability.

FBS is contraindicated where there is a risk of infection transmitted from the mother (e.g. HIV, hepatitis B, herpes or group B β-haemolytic streptococci), a fetal bleeding diathesis (e.g. Von Willebrand's disease) and in severe prematurity (e.g. before 32–34 weeks).

Method of fetal blood sampling

The mother is placed in the lithotomy position with 15° lateral tilt (or in the left lateral position if approaching full dilatation). An amnioscope appropriate for the dilatation is inserted and the scalp is dried with a sponge or swab on long sponge-holders. The scalp is then sprayed with ethyl chloride to induce hyperaemia

and the area is covered with a thin layer of paraffin jelly (so that the blood will form a blob and not run). A blade is used to make a small nick in the scalp and the blob is touched with the capillary tube (touching the scalp directly may occlude the tube). If possible, three samples are taken to ensure consistency of results.

Interpretation of results

The scalp blood pH reflects the state of the fetus only at the time of the sample, while the 'base excess' reflects a change over a longer period. The pH is plotted on a logarithmic scale whereas base excess is on a linear scale, e.g. a fetus with a pH of 7.22 and a base excess of –12 mEq/l is more likely to be at risk than one with a similar pH and base excess of –6 mEq/l. The correlation between CTGs and scalp pH is not precise but as a general rule:

- If all four components of the CTG are normal, the risk of a pH < 7.20 is ≈ 2%.
- With one or two components of the CTG abnormal, the risk of a pH < 7.20 is ≈ 20%.
- With two to four components of the CTG abnormal, the risk of a pH < 7.20 is ≈ 50%.

It is common practice to deliver the baby if the pH is < 7.20, although it may be the rate of fall in pH rather than the absolute value which is relevant. See Tables 44.2 and 44.3.

Table 44.2
pH results following fetal blood sampling

pH		
> 7.25	Normal	No action
7.20–7.25	Borderline	Repeat in 30–60 minutes if not delivered
< 7.20	Abnormal	Deliver by forceps, ventouse or caesarean section as appropriate

Table 44.3
Base excess results following fetal blood sampling

Base excess	
< –6 mEq/l	Normal
–6.1 to –7.9 mEq/l	Borderline
> –8 mEq/l	Metabolic acidosis

Clinical examples of fetal monitoring scenarios with corresponding CTGs

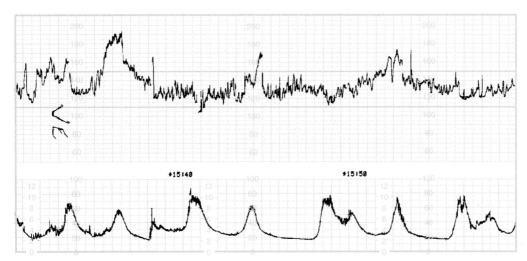

Fig. 44.1 **A 29-year-old para 2, with a history of two previous normal deliveries, was admitted with apparently good contractions.** The cervix was 3 cm dilated and fully effaced, but there was thick meconium staining. The CTG, however, was reassuring with a baseline of 130 b.p.m., good beat-to-beat variability and accelerations. She was given pethidine 100 mg for pain relief.

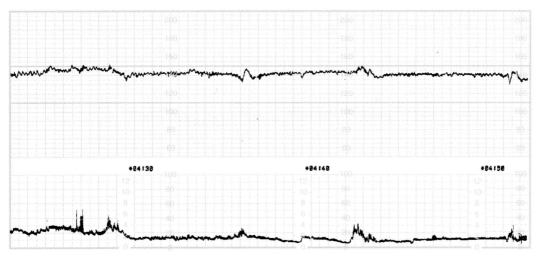

Fig. 44.2 **After a further 2 hours, however, there was loss of baseline variability.** Although there were no decelerations, it was recognized that meconium is a marker for fetal compromise and it was decided to perform fetal blood sampling. The pH was within the normal range at 7.31 and she went on to have a normal delivery 3 hours later.

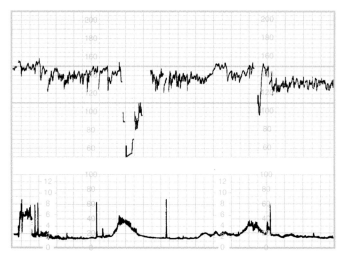

Fig. 44.3 **A 40-year-old primigravida was admitted after spontaneous rupture of membranes.** The liquor was clear and she was having mild contractions once every 8 minutes. The CTG baseline was 130–140 b.p.m. with good reactivity but there were variable decelerations. These are not uncommon after membrane rupture as liquor cushions the baby and cord compression is less likely. Because the rest of the CTG was reassuring, she was allowed to establish in labour spontaneously. The decelerations resolved, but she required a caesarean section for failure to progress beyond 8 cm despite Syntocinon. The baby was in an occipitoposterior position.

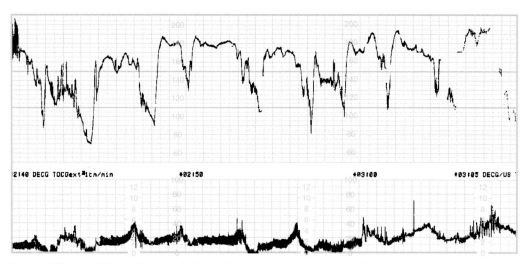

Fig. 44.4 **This is the CTG of a 27-year-old primigravida who was induced at term +12 days as she was 'post-dates'.** After prostaglandin gel was given vaginally the cervix was suitable for membrane rupture and the induction was continued with Syntocinon. This trace is at 6 cm and it shows a baseline around 180 b.p.m. with reduced variability and late decelerations. Fetal blood sampling showed a pH of 7.28, but on repetition 30 minutes later it was 7.19. By this stage the cervix was fully dilated and she had an uneventful ventouse delivery.

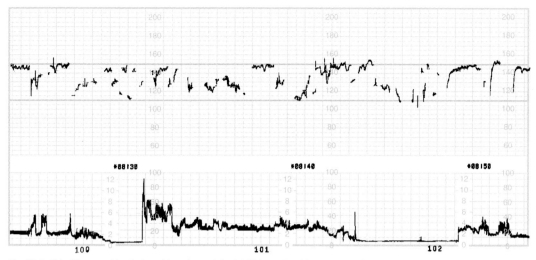

Fig. 44.5 **This 19-year-old primigravida, who weighed 105 kg at booking, was admitted in early labour.** The CTG shows poor pick-up from the abdominal Doppler probe and, after the membranes were ruptured, a scalp clip was applied. The subsequent traces were reassuring and she had a normal delivery.

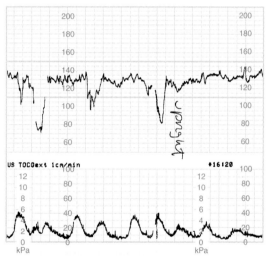

Fig. 44.6 **A 26-year-old primigravida was induced at 33 weeks for worsening pre-eclampsia.** The baby's estimated weight was on the 10th centile but liquor volume, biophysical profile and CTG were all normal. 8 hours after administration of the prostaglandin gel, with the cervix still closed, there were three unprovoked variable decelerations. While the relatively reassuring baseline variability might have warranted more conservative management in a normally grown term fetus the underlying factors were felt sufficient to warrant caesarean section. The baby, weighing 1.6 kg, had Apgar scores of 9 and 10 at 1 and 5 minutes and made uneventful progress.

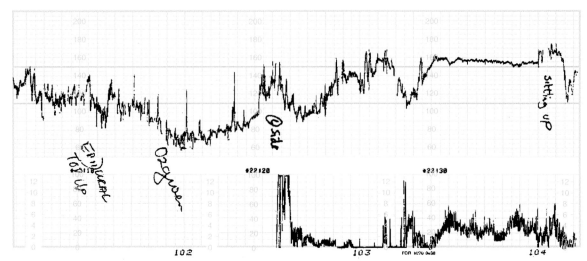

Fig. 44.7 This is the CTG of a 34-year-old primigravida at 4 cm who had just had an epidural sited. After epidural top-up there was a baseline bradycardia, which recovered to a tachycardia and settled again to normal. It is recognized that the peripheral hypotension associated with regional anaesthesia leads to placental hypoperfusion and fetal bradycardia. The bradycardia usually resolves spontaneously.

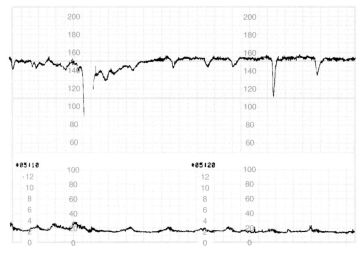

Fig. 44.8 This primigravida was admitted from home at 8 cm dilatation. She had been quite sore at home, but was not expecting to be at such an advanced stage of labour. The CTG had virtually no beat-to-beat variability and there were shallow late decelerations. A fetal blood sample showed a pH of 7.09 and a caesarean section was carried out. The baby had Apgar scores of 3 at 1 minute and 7 at 5 minutes, and weighed only 2.23 kg at 37 weeks' gestation. It made excellent progress.

Long-term prognosis following delivery

There are two questions to be considered under this heading:

- The first is whether a particular infant, born with apparent compromise, will later turn out to be neurologically normal, i.e. prospective prediction.
- The second is whether an infant, later discovered to be affected by cerebral abnormality, sustained its injury prior to the onset of labour or as the result of some intrapartum insult, i.e. retrospective evaluation.

Before considering these two overlapping issues, it should be noted that the term 'birth asphyxia' is best avoided as it is rarely possible to prove that 'asphyxia' occurred and even more difficult to time this to the birth. There is also a trend away from the term 'fetal distress' towards the phrase 'non-reassuring fetal status'.

Prospective prediction

The actual length of time and degree of hypoxia required to produce cerebral palsy in a previously healthy fetus are unknown but there are specific mechanisms which protect the fetus for considerably longer than an adult with similar blood gas concentrations. Nonetheless hypoxia, whether of antenatal or intrapartum origin, can cause cerebral injury, and attempts have been made to correlate status at delivery with long-term neurological outcome. CTG abnormalities, Apgar scores, neonatal behaviour and neonatal brain imaging have all been evaluated.

CTGs and Apgar scores are of very limited value in assessing long-term prognosis. There is a high incidence of non-reassuring CTGs in what are later shown to be normal infants. The same is true for Apgar scores, which are essentially a guide to stages of resuscitation rather than hypoxic injury. Low Apgar scores do not indicate the cause of the baby's poor condition, and are simply a reflection of its immediate status. Prolonged low values, however, are a more useful guide. Of those babies with an Apgar score < 3 at 10 minutes, two-thirds usually die within 1 year and, of the survivors, 80% are normal.

Abnormal neonatal behaviour, referred to as 'neonatal encephalopathy', is considerably more useful. Neonatal encephalopathy is a clinically defined syndrome of disturbed neurological function occurring during the first week after birth characterized by difficulty with initiating and maintaining respiration, depression of tone and reflexes, altered level of consciousness, and seizures. There are three grades:

1. Hyper-alert and jittery with reduced tone and dilated pupils. This usually resolves within 24 hours without problems.
2. Lethargic, with seizures and a weak suck. There is a 15–27% chance of severe sequelae.
3. Flaccid, no suck, no Moro reflex and prolonged seizures. The chance of severe sequelae is nearly 100%.

The prognosis is generally good if the baby does not develop Grade 3 neonatal encephalopathy, or if Grade 2 neonatal encephalopathy lasts less than 5 days.

Radiological assessment is also of value in assessing long-term neurological function. The prognosis is good if a CT or MRI scan appears normal but is less good if there is evidence of cerebral damage. This damage is most obvious in the periventricular area, an area particularly susceptible to insult, and appears radiologically as periventricular leucomalacia. Early cerebral oedema suggests a recent event, as oedema usually appears within 6–12 hours of an insult and clears by 4 days

afterwards. Further clinical evaluation may be available from an electroencephalograph (EEG). The incidence of death or handicap is low if the EEG is normal. Often, however, despite these measures the prognosis can often not be defined with accuracy and only long-term follow-up will reveal the true clinical picture.

Retrospective evaluation

Cerebral palsy, which is characterized by non-progressive abnormal control of movement or posture, is usually not diagnosed until months or years after birth and it is often at this point, retrospectively, that questions are asked about whether the cause lay in some obstetrical difficulty with the delivery. In many instances it is impossible to say whether the cerebral insult was antenatal in origin or whether it truly occurred in labour, but this apparently academic point has two important implications. Firstly, if most cases of cerebral palsy are antenatal in origin then no amount of intrapartum monitoring will affect the eventual outcome. Secondly, there may be major medicolegal ramifications. If a cerebral insult is found to have occurred as the result of negligence during labour, a potentially very large sum of money may need to be paid in compensation.

Epidemiological studies suggest that in about 90% of cases the cerebral injury are antenatal in origin, and that in the remaining 10% the problems may have been the result of either antenatal or intrapartum difficulties. In particular there is a strong association with prematurity, fetal growth restriction, intrauterine infection, fetal coagulation disorders, antepartum haemorrhage, and chromosomal or congenital anomalies. Many are idiopathic. Intrapartum complications appear to play only an infrequent role in the causation of cerebral palsy. Reduced CTG variability, meconium staining, low Apgar scores and neonatal encephalopathy may all reflect pre-existing cerebral injury from some earlier antenatal event.

There are many conflicting views about the criteria required to implicate intrapartum events as the cause of cerebral injury. One set of views is expressed in Box 44.2, but while accepted by many, they are not the universal views of all clinicians.

In summary, therefore, research strongly suggests that the large majority of neurological pathologies causing cerebral palsy occur as a result of multifactorial and mostly unpreventable reasons during either fetal development or the neonatal period. This, however, should not be an excuse for careless intrapartum care and every effort should still be made to identify and act upon identifiable causes of potential cerebral injury.

Box 44.2

CRITERIA TO DEFINE AN ACUTE INTRAPARTUM HYPOXIC EVENT AS THE CAUSE OF LATER CEREBRAL INJURY

- Evidence is required of a metabolic acidosis in an intrapartum fetal blood sample, umbilical arterial cord, or in very early neonatal blood. Metabolic acidaemia at birth is, however, comparatively common (2% of all births), and the vast majority of these infants do not develop cerebral palsy. An appropriate cut-off point that correlates with a risk of neurological deficit may be a pH of less than 7.00 and a base deficit of less than −16 mmol/l.

- There should be early onset of severe or moderate neonatal encephalopathy. It should be noted that over 75% of cases of neonatal encephalopathy have no other clinical signs of intrapartum hypoxia.

- Cerebral palsy should be of the spastic quadriplegic or dyskinetic type. Spastic quadriplegia and, less commonly, dyskinetic cerebral palsy are the only subtypes of cerebral palsy associated with acute hypoxic intrapartum events. Hemiplegic cerebral palsy, spastic diplegia, and ataxia do not have this association.

Key points

- The purpose of monitoring the fetus is to try to identify those which might be of risk of hypoxic injury so that delivery can then be expedited and potential problems prevented. This process of monitoring usually involves some form of fetal heart rate assessment either with intermittent auscultation or by continuous electronic measurement (cardiotocography). Fetal blood sampling is also useful.

- Any interpretation of a CTG has to take account of the full clinical situation rather than just the isolated CTG itself.

- Meconium (fetal stool) staining of the liquor increases the chance that there is underlying fetal compromise. A normal CTG, however, is usually reassuring.

- Cerebral palsy is often the result of antenatal factors rather than intrapartum problems. This, however, should not be an excuse for careless intrapartum care and every effort should still be made to identify and act upon identifiable causes of potential cerebral injury.

45

Induction of labour

Induction of labour is indicated when the risks of continuing the pregnancy are felt to be greater than the risks of ending the pregnancy. Induction is usually carried out in the interest of fetal well-being and less commonly for maternal reasons. The decision is often difficult, particularly at preterm gestations, and many factors, including the availability of neonatal facilities, need to be considered. Labour should not be induced unless there are good medical reasons to do so.

It should be noted that 'induction' is different from 'augmentation'. Induction refers to the process of starting labour and can only be applied to a mother who is not already in labour. Augmentation describes the process of accelerating labour after it has already started.

Fetal indications

- Post-dates – usually > 10 days past the expected due date (p. 317).
- Fetal growth restriction with risk of fetal compromise (based on estimated growth and fetal monitoring, see p. 359). There may be associated pre-eclampsia.
- Certain diabetic pregnancies (p. 327).
- Deteriorating haemolytic disease of the newborn (rare).
- Worsening fetal abnormalities (rare), e.g. cardiac lesions, hydrops or twin–twin transfusion syndrome.

Maternal indications

- Pre-eclampsia. This is a condition in which both maternal and fetal interests are relevant. While it may, for example, be appropriate to induce for mild pre-eclampsia at term, the pre-eclampsia would need to be severe in a markedly preterm infant.
- Deteriorating medical conditions (cardiac or renal disease, severe systemic lupus erythematosus (SLE)).
- In very rare situations in which treatment is required for malignancy.

The decision to induce labour depends on the balance between the risks of ongoing fetal surveillance and the risks of induction and preterm delivery. Induction risks are largely related to the use of 'oxytocics', the preparations that are used to stimulate uterine activity

415

Table 45.1
Oxytocics

	Route	Type of drug	Dose	Use	Side-effects
Syntocinon	i.v. infusion	Synthetic oxytocin – an octapeptide	Infusion up to 12 milliunits/min	To induce or augment labour	Risk of hyperstimulation and rupture
Syntocinon	i.v or i.m. bolus	Synthetic oxytocin – an octapeptide	10 IU	Treat or prevent postpartum haemorrhage	
Ergometrine	i.v. or i.m. bolus	Ergot derivative	500 μg	Treat postpartum haemorrhage	Causes nausea, vomiting and hypertension. Contraindicated in hypertension and cardiac disease
Syntometrine	i.v. or i.m. bolus	Combination	10 IU of Syntocinon + 500 μg of ergometrine = 1 ml	Treat or prevent postpartum haemorrhage	See ergometrine
Carboprost	i.m. or intramyometrial	Prostaglandin	250 μg	Treat or prevent postpartum haemorrhage	Causes GI upset, particularly diarrhoea, and pyrexia. Contraindicated with cardiac, pulmonary, renal or hepatic disease

(Table 45.1). The side-effect of greatest concern is that of uterine hyperstimulation, which carries significant risks of fetal compromise. The process of induction is also associated with increased obstetric intervention, particularly if carried out before 41+ weeks' gestation. Finally, induction may be unsuccessful and the obstetrician may feel compelled to undertake a caesarean section that would not otherwise have been necessary.

Before induction, the gestation should again be confirmed, the presentation checked and any contraindications (e.g. placenta praevia) excluded. It is important to note that caution is required in those who have had a previous caesarean section or previous uterine surgery, as induction carries an increased risk of uterine scar rupture. In addition, grand multiparity or a history of previous precipitate labour also carry increased risks of hyperstimulation.

The decision about which technique is the most appropriate depends on the favourableness of the cervix as assessed by Bishop's scoring system (Table 45.2). This

> **Box 45.1**
>
> *OVERVIEW OF INDUCTION*
>
> - Confirm that the indications for induction are appropriate and that there are no contraindications
> - Cervix unfavourable (Bishop's score ≤ 6) → 'ripen' with a vaginal prostaglandin preparation
> - Cervix favourable (Bishop's score > 6) → artificial rupture of the membranes ± Syntocinon

guides the decision on the most appropriate method of induction (Box 45.1).

- If the score is ≤ 6, the cervix should be 'ripened' with prostaglandins (e.g. gel or pessary).
- If > 6, either prostaglandins or artificial rupture of the membranes ± Syntocinon may be considered (there may be greater patient satisfaction with the former, but the latter may allow more control).

Unfavourable cervix

Prostaglandins

As discussed on page 395, prostaglandins promote cervical ripening and stimulate uterine contractility. They have been administered by the oral, parenteral and vaginal routes as well as directly through the cervix

Table 45.2
Bishop's scoring system for cervical assessment

Score	0	1	2
Cervical dilatation (cm)	< 1	1–2	3–4
Length of cervix (cm)	> 2	1–2	< 1
Station of presenting part (cm)	Spines –3	Spines –2	Spines –1
Consistency	Firm	Medium	Soft
Position	Posterior	Central	Anterior

and infused into the extra-amniotic space. The main side-effect is of gastrointestinal upset with nausea, vomiting and diarrhoea which may occur in up to 50% of instances depending on the route of administration. Vaginal preparations have fewer side-effects than oral or parenteral preparations. Administration directly into the cervix has been associated with higher failure rates than other routes.

Prostaglandin E_2 (PGE$_2$) and misoprostol (a methyl ester of prostaglandin E$_1$) are used in clinical practice. The gel or tablet is inserted into the posterior fornix and, if there is no uterine activity, the cervix is reassessed after 6 hours. If the Bishop's score is < 7 further prostaglandin is given and the cervix reassessed again 6 hours later. Further doses may then be given or the patient left for 12–18 hours (e.g. overnight). If at any stage the Bishop's score is > 6 an artificial rupture of the membranes may be performed, reassessment made in a further 2 hours and Syntocinon started if there is still no change. Prostaglandins should not be given if there is regular uterine activity.

Sustained-release preparations are also available in the form of a polymer-based vaginal insert containing PGE$_2$, with retrieval thread. The preparation is placed in the posterior fornix for 12 hours, after which it is removed. This technique has the advantage that the insert can be removed if hyperstimulation develops, and trials indicate that it is as safe as other topical preparations. It has not, however, been shown to be superior to gel or tablets.

Favourable cervix

If the cervix is favourable, the choice is between:

- prostaglandin
- artificial rupture of the membranes
- artificial rupture of the membranes and Syntocinon.

It remains unclear which of these is the superior induction method, but there is some evidence that maternal satisfaction is greater with prostaglandins. The requirement for analgesia and the rates of postpartum haemorrhage may be lower in this group as well. On the other hand, almost 90% of women suitable for artificial rupture of membrane will enter labour spontaneously following the procedure.

Artificial rupture of the membranes (ARM)

Artificial rupture of the membranes (or 'amniotomy') may be used to induce labour in those with a sufficiently favourable cervix and is also used for augmentation of labour. It probably works by a combination of uterine decompression and local prostaglandin release. Another advantage is that it allows assessment of the colour of the liquor (see Meconium staining of the liquor, p. 406).

ARM has been advocated by some for all labours, spontaneous or induced. This is surrounded by a degree of controversy as it can be argued that there is less cushioning of the fetal head and therefore a greater incidence of fetal heart rate decelerations. Trials suggest that early artificial rupture of the membranes and Syntocinon probably do not confer benefit over conservative management in nulliparous women with mild delays in early spontaneous labour.

Before ARM, vaginal examination is performed. The fetal head should be well applied to the cervix to minimize the risk of cord prolapse. With asepsis, the tips of the index and middle fingers of one hand should be placed through the cervix onto the membranes (Fig. 45.1). The amniotomy hook should be allowed to slide along the groove between these fingers (hook pointing towards the fingers) until the cervix is reached. The point is then turned upwards to break the membrane sac. Liquor is usually seen, but may be absent in oligohydramnios or with a well-engaged head. Cord prolapse should be excluded before removing the fingers and then the fetal heart should be rechecked. Absent liquor following artificial rupture of the membranes should be treated in the same way as meconium staining, with careful monitoring of the fetal condition.

Syntocinon

This may be used for induction after ARM with a favourable cervix, or for augmentation of a slow non-obstructed labour. It should only be started after membrane rupture, and continuous CTG monitoring is

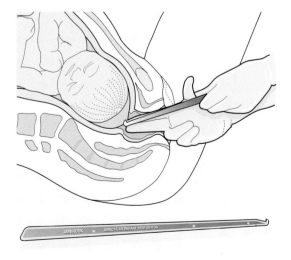

Fig. 45.1 **Artificial rupture of the membranes can be used to induce or augment labour.** (From Greer et al 2003.)

mandatory. The dose should be titrated against the contractions, aiming for not more than 6–7 contractions every 15 minutes.

In induction, the use of Syntocinon immediately after ARM reduces the time to delivery, the rate of postpartum haemorrhage and the need for operative delivery. Nevertheless, without Syntocinon labour will begin within 24 hours of ARM in 88% of cases, so it is unclear whether these advantages outweigh the maternal inconvenience of an intravenous infusion, restricted mobility and continuous fetal monitoring. An individual approach is advised.

Other methods of induction

Membrane sweep

This involves performing a vaginal examination and inserting a finger through the internal cervical os to separate the membranes from the uterine wall, thus releasing endogenous prostaglandins (Fig. 45.2). It is often uncomfortable for the mother. If a sweep is carried out once after 40 weeks' gestation, it doubles the incidence of spontaneous labour over controls, especially in those with a low Bishop's score. The risk of infection is considered to be minimal.

Antiprogesterones

Mifepristone, a progesterone antagonist, has been studied in early pregnancy and has been shown to increase uterine activity and lead to cervical softening. Research into its use as an induction agent later in pregnancy has shown promising results, but it is not yet in clinical use.

Extra-amniotic saline

This involves passing a Foley catheter through the cervix and infusing normal saline into the extra-amniotic space. The infusion volume should be limited to 1500 ml. Success at cervical ripening has been shown to be similar to that of PGE_2 but the process carries a small risk of introducing infection. It is a much cheaper technique than using PGE_2 and this, together with the fact that PGE_2 needs to be refrigerated, may make it a more suitable method for less affluent countries. It has not yet been compared in studies to misoprostol, a much cheaper prostaglandin preparation than PGE_2.

Failed induction

Despite the above techniques, induction of labour is sometimes unsuccessful. The plan then depends on the reason for the induction. If it was for some significant fetal or maternal indication, there is probably little choice but to consider caesarean section. If, on the other hand, the induction was for some epidemiological reason (e.g. for post-dates), then it may be reasonable to consider a more conservative approach. This would depend on an informed discussion with the patient and her partner.

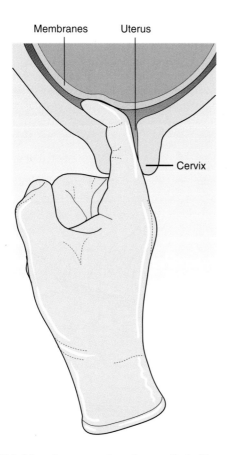

Membranes   Uterus

Cervix

Fig. 45.2 **A 'membrane sweep' may increase the incidence of spontaneous labour.**

Key points

- The risks of induction need to be balanced against the risks of letting the pregnancy continue.
- The use of oxytocics carries the risk of uterine hyperstimulation. Close fetal monitoring is important.
- If the cervix is unfavourable, prostaglandins should be used for ripening. If favourable, artificial rupture of the membranes ± Syntocinon is favoured by most.
- Newer methods of induction are being evaluated.

46

Pain relief in labour

Introduction

Labour can be an intensely painful experience and descriptions of analgesic methods date back thousands of years. Many different forms of analgesia are available. Although all mothers do not necessarily wish to strive for a completely painless delivery, most women want to be comfortable, in control and actively participating in the birth of their babies.

Factors influencing pain

Maternal perceptions of labour pain vary widely depending on obstetric factors, the environment and the mother's psychological perception of the situation. Parity has a significant effect, with higher verbal pain scores for primigravid labours (Table 46.1).

Long labours are perceived as being more painful, and fatigue will lower the pain threshold further. Labour is also reported to be more painful with fetal malposition, and a woman whose baby is in an occipito-posterior position in particular may experience continuous backache. Psychological support is extremely valuable, and the continuous presence of a supportive companion (who need not necessarily be a qualified practitioner, or the woman's partner) has been shown to significantly reduce the analgesic requirements.

Methods of pain relief

Various methods of pain relief are available and are summarized in Box 46.1.

Table 46.1
The labour of a primigravid woman is, in general, more painful than that of a multigravida

Pain	Primigravidae (% of women asked)	Multigravidae (% of women asked)
Mild	9	24
Moderate	30	30
Severe	38	35
Extremely severe	23	11

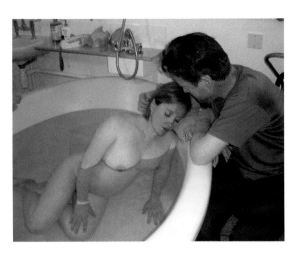

Fig. 46.1 **A birthing pool.** The environment for labour and delivery is important in reducing the need for pharmacological intervention. (With permission)

Non-pharmacological methods

Psychoprophylaxis

A woman who enters labour calmly, and who views the birth of her child as a happy event, is likely to require less pharmacological intervention. This may be enhanced by a positive attitude from any birth partner she may have as well as from the midwives, doctors or medical students involved in the labour.

Maternal education usually includes antenatal classes to prepare for childbirth. Antenatal relaxation training may engender calm, thus conserving energy, but false expectations may result in disappointment. Techniques taught at antenatal classes include:

- Breathing exercises. These do not reduce pain, but allow a feeling of greater control.
- Distraction techniques. Music, aromatherapy, reciting poetry, back rubbing, ambulation and warm baths may all have a role to play.

Environment in labour

The physical environment for labour and delivery is also important in reducing the need for pharmacological intervention. Birthing rooms with subdued lighting and options for alternative positions such as a squatting, all fours, or a birthing chair may reduce the need for pharmacological pain relief. The use of birthing pools for labour or delivery has grown in popularity (Fig. 46.1).

Transcutaneous electrical nerve stimulation (TENS)

This involves high-frequency low-intensity stimulation of the dorsal columns in the spinal cord by passing an electrical current through the intact skin. Two electrodes are placed over the dermatomes of T11–L1 and two over S2–S4. The mother can then control the frequency and intensity of a battery-operated electrical generator with oscillating currents varying from 0–40 mA at 40–150 Hz. It is believed that low-intensity signals cause the release of endorphins and high-frequency signals close the spinal neuronal gate, thus blocking painful stimuli. TENS is most useful in early labour.

Complementary medicine

Complementary medicine is the treatment and prevention of disease by techniques regarded by western medicine as scientifically unproven or unorthodox. While sceptics argue that any apparent benefits are simply the effect of placebo, others believe that many therapies have important roles, and some encouraging research is beginning to emerge. A few of these complementary techniques are outlined below.

Homeopathy dates from the early 19th century and is a system of medicine whose fundamental principle is the law of similars, in that 'like' is cured by 'like'. When a drug was found to produce the same symptoms as did a certain disease, it was then used in much smaller doses to treat that disease. It had been observed, for example, that quinine given to a healthy person caused similar symptoms to malaria, and quinine therefore became a malaria treatment. The principle of homeopathy is that the smaller the dose, the greater the effect, and most potencies are administered in such minute doses as to contain fewer than a small number of molecules, if any at all.

Acupuncture is a technique of traditional Chinese medicine dating back 5000 years in which a number of very fine metal needles are inserted into the skin at specifically designated points. These points are not distributed at random but follow a prescribed pattern, and the lines that link these points to each organ system are referred to as meridians. Research has suggested that acupuncture may work by stimulating or repressing the autonomic nervous system, and may affect endorphin release. It has been used extensively antenatally with some success, as well as for induction of labour and for pain relief in labour itself.

Herbal medicine, the use of natural plant substances to treat disease, has existed since prehistoric times and is the primary form of medicine for around 80% of the world's population. Over 80 000 species of plants are regarded as having useful properties. Use in obstetrics, including labour, is widespread but there is little supportive research to suggest benefit or otherwise. Caution is always required in administering any preparation in pregnancy that may carry the potential for adverse fetal affects.

Other techniques include hypnosis, massage treatments and various 'New Age therapies' such as guided imagery and naturopathy.

Injectable drugs

Systemic opioid analgesia

The basis of pharmacological pain relief is systemic opioids with or without sedatives or anti-emetics. Pethidine 50–150 mg i.m. is favoured by many and, although it does not reduce the pain score in labour, many women feel that they find the pain more bearable. Some women, however, seem to feel disorientated and experience loss of control. Diamorphine 5–10 mg i.m. is also popular in a few centres.

Pethidine and diamorphine can also be administered i.v. to give a more rapid onset of effect, but at the expense of more side-effects (Box 46.2). It is good practice to prescribe an anti-emetic at the same time. Patient-controlled analgesia with pethidine or morphine is used for very painful labours if regional analgesia is not available or is contraindicated (for example because of coagulation problems). Babies may require to be given naloxone immediately postnatally (see below).

Supportive drugs

Anti-emetics, such as prochlorperazine, may be useful to counteract the nausea associated with the opioids. Sedatives, such as one of the benzodiazepines, have only a limited role but may be useful if a mother is extremely anxious in early labour.

Naloxone (*Narcan*) is a pure opioid antagonist which is used to treat respiratory depression caused by opioid use. Neonatal respiratory depression is unpredictable and naloxone is administered only if clinically indicated.

Box 46.2

SIDE-EFFECTS OF SYSTEMIC OPIOIDS IN LABOUR

Maternal
- Nausea and/or vomiting
- Gastric stasis
- Hypotension
- Respiratory depression
- Inadequate analgesia

Fetal
- Decrease of beat-to-beat variability on cardiotocograph

Neonatal
- Decreased Apgar score
- Respiratory depression
- Decreased neurobehavioural score

Inhalation analgesia

Nitrous oxide is an analgesic if given in subanaesthetic doses and, as it is relatively insoluble in blood, it achieves an analgesic concentration in the brain after only five or six breaths. It is mixed with oxygen in a 50 : 50 ratio as 'Entonox' and can be either stored in a cylinder (blue with white shoulders), or piped directly to the delivery room. The mother is able to self-administer under supervision through a face-mask or via a mouthpiece as required.

As it takes 45 seconds or so to attain maximal analgesic effect, inhalation should begin as soon as the contraction begins so that the concentration will be analgesic at the contraction's peak. It should be stopped as the pain of the contraction begins to cease and its effects should have worn off by the end of the contraction.

Pudendal analgesia

The pudendal nerve, derived from the second, third and fourth sacral nerve roots, supplies the vulva and perineum. It crosses the sacrospinous ligament behind the ischial spine along with the pudendal artery (p. 74), and local infiltration at this point may provide useful perineal analgesia for a low outlet forceps or ventouse delivery. A pudendal needle is inserted through the sacrospinous ligament and, after aspirating to ensure that the injection is not intravascular, a local anaesthetic is injected behind the ligament on that side (Fig. 46.2).

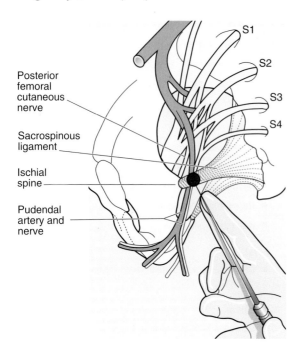

Posterior
femoral
cutaneous
nerve

Sacrospinous
ligament

Ischial
spine

Pudendal
artery and
nerve

S1
S2
S3
S4

Fig. 46.2 **The pudendal nerve runs behind the sacrospinous ligament.**

The injection is repeated on the other side and it is usual to infiltrate the perineum directly at the same time.

Regional analgesia

It is likely that the increased use of regional blockade in the UK, and therefore reduction in use of general anaesthesia, has contributed to the marked reduction in anaesthetic-related maternal deaths over the past 20 years.

Lumbar epidural analgesia

This method of pain relief has become increasingly popular over the last 25 years and many obstetric units now have an 'on-request' epidural service. Because of the potential risks of this method, however, it should be provided in units with trained resident anaesthetic staff.

Lumbar epidural analgesia provides superior pain relief in labour with no concomitant sedation. The block can be extended to provide anaesthesia for operative delivery by forceps or caesarean section, although spinal analgesia may be preferable in some instances (see below). Regional anaesthesia for caesarean section avoids the risks of general anaesthesia, particularly the aspiration of gastric contents (Mendelson's syndrome). The most important disadvantage of epidural analgesia is that the woman is immobilized during labour, although work is under way with 'walking epidurals'.

The main indication for epidural analgesia is that a woman requests it and the request is felt to be appropriate. This may particularly be the case with a long slow labour. An epidural is also useful in multiple pregnancy to allow easier manipulation of the second twin if necessary. As regional anaesthesia leads to distal vasodilatation following concomitant sympathetic blockade, it is contraindicated with hypovolaemia secondary to haemorrhage as the blood pressure may fall precipitously. This hypotensive effect may be therapeutically useful to control severe hypertension in pre-eclampsia providing that a clotting screen is normal prior to insertion.

An intravenous infusion is set up and the mother given a 'preload' of 500–1000 ml of crystalloid fluid. The epidural catheter is then sited and a 'test-dose' of a short-acting anaesthetic (usually lidocaine (lignocaine)) is given. Profound hypotension following the test dose suggests inadvertent subarachnoid placement, and circumoral tingling or a metallic taste in the mouth suggests inadvertent intravenous placement. Providing all is well, repeated doses or a continuous infusion of a longer-acting anaesthetic agent (usually bupivacaine) can be given to maintain anaesthesia, while monitoring the mother for hypotension and the baby for signs of distress. The level of block can be checked by pin-prick or cold stimulus, e.g. with ethyl chloride spray, aiming for diminution of sensation to T10 (i.e. the umbilicus).

Excessive hypotension following peripheral vasodilatation can be treated with intravenous ephedrine as well as with a bolus of intravenous crystalloid or colloid. There may possibly be a higher incidence of forceps delivery with epidural anaesthesia, perhaps because fetal head rotation is less likely with a relaxed pelvic floor. The analgesic effects may also reduce the mother's urge to push. Inadvertent dural puncture may lead to a CSF leak and 'spinal' headache in the immediate puerperium. Postnatal urinary retention is not common but extradural haematomata and abscesses are very rare.

These complications indicate the importance of obtaining informed consent before epidural insertion. Nevertheless, it is very important to compare side-effects of epidural analgesia with side-effects of conventional analgesia, and to balance their advantages and disadvantages.

Spinal analgesia

A single injection of local anaesthetic into the subarachnoid space provides a dense block for 2–4 hours which is particularly useful for caesarean section or some instrumental deliveries (Fig. 46.3). The contraindications for spinal analgesia are as for epidural analgesia, and ways in which spinal and epidural analgesia differ are listed in Table 46.2.

General anaesthesia

There has been a trend over the past 20 years away from the use of general anaesthesia for caesarean

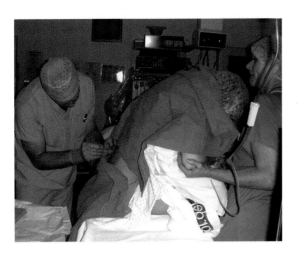

Fig. 46.3 **Spinal anaesthesia provides a dense block which is particularly useful for caesarean section and some instrumental deliveries.**

Table 46.2
Differences between epidural and spinal analgesia

Epidural	Spinal
Extradural catheter placement	Subarachnoid injection
Cannula allows top-up for prolonged use	One-off injection lasting 2–4 hours
Analgesic effect may be patchy	Dense and relatively reliable anaesthetic blockade

sections and towards the regional techniques discussed above. General anaesthesia in pregnancy carries greater risks than in non-pregnant patients, mainly because of the increased chance of aspirating gastric contents which can cause a potentially serious pneumonitis. Progesterone, acting as a smooth muscle relaxant, reduces lower oesophageal sphincter tone and makes reflux more likely to occur, an effect exacerbated by increased abdominal pressure from the enlarged uterus. In addition, as the gastric contents are more acidic in pregnancy, any aspiration is more likely to lead to pneumonitis.

The main indications for general anaesthesia are:

- a need to deliver the baby with immediate urgency on account of acute distress, for example with a cord prolapse or sudden abruption
- in the presence of a maternal coagulopathy, where regional techniques carry the risk of an extradural haematoma
- where there is severe haemorrhage, as regional blockade may exacerbate systemic hypotension.

Pre-oxygenation is important, if time allows, as is aspiration prophylaxis with an antacid (e.g. sodium citrate) or an H_2 antagonist. Cricoid pressure should be applied during induction and there should be a clear 'failed intubation drill'. Thiopental is commonly used as the induction agent along with a neuromuscular blocking agent (e.g. suxamethonium) to facilitate intubation. There is minimal fetal exposure to either of the agents. Ketamine is a safer agent in terms of airway management and its sympathomimetic action may be useful in major haemorrhage, but recovery may be complicated by hallucinations and other psychotic sequelae. It is often used in less-affluent settings in which there are fewer facilities for secure airway management.

Future developments in analgesia for labour

It is important to encourage women to attend antenatal classes and to ensure optimal continuous midwifery support during labour. Anaesthetists, obstetricians and midwives should take cognisance of the non-pharmacological methods of pain relief.

The management of epidural analgesia may be refined to achieve 'comfort' rather than a completely 'pain-free' labour. It may become possible to provide the same benefits with small mixed doses of agents which are complementary and additive, for example local anaesthetics, opioids and alpha-adrenergic agents like clonidine. This has the potential to maximize benefits and minimize side-effects.

Continuous subarachnoid analgesia with small doses of hyperbaric bupivacaine, with or without an opioid, administered via a microcatheter may also prove to combine the benefits of the spinal and epidural techniques.

Key points

- Different women have different pain thresholds and different labours produce different pain. A mother should ideally be aware of her choice of analgesic methods.

- Non-pharmacological methods of pain relief include breathing exercises, distraction techniques, alternative positions, transcutaneous nerve stimulation and complementary therapies.

- Inhalational analgesia with Entonox is very safe.

- The main pharmacological method of pain relief is systemic opioid analgesia.

- Lumbar epidural analgesia and spinal anaesthesia have important and differing indications.

47

Precipitate labour and slow labour

Introduction

Abnormal uterine activity has no clear definition, partly because the range of normal uterine activity itself has no clear definition. It is reasonable to refer to uterine 'overactivity' as that which results in labour progressing too quickly, and 'inadequate' uterine activity as that which is insufficient to provide adequate progress, but the rate of progress has no precise definition either. In practice, overactivity presents as rapid painful contractions often associated with fetal distress, and inadequate uterine activity as absent or slow cervical dilatation.

Precipitate labour results from uterine overactivity. Slow labour may result from inadequate uterine activity, cephalopelvic disproportion, or a combination of the two.

Cephalopelvic disproportion refers to how well the fetal head fits through the pelvis and may occur if the fetal head is too big or the pelvis too small. It is subdivided into 'true' cephalopelvic disproportion if the head is in the correct position and 'relative' cephalopelvic disproportion if the obstruction is caused by the head presenting in some less favourable position.

Precipitate labour

Spontaneous hypercontractility is rare, perhaps occurring in only 1 : 3000 pregnancies. The contractions may be excessively long or be excessively frequent and there is a risk of fetal hypoxia due to interference with the placental blood supply.

Uterine hyperstimulation occurs much more commonly, however, and by definition is caused by the use of oxytocics. Both Syntocinon and prostaglandins may be implicated. The choice of dosage regimens for each represents a compromise between efficacy and the risk of hyperstimulation. The appropriate dose of Syntocinon remains controversial, but there is good evidence for starting at a low dose, around 0.5–1 mU/min, and increasing over 4 or 5 hours to 12 mU/min. Some clinicians support the use of regimens up to 40 mU/min.

With prostaglandins, hyperstimulation is also a significant risk but is less likely if their administration is intravaginal, rather than oral, intracervical or directly extra-amniotic.

Precipitate labour resulting from either spontaneous hypercontractility or uterine hyperstimulation may lead

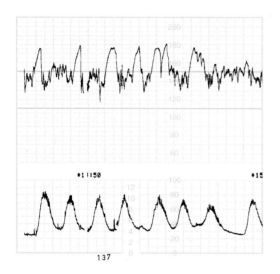

Fig. 47.1 **Cardiotocograph trace in precipitate labour.** There is hyperstimulation secondary to Syntocinon administration with 5 contractions occurring every 10 minutes. Despite this, there are reassuring fetal accelerations.

to fetal distress. Placental blood supply is via intramyometrial blood vessels which are constricted during the contraction, and excessively long or frequent contractions reduce the chance of recovery in the short times when blood flow is returned (Fig. 47.1). Precipitate labour may also predispose to uterine rupture in parous women, particularly if there is a pre-existing caesarean section scar.

Management of precipitate labour is largely dependent on the fetal condition. If a Syntocinon infusion is running it should be stopped and the mother given a tocolytic, e.g. a bolus of subcutaneous terbutaline or intravenous ritodrine. If severe fetal distress is apparent it may be necessary to delivery the baby either instrumentally or by caesarean section depending on the dilatation of the cervix. If a caesarean section is arranged it is worth carrying out a vaginal examination prior to starting the operation as the cervix may dilate rapidly during the time taken in the transfer to theatre.

It is important to note that frequent uterine contractions are also a feature of placental abruption. Contractions with a frequency of more than one every 2 minutes are highly suggestive of this problem and these frequent contractions may increase the distress of a fetus already compromised by partial placental separation. The diagnosis of placental abruption is even more likely if there is associated lower abdominal pain, backache or vaginal bleeding. Tocolytics are contraindicated as uterine relaxation may exacerbate the bleeding and precipitate further placental separation.

Slow labour

As discussed on page 401, it is important to monitor labour with a partogram in order to identify abnormalities in the progress of labour at the earliest stage. Early correction of abnormal labour reduces its duration and makes it more likely that the mother will achieve a vaginal delivery.

Slow labour is associated with:

- eventual fetal 'distress' and risk of fetal hypoxic injury
- an increased risk of intrauterine infection leading to fetal and maternal morbidity
- maternal anxiety and longer-term 'psychological' scarring
- loss of confidence in those providing maternity care.

These in turn are associated with a greater chance of the mother being delivered by caesarean section or requiring an instrumental delivery. The causes of slow labour are summarized in Table 47.1 and the outcome in Table 47.2.

Table 47.1
Clinical classification of slow labour

Clinical features	Caused by
Prolonged latent phase	Idiopathic
Prolonged active phase and secondary arrest	Inadequate uterine activity: • Hypoactive • Incoordinate
	Obstruction (cephalopelvic disproportion): • True cephalopelvic disproportion (head too big or pelvis too small) • Relative cephalopelvic disproportion (malposition of the head increases the diameter of the presenting part)

Table 47.2
Outcome of delivery based on pattern of labour

	% of cases	Spontaneous vertex delivery %	Instrumental delivery %	Caesarean section %
Normal pattern	65–70	80	18	2
Prolonged latent phase	2–5	75	10	15
Prolonged active phase	20–30	55	30	15
Secondary arrest	5–10	40	35	25

Prolonged latent phase

Chapter 43 describes how the first stage of labour is divided into two parts, the latent phase (from the onset of contractions until the cervix is fully effaced) and the active phase (when the cervix begins to dilate). The latent phase is most likely to be prolonged in those whose cervix is unfavourable, and prolonged latent phase is therefore much more common in primigravidae (Fig. 47.2).

There is rarely any serious cause for a prolonged latent stage. Cephalopelvic disproportion usually presents at more advanced stages of cervical dilatation. Only very rarely are the symptoms mimicked by dehiscence of a previous caesarean section scar. With a prolonged latent stage, the mother often becomes weary and exhausted from what can sometimes be discomfort over a number of days. Within reason, it is important to resist the temptation to actively intervene by artificially rupturing the membranes, at least until the cervix is 2 or 3 cm dilated and fully effaced with a well-applied presenting part. Administration of oxytocics may prolong the delay and therefore increase the risk of further obstetric intervention in what might, with patience,

have been an uneventful labour. Reassurance, encouragement and appropriate analgesia over this time are extremely important.

Prolonged active phase and secondary arrest

The active phase may be prolonged because of inadequate uterine activity or cephalopelvic disproportion (Fig. 47.3).

Inadequate uterine activity

The uterus may be hypoactive or incoordinate. A hypoactive uterus is one with low resting tone and only weakly propagated contractions. There is often a longer interval between contractions and the contractions are not particularly painful.

Incoordinate uterine activity may occur because of inadequate 'fundal dominance'. As noted on page 394, normal uterine contraction begins at a pacemaker point close to the junction of the uterus and the fallopian tube. It spreads from this point downwards with its maximal

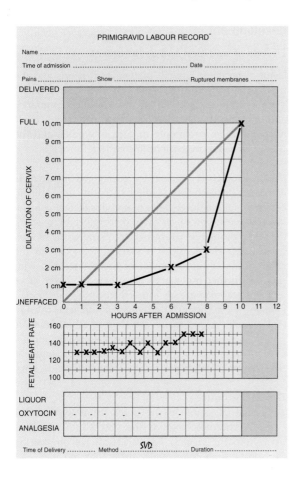

Fig. 47.2 **Partogram with prolonged latent phase.**

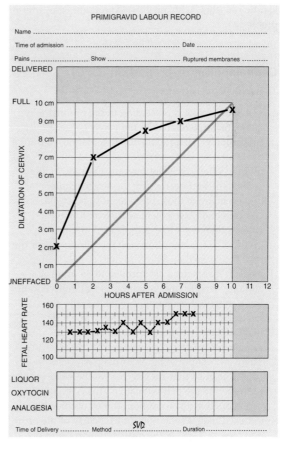

Fig. 47.3 **Partogram with prolonged active phase.**

intensity at the fundus (where the muscle is thickest), its intensity intermediate at the mid-zone and least at the lower segment. With incoordinate uterine activity, however, the intensity profile appears to be reversed with the maximal intensity in the lower segment (where the muscle is thinnest) and weakest at the fundus. This is much less efficient. The resting tone is also found to be increased throughout and the threshold for pain is therefore reached earlier in the contraction.

Inadequate uterine activity has no specific cause, but is much commoner in primigravidae. It may simply be a developmental feature of the uterine muscle and there is evidence that many will resolve spontaneously given sufficient time. There is also some evidence that inadequate uterine activity is associated with cephalopelvic disproportion. This is because cervical dilatation itself may improve uterine activity, but is less likely to occur if the presenting part is pressing less firmly on the cervix.

If progress is satisfactory, there is no need to consider treatment of inadequate uterine activity. Most will respond well to oxytocics, usually given by a stepwise i.v. Syntocinon infusion as described above. As labour is likely to be prolonged, care should be taken to make sure that the mother does not become dehydrated or ketotic as this will further exacerbate the uterine problem.

Cephalopelvic disproportion (CPD)

This may occur because:

1. The baby's head is presenting in the optimal way but is too large relative to the pelvis ('true' cephalopelvic disproportion). It is diagnosed only if the head does not become engaged despite adequate uterine activity. It is not possible to predict CPD antenatally and even using the strictest antenatal criteria many of those considered to be at risk by clinical pelvic assessment will go on to have a vaginal delivery. More complicated attempts to predict CPD using ultrasound measurements of the fetal head together with X-ray or CT pelvimetry measurements have also proved to be unreliable and only lead to unnecessary surgical intervention. Even short stature should not necessarily be regarded with suspicion as these women are more likely to have smaller babies. The only true pelvimeter is labour.
2. There is a malpresentation or malposition of the baby's head so that a wider part of the head is being presented to the pelvis (p. 432). This is 'relative' cephalopelvic disproportion. It may occur with deflexed malpresentations (particularly of the brow and face, p. 431) but the most common cause of relative CPD occurs when the head rotates to the occipitoposterior (p. 436) rather than the occipitoanterior position. The first stage and second stage progress more slowly and, although spontaneous delivery is quite possible with the head coming out 'face to pubis', secondary arrest is not uncommon.
3. There is some form of pelvic abnormality. Major abnormalities are uncommon, particularly in the developed world, and are usually associated with disease, injury or severe nutritional problems. The obstetric classification is based on the shape of the pelvic brim as it is the pelvic inlet which seems to be the major determinant of successful delivery (Fig. 47.4).

Pelves with normal shape and bone development

The round 'gynaecoid' pelvis is the commonest and, as would be teleologically predicted by the theory of natural selection; it is obstetrically ideal. The long oval 'anthropoid' pelvis is also relatively common but is associated with occipitoposterior presentation.

Pelves with abnormal shape and bone development

Defects of nutrition and environment

Minor The flat-brimmed 'platypelloid' pelvis and the triangular 'android' pelvis are considered to be minor variations associated with adverse nutrition in infancy and childhood. The flat-brimmed pelvis is found relatively more commonly in African women and the triangular pelvis in those from southern Europe.

Major Rickets is caused by prolonged vitamin D deficiency in early life leading to poorly mineralized bones containing large areas of soft uncalcified osteoid. Weight bearing produces bony deformities by pushing the sacral promontory forward and pivoting the sacrum backwards. The result is a marked reduction in the anteroposterior measurement of the pelvic brim with possible further mid-cavity narrowing in severe cases as the acetabulae are also forced inwards. As the diet in many western countries contains adequate calcium and vitamin D, and many 'developing' countries have plenty of exposure to sunshine, rickets is uncommon. Osteomalacia – caused by adult calcium deficiency – is rare, except in certain parts of northern India and China.

Disease or injury

Abnormal pressure on the pelvis from kyphosis or scoliosis gradually moulds the pelvis into funnelled or asymmetric shapes. Asymmetrical weight bearing from polio or a congenitally dislocated hip may also mould the pelvis to less favourable proportions. Pelvic fractures may leave the pelvis asymmetrical, and

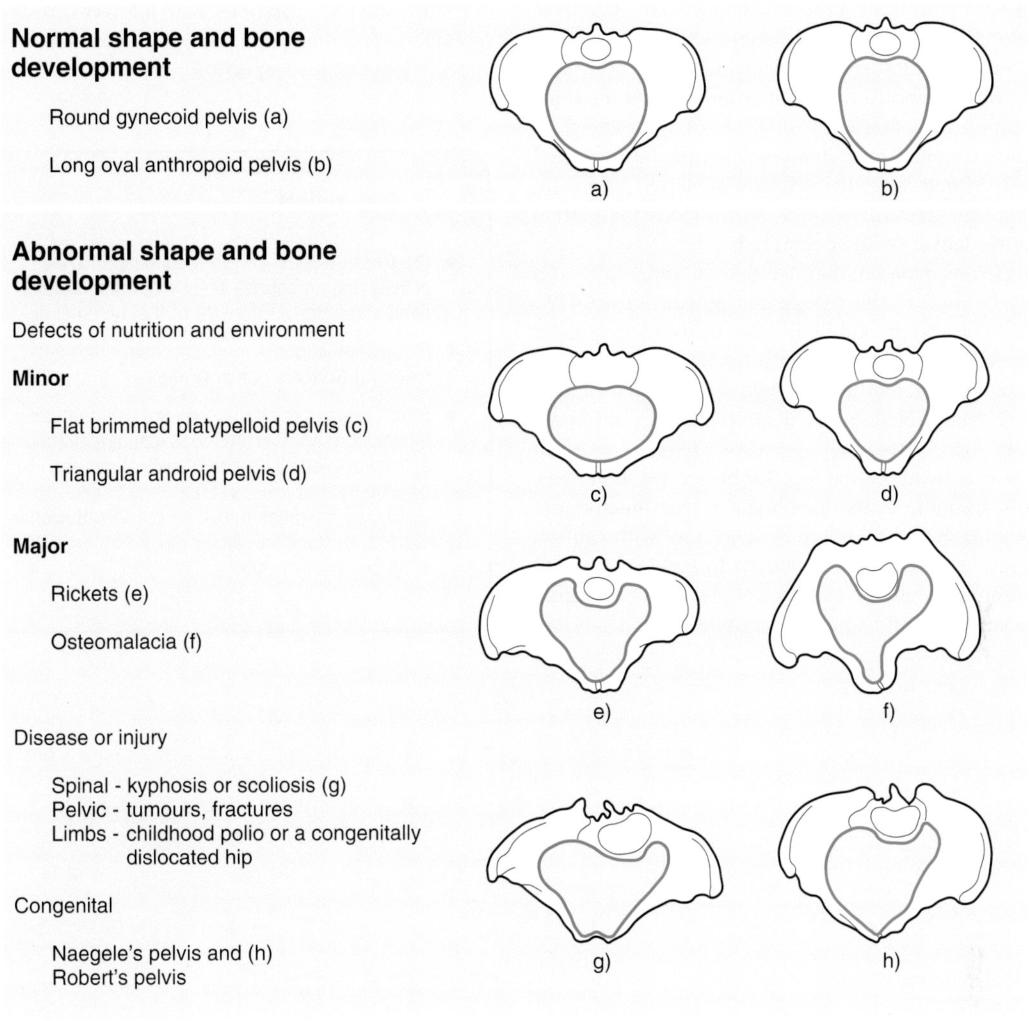

Normal shape and bone development

Round gynecoid pelvis (a)

Long oval anthropoid pelvis (b)

a)   b)

Abnormal shape and bone development

Defects of nutrition and environment

Minor

Flat brimmed platypelloid pelvis (c)

Triangular android pelvis (d)

c)   d)

Major

Rickets (e)

Osteomalacia (f)

e)   f)

Disease or injury

Spinal - kyphosis or scoliosis (g)
Pelvic - tumours, fractures
Limbs - childhood polio or a congenitally
       dislocated hip

Congenital

Naegele's pelvis and (h)
Robert's pelvis

g)   h)

Fig. 47.4 **Classification of pelvic shapes.**

excessive bone formation at the fracture site may further narrow the passage.

Congenital malformations

Congenital absence of one or both sacral masses results in direct fusion of the sacrum to the ilium and marked narrowing – Naegele's pelvis and Robert's pelvis.

Management of slow labour

When progress is slow or when there is secondary arrest it is important to distinguish whether the cause is inadequate uterine activity or cephalopelvic disproportion.

The strength of contractions is difficult to assess reliably. Direct intrauterine pressure monitoring is essentially only a research tool. Some idea of the strength can be gained through maternal observation and abdominal palpation. With an experienced observer, this can provide useful clinical information. In the presence of cephalopelvic disproportion there will be caput and moulding, and malposition or malpresentation may be identified by careful vaginal examination.

In practice the clinical decision is whether or not to start a Syntocinon infusion.

The main risks of starting Syntocinon are of:

- hyperstimulation of the uterus and subsequent fetal distress
- rupture of the uterus (this applies to multiparous mothers only and particularly to those with a previous caesarean section scar).

In primigravidae with slow progress or secondary arrest who do not have a prohibitive malpresentation (e.g. brow presentation) it is reasonable to start Syntocinon.

This is not appropriate if there is suspected fetal distress and should only be after the membranes have been ruptured or have ruptured spontaneously. The aim is to titrate the infusion to the point where the contractions are coming at a frequency of three or four every 10 minutes. Vaginal examinations should be repeated every 2–3 hours after the infusion is started to ensure adequate progress. If progress is still inadequate, then operative delivery will be required.

In parous women the decision is more difficult, mainly because of the risk of uterine rupture (p. 449). Rupture can occur suddenly and leads to expulsion of the fetus into the peritoneal cavity. Fetal death is common. If the mother has had a previous vaginal delivery, true cephalopelvic disproportion is extremely unlikely, but if the only previous delivery was an elective caesarean section (e.g. for breech presentation), there is no guide to the likelihood of true obstruction. Syntocinon should therefore be used only with caution and only in those women thought to have inadequate uterine activity with no evidence of obstruction. Vaginal examinations should again be repeated every 2–3 hours to ensure adequate progress, with a lower threshold for caesarean section in those thought to have some degree of cephalopelvic disproportion.

Key points

- Progress in labour requires adequate uterine activity and an appropriately proportioned fetal head compared to the size of the maternal pelvis.

- Precipitate labour is most commonly iatrogenic following oxytocic administration.

- Slow progress is often corrected with the use of Syntocinon, whether due to inadequate uterine activity or a small degree of cephalopelvic disproportion. Care must be taken to exclude a significant malpresentation before the infusion is started. Syntocinon carries a risk of uterine rupture in parous women only.

48

Malpresentations and malpositions

In the third trimester of pregnancy abdominal palpation should aim to define the lie, presentation, and position of the fetus, in that order. The *lie* refers to the long axis of the fetus in relation to the long axis of the uterus. Usually the fetus is longitudinal, but occasionally it may be transverse or oblique. The *presentation* is that part of the fetus which is at the pelvic brim, in other words the part of the fetus presenting to the pelvic inlet. Normal presentation is the vertex of the fetal head and the word 'malpresentation' describes any non-vertex presentation. This may be of the face, brow, breech or some other part of the body if the lie is oblique or transverse.

The *position* of the fetus refers to the way in which the presenting part is positioned in relation to the maternal pelvis. Strictly speaking this refers to any presenting part, but here it will be considered in relation to those fetuses presenting head first (cephalic). As we have seen, the head is usually occipitotransverse at the pelvic brim and rotates to occipitoanterior at the pelvic floor. 'Malposition' is when the head, coming vertex first, does not rotate to occipitoanterior, presenting instead as persistent occipitotransverse or occipitoposterior.

Malpresentation

Those with a deflexed or brow presentation offer a wide diameter to the pelvic inlet (Fig. 48.1).

Face presentation

This occurs in about 1 : 500 births (Fig. 48.2a). It is associated with anencephaly but this is a rare cause even in an unscreened population. Face presentation is usually only recognized after the onset of labour and, if the face is swollen (Fig. 48.2d), it is easy to confuse this presentation with that of a breech. The position of the face is described with reference to the chin, using the prefix 'mento-'.

The face usually enters the pelvis with the chin in the transverse position (mentotransverse) and 90% rotate to mentoanterior so that the head is born with flexion (Fig. 48.2b). If mentoposterior, the extending head presents an increasingly wider diameter to the pelvis leading to worsening relative cephalopelvic disproportion and impacted obstruction (Fig. 48.2c). A caesarean section is usually required.

431

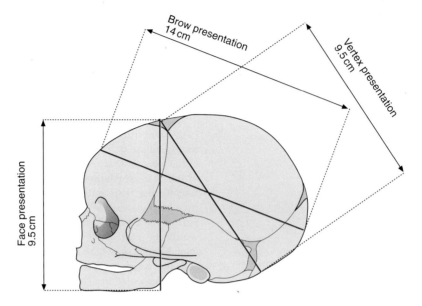

Fig. 48.1 **The presenting diameter is dependent on the degree of flexion or extension of the fetal head.**

Brow presentation

This occurs in only approximately 1 : 1500 births and is the least favourable for delivery. The supraorbital ridges and the bridge of the nose will be palpable on vaginal examination. The head may flex to become a vertex presentation or extend to a face presentation in early labour. If the brow presentation persists, a caesarean section will be required.

Breech presentation

Breech presentation describes a fetus presenting bottom-first. The incidence is around 40% at 20 weeks, 25% at 32 weeks and only 3% at term. The chance of a breech presentation turning spontaneously after 38 weeks is less than 4%. Breech presentation is associated with multiple pregnancy, bicornuate uterus, fibroids, placenta praevia, polyhydramnios and oligohydramnios. It may also rarely be associated with fetal anomaly, particularly neural tube defects, neuromuscular disorders and autosomal trisomies. At term, 65% of breech presentations are frank (extended) with the remainder being flexed or footling (Fig. 48.3). Footling breech carries a 5–20% risk of cord prolapse (p. 442).

Mode of delivery

There has been extensive debate about the safest route of delivery – whether it should be vaginal or by caesarean section. The risks of vaginal delivery are small, but include intracranial injury, widespread bruising, damage to internal organs, spinal cord transection, umbilical cord prolapse and hypoxia following obstruction of the after-coming head. The risks of caesarean section are largely maternal and related to surgical morbidity and mortality. There is now evidence that planned caesarean section is associated with less perinatal mortality and less serious neonatal morbidity than planned vaginal birth at term. The risks of serious maternal complications are much about the same, partly because planned vaginal delivery often ends with an intrapartum caesarean section and such caesarean sections carry greater risks than planned elective sections. The problem of delivery can be removed if it is possible to turn the baby prior to the onset of labour. This process is called external cephalic version.

External cephalic version (ECV)

All women with an uncomplicated breech pregnancy at term should be offered ECV at around 38 weeks' gestation. There is no point in attempting ECV with a significant placenta praevia, as a caesarean section will still be required, and version is also contraindicated with multiple pregnancies and those whose pregnancies have been complicated by an abruption. It is relatively contraindicated in those with pre-eclampsia and fetal growth restriction.

Procedure

A cardiotocograph and ultrasound scan should be checked. Some obstetricians like the patient to be fasted

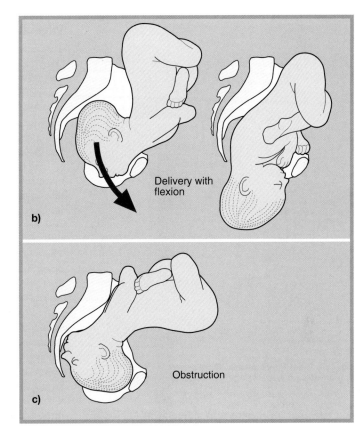

Delivery with flexion

b)

Obstruction

c)

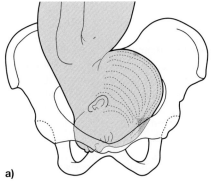

a)

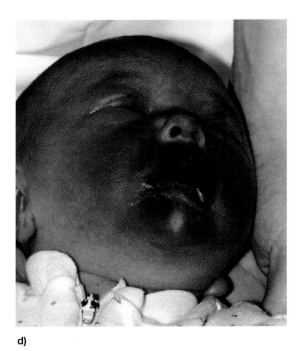

d)

Fig. 48.2 **Face presentation. (a)** The head enters the pelvic brim in the transverse position. **(b)** Most rotate to the mentoanterior position and deliver without problems. **(c)** Those that rotate to mentoposterior will obstruct. **(d)** Face presentation is often associated with oedema and bruising. This baby recovered without problems.

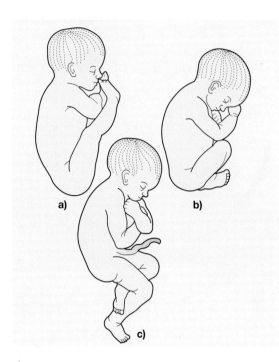

Fig. 48.3 **Breech presentation.** Those presenting by the breech may be **(a)** extended (or frank); **(b)** flexed; or **(c)** footling.

and prepared for theatre, and although this is usually not necessary, it is reasonable to have access to theatre close at hand. ECV is most likely to be successful when the presenting part is free, the head is easy to palpate and the uterus feels soft.

Ask the mother to lie flat with a 30° lateral tilt. If the uterus is not soft, establish an intravenous infusion of ritodrine at 200 μg/min for 15 minutes. Applying scanning gel to the abdomen allows easier manipulation and permits scanning during the procedure if required. Disengage the breech with the scan probe or hands, and then attempt to rotate in the direction in which the baby is facing (i.e. forward roll/somersault). Check the fetal heart every 2 minutes. If unsuccessful, return the fetus to breech rather than leave it transverse. Give anti-D 500 IU i.m. if rhesus negative. The success rate of version is ≈ 30% for primigravidae and ≈ 50% for parous women.

Caesarean section for breech presentation

The evidence quoted above considers term pregnancies only. It is probably also advisable to carry out a caesarean section in preterm deliveries, as there is the additional risk of the cervix closing around the neck after delivery of the breech. Whether caesarean section is also appropriate in extreme prematurity is more difficult to assess, as the delivery may still be traumatic for the baby. In this instance, the operation should be performed by an experienced obstetrician.

Vaginal delivery for breech presentation

This may occasionally still be considered appropriate by some clinicians if the estimated fetal weight is < 3.8 kg and there is no fetal compromise, pre-eclampsia or placenta praevia. Ideally the onset of labour should be spontaneous, the breech frank or flexed (but not footling) and the liquor volume normal. Those not assessed antenatally and presenting in advanced labour with an engaged breech usually deliver without adverse consequences.

The first stage is managed with caution. The role of epidural analgesia is controversial – its use may facilitate manipulation of the fetus, but its presence may inhibit the desire to push, which is important in breech delivery. Augmentation must only be used if disproportion has been excluded and even then with caution. There is no contraindication to a fetal 'scalp' electrode being applied to the breech providing care is taken to avoid genital injury.

The bitrochanteric diameter engages in the pelvic brim in the transverse position (much as the sagittal suture is transverse with cephalic presentation). As the breech descends it rotates to anteroposterior and advances over the perineum with pushing. An episiotomy is performed and the temptation to pull must be resisted. If the breech is frank, the knees should be flexed to deliver the legs (Fig. 48.4a,b) and it is then important to wait for the body to advance further. The anterior shoulder is delivered under the symphysis (Fig. 48.4c,d). If this is not possible, the posterior shoulder may be delivered first by rotating the back 180° (anteriorly) bringing the shoulder anteriorly under the symphysis. The baby is then rotated 180° back again (again with the back anteriorly) for the remaining shoulder (Lovset's manoeuvre, Fig. 48.4e). The breech should be allowed to hang in order for the head to flex. The whole body can then be lifted vertically by the legs, and an assistant should hold the legs in that position. The head can then be delivered by outlet forceps (Fig. 48.4h), or by gently putting the index finger of one hand in the baby's mouth (avoid traction on the jaw) and with the index and middle fingers of the other hand on the occiput the head can be delivered by flexion (Mauriceau–Smellie–Veit manoeuvre, Fig. 48.4g).

Should the head of a preterm breech become entrapped behind an incompletely dilated cervix, it should first be flexed as far as is possible to narrow the presenting diameter. Failing this, the options are then to incise the cervix at the 4 and 8 o'clock positions (risking massive, potentially fatal maternal haemorrhage) or to push the fetus back up and perform a caesarean section (very difficult). Because such interventions are very risky to the mother, it may be preferable to await spontaneous delivery.

All babies presenting by the breech should be checked for developmental dysplasia of the hip (p. 474) and Klumpke's paralysis (p. 475).

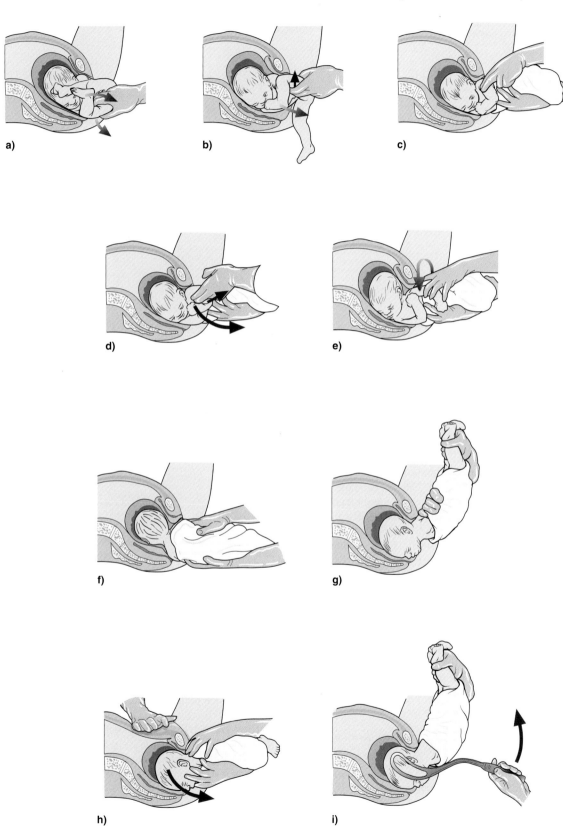

a)

b)

c)

d)

e)

f)

g)

h)

i)

Fig. 48.4 **Vaginal breech delivery.**

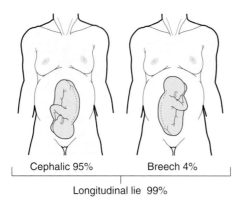 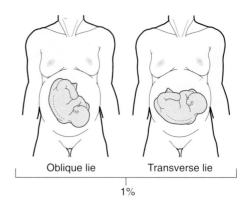

Fig. 48.5 **Fetal lie at term.**

Transverse lie and oblique lie

These are uncommon, occurring in less than 1% of deliveries at term (Fig. 48.5). Usually there is no specific cause but abnormal lie is more common in multiparous women, multiple pregnancies, preterm labour and polyhydramnios. It may also be associated with placenta praevia, congenital abnormalities of the uterus and lower uterine fibroids.

If transverse lie is identified antenatally a scan should be undertaken to exclude placenta praevia, polyhydramnios, lower uterine fibroids and a pathologically enlarged fetal head. External cephalic version is usually possible (see above), and the mother should be reviewed a few days later to ensure that the lie is still cephalic. She should be advised to come to hospital if there is any suspicion of early labour as it may still be possible to carry out an external cephalic version at that stage providing the membranes are still intact. She should also particularly be advised to present if there is any suspicion of membrane rupture, as there is a risk of cord prolapse (Fig. 48.6a).

If the lie is transverse in established labour, particularly after membrane rupture, a caesarean section will be required (Fig. 48.6b). A vertical uterine incision may be necessary to allow adequate access for delivery.

Unstable lie

An unstable lie is one that varies from examination to examination. The options are:

● Manage conservatively, with repeated ECVs as required, and await the spontaneous onset of labour. Should the membranes rupture with the fetus in a non-cephalic presentation there may be a risk of cord prolapse, and inpatient management is considered appropriate by some.

● Arrange to turn the baby to cephalic presentation and then induce labour. This is sometimes referred to as a 'stabilizing induction'. The disadvantage is that the induction itself is not without risks, and the lie may become unstable again even after the membranes have been ruptured.

● Carry out a caesarean section. This has the surgical disadvantages discussed on page 457.

Malposition

Normally the head engages at the pelvic brim in the occipitotransverse position, flexing as it descends into the pelvic cavity and rotating to occipitoanterior (OA) at the level of the ischial spines. The head then extends as it descends, distending the vulva until it is delivered. In about 10% of pregnancies, the fetal head enters the pelvis in a more occipitoposterior (OP) position than transverse or anterior, either by chance, or in association with an abnormally shaped pelvis, particularly the long oval 'anthropoid' pelvis. The baby is then in a direct occipitoposterior position (DOP), or with the occiput to the right or left of the midline, referred to as right or left occipitoposterior (ROP or LOP).

There are then three main possibilities (Fig. 48.7a):

● the occiput will rotate anteriorly (through approximately 135°) to occipitoanterior, and then (usually) deliver normally (65%)
● it will partially rotate to occipitotransverse and not deliver (20%), or
● it will rotate more posteriorly to occipitoposterior (15%).

Those that remain OP have greater difficulty negotiating the birth canal and are less likely to deliver spontaneously. The normal mechanism of delivery involves extension of the head to OA, but extension is not possible in the OP position and a wider diameter is presented to the outlet (Fig. 48.7b,c). With malposition, the first and second stages of labour are usually longer, partly because of the greater presenting diameter (relative cephalopelvic disproportion) and partly because the head is less well applied to the cervix and therefore less able to encourage its dilatation. Back pain in labour is common with OP position. The mother is more likely to request an epidural, is more likely to experience secondary arrest due to relative cephalopelvic disproportion, and more likely to require augmentation with Syntocinon.

If the cervix does not reach full dilatation despite Syntocinon, a caesarean section will be required. If full dilatation is reached, it is quite possible for a baby to deliver in the OP position (with the head coming out 'face to pubis'), but not uncommonly manual rotation, rotational ventouse, or Kielland's rotational forceps delivery will be required (p. 455).

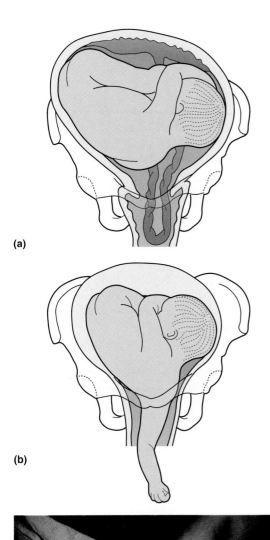

(a)

(b)

(c)

Fig. 48.6 **Transverse lie is associated with (a) cord prolapse, (b) obstructed labour, (c) arm prolapse.**

> ### Key points
>
> - Normal presentation is with the vertex of the fetal head, and the word 'malpresentation' describes any non-vertex presentation. It may be of the face, brow, breech or some other part of the body if the lie is oblique or transverse. Those who are presenting by the brow usually become obstructed, and those who are lying transversely always become obstructed. Babies presenting by the breech can often deliver vaginally, but there is a small risk of intrapartum injury. Babies with a face presentation usually deliver without significant problems.
>
> - The term 'malposition' refers to the situation when the head, coming vertex first, does not rotate to occipitoanterior, and presents instead as persistent occipitotransverse or occipitoposterior. It is associated with prolonged labour and relative cephalopelvic disproportion.

Pregnancy and the puerperium

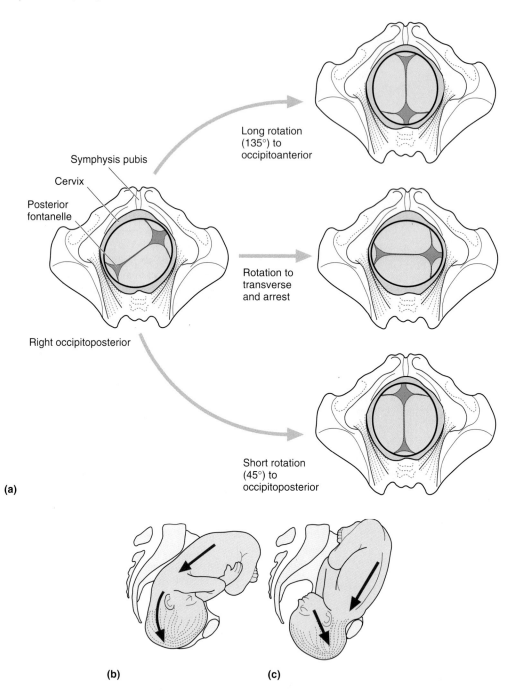

Symphysis pubis

Cervix

Posterior
fontanelle

Long rotation
(135°) to
occipitoanterior

Rotation to
transverse
and arrest

Right occipitoposterior

Short rotation
(45°) to
occipitoposterior

(a)

(b)   (c)

Fig. 48.7 **Occipitoposterior position (a).** Compared to an occipitoanterior position **(b)**, there is a wider presenting diameter **(c)**.

49

Obstetric emergencies

Worldwide, one woman dies every minute of every day from a complication of pregnancy. In developed countries maternal death is uncommon, but evidence from the UK Confidential Enquiry into Maternal Deaths found substandard care in around two-thirds of cases. This is partly due to the fact that most obstetrical emergencies are rare and often unfold with such rapidity that junior medical staff can find themselves facing potentially catastrophic conditions that they may never have seen before, let alone have treated.

This chapter will examine the obstetrical emergencies listed below, but see also haemorrhage (p. 351), eclampsia (p. 372) and pulmonary embolism (p. 329):

- unexpected collapse
- amniotic fluid embolism
- prolapsed umbilical cord
- retained placenta
- shoulder dystocia
- uterine inversion
- uterine rupture.

Principles of management

Anticipation and preparation are essential – and they may lead to prevention. For example, if the mother has a history of postpartum haemorrhage, anticipation with i.v. access and blood sent for group and save in early labour may make an important difference to the outcome should the problem recur. If there are risk factors for shoulder dystocia, such as a presumed large fetus in a mother with diabetes and a long first stage of labour, it is important to ensure that senior medical staff are present on the labour ward at the time of delivery.

In addition, as life-threatening emergencies are relatively rare it is important that there should be regular 'fire drills' of obstetrical emergencies to ensure that all staff are fully prepared and that the equipment is fully functional. It should also be remembered that emergencies can arise anywhere in the unit, not just in the labour ward.

The principles outlined in Box 49.1 can be adapted for initial resuscitation in all obstetric emergencies which involve maternal compromise. Remember that there are often two lives at stake and in most emergencies minutes or even seconds count. Remember too, however, that panicking is never helpful.

Box 49.1

ON IDENTIFICATION OF AN EMERGENCY

1. Call for help. **Emergency bleep** the obstetrical emergency team. This should include a senior obstetrician and anaesthetist, the theatre team, a paediatrician, midwifery sister, a porter and the junior medical staff.
2. Apply ABC if appropriate:

   - **Airway**: Place patient head down, maintain airway patency, Give O₂ (15 l/min) via face-mask, attach pulse oximeter.
   - **Breathing**: Assess, monitor respiratory rate, ventilate if indicated.
   - **Circulation**: Insert two grey/brown i.v. cannulae, Take full set of bloods (FBC, coagulation, crossmatch, urea and electrolytes, and liver function tests). In all cases of severe haemorrhage give 1 litre 0.9% saline stat.
3. Check maternal observations as appropriate, e.g. pulse, blood pressure, O₂ saturation monitoring, and bladder catheter for urinary output measurement.

   At this point see the appropriate management guidelines for the particular emergency as well as:

4. Considering an ECG, blood glucose measurements, central venous monitoring and an arterial line.
5. Using a compression cuff and warmer to give fluids if rapid administration is indicated.
6. Remembering to document fully in the notes all observations, procedures and actions with date, timings, a signature and a printed name.
7. Remembering the mother's partner. Although some partners might wish to wait outside, others may prefer to stay in the room.

It should be noted that an obstetrical emergency can cause profound lifelong psychological problems for both the mother and her partner. This can manifest itself as postnatal depression, post-traumatic stress syndrome and a real fear of becoming pregnant again. Counselling and debriefing after such experiences should be encouraged both whilst the woman is in hospital and some weeks later.

Unexpected collapse – diagnosis

In such situations, in which logical thinking may be hampered, recourse to a mnemonic such as 'I'D SCREAM HELP' may be of benefit to exclude causes that otherwise may be missed (Table 49.1).

Amniotic fluid embolism

Epidemiology

This is one of the most catastrophic conditions that can occur in pregnancy. It is rare, with an incidence somewhere between 1 : 8000 and 1 : 30 000, and until recent years the mortality at 30 minutes was around 85%. Although improved ITU facilities and improved understanding of the condition have reduced this mortality, it still remains the third highest cause of maternal death within the UK.

Aetiology

The exact pathophysiology remains unclear. It was formerly thought that some breakdown occurred in the physiological barrier separating the mother and fetus, allowing a bolus of amniotic fluid to enter the maternal circulation. This bolus moved to the pulmonary circulation and produced massive perfusion failure, bronchospasm and shock. More recently it has been suggested that the underlying mechanism may be an anaphylactoid reaction to fetal antigens entering the maternal circulation and individual variations in sensitivity to these antigens are reflected by the severity of the resulting clinical picture.

Risk factors

Amniotic fluid embolism can occur at any time in pregnancy but it most commonly occurs in labour (70%), after vaginal delivery (11%), and following caesarean section (19%). The following risk factors have been identified:

- multiparous
- placental abruption
- intrauterine death
- precipitate labour
- suction termination of pregnancy
- medical termination of pregnancy
- abdominal trauma
- external cephalic version
- amniocentesis.

Clinical features

The clinical picture usually develops almost instantaneously and the diagnosis must be considered in all collapsed obstetric patients. The mother may demonstrate some or all of the signs and symptoms listed in

Table 49.1
I'D SCREAM HELP – POTENTIAL CAUSES OF OBSTETRICAL COLLAPSE

		Clinical features	Page
I	Inversion of uterus	Occurs in the third stage only. It may lead to profound hypotension (There may be only a partial inversion and therefore the diagnosis may not be obvious)	448
D	Drugs	If opiates, give naloxone	
S	Sepsis	Vasodilated, tachycardia, cyanosis, pyrexia	
C	CVA	May be past history of intracranial problems (e.g. previous subarachnoid haemorrhage). Nausea and vomiting with headache. May have been evidence of pre-eclampsia	
R	Rupture of uterus	Sudden abdominal pain; vaginal bleeding; fetal compromise; laparotomy required	449
E	Embolism	Amniotic fluid: associated with multiparity, precipitate labour, uterine stimulation and caesarean section. There is sudden dyspnoea, fetal distress and hypotension followed within minutes by cardiorespiratory arrest ± seizures	440
		Pulmonary: pleuritic chest pain, sudden dyspnoea, cough, haemoptysis and collapse	329
A	Anaphylaxis	There may be cyanosis, hypotension, wheezing, pallor, prostration and tachycardia ± urticaria	
M	Myocardial infarction	May be past history of heart disease. Chest pain	
H	Haemorrhage	May be antepartum or postpartum. Bleeding may be underestimated, particularly in concealed abruption (hard painful uterus) or uterine rupture (shock, cessation of contractions, disappearance of presenting part from pelvis and fetal distress)	351
E	Eclampsia	There is a tonic–clonic seizure (history should differentiate from epilepsy and amniotic fluid embolism)	372
L	Low glucose (diabetics)	History of diabetes. Pale and clammy. Give glucagon or dextrose	
P	Placental abruption	Abdominal pain ± vaginal bleeding, coagulopathy and fetal distress	351

Box 49.2 but classically a woman in late stages of labour or immediately postpartum starts to gasp for air, starts fitting and may have a cardiac arrest. There is often a profound disseminated intravascular coagulopathy (DIC) with massive haemorrhage, coma and death. There is inevitable fetal distress.

Diagnosis

The definitive diagnosis is usually at post-mortem and is made by confirming the presence of fetal squames in the pulmonary vasculature. It is also possible to confirm the diagnosis in a surviving patient, again by finding fetal squames in washings from the bronchus or in a sample of blood from the right ventricle. In the acute situation, as there is no single clinical or laboratory finding which can diagnose or exclude amniotic fluid embolism, the diagnosis is clinical and by exclusion (see Table 49.1).

Management

This is primarily supportive and should be aggressive. There is, however, no evidence that any specific type of intervention significantly improves maternal prognosis.

Initial therapy is aimed at supporting cardiac output and management of DIC. If the woman is undelivered, an immediate caesarean section may be appropriate, providing the mother can be stabilized.

A chest X-ray will often show pulmonary oedema, and an increase in right atrial and right ventricular size. The ECG demonstrates right ventricular strain and there is a metabolic acidosis (reduction of Pa_{O_2} and Pa_{CO_2}).

In addition to the initial management of an obstetrical emergency (Box 49.1), therapy may include:

1. aggressive fluid replacement
2. maintenance of cardiac output with a dopamine infusion
3. treatment of anaphylaxis with adrenaline (epinephrine), salbutamol, aminophylline and hydrocortisone
4. treatment of DIC with fresh frozen plasma and cryoprecipitate
5. treatment of haemorrhage after delivery with Syntocinon, ergometrine, Haemabate, and uterine massage (p. 351)
6. early transfer to an ITU for central monitoring, respiratory support and other therapy as appropriate.

Box 49.2

SYMPTOMS AND SIGNS OF AMNIOTIC FLUID EMBOLUS

Symptoms
- Chills
- Shivering
- Sweating
- Anxiety
- Coughing

Signs
- Cyanosis
- Hypotension
- Bronchospasm
- Tachypnoea
- Tachycardia
- Arrhythmias
- Myocardial infarction
- Seizures
- Disseminated intravascular coagulopathy

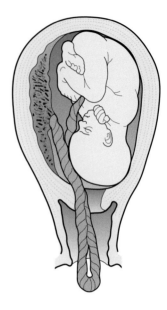

Fig. 49.1 **Umbilical cord prolapsing through incompletely dilated cervix.** This is due partially to a high presenting part.

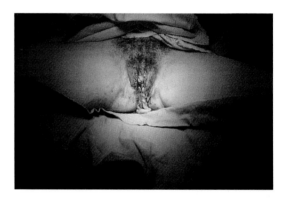

Fig. 49.2 **The umbilical cord is visible at the introitus.** This fetus requires immediate delivery. (Reprinted from *Picture Tests Obstetrics and Gynaecology*, Rymer J, Fig. 155, p. 78, 1995, by permission of the publisher Churchill Livingstone.)

Prognosis

The outcome for the baby is appalling with a perinatal mortality rate of approximately 60% and most survivors usually suffering neurological impairment. Maternal outcome in mothers who have suffered a cardiac arrest is complicated by the fact that many are left with serious neurological impairment.

Prolapsed umbilical cord

Definition

'Cord presentation' is defined as the presence of the cord between the membranes and the presenting part prior to membrane rupture. 'Prolapsed umbilical cord' refers to the same situation after membrane rupture. The cord can remain in the vagina (occult prolapse) or can prolapse through the vagina to the perineum (Figs 49.1 and 49.2). It is a true obstetrical emergency requiring immediate action.

Epidemiology

The incidence is related to presentation (Table 49.2). Any obstetrical condition that precludes a close fit

Table 49.2
Incidence of cord prolapse in relation to presentation

Presentation	Incidence
Vertex	0.4%
Frank breech	0.5%
Flexed breech	4–6%
Footling breech	15–18%

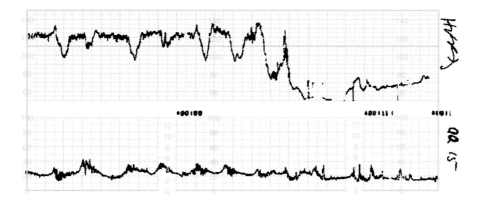

Fig. 49.3 **In an occult umbilical cord prolapse the only indication may be CTG abnormalities which should mandate a vaginal examination.**

between the fetus and the pelvic inlet makes a cord prolapse more likely, particularly breech presentation, malposition, prematurity, polyhydramnios, fetal growth restriction and placenta praevia. Other predisposing factors include a long umbilical cord, artificial rupture of membranes, and being a second twin.

Clinical features/investigation

There are two main insults to the cord, both of which may lead to cessation of fetal blood flow and fetal death. Firstly there is direct compression by the fetal body against the maternal pelvis and secondly there is likely to be cord spasm from exposure to the cool external atmosphere.

Cardiotocography (CTG) usually indicates fetal distress in the form of deep decelerations or a single prolonged deceleration (Fig. 49.3).

In some instances the cord is clearly visible protruding through the vagina, but it may be found at a vaginal examination, perhaps carried out in response to some CTG abnormality. It is important to routinely exclude cord prolapse following artificial rupture of the membranes.

Management

Seconds count. If there is any possibility that a fetal heartbeat is still present, the baby should be delivered immediately. If the cervix is fully dilated this should be by forceps or ventouse; if not, by immediate caesarean section under general anaesthesia.

To protect the cord from occlusion during the transfer to theatre the woman should be placed in the head-down position and a hand placed in the vagina to lift up the presenting part off the cord and prevent cord compression. An alternative is the knee–chest position (Fig. 49.4). The cord should be kept within the vagina and handled as little as possible to avoid spasm.

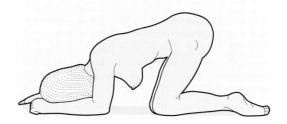

Fig. 49.4 **The knee–chest position should be adopted on the way to theatre.** Gravity ± an assistant's hand displace the presenting part away from the umbilical cord.

A tocolytic, e.g. terbutaline 0.25 mg s.c., can be given to minimize contractions.

If there is doubt as to fetal viability, for instance if the cord has prolapsed at home or silently on the antenatal ward, it is important to establish fetal viability before rushing to unnecessary surgical intervention. The absence of cord pulsation does not necessarily indicate fetal death, particularly if the prolapse is acute, and the fetal heart should be assessed, ideally by ultrasound. If fetal death has occurred the mother should be allowed to labour.

Prognosis

Fetal mortality has been reduced over the years with the increasing use of caesarean section and improvement in neonatal ITU but still remains around 10%.

Retained placenta

Definition

Retained placenta is defined as failure to deliver the placenta within 30 minutes of delivery of the fetus.

A retained placenta increases the risk of postpartum haemorrhage by a factor of 10 owing to the inability of the uterus to contract down completely. This risk appears to be maximal at 40 minutes after delivery. Such haemorrhage can be severe and life-threatening.

Epidemiology

Retained placenta occurs in 2–3% of all vaginal deliveries and is more likely with preterm gestations: if the baby is delivered before 37 weeks the incidence increases by a factor of three and if delivered at 26 weeks the risk is increased by a factor of 20.

Pathology

During normal childbirth 90% of placentas are usually delivered within the first 15 minutes. Placental delivery is usually preceded by signs of placental separation, i.e. lengthening of the cord, a sudden small gush of dark blood and increased mobility of the uterus. Failure of the placenta to deliver may occur because of an unusually adherent unseparated placenta, or because the placenta has separated successfully but is retained within the uterus by a partially closed cervix. Failure of separation is much the more worrying of these two situations.

An adherent placenta is the result of abnormal placental implantation during the first trimester. Normally the invading fetal trophoblast cells are arrested by the maternal decidual barrier, probably by the action of a specific form of leucocyte. If this maternal decidual layer is in some way ineffective, the trophoblast cells may invade further than usual and may extend through the myometrium or even as far as the outer serosal layer. The decidual barrier may be rendered ineffective by a number of factors and is, for example, often thin and scarred following caesarean section. When over-invasion occurs, the placenta becomes abnormally adherent and is referred to as placenta accreta (Box 49.3).

Placenta accreta is subdivided into placenta increta and placenta percreta depending on the depth of invasion (see Table 49.3). There is loss of the physiological cleavage plane so that the placenta is unable to separate

---

Box 49.3

RISK FACTORS FOR PLACENTA ACCRETA

- Previous retained placenta
- High parity
- Advanced maternal age
- Placenta praevia
- Previous caesarean section
- History of dilatation and curettage or suction termination of pregnancy
- Previous postpartum endometritis

---

after delivery of the baby, and partial separation or iatrogenic effort at separation may lead to profound haemorrhage.

A particular problem is the increasing prevalence of mothers who have had previous caesarean sections. If there is a low anterior placenta in a subsequent pregnancy there will be a significant risk of placenta accreta and subsequent haemorrhage.

Management

If the patient is bleeding heavily, a retained placenta is an obstetrical emergency and treatment must be immediate. Aside from the initial resuscitation measures (above) the patient should be transferred to theatre for a manual removal of placenta.

If there is no bleeding an initial conservative approach can be adopted. Although intravenous access should be established and crossmatch arranged in case bleeding begins, it is reasonable to wait an hour or so for spontaneous expulsion of the placenta to occur. In the interim the use of Syntocinon, the 'rubbing-up' of a contraction, or breast-feeding, with its resultant physiological release of oxytocin, may help to aid expulsion.

If the placenta is still retained after 1 hour, the mother should be transferred to theatre for regional or general anaesthesia. Then, under aseptic conditions, a hand is passed into the uterus through the cervix in order to identify the cleavage plane between the placenta and the uterine wall. The placenta can then be gently stripped off the uterine wall and delivered (Fig. 49.5). Once it is out, a contraction should be 'rubbed-up' and a bolus of Syntocinon given i.v. to reduce the risk of postpartum haemorrhage due to an atonic uterus. The procedure must be covered with antibiotics as there is a significant association between

---

Table 49.3
Classification of abnormal placental attachment (placenta accreta)

Type	Pathology
Placenta increta	Invades the myometrium
Placenta percreta	Invades through the myometrium and penetrates the outer serosal layer of the uterus. It may invade adjacent structures including bladder and bowel

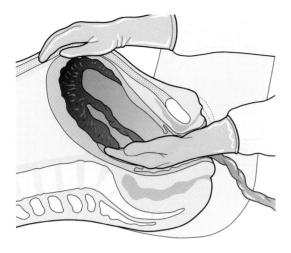

Fig. 49.5 **Manual removal of the placenta.** A cleavage plane is identified with the fingers, which then continue along the plane until the placenta is fully separated from the uterine wall.

manual removal of the placenta and postpartum endometritis.

If the cleavage plane cannot be found and the placenta is so firmly adherent to the uterine wall as to make removal impossible or dangerous (uterine rupture) the clinical diagnosis is of placenta accreta. Subsequent management then depends on the degree of haemorrhage. If there is persistent uncontrollable haemorrhage a hysterectomy will be required but if there is no active haemorrhage, suction curettage or conservative management are options. With conservative management, when the placenta is left in situ to be absorbed over time, there is a significant incidence of major complications.

Shoulder dystocia

Shoulder dystocia is one of the most frightening and threatening obstetrical emergencies. There is a need to act quickly in order to prevent serious fetal morbidity and mortality.

Definition

The fetal anterior shoulder becomes impacted behind the symphysis pubis, preventing delivery (Fig. 49.6a). Clinically it is defined as difficulty delivering the shoulders such as to require some obstetrical intervention beyond episiotomy and downward traction. Although the incidence overall is around 0.2%, it rises to 0.5% with a fetal weight of over 3.5 kg and 10% with a weight of over 4.5 kg. Shoulder dystocia accounts for 8% of all intrapartum fetal deaths.

> **Box 49.4**
>
> *RISK FACTORS FOR SHOULDER DYSTOCIA*
>
> **Antepartum**
> - Macrosomia
> - Past history of dystocia
> - Diabetes
> - Post-dates
> - Obese mother
> - High parity
> - Male fetus
>
> **During first stage of labour**
> - Prolonged first stage
> - Secondary arrest > 8 cm
> - Mid-cavity arrest
> - Forceps/ventouse delivery
>
> **During second stage of labour**
> - Difficulty delivering chin

Risk factors

Although risk factors have been identified (Box 49.4) they have only very limited predictive value. 50% of shoulder dystocias occur in normal-size fetuses and 98% of large fetuses do not have dystocia. It is estimated that 3695 elective caesarean sections would have to be performed in non-diabetic mothers with babies estimated to weigh more than 4.5 kg in order to avoid one permanent brachial plexus injury.

Clinical features

The baby's head is often delivered as far as the chin and the fetal body is in the pelvis.

The umbilical cord is trapped and occluded between the fetal trunk and the maternal pelvis leading to rapid fetal hypoxia and death. The pH drops by an estimated 0.04 per minute and it therefore takes around 7 minutes for the pH of a previously uncompromised fetus to fall below 7.00. It is estimated that 50% of deaths occur within 5 minutes.

Another problem is that of brachial plexus damage due to excessive downward traction of the head during attempts at delivery. It is possible to damage nerve roots between C5–T1, C5–6 (Erb's palsy, Fig. 49.6i) or C7–T1 (Klumpke's palsy).

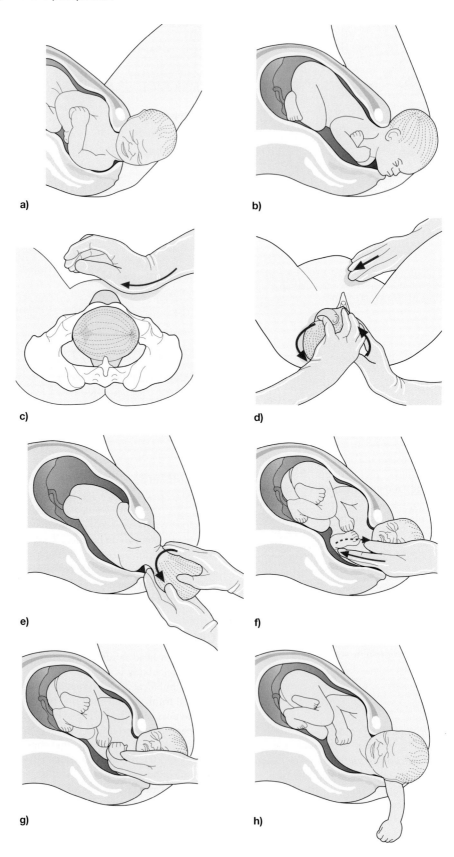

a)

b)

c)

d)

e)

f)

g)

h)

Fig. 49.6a–h **(continues next page)**

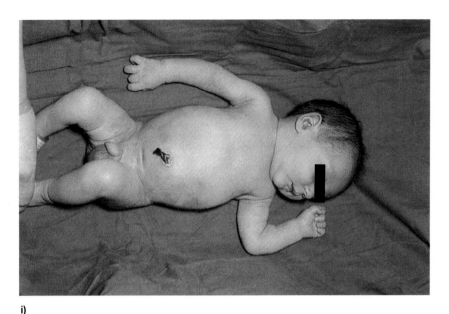

i)

Fig. 49.6 **Shoulder dystocia. (a)** The anterior shoulder becomes impacted behind the symphysis pubis. **(b)** McRoberts' position. **(c)** Suprapubic pressure to rotate the shoulder under the symphysis pubis. **(d,e)** The Woods' screw manoeuvre. **(f,g,h)** Delivery of the posterior shoulder. **(i)** There is a right-sided Erb's palsy following a shoulder dystocia. The baby was otherwise well. (Part (i) reprinted from *Picture Tests Obstetrics and Gynaecology*, Rymer J, Fig. 168, p. 85, 1995, by permission of the publisher Churchill Livingstone.)

While the main concern about shoulder dystocia relates to the fetus, there may also be the maternal complications of genital tract trauma and postpartum haemorrhage secondary to uterine atony. Uterine rupture is rare.

Shoulder dystocia remains an extremely serious, unpredictable and relatively rare event. Fetal survival and neurological normality are proportional to the speed of successful resolution.

Management

This is an obstetrical emergency where, again, seconds count. The aim is to disimpact the anterior shoulder and allow the fetus to be delivered.

The mnemonic 'HELPERR' is useful to help the clinician through a set of detailed manoeuvres in a calm logical way. Each manoeuvre is attempted for a maximum of 30 seconds before moving to the next (Table 49.4).

If all else fails there are three 'last resort' measures. These are described in brief:

1. Symphysiotomy: the symphyseal joint is split with a scalpel, thereby increasing the pelvic diameters (Fig. 49.7).
2. The anterior clavicle of the fetus is deliberately fractured to reduce the bisacromial distance.
3. The Zavanelli manoeuvre: this involves replacing the head with flexion and rotation, and then delivering by caesarean section. In the largest series to date, out of 59 such procedures 53 were successful.

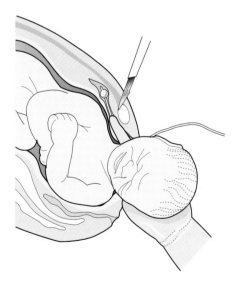

Fig. 49.7 **Symphysiotomy.** The left forefinger is shown displacing the urethra to the maternal left. A scalpel is positioned above the pubic symphysis and the joint divided anterior to posterior.

Table 49.4
HELPERR

H	Help	As with all obstetric emergencies the first response is to crash bleep the emergency team
E	Episiotomy	This allows room for imminent internal manoeuvres and reduces the frequency of vaginal lacerations
L	Legs	Known as the McRoberts' manoeuvre. With one midwife to each leg, the mother's legs are flexed hard against her abdomen and at the same time abducted outwards. This straightens the sacrum relative to the lumbar vertebrae and rotates the symphysis towards the maternal head, allowing the baby's shoulder to pass under by continuous traction on its head. This manoeuvre may be successful in 40–60% of cases (Fig. 49.6b)
P	Pressure	With the legs in the McRoberts' position, suprapubic pressure is applied to push the anterior fetal shoulder (CPR style) downwards towards the fetal chest in an attempt to rotate the shoulder into the oblique, and also to reduce the bisacromial diameter (Fig. 49.6c). This is used in conjunction with continuing head traction. If constant pressure fails, a rocking movement may be tried
E	Enter	Also known as the Woods' screw manoeuvre. The attendant's hand enters the vagina. The middle and index fingers are placed on the posterior aspect of the anterior shoulder and an attempt is made to rotate the shoulder forwards (Fig. 49.6d,e). If this fails, those fingers are kept static and the index and middle finger of the other hand are placed on to the anterior aspect of the posterior shoulder. Both sets of fingers are again used to attempt rotation. If this fails, the reverse Woods' screw manoeuvre is attempted. The fingers on the posterior shoulder are withdrawn completely. The fingers on the anterior shoulder slide down the fetal back to the posterior aspect of the posterior shoulder and rotation is attempted again
R	Remove the posterior arm	The hand of the operator is passed into the hollow of the sacrum, the fetal elbow identified, the forearm flexed and then delivered by sweeping it across the fetal chest and face (Fig. 49.6f,g,h). Fractures of the humerus are not uncommon with this manoeuvre
R	Roll over	It is possible to displace the anterior shoulder during the act of turning the mother over into the all fours position. If not, an attempt can be made to deliver the posterior shoulder first, i.e. the shoulder nearest the ceiling. It is possible to try all the above manoeuvres again in this new position

Uterine inversion

Definition

Uterine inversion is rare, occurring in 1/2000–1/20 000 pregnancies, but as it may lead to rapid maternal death, it is an extremely significant third stage complication. The uterus may undergo varying degrees of inversion and, in its extreme form, the fundus may pass through the cervix such that the whole uterus is turned completely inside out (Fig. 49.8a). As there is a rich vagal supply to the cervix the inversion leads to profound vasovagal shock, and this may be exacerbated by massive postpartum haemorrhage secondary to uterine atony.

Pathology

Inversion occurs with active management of the third stage, that is to say it is iatrogenic (Fig. 49.9). It is the result of traction on an umbilical cord attached to a fundal placenta and is more likely in association with the factors listed in Box 49.5.

Clinical presentation

With complete inversion, the uterus will appear as a bluish-grey mass protruding from the vagina, and in extreme cases there may also be vaginal inversion. The placenta remains attached in about 50% of cases. If the inversion is partial the only obvious sign may be that of profound shock out of proportion to any blood loss. The diagnosis will require a vaginal examination. Rarely the presentation is sudden death following neurogenic shock (Fig. 49.10).

Management

90% of patients will have immediate life-threatening haemorrhage. In order to minimize vasovagal-induced shock and minimize the haemorrhage it is imperative

---

Box 49.5

FACTORS ASSOCIATED WITH UTERINE INVERSION

- Previous history
- Fundal placental implantation
- Uterine atony
- Improper management of the third stage

a)   b)   c)

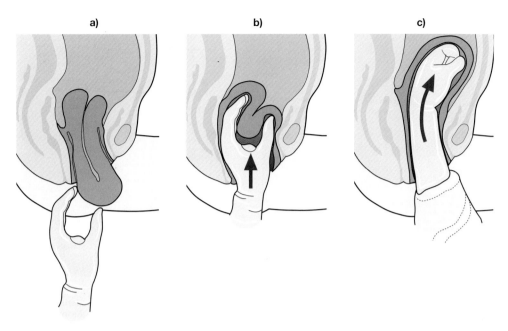

Fig. 49.8 **Replacing an inverted uterus. (a)** Recognition of uterine inversion. **(b)** Replacement of the uterus through the cervix. **(c)** Restitution of the uterus.

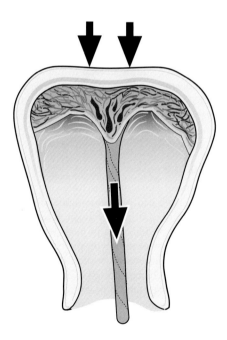

Fig. 49.9 **Undue traction on a fundally sited placenta without guarding the uterus may result in uterine inversion.**

to replace the uterus as quickly as is practicable. Immediate resuscitation is required (Box 49.1) and should involve all available obstetrical and anaesthetic help. Simultaneous attempts should be made to replace the uterus. No attempt should be made to separate the placenta as this may exacerbate the haemorrhage.

One method of reduction is to grasp the uterine fundus with the fingers directed towards the posterior fornix and replace the uterus back into the vagina, pushing the fundus towards the umbilicus and allowing the uterine ligaments to pull the uterus back into position (Fig. 49.8b,c). Alternatively the centre of the uterus may be indented with three or four fingers and only the centre of the fundus pushed up until it re-inverts. Once re-inversion has occurred, the hand inside the uterus should maintain pressure on the uterine fundus until oxytocics have been given in order to maintain a contracted uterine state and prevent recurrence.

Should these methods fail O'Sullivan's technique should be employed. This involves passing 2 litres of warmed fluid into the vagina using either a ventouse cup or anaesthetic gas tubing. The resulting vaginal distension, especially at the vault, is extremely effective at allowing the uterus to return to the normal position. If successful, the fluid should be allowed to drain and oxytocics given as above.

Should all of these attempts fail, a laparotomy is required to aid re-inversion. An incision may be required at the rim of the inversion (Fig. 49.11). Hysterectomy is an option.

Uterine rupture

Loss of the integrity of the wall of the uterus may occur either suddenly, or more gradually during the progress of labour. The uterine cavity may communicate directly with the peritoneal cavity (a complete uterine rupture,

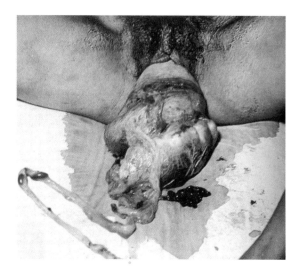

Fig. 49.10 **A fatal uterine inversion with the placenta still attached.** (Reprinted from *Williams Obstetrics*, Cunningham FG, Wenstrom KD, Gilstrap LC et al, Fig. 32-25, p. 768, 2001, with permission of The McGraw-Hill Companies.)

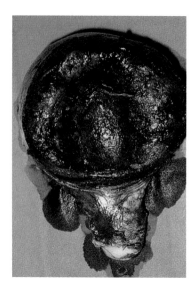

Fig. 49.12 **A complete rupture of the uterus from the lower uterine segment towards the fundus.** (Reprinted from *Obstetrics Colour Guide 2E*, James M, Fish ANJ, Chapman M, Fig. 239, p. 136, 1998, by permission of the publisher Churchill Livingstone.)

Fig. 49.12) or be separated from the peritoneal cavity by the visceral peritoneum of the uterus (incomplete uterine rupture or uterine dehiscence).

A complete uterine rupture is a life-threatening emergency often resulting in fetal death, and may lead to maternal death from massive intra-abdominal haemorrhage. Early recourse to caesarean section in 'high-risk' parous labours with signs of obstruction is likely to reduce the incidence.

Epidemiology

This obstetrical emergency is rare in multiparous women who have had previous vaginal deliveries and virtually unheard of in primigravida. It does, however, complicate 0.6% of deliveries in those who have had a previous caesarean section, with the rupture occurring at the site of the caesarean section incision. This risk increases further when oxytocics, such as prostaglandins or oxytocin, are used, and it is assumed that the consequent powerful contractions place a greater strain on the scar. The risk of rupture is increased yet again if the previous caesarean section was 'classical' rather than 'lower segment' (i.e. midline rather than low transverse) and up to a third of pregnancies with classical incisions may be complicated by rupture even several weeks before term. Most obstetricians would offer those with a midline scar an early elective caesarean section.

Pathology

With complete rupture, the fetus may be extruded into the abdominal cavity. As the rupture can extend

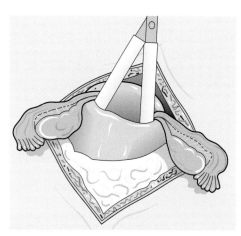

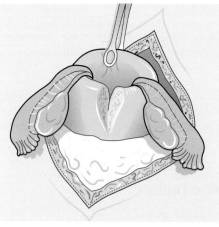

Fig. 49.11 **It may be impossible to reduce the inversion with division of the involuted rim at laparotomy.**

laterally into the uterine arteries or broad ligament plexus of veins there is often severe haemorrhage. Even less commonly, rupture may occur following direct abdominal trauma, for example a road traffic accident.

In caesarean section scar dehiscence, the fetal membranes remain intact. There is usually minimal bleeding and the rupture does not usually involve the entire scar length. Occasionally these are found incidentally at caesarean section carried out for other clinical reasons.

Risk factors

There are many risk factors which increase the risk of uterine rupture (Box 49.6), and most of the intrapartum causes are the consequence of increased force being applied to the uterine muscle.

Box 49.6

RISK FACTORS ASSOCIATED WITH UTERINE RUPTURE

Antepartum
- Certain congenital malformations of uterus
- External trauma
- Classical caesarean section
- Lower segment caesarean section
- Previous uterine trauma/surgery
- External cephalic version

Intrapartum
- Induction with previous caesarean
- Oxytocin in the multiparous mother
- Precipitate delivery
- Obstructed labour
- Forceps, especially Kielland's
- Shoulder dystocia
- Breech extraction
- Difficult manual removal of placenta

Clinical features

The most common sign of uterine rupture is that of fetal distress identified by CTG. This occurs in 70%. Other features include vaginal bleeding (4%), abdominal pain (8%), and easily palpable fetal parts per abdomen. Occasionally the fetal head is felt to have risen higher on vaginal examination. Dehiscence or rupture may occasionally be identified at a vaginal examination for postpartum haemorrhage. In severe instances there may be cardiovascular collapse.

Management

If uterine rupture is suspected the initial drill of summoning immediate help and resuscitation is followed by an immediate emergency laparotomy to deliver the baby. At the time of laparotomy it may be possible to repair the defect, especially if this is simple dehiscence of a previous caesarean section scar. If there is massive haemorrhage (more likely if the rupture is complete), or if it does not involve a previous scar, or has led to extension of a scar, an emergency hysterectomy is likely to be required. Most cases of uterine rupture are not identified at the time of rupture and only become apparent at caesarean section for fetal distress.

Prognosis

With complete rupture and expulsion of the fetus into the abdominal cavity the perinatal mortality rate approaches 75%. If untreated, most women would die from haemorrhage and infection.

Key points

- Obstetrical emergencies are rare and often unfold rapidly. They are often very frightening for everybody.
- It is extremely important to be prepared to act promptly and to know exactly what to do and when to do it.

50

Operative delivery

The phrase 'operative delivery' is used to describe both caesarean section and instrumental vaginal delivery. It may be indicated to expedite delivery in the presence of fetal distress, or for 'delay' or failed progress despite good contractions and maternal effort. The choice between caesarean and instrumental delivery depends partly on the stage of labour, with instrumental delivery possible only in the second stage; even then, specific criteria must be met. Caesarean section can be used in both the first and second stage of labour.

Instrumental vaginal delivery

The most common indications for instrumental delivery are presumed fetal distress and second stage delay. The criteria in Box 50.1 must be fulfilled before the procedure can be carried out.

Very careful assessment is required prior to instrumental delivery, beginning with abdominal palpation. There should be no head palpable above the symphysis although occasionally one-fifth is palpable in occipitoposterior positions. One of the most difficult parts of an instrumental delivery is being completely certain of the fetal position prior to applying the forceps or ventouse. If there is a suspicion from palpation of the sutures that the fetal head is occipitotransverse, it is

---

Box 50.1

CRITERIA FOR INSTRUMENTAL VAGINAL DELIVERY

- The cervix fully dilated with the membranes ruptured

- The head at spines or below, with no head palpable abdominally

- The position of the head known

- The bladder empty

- Analgesia satisfactory (perineal infiltration and pudendal blocks usually suffice for mid-cavity and ventouse deliveries but spinal or epidural analgesia is required for Kielland's rotational forceps)

often helpful to try to feel for an ear anteriorly under the symphysis pubis.

The choice is between forceps and the ventouse.

Forceps delivery

There are three main types of obstetric forceps (Fig. 50.1):

- low-cavity outlet forceps (e.g. Wrigley's), which are short and light, and are used when the head is on the perineum
- mid-cavity forceps (e.g. Haig Ferguson, Neville–Barnes, Simpson's) for use when the sagittal suture is in the anteroposterior plane (usually occipitoanterior)
- Kielland's forceps for rotational delivery to an occipitoanterior or occipitoposterior position. The reduced pelvic curve allows rotation about the axis of the handle.

Low- or mid-cavity non-rotational forceps

The mother should be placed in the lithotomy position with her bottom just over the edge of the bed (the bottom half of the bed often lifts away). Using an aseptic technique, the perineum is cleaned and draped, the bladder emptied and the vaginal examination findings rechecked. A pudendal block (p. 421) and perineal

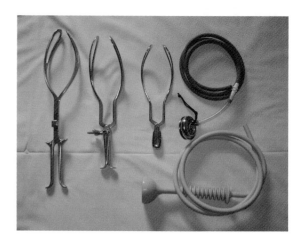

Fig. 50.1 **Selected types of forceps and ventouse cups.** The forceps, from left to right, are Kielland's, Haig Ferguson's and Wrigley's. The orange tubing is attached to an O'Neill occipitoanterior metal cup, and the blue ventouse is a 'Silc' cup.

infiltration are inserted if required, and the forceps assembled discreetly in front of the perineum before application, care being taken to ensure that the pelvic curve will be sitting over the malar aspect of the baby's head, convex towards the baby's face. The rest of the technique is shown in Figure 50.2.

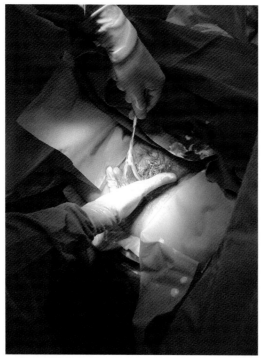

(a)

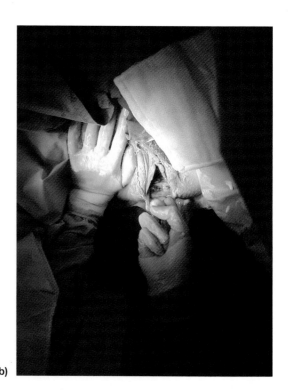

(b)

Fig. 50.2 **(a) and (b).**

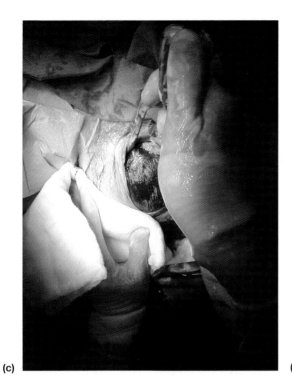

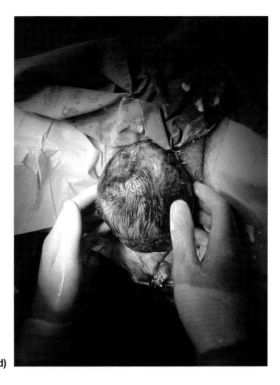

(c)   (d)

Fig. 50.2 **Outlet forceps delivery with Wrigley's forceps.** The handle in the operator's left hand is inserted to the mother's left side by placing the right hand into the vagina to prevent injury and slipping the blade between the hand and baby's head between contractions **(a)**. Opposite hands are used to insert the right blade, and the blades are locked into position by lowering the handles and allowing articulation to occur gently. Traction is applied by pulling initially downwards at an angle of ≈ 60° (maternal pelvis to obstetrician's pelvis if the obstetrician is sitting **(b)**), with the direction of traction becoming horizontal and then upwards as the baby's head advances over the perineum **(c)**. It is usual to perform an episiotomy as the vulva stretches but occasionally, as here, this may not be necessary especially in a parous woman. The forceps are removed after delivery of the baby's head and the remainder of the baby delivered as normal **(d)**.

Rotational forceps

These forceps, known as Kielland's forceps (Fig. 50.3), lack the pelvic curve of non-rotational forceps and can be applied directly to the baby's head, if occipito-posterior, to allow gentle rotation to occipitoanterior. After rotation, delivery is as for the mid-cavity forceps.

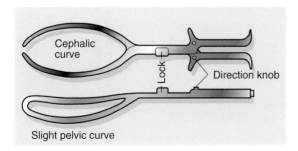

Fig. 50.3 **Kielland's forceps for rotational delivery.**

If the baby's head is occipitotransverse, the blades may be applied directly or the anterior blade applied posteriorly before being 'wandered' past the baby's face to the anterior position (Fig. 50.4). These forceps require considerable skill and may be associated with greater maternal injury than rotational ventouse. They should only be used by experienced obstetricians.

'Manual rotation' of the head is sometimes possible, and it is usual to use the right hand for left occipito-transverse (LOT) positions (Fig. 50.5) and the left hand for right occipitotransverse (ROT) positions. The head is grasped transversely and rotated with a pronation movement. Alternatively, it may be possible to achieve purchase on the head using the fingertips in the lamb-doid sutures. Some operators prefer to rotate during a contraction to minimize the risk of pushing the head up out of the pelvis. If rotation is successful, it is almost always necessary to hold the new position with one hand while applying non-rotational forceps with the other to prevent the head rotating back again. Delivery with forceps is then completed in the usual way.

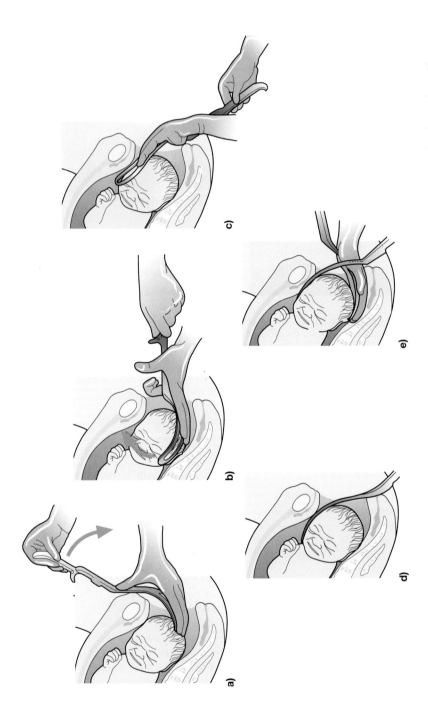

Fig. 50.4 **Delivery with Kielland's rotational forceps. (a)** The anterior blade is initially applied posteriorly. **(b,c,d)** It is then 'wandered' to the anterior position across the baby's face. **(e)** The posterior blade can then be applied and the baby's head rotated to the occipitoanterior position.

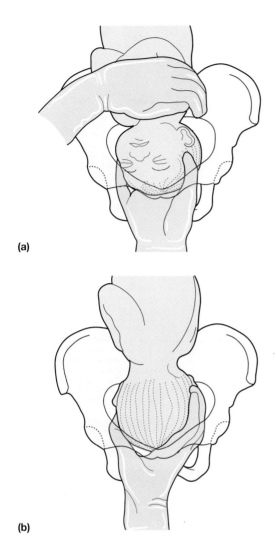

(a)

(b)

Fig. 50.5 **Manual rotation from left occipitoposterior (LOP) to direct occipitoanterior (DOA) position using the right hand.**

Ventouse

Whether to use ventouse or forceps remains an area for debate, but depends to a significant degree on operator experience and familiarity. Ventouse has the theoretical advantage that less pelvic space is required – with forceps the diameter of the presenting part includes both the fetal head and the width of the forceps, whereas with the ventouse it is only the diameter of the head which needs to be delivered.

The use of ventouse compared to forceps is associated with an increased risk of failure, less anaesthesia requirements, less maternal perineal or vaginal trauma, more cephalhaematomata, more retinal haemorrhages, and more low Apgar scores at 5 minutes. No differences between ventouse and forceps deliveries were found in the one study that followed-up mothers and children for 5 years. The use of a soft Silastic cup rather than

a metal vacuum extractor cup is associated with more failures but fewer neonatal scalp injuries. Silastic cups are therefore often used for occipitoanterior deliveries and a metal occipitoposterior cup for transverse and posterior malpositions. The same criteria for use apply to ventouse delivery as to forceps (Box 50.1).

Ideally the cup should be placed in the midline overlying, or just anterior to, the posterior fontanelle. Suction is applied, care being taken to ensure that the vaginal skin is not included under the cup. Traction is also applied downwards as for forceps, but delivery is much more likely to be successful if traction is timed with contractions and maternal effort (Fig. 50.6). The risk of significant fetal injury is increased with the duration of application (p. 475).

Although it has been suggested that it should not be used at gestations of less than 36 weeks because of the risk of cephalhaematoma and intracranial haemorrhage, a case control study suggests that this restriction may be unnecessary. Nonetheless, caution is probably still required. There is minimal risk of fetal haemorrhage if the extractor is applied after fetal blood sampling or application of a spiral scalp electrode. No significant scalp bleeding was reported in two randomized trials comparing forceps and ventouse. The ventouse is contraindicated with a face presentation.

Forceps delivery before full dilatation of the cervix is contraindicated and ventouse delivery before full dilatation should only be considered in special circumstances and with a very experienced operator.

Caesarean section

Caesarean section may be:

1. pre-labour – this can be 'electively', for example with placenta praevia, severe fetal growth restriction, severe pre-eclampsia, transverse lie, breech presentations, or as an emergency, for example following a large abruption
2. in labour (i.e. 'emergency'), usually for the reasons listed under 'forceps', if the cervix is not fully dilated or the mother is unsuitable for vaginal delivery.

Maternal mortality is higher for emergency caesarean section than for elective. Overall there is also significant morbidity from thromboembolic disease, haemorrhage and infection. Deaths from thromboembolism have been dramatically reduced by the widespread use of appropriate thromboprophylaxis.

Lower uterine segment caesarean section is by far the most commonly used technique and has a lower rate of subsequent uterine rupture, together with better healing and fewer postoperative complications. A 'classical' caesarean section (vertical uterine incision) will provide better access for a transverse lie following

Pregnancy and the puerperium

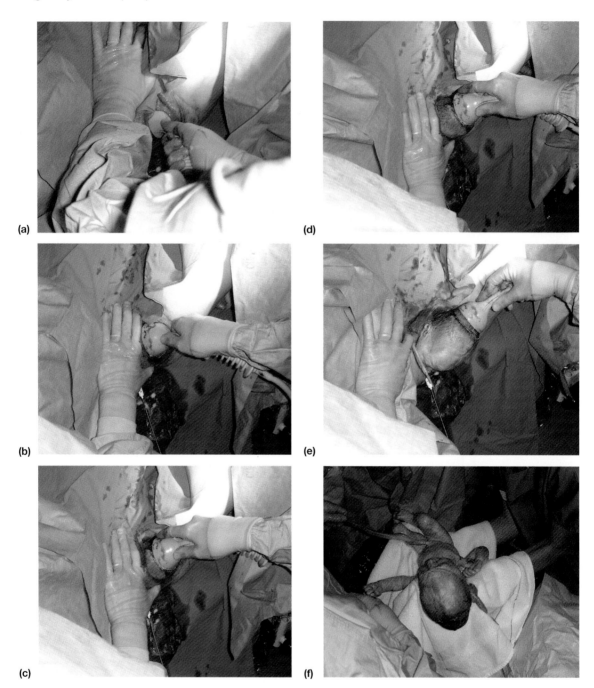

Fig. 50.6 **Ventouse delivery.** The ventouse cup is applied in the midline overlying, or just anterior to, the posterior fontanelle, care being taken to ensure that the vaginal skin is not included under the cup. Traction is then applied to coincide with maternal effort.

Fig. 50.7 **Delivery by caesarean section.** The table should be tilted 15° to the left side (to reduce aortocaval compression) and a lower ▶ abdominal transverse incision made, cutting through the fat **(a)** and the rectus sheath **(b)** to open the peritoneum. The bladder is freed **(c)** and pushed down, and a transverse lower segment incision is made in the uterus **(d)**. If the presentation is cephalic the head is then encouraged through the incision with firm fundal pressure from the assistant. Wrigley's forceps are occasionally required. If the baby is presenting by the breech, traction is applied to the baby's pelvis by placing a finger behind each flexed hip to deliver the bottom first **(e)**. If transverse, a leg should be identified and pulled to deliver the baby (i.e. internal podalic version). After delivery Syntocinon is given intravenously and after uterine contraction the placenta is delivered **(f)**. Haemostasis is obtained with clamps and a check is made to ensure that the uterus is empty and that there are no ovarian cysts. The incision is closed with two layers of dissolving suture to the uterus, one layer to the rectus sheath **(g)** and one layer to the skin **(h)**.

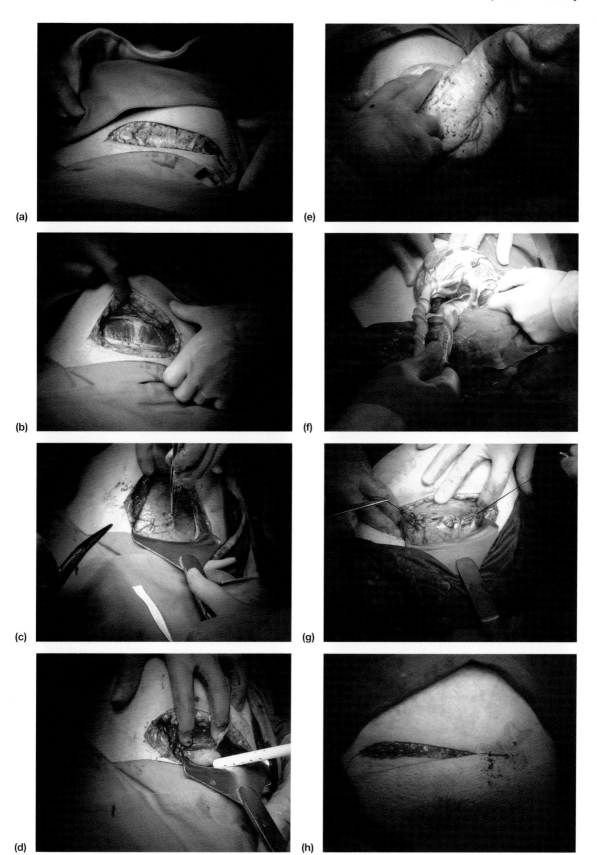

(a)

(b)

(c)

(d)

(e)

(f)

(g)

(h)

ruptured membranes, or with very vascular anterior placenta praevias, very preterm fetuses (particularly after spontaneous rupture of the membranes (SRM)), or large lower-segment fibroids. The chance of scar rupture in subsequent pregnancies following a vertical uterine incision is, however, much greater than with the transverse incision.

Preparation includes i.v. access, group and save, sodium citrate ± ranitidine (to reduce the incidence of Mendelson's syndrome), appropriate thromboprophylaxis, antibiotic prophylaxis, anaesthesia (spinal, epidural or general), and bladder catheterization. The details of the operation are outlined in Figure 50.7.

Caesarean section on request

Women who have had a previous difficult instrumental delivery usually have a much more straightforward delivery next time around, but may occasionally request an elective caesarean section. This is controversial and careful consideration of the advantages and disadvantages is required. In general, those with a previous caesarean section for a non-recurrent indication, e.g.

breech, fetal distress or relative cephalopelvic disproportion secondary to fetal malposition should be offered a trial of labour, but repeat elective caesarean section may be considered in certain circumstances.

Others may also request an elective caesarean section for a first delivery, even if there are no complications. Again, the advantages and disadvantages need careful consideration before an informed decision is reached.

Key points

- Forceps may be low-cavity (outlet), mid-cavity or rotational (Kielland's).

- The use of ventouse compared to forceps is associated with less maternal perineal trauma, more cephalhaematomata and more retinal haemorrhages.

- Maternal morbidity is higher for emergency caesarean section than for elective.

51

Stillbirth and neonatal death

Introduction

Loss of a baby at any stage of pregnancy is an extremely distressing event for parents. Among supporting staff, it may also engender feelings from profound sadness to a sense of personal failure. This sudden bereavement is a very challenging aspect of obstetric care through which to guide parents successfully, and this chapter will consider stillbirth and its immediate management.

Neonatal mortality, the loss of a live baby within the first 4 weeks of life, is also extremely tragic. This will also be considered in detail, focusing particularly on the differences between western care and care in less affluent countries.

The definitions of terms used in this chapter are in Table 51.1.

Stillbirth

Immediate management of in-utero fetal demise

In the absence of some obvious precipitating event, the diagnosis is often first suspected because of reduced fetal movements. Further suspicions are raised when the fetal heart is not heard with the Pinard stethoscope or Doppler probe, and the diagnosis of fetal death is usually confirmed by ultrasound scan. It is worth taking a short time to exclude any obvious fetal

Table 51.1
Definitions

Stillbirth	Any fetus born with no signs of life, after 24 weeks of gestation
Early neonatal death	Death in the first 6 days of life
Late neonatal death	Death from age 7 days to 27 completed days of life
Perinatal deaths	All stillbirths, plus deaths in the first week of life
Perinatal mortality rate (PNMR)	The number of perinatal deaths per 1000 live and stillbirths
Post-neonatal death	Deaths at and beyond 28 days, but under 1 year
Infant death	Deaths at age under 1 year

abnormality on the scan in case post-mortem is declined, but in reality, time is limited by the pressure to break the news. There is no easy way to do this, but it is essential to allow the parents to control the pace of subsequent events. The temptation to deliver a long speech on further management should be resisted until they are ready to begin asking the questions. The parents may need to be alone for a short time, and a room should be organized for them, ideally well away from the noise of a ward or clinic.

Labour will need to be induced. The technique is much the same as for any labour induction, although there is probably a useful role for 48 hours of pre-labour preparation with mifepristone. Some parents may not want this delay, while others may value a day or two at home before having to undergo such a physically and emotionally draining time.

All appropriate analgesia should be offered and experienced supportive midwifery care is vital. In general it is preferable to delay membrane rupture as long as reasonably possible as the risk of chorio-amnionitis is probably increased in comparison to live births. After delivery, the parents should be encouraged to see and hold their baby. This is a very impressionable time for the couple (Box 51.1). Parents often find it useful to have photographs of the baby, as well as hand-prints, foot-prints and a lock of the baby's hair.

Some hospitals have a bereavement counsellor, whose role it is to explain the legal requirement of registration and discuss funeral arrangements, and some units are fortunate enough to have counsellors who will follow-up the parents at home. Most hospitals, however, do not. It is essential that the general practitioner and community midwife are informed before the woman is discharged from hospital. The couple should also be provided with a booklet containing information on, and contact numbers for, any local support groups, for example SANDS – the Stillbirth and Neonatal Death Society.

Investigation

All parents will ask the question 'why?' and most will want a full range of investigations to be carried out in order to establish both diagnosis and prognosis.

Maternal blood tests should be sent to look for:

- Evidence of congenital infection with toxoplasmosis, rubella, cytomegalovirus or human parvovirus.
- Lupus anticoagulant and antiphospholipid antibodies. These are associated with recurrent miscarriage, stillbirth, arterial and venous thrombosis, fetal growth restriction, pre-eclampsia and thrombocytopenia. There is now evidence that giving low-dose aspirin throughout pregnancy increases the incidence of live births.

Box 51.1

A MOTHER'S STORY

When a child dies you can't, as with other deaths, adapt. You can't dismantle the connection you shared and eventually come to accept the world without them. For me, my child will always exist. Not because I dwell on his death, but because I was – I still am – his mother.

We already had one healthy son. When I found out I was pregnant for the second time, I was thrilled. I'd somehow imagined that I wouldn't have enough love for another child but it turns out that, where children are concerned, we do. On some deep level I trusted my body to bring this child into being – it was just a case of counting down the months. But then he ran into very serious problems. Sitting in the specialist's waiting room I looked at the walls covered with letters of thanks, photos of tiny babies that this man had saved. 'Maybe,' I thought, 'just maybe.'

'I'm sorry,' he said 'I don't think he's going to make it.' A million moments pass us all the time – minutes of no import, filled with the ordinary everyday. And then one comes along and, on that pinprick of time, you trip and tumble. Then you fall and fall, because there is no floor. I know I wanted to give way, to allow the pain to become real. But I just froze. The baby was still in me, dying instead of growing. Things would have to happen – dreadful things – and I shut down. I lay for two days, waiting for him to die. Outside it was a blazing summer day, but we closed the curtains. On the Sunday morning I knew it was over. I didn't say at first, I needed time to absorb it. At lunchtime I told my husband 'I know he has died.'

The prospect of going through labour seemed macabre. Finally after 7 hours he arrived. How else can I describe it? He wasn't born, he was just there, silent and still, not breathing. I wanted to scream out 'open your eyes!' But there was none of that and it just felt so wrong. His still-warm weight on me; knowing that those moments were all we had.

The despair that followed was deeper than I could ever have imagined. I came home without my baby, empty armed – and everything felt wrong. Upturned. When an adult dies there is a space in the house, but we hadn't even prepared the nursery. 'Keep talking,' we were advised, and we did. But what was there to talk about? Our son, after all, had no history; we'd made no memories with him. But we had had that love for him, the portion of love we'd set especially aside for our son. When I got pregnant again, the 9 months were nightmarish, charged with the fear that we'd lose this one too. When they handed him too me, he let out a cry and it was the most wonderful thing I have ever heard.

We're through it. It's not behind us, but it's with us. We have made it part of our lives, because he *is* part of our lives.

- Diabetes, either with a random blood glucose or HbA$_{1c}$.
- Fetomaternal haemorrhage, with a Kleihauer test.
- Isoimmunization, either rhesus or non-rhesus.

A post-mortem examination is extremely important. It is very rare for parents to regret this being carried out and it is not possible to have a useful post-mortem at some later stage if the parents change their minds. The request must be handled as delicately as possible, and if the parents decline it may be worth offering a more restricted post-mortem, biopsies or radiological investigations.

The post-mortem will include measurements of the baby's length and weight, and a detailed external inspection, particularly of the limbs and face. A systematic internal examination is then carried out to look for any malformations of the viscera, limbs or genitalia. Genetic advice may be sought and a karyotype is often checked using samples of skin or blood. Histology is usually carried out on significant organs, and X-rays taken if there is a suspicion of a skeletal dysplasia.

Placental examination, both macro- and microscopic, can provide useful information as to the cause of death. There may be a retroplacental clot indicating a placental abruption, or the aberrant vascular supply of vasa praevia. Atheromatous deposits throughout the placenta may be indicative of poor placentation and may explain fetal growth restriction or hypoxia as a cause of death.

Photographs are usually taken throughout as a record of any abnormality.

Causes of stillbirth

Rates in many western countries have fallen over the past 50 years to a level around 6/1000 births, probably because of improved overall maternal health, better nutrition and wider education. An important, though probably lesser, role has been associated with improved obstetric care.

The obstetrical classification of stillbirths is summarized in Table 51.2. Congenital anomaly and the much larger 'unexplained' stillbirth categories are considered below. For antepartum haemorrhage, hypertension, medical disorders and isoimmunization see relevant Chapters.

Congenital abnormalities (see also p. 476)

These may or may not have been diagnosed antenatally (Table 51.3).

Despite antenatal screening for structural defects, many cardiovascular conditions remain unrecognized. Detailed ultrasound views of the heart can be difficult to assess with repeatable accuracy, and cardiac abnormalities make up the largest group of lethal congenital anomalies.

The incidence of neural tube defects (NTDs) among neonates seems to be falling. This can in part be explained by an increased number of earlier terminations following antenatal diagnosis with either alpha-fetoprotein or ultrasound, but there is probably a background reduction that is independent of this. As there is now good evidence that daily folic acid in the first weeks of pregnancy also reduces the incidence of NTDs, an argument can be put forward for routine supplementation of commonly eaten foodstuffs, for example bread or cereals.

Unexplained stillbirth

It is frustrating and disappointing that this group still accounts for so many stillbirths, and it remains difficult to know how to move forward in reducing the number. Whether a cause has been identified or not, all those who have lost a baby should be offered a follow-up appointment.

Table 51.2
Obstetrical classification of stillbirth – Scottish figures 1999

Classification	Notes	Frequency
Unexplained < 2500 g	Often associated with prematurity	38%
Unexplained ≥ 2500 g		24%
Antepartum haemorrhage	Abruption and placenta praevia	16%
Congenital anomaly	Any structural, genetic or biochemical cause	9%
Hypertension of pregnancy		7%
Maternal disorder	e.g. maternal trauma, diabetes, surgery	3%
Miscellaneous		2%
Isoimmunization	Rhesus or non-rhesus	< 1%
Trauma/mechanical	e.g. uterine rupture, birth trauma, cord prolapse	< 1%

Table 51.3
Examples of potentially lethal congenital anomalies by system

System	Examples	Diagnosis
CNS	Anencephaly	Ultrasound scan
Cardiovascular	Ventricular hypoplasia, valvular incompetence and arrhythmias	Ultrasound scan
Renal	Infantile polycystic kidney disease, posterior urethral valves, Potter's syndrome	Ultrasound scan
Alimentary	Diaphragmatic hernia	Ultrasound scan
Chromosomal	Turner's syndrome (45XO), Down's syndrome (47 +21), Edward's syndrome (47 +18) and Patau's syndrome (47 +13)	While around two thirds of fetuses with Down's syndrome will look normal at 18 weeks, most with Edward's and Patau's syndromes do show some abnormality, even though these are often not specific or diagnostic. An amniocentesis is therefore required to establish the diagnosis with certainty. (For screening, see p. 341)
Respiratory	Pulmonary hypoplasia (e.g. following very early preterm rupture of the membranes or Potter's syndrome)	Ultrasound scan
Skeletal	Thanatophoric dysplasia, achondrogenesis, osteogenesis imperfecta type II	Ultrasound scan
Multiple abnormalities	Cystic hygroma (particularly if associated with aneuploidy)	Ultrasound scan
	VATER association – this refers to a condition in which there are Vertebral, Anal, Tracheal or oEsophageal and Renal lesions. (Also extended to VACTERL by adding Cardiac and Limb abnormalities)	

Follow-up and subsequent pregnancy

The appointment should be in a suitable clinic some 4–8 weeks after the delivery, depending on when any results are expected to be available. This enables the obstetrician to discuss all the factors involved, provide information on likely recurrence, and consider the appropriateness of any antenatal testing in a future pregnancy.

The consultation can be difficult, particularly in the 'unexplained' group. The chance of unexplained stillbirth in a subsequent pregnancy is low, probably less than 5%, and the couple should be reassured about this. In the absence of any identifiable cause, however, it is difficult to monitor for problems. Screening for chromosomal abnormalities and carrying out an ultrasound scan for structural abnormality may provide reassurance, but it is likely that both of these would have been normal with the pregnancy that was lost. More frequent antenatal visits may also provide reassurance, particularly with growth scans every few weeks from 24 weeks onwards. It would also be relevant to check the liquor volume and umbilical artery Doppler flow as pregnancy advances.

Throughout, it is important to offer easy access to professional advice and support at times of anxiety, particularly if there are worries about fetal movements. There should be an easy point of contact at any time if problems do occur.

By 38–39 weeks, many couples will be extremely anxious, and are often keen to have labour induced. Induction carries the risks of fetal distress and hyperstimulation, and conservative management carries the risk, albeit small, of further in-utero demise. The pros and cons of these two should be discussed with the couple and an informed decision reached. Induction at this stage would not be an unreasonable course of action to minimize parental anxiety.

Neonatal mortality

Neonatal mortality is the loss of a live-born baby within the first 4 weeks of life. Perinatal mortality is the sum of stillbirths and early neonatal mortality (within the first 7 days from birth).

Western causes of neonatal mortality

These are outlined in Figure 51.1. Although only about 8% of babies are born prematurely, this group contains

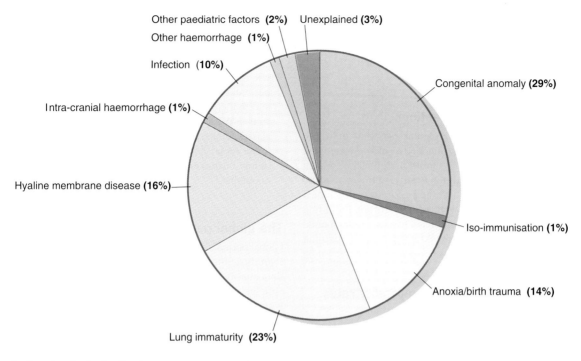

Fig. 51.1 **Paediatric classification of neonatal deaths – Scottish figures 1999.** The overall rate is 3.5/1000 live births.

almost 80% of the perinatal deaths. The causes of death amongst this group are varied but the majority are from:

- respiratory distress syndrome secondary to lung immaturity
- neonatal infection.

Advances in neonatal care have improved the survival of many premature infants, but particularly with the development of improved ventilation techniques and exogenous surfactant administration, it is now accepted practice to resuscitate babies at even earlier gestations than in the past. Survival below 24 weeks, however, is very rare (Table 51.4).

Epidemiologists associate perinatal mortality with three factors: maternal age, parity and socio-economic class. Although they are considered separately here, this is not so in practice. For example, higher parity is usually associated with increase in maternal age.

Table 51.4
Approximate neonatal mortality/1000 live births for western countries by gestation

Gestation	Neonatal mortality/1000 live births (approx.)
24 weeks	800
28 weeks	180
32 weeks	44
36 weeks	10

Maternal age
The safest time to have children has traditionally been between 25 and 29 years. The highest rates of neonatal mortality are in babies born to women under the age of 20 and over the age of 35. These increases at the extremes of reproductive life are due to:

- the higher incidence of medical conditions and higher parity in women over 35, and
- the lack of antenatal care and support that often occurs in women under the age of 20.

Parity
The safest pregnancies appear to be the second and third. First pregnancies are associated with a higher incidence of problems such as proteinuric hypertension and obstructed labour. As mentioned above, higher parity is often a reflection of increasing maternal age, and medical complications are more common.

Social class
There is a steady increase in neonatal mortality as social class falls.

Other factors

- Reproductive history. The risk of a perinatal death is increased if the previous pregnancy ended in premature birth, miscarriage or perinatal death.
- Ethnic factors are also important and are in themselves multifactorial. Some women from ethnic

465

minorities may experience communication problems, may have had inadequate antenatal care, may be at increased risk because of consanguinity and are more likely to decline termination of a diagnosed lethal anomaly.

Perinatal mortality meetings

Most obstetric units hold regular perinatal mortality meetings. They are usually attended by all those involved in perinatal care and allow a multidisciplinary approach to the case review. In addition to striving for an accurate diagnosis, the meeting also addresses ways in which such a death may be prevented in the future. Providing this learning process is conducted in a non-judgemental atmosphere, it can be an extremely useful learning exercise for all concerned.

Comparison of perinatal mortality rates (PNMR) in different areas

International comparisons of PNMR can be misleading. For example:

- Different countries have minor variations in the definition and therefore differences in inclusion criteria.
- Countries such as Sweden have a more homogeneous population with an overall higher social class.
- There may be different reproductive patterns – for example in China, where many couples have only one baby.

- There may be differing rates of fetal abnormality, for example the UK has a high incidence of neural tube defects.
- Differences can also be seen within a country. In the UK, again as an example, there is a tendency for the perinatal mortality rate to be lowest in the south east and to increase towards the north west. This trend runs in parallel with the proportion of lower social classes, which follows a similar distribution. In the lower social classes there is an increased incidence of low-birth-weight babies and congenital anomalies.

The global perinatal mortality problem

Global perinatal statistics are more difficult to determine than those for western countries (Fig. 51.2). In general, data quality is likely to be worse for countries that have suffered recent disruptions in infrastructure because of war or natural disasters. Deaths during the neonatal period account for almost two-thirds of all deaths in the first year of life, and 40% of deaths before the age of 5 (see Box 51.2; the 'two-thirds' rule). Current estimates suggest that 34 out of every 1000 babies born in developing countries die before they reach 1 month of life.

A disturbing feature of newborn mortality is the marked variation in rates between low-income and high-income countries. For example the neonatal mortality rate (NMR) in Mali is about 60 per 1000 live births compared to Sweden, where the rate is less than 3 per 1000 (Table 51.5). The disparity between regions is even

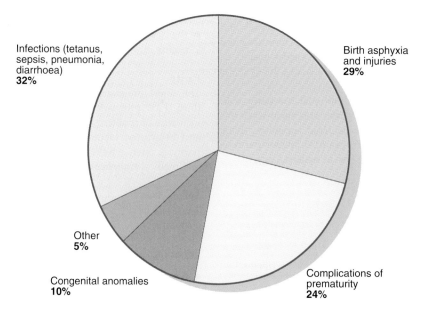

Fig. 51.2 **Paediatric classification of neonatal deaths (WHO) – global figures 1999.** The overall rate is 31/1000 live births.

Table 51.5
World neonatal mortality rates by region

	Estimated number of live births per year (thousands) 1999	Estimated neonatal mortality rate per 1000 live births circa 1999	Lifetime risk of a mother experiencing a neonatal death (%) calculated
Africa	28 685	42	21
Asia	76 090	34	9
Latin America/Caribbean	11 553	17	5
Europe	7 374	6	< 1
World	129 596	31	8

Box 51.2

THE 'TWO-THIRDS RULE' OF GLOBAL INFANT MORTALITY RATES (THIS RULE APPLIES ONLY TO THE WORLD AVERAGE)

- More than seven million infants die each year between birth and 12 months
- Almost two-thirds of infant deaths occur in the first month of life
- Among those who die in the first month of life, about two-thirds die in the first week of life
- Among those who die within the first week, two-thirds die in the first 24 hours of life

---

wider when we use the lifetime risk of a mother experiencing a neonatal death as the standard of comparison. Family size is larger in developing countries and a mother in western Africa, for example, has an approximately 30% risk of one of her babies dying in the first month, compared to a mother in Western Europe or North America where the likelihood is less than 1%. Almost a third of mothers in western Africa have lost at least one newborn baby.

The neonatal mortality rate (42 per 1000) and the perinatal mortality rate (76 per 1000) are highest in Africa, and neonatal mortality is highest of all in West Africa, at 54 per 1000 live births. Asia has a lower average neonatal death rate (34 per 1000), but because of that region's higher population, it accounts for 60% of the world's neonatal deaths.

The family incurs the cost of healthcare during pregnancy and delivery, and if the newborn dies, the additional costs of the funeral and burial. Caring for a disabled or sick child can consume the family budget and, in many cases, is an added burden on family members who would otherwise work and make money. Disabled and sick newborns add to local and national healthcare costs, stretching already scarce resources. The social costs are harder to quantify. A newborn death is an extremely distressing emotional experience for the new mother and her family, and it is also a social stigma in many cultures.

Global causes of neonatal deaths

Determining why newborns die in developing countries is difficult because most deaths occur at home, and families are often reluctant to seek outside help for a variety of sociocultural, logistical and economic reasons (Fig. 51.3). The data, however, point to four main causes of neonatal death:

1. infection (tetanus, sepsis, pneumonia, diarrhoea)
2. complications during delivery (leading to birth asphyxia and birth injuries)
3. complications of prematurity
4. congenital anomalies.

Infections

Every year, an estimated 30 million newborns acquire a neonatal infection, and between one and two million of those infected die. The most common of these infections lead to neonatal tetanus, sepsis, pneumonia and diarrhoea, which together account for around 30% of neonatal deaths. Where hygiene is poor, newborns may become infected with bacteria leading to serious infections in the skin, umbilical cord, lungs, gastrointestinal tract, brain, or blood.

Neonatal tetanus has been eliminated today in over 100 countries through immunizing mothers with tetanus toxoid, ensuring clean delivery practices, and maintaining clean care of the umbilical cord stump. Early and exclusive breast-feeding also contributes to reduced neonatal mortality from infections. Tetanus toxoid is one of the cheapest, safest, and most effective vaccines. It costs about US$1.20 – a sum that includes the purchase and delivery costs of three doses of vaccine. Three doses of tetanus toxoid ensure 10–15 years' protection for a woman and immunity for her newborns during the critical first 2 months of life. Five doses ensure a

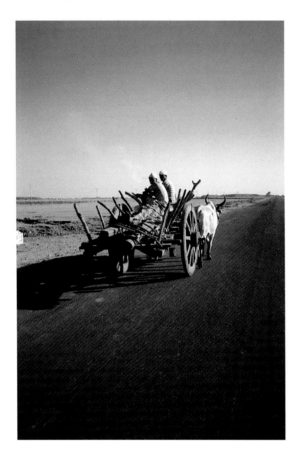

Fig. 51.3 **Even if obstetric facilities are available, many people have to travel long distances to reach them.**

lifetime of protection for the mother, yet only around 50% of pregnant women in developing countries are fully immunized.

Malaria is also associated with an increased risk of spontaneous miscarriage and stillbirths and is linked with maternal anaemia. These complications can be reduced by providing antimalarial treatment and iron supplements antenatally. Use of bed-nets impregnated with insecticide has also been proven to be effective in preventing malaria.

Complications during delivery

The WHO estimates that between four and nine million newborns suffer birth asphyxia each year. Of these, an estimated 1.2 million die and at least the same number develop severe consequences such as cerebral palsy and mental impairment. Prompt detection and management of obstetric complications could prevent many of these deaths and disabilities.

Historically, skilled care at delivery has been associated with lower neonatal death rates. Skilled attendants at birth must be able to manage normal deliveries,

and diagnose and manage, or refer, complicated cases. On average around 60% of births occur in the home and only 50% of all births are attended by a health worker with appropriate skills. In other words, 53 million women each year give birth without the help of a trained professional. In some countries the incidence of skilled care at deliveries is much lower; 2% in Somalia, for example, and 9% in Nepal. Even in those cases where skilled healthcare is available, ongoing training and supervision of personnel and quality referral care for obstetric emergencies must be ensured.

Complications of prematurity

There is some evidence that the incidence of premature labour becomes less with improved maternal health.

Congenital anomalies

Congenital anomalies are the fourth most common cause of newborn deaths, a category that includes

---

Box 51.3

POTENTIAL DEVELOPMENTS TO IMPROVE PERINATAL CARE

Care during pregnancy

- Improve the nutrition of pregnant women
- Immunize against tetanus
- Screen and treat infections, especially syphilis and malaria
- Improve communication and counselling: birth preparedness, awareness of danger signs, and immediate and exclusive breast-feeding
- Monitor and treat pregnancy complications, such as anaemia, pre-eclampsia, and bleeding
- Promote voluntary counselling and testing for HIV
- Reduce the risk of mother-to-child transmission of HIV

Care at time of birth

- Ensure skilled care at delivery
- Provide for clean delivery: clean hands, clean delivery surface, clean cord cutting, tying and stump care, and clean clothes
- Keep the newborn warm: dry and wrap baby immediately, including head cover, or put skin-to-skin with mother and cover
- Initiate exclusive breast-feeding within the first hour
- Give prophylactic eye care, as appropriate

neural tube defects, cretinism, and congenital rubella syndrome. Cretinism can be avoided by providing mothers with adequate iodine, and congenital rubella syndrome can be prevented by immunizing mothers against rubella.

Cost-effective solutions

If improving newborn health were a matter of making medical or scientific breakthroughs, building expensive healthcare infrastructures, or purchasing expensive high-tech ventilators and incubators, then the reluctance to take up the cause of newborns might be more understandable. But it is not. Experience in developed nations has shown that neonatal and perinatal mortality rates fell most dramatically long before neonatal intensive care units came into existence, thanks to relatively simple, low-cost interventions such as better maternal and obstetric care, better routine newborn care, and the introduction of antibiotics (Box 51.3).

Low-cost, proven interventions can be carried out entirely within the framework of existing maternal and child health programmes. Current reviews indicate that essential care during pregnancy, childbirth, and the newborn period costs an estimated US$3 a year per capita in low-income countries.

Key points

- The loss of a baby at any stage of pregnancy is an extremely distressing event for parents.

- A stillbirth may occur for a large number of reasons, including antepartum haemorrhage, congenital anomaly or hypertensive disorders of pregnancy. The majority, however, are unexplained.

- In western countries, the majority of neonatal deaths occur in association with prematurity. Worldwide, infection and birth injury are more common than the complications of preterm birth.

Neonatal care

Introduction

Good-quality neonatal care is extremely important, and may have key implications for the rest of a baby's life. Those born prematurely need skilled intensive support, and those born with presumed hypoxia need appropriate resuscitation. The early neonatal period is often the time when congenital abnormalities become apparent and precise diagnosis and management can make a difference to the quality of life, or even influence whether the baby will live or die. The aim of this chapter is not to provide a comprehensive guide to neonatal care, but rather to highlight some of the more common neonatal problems which can occur.

It is essential that the obstetrician, midwife, paediatrician, radiologist, neonatologist and neonatal nurse collaborate closely as a team. High-quality communication is essential if decision-making is to be optimized.

The transition at birth

The apparent ease with which most babies make the transition from fetal to neonatal life conceals a host of complex physiological changes in virtually every system. Several relatively common neonatal disorders are related to difficulties with this transition.

Respiratory system

The fetal lung at term contains about 100 ml of liquid. This equals the functional residual capacity and in a sense the fetal lung can be said to form around a liquid cast of the future air spaces. Lung fluid is formed by alveolar cells, and fluid is essential for normal lung growth and development.

The fluid must be cleared at birth to make way for air, and failure to do so leads to breathlessness. This is known as transient tachypnoea of the newborn (TTN). It may last for a day or two, and is commoner after elective caesarean section.

Respiratory distress syndrome (RDS) is caused by a deficiency of surfactant and is commoner in preterm infants (0.1% at term vs 30% at 28 weeks). Surfactant, a complex lipoprotein consisting largely of phosphatidyl choline, is synthesized by type II pneumocytes within the alveoli and is important in allowing the alveolus to expand. Hypoxia, acidosis and hypothermia reduce surfactant production; antenatal steroids increase

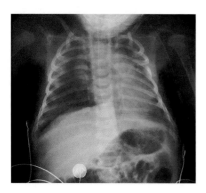

Fig. 52.1 **Respiratory distress syndrome following emergency caesarean section.** The mother had diabetes which predisposes to respiratory distress syndrome. Note the ground-glass appearance of the lungs.

production and thereby reduce the incidence of RDS. Clinically there is tachypnoea, grunting and intercostal recession commencing within the first 4 hours of life, and the chest X-ray demonstrates a generalized reticulo-granular appearance referred to as like 'ground glass' (Fig. 52.1). Treatment is with oxygen ± supportive ventilation and often includes giving artificial surfactant through an endotracheal tube.

Meconium aspiration syndrome is also a potentially serious respiratory complication. In utero, meconium is usually retained within the colon. Although it may be passed through the sphincter under physiological conditions, particularly after 40 weeks, it also has an association with fetal hypoxic stress. Meconium is irritant to the neonatal lungs and may lead to a pneumonitis, the meconium aspiration syndrome (Fig. 52.2). Clinical features range from mild neonatal tachypnoea to severe respiratory compromise. The incidence is probably unrelated to fetal pH (and indeed the majority of babies with meconium aspiration syndrome are not acidotic

at delivery) but the syndrome is more likely to be severe if there is associated acidosis. It is also more severe when the meconium is thick. Treatment is with oxygen, mechanical ventilation and, if very severe, extracorporeal membrane oxygenation.

Cardiovascular system

The switch from fetal to neonatal circulation is normally made rapidly after birth. The key event is relaxation of the smooth muscle in the pulmonary blood vessels, which is triggered by the entry of oxygen into the lung with the first breath (note this paradoxical response to oxygen which is the opposite of all other blood vessels).

In some babies, especially when there has been prolonged fetal hypoxia, this circulatory switch does not occur and may itself lead to further hypoxia. This condition is known as persistent fetal circulation and is difficult to distinguish clinically from congenital cyanotic heart disease.

Genitourinary system

Although the fetal kidney is important in maintaining the amniotic fluid volume, it has a negligible role in the excretion of waste products. After birth, the kidney must excrete all the body's waste as well as conserve fluid. In a baby born at term, the kidney is just able manage this role although there is always an initial rise in the blood urea and creatinine concentrations. The maximum urine osmolality which the newborn can attain is about 600 mOsm/kg (compared with 1800 mOsm/kg in the adult) and it is therefore not surprising that dehydration and electrolyte disturbances are common complications of neonatal illness.

Gastrointestinal system

The fetus swallows amniotic fluid at about the same rate as it is produced, and deficiencies in fetal swallowing result in polyhydramnios. If there has been polyhydramnios, the baby should be checked for swallowing problems and should have an orogastric tube passed in order to exclude complete oesophageal atresia.

Haematological system

The term fetus has a high haemoglobin concentration, at around 18 g/dl. This is a response to the low arterial oxygen tension (3–4 kPa) which characterizes the latter part of intrauterine life. Once the oxygen tension rises after birth, this high haemoglobin is no longer needed and has fallen to around 10 g/dl by about 8 weeks of age.

The white cell count at birth is high (12–20 × 10^9/l) and polymorphs predominate. By 4 days of age, it is usually in the range 7–12 × 10^9/l and is mainly lymphocytic.

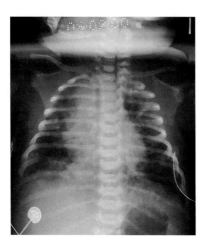

Fig. 52.2 **Meconium aspiration syndrome.** Note the widespread patchy shadowing in both lungs.

Table 52.1
The Apgar score (slightly simplified)

Feature	Score 0	Score 1	Score 2
Breathing	None	Gasping	Vigorous
Heart rate	None	< 100 b.p.m.	> 100 b.p.m.
Skin colour	White	Blue	Pink
Muscle tone	None	Poor	Good
Response to stimulation	None	Minimal	Vigorous

Interpretation: Maximum score = 10; most well babies score 7 or more.

Box 52.1

HEAT BALANCE AT BIRTH

Mechanisms of heat loss (in priority order)
- Evaporation of water from wet skin
- Convective loss due to air currents
- Radiation to cold surfaces
- Conductive loss to cold mattress

Mechanisms of heat gain
- Oxidation of brown fat (plentiful in newborn)
- Muscular activity
- Radiant heater over cot or Resuscitaire
- Warm mattress

Routine care at birth

There are several routine observations and procedures to perform on the newborn shortly after birth but none of them should be allowed to prevent the mother from seeing and holding her baby as soon as possible.

Assessment

The baby's condition at 1 minute and 5 minutes of age is assessed by means of the Apgar score – see Table 52.1. The purpose of this is to have a reasonably objective record of how the baby initially responded to the challenge of extrauterine life. It serves as a guide to the need for resuscitation but, unless the score fails to improve with resuscitation, it has very little predictive value for later disability (p. 412). A low Apgar score is not synonymous with birth asphyxia. It could, for example, be a reflection of a pre-existing fetal problem or sedation caused by the maternal drug administration.

Preventing hypothermia

Newborn babies can lose heat faster than they can generate it (Box 52.1). Hypothermia is dangerous and must be prevented. The delivery room must be warm and draughts kept to a minimum. The baby should be dried at once, especially the top of the head from which most heat is lost, and wrapped in dry towels or blankets. If resuscitation is required, it should be performed under a radiant heater. Increasingly, neonatologists are putting babies into polythene bags even prior to intubation to minimize evaporative losses and improve temperature control.

Examination

Providing all appears well, all that is needed in the labour ward is a quick check for any obvious external abnormalities. A full routine examination should be deferred until later.

Weighing and measuring

Weight, length and head circumference measurements provide an assessment of how well the baby has grown in utero and are a baseline against which to judge subsequent growth. Table 52.2 gives some normative term data and such data are available for neonates born at earlier gestations.

The umbilical cord

The cord should be checked to see whether it contains the usual two arteries and one vein. A single artery has a 20% association with congenital abnormalities, mainly of the genitourinary system. A plastic cord clamp should be fixed so as to leave about 2 cm of cord proximally. Subsequent care of the cord is controversial. Some authorities advocate no specific measures, whereas most like to apply an antiseptic agent, such as chlorhexidine powder. If the baby is likely to need intensive care, the cord should be left longer to allow arterial and venous cannulation.

Table 52.2
Some dimensions of a 'normal' male* infant at 40 weeks

Weight	3500 g
Length	50 cm
Head circumference	35 cm
Brain weight	400 g (12% of body weight)
Blood volume	280 ml (80 ml/kg)

* Females are about 10% smaller.

Preventing haemorrhagic disease of the newborn

Vitamin K does not cross the placenta well and newborn babies have low serum concentrations and poor stores. They do not have gut bacteria to synthesize it for them, and human milk is a relatively poor source of the vitamin. Lack of vitamin K leads to shortage of clotting factors II, VII, IX and X and about 1 in 1000 breast-fed babies will experience serious bleeding, a condition known as haemorrhagic disease of the newborn. The classical form occurs between days 1–7, although an early form occurs in infants born to mothers taking anticonvulsants and a late (and sometimes more serious form) may also occur, even up to 12 weeks after delivery. Bottle-fed babies are much less at risk because formulae are supplemented with vitamins.

Almost complete protection is given by the administration of vitamin K 1 mg i.m. at the time of birth, and possibly less-complete protection is provided by giving 2 mg vitamin K p.o. twice in the first week (with a further oral dose at 1 month). Some epidemiological studies have found an association between i.m. vitamin K (as opposed to oral vitamin K) and childhood leukaemias, resulting in a swing away from treatment. Subsequent studies have failed to prove the connection.

Perinatal asphyxia

Evolution has equipped the fetus with a remarkable ability to tolerate asphyxia without adverse problems, to the extent that sometimes 10 or 15 minutes of absolute anoxia can be compatible with normal survival. In practice, absolute anoxia only occurs with rare events such as massive placental abruption or cord prolapse. Asphyxia may lead to cerebral palsy, essentially a motor disorder affecting posture and movement which is variably accompanied by mental impairment, epilepsy or sensory defects. Despite popular belief, it is likely that less than 10% of cerebral palsy is caused primarily by perinatal asphyxia.

Neonatologists are wary of making a diagnosis of perinatal asphyxia unless there is a good antenatal history (e.g. abruption) together with neonatal 'depression' (e.g. poor Apgar scores) and evidence of subsequent multiorgan failure. Such multiorgan failure may present with seizures, cerebral oedema, oliguria, haematuria, coagulopathy, jaundice or occasionally pulmonary haemorrhage. The question of predicting the likelihood of neurological injury following a specific birth and the question of whether a subsequent cerebral abnormality was caused by a specific intrapartum insult are discussed on page 412.

Resuscitation

Babies with low Apgar scores require resuscitation – they may be apnoeic, atonic, pale, unresponsive and have low heart rates. It is sometimes difficult to know when to intervene in those with intermediate Apgar scores, but as a general guide, those who do not breathe within 30 seconds of birth usually need some help, especially if the heart rate remains below 100 beats per minute.

Effective ventilation of the lungs is the key to neonatal resuscitation and usually little else is needed. Ventilation can be accomplished using a well-fitting face mask and a resuscitation bag incorporating a pressure-release valve, set appropriately for the gestation of the baby. The usual response to effective resuscitation is a rapid improvement in heart rate and skin colour. Intubation is more efficient but is a skill which must be acquired and maintained.

Neonatal examination

Sometime during the first day or two of life all newborn babies should be carefully and systematically examined, for the reasons outlined in Box 52.2. The technique for this examination must be learned, as must the range of normal findings. It is probably better to follow an anatomical progression from head to toe (Table 52.3) rather than to adopt a system-orientated approach.

Developmental dysplasia of the hip

Developmental dysplasia of the hip (previously referred to as 'congenital dislocation of the hip') has an overall incidence of approximately 1%, but is commoner in

---

Box 52.2

REASONS FOR PERFORMING THE ROUTINE NEWBORN EXAMINATION

- To detect abnormalities for which early diagnosis and treatment offer an improved prognosis, e.g., congenital hip dysplasia

- To detect abnormalities early in order to plan therapy, follow-up or genetic counselling, e.g., cardiac abnormalities, Down's syndrome

- To reassure parents that their baby appears to have no serious problem

- It is an opportunity to provide health education

Table 52.3
Key abnormalities in routine newborn examination

Head	Abnormal size or shape Raised anterior fontanelle tension
Face	Dysmorphic features, facial nerve palsy
Eyes	Asymmetry, lens opacities
Mouth	Cleft-palate, thrush
Jaw	Micrognathia
Neck	Goitre, sternomastoid nodules
Chest	Breathlessness
Heart	Murmurs or signs of overactivity
Abdomen	Enlarged kidneys or other masses
Umbilicus	Signs of sepsis
Groins	Herniae
Genitalia	Ambiguity of sex. Undescended testes or urethral abnormalities in the male, bulging of the hymen or bleeding in the female
Anus	Imperforate
Spine	Abnormal curvature or any surface lesion
Hips	Signs of dysplasia
Feet	Talipes (twisting of feet and ankles)
CNS	Abnormal tone, lack of movement or reduced responsiveness

breech presentation, oligohydramnios, firstborn females and those with a family history. Early neonatal diagnosis carries an excellent prognosis as most respond to several months in a versatile harness (the Pavlik harness – pronounced 'Pau-lick'). Those in whom the diagnosis is delayed rarely attain normal hip development. Clinical screening with Ortolani's test may miss a significant proportion of cases. Ultrasound is likely to detect a greater proportion and, although commonly only used in higher-risk neonates, it may become part of the routine screening process.

Biochemical screening

As well as screening by physical examination, babies in the UK are screened biochemically for a number of different disorders by checking a heel-prick blood sample on about the 7th day of life. The disorders assessed vary in different regions, but may include phenylketonuria, congenital hypothyroidism, cystic fibrosis and galactosaemia.

Physical birth injury

Serious injury to the baby during birth is rare in western practice. Injuries are most likely to occur when there is absolute or relative disproportion between the size of the baby and the maternal pelvis, or following malpresentation or instrumental delivery. Preterm babies are more easily damaged than those at term.

Nerve palsies

These are due either to overstretching of the nerve or to direct external pressure on the nerve. In more than 85% of instances, the nerve fibres remain intact and full recovery occurs. Nerve disruption may result in permanent disability.

Brachial plexus

Erb's palsy is caused by injury to roots C5 and C6 and produces a limp arm, held alongside the body with the forearm pronated – 'waiter's tip' posture (Fig. 49.6i). Klumpke's palsy is rarer, involves C8 and T1, and mainly affects the wrist extensors and the small hand muscles. Injury to the phrenic nerve is rare. It is associated with brachial plexus injury and can cause marked respiratory difficulty.

Facial nerve

This is a lower motor neuron lesion due to compression of the facial nerve by maternal pelvic bones or forceps. Minor, transient cases are quite common but permanent weakness is seen in only about 5% of instances.

Skeletal injury

Although the skull often undergoes marked distortion during delivery, fractures are very uncommon and usually cause no trouble. Fractures of the clavicle are not infrequently seen even after normal delivery and usually heal very well, although sometimes with massive callus formation. Fractures of other bones are rare and suggest significant trauma at delivery.

Soft tissue injury

This is rarely of any serious consequence but may be distressing for parents as well as for whoever conducted the birth.

Caput succedaneum

Essentially oedema of the 'presenting' scalp, this disappears rapidly after birth and requires no treatment.

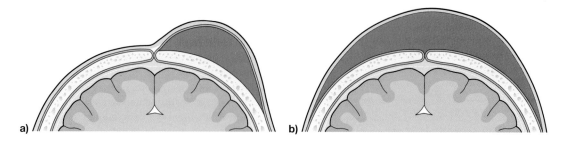

Fig. 52.3 **Comparison of cephalhaematoma and subaponeurotic haemorrhage. (a)** The space under a cephalhaematoma is relatively small and major blood loss is unlikely. **(b)** There is a much larger potential space under the aponeurosis, and there may be serious blood loss.

Chignon

This is the name given to the swelling produced by a ventouse vacuum extractor. There are usually no complications, but infection and necrosis of the skin can occur.

Cephalhaematoma

Bleeding between a skull bone and its overlying periosteum occurs in about 1% of babies. The lesion is confined to the margins of the bone by attachment of the periosteum, which prevents the amount of blood loss from becoming significant (Fig. 52.3a). It is almost always parietal, but can occasionally be occipital. Palpation around the edge of the lesion often gives the impression of an associated depressed fracture but this is an illusion. In 5% of cases there is an inconsequential linear fracture of the underlying bone. Spontaneous regression occurs and no treatment is required.

Subaponeurotic haemorrhage

This is much rarer than cephalhaematoma, but may lead to serious blood loss and can be fatal. There is bleeding into the potentially very large space between the skull and the overlying occipitofrontalis aponeurosis (Fig. 52.3b).

Sternomastoid tumour

This is a fibrous lump in the sternomastoid muscle, probably secondary to compression of the muscle leading to ischaemia. It settles spontaneously but can cause torticollis.

Congenital abnormalities

Approximately 2% of newborn babies have a serious abnormality detectable at, or soon after, birth. Some of the more serious abnormalities may have been identified antenatally following appropriate screening, particularly neural tube defects, renal agenesis, diaphragmatic herniae and some cardiac problems. In addition to these major abnormalities, 2–3% more babies may have some minor abnormality. Congenital abnormalities are discussed in more detail in Chapter 36.

Feeding

At term, human milk has considerable advantages over a cow's milk-based formula (see Box 52.3). In addition, breast-feeding is psychologically advantageous to both mother and baby, and also confers physiological and disease-prevention benefits on the mother. Mothers should be encouraged to put the baby to the breast soon after birth and thereafter the baby should be fed on demand. In many 'developed' countries the prevalence of breast-feeding remains low, and marketing from artificial feed companies is intense.

Correct reconstitution of powdered milk formulae is essential for safe artificial feeding, as babies do not tolerate excessive osmolar loads (see Table 52.4). Whichever way the baby is fed, a close watch must be kept on

---

Box 52.3

ADVANTAGES OF HUMAN MILK

- It contains IgA, lactoferrin and other proteins which protect against infection
- It is not allergenic
- It is easily digested and meets the nutritional needs of the newborn
- It is normally uncontaminated by pathogens
- It partially protects against necrotizing enterocolitis

Table 52.4
Recommended feed volumes for term newborn infants

Day 1	60 ml/kg
Day 2	75 ml/kg
Day 3	90 ml/kg
Day 4	120 ml/kg
Day 5	150 ml/kg

the adequacy of weight gain. Between 170 g and 200 g per week is appropriate for a neonate at term during the first few weeks of life.

Special formulae are available for preterm babies, and have higher levels of protein, sodium, calcium and phosphate. Preterm babies should gain weight at about 12 g/kg/day. 'Special' milks, such as those based on soya, should only be used when there are clear medical indications.

Signs of illness

Newborn babies have a very limited number of ways to show that they are ill (Box 52.4). These signs may be subtle and most often are first noticed by the mother or the nursing staff. The signs may occasionally be non-specific, so that a baby with an infection may initially be clinically indistinguishable from one with a metabolic disorder or even cardiac disease. This, coupled with the speed with which newborn babies deteriorate during serious illness, means that a very high index

---

Box 52.4

SIGNS OF ILLNESS IN THE NEWBORN

- Excessive sleepiness and lack of interest in feeding
- Slow feeding
- Diminished or, occasionally, excessive crying
- Poor muscle tone, with limbs held extended rather than flexed
- Skin pallor or slaty-grey coloration with mottling
- Temperature instability
- Vomiting and abdominal distension
- Episodes of apnoea
- Tachypnoea and tachycardia
- Grunting respirations

---

of suspicion and a low threshold for investigation are appropriate.

When a baby shows some of the features listed in Box 52.4, infection is by far the likeliest cause and the following approach should be pursued:

- Take a history, considering particularly:
  - maternal health during pregnancy
  - risk factors for infection, such as prolonged rupture of the membranes, maternal illness or nursery contact with sick babies
  - family history of neonatal illness or neonatal death.
- Examine the baby. As well as assessing the severity of illness the examination should seek signs of superficial infection, which might have led to septicaemia, and signs of organ dysfunction.
- Investigate as follows:
  - blood culture
  - full blood count and film
  - blood glucose – by stick test
  - arterial blood gas, if the baby is breathless or seriously ill
  - C-reactive protein
  - urine culture
  - swabs, from any inflamed lesions
  - chest X-ray
  - stool culture if stools abnormal
  - lumbar puncture if sepsis is suspected and the source is unclear.
- Treat. If infection seems a possibility, broad-spectrum antibiotic therapy should be started, for example a combination of ampicillin and gentamicin or a third-generation cephalosporin. The results of investigations will allow the rationalization of treatment.

Jaundice

Clinically apparent jaundice (serum bilirubin greater than about 75 µmol/l) affects more than half of all newborns during the first week of life.

Physiological jaundice

Almost all jaundiced babies will have a harmless physiological jaundice which is part of the normal transition from fetal to postnatal life. The fetal liver does not handle unconjugated bilirubin but rather leaves it to cross the placenta to be conjugated and excreted by the mother. Following birth, the neonatal liver must handle all of the unconjugated bilirubin produced but cannot do so immediately. During the first few days of life, liver function improves rapidly but while this is happening the serum unconjugated bilirubin invariably rises.

Unconjugated bilirubin can cross the blood–brain barrier and is toxic to the central nervous system, especially the basal ganglia and the auditory pathways. Bilirubin encephalopathy, or kernicterus, may lead to an athetoid cerebral palsy, deafness, and may even be lethal. The unconjugated serum bilirubin concentration probably needs to exceed 500 µmol/l in order to injure the brain of a healthy term infant and this never occurs with physiological jaundice.

Pathological jaundice

The main problem with physiological jaundice is that it makes it difficult to spot the very few infants with pathological jaundice due to the causes in Box 52.5. Some of these conditions are important in their own right, while others pose a risk of kernicterus. Jaundice which fulfils any of the criteria listed in Box 52.6 should be regarded as potentially pathological.

Most of the pathological causes of jaundice are easy to understand and it is relatively easy to reach a diagnosis if a systematic approach is adopted. Box 52.7 lists the main tests to be performed.

Breast milk jaundice

Breast milk jaundice is still not completely understood but it is thought that compounds in the milk of some women interfere with conjugation of bilirubin in the baby's liver. It is a harmless condition but problematic because there is no specific test for it. It presents as persistent jaundice which is mainly unconjugated in nature. Other more serious causes of persistent jaundice,

---

Box 52.5

MAJOR PATHOLOGICAL CAUSES OF NEONATAL JAUNDICE

1. **Excessive production of bilirubin:**
   a. Intravascular haemolysis due to rhesus or ABO incompatibility or inherited red cell defects
   b. Bruising
   c. Polycythaemia

2. **Diminished conjugation:**
   a. Breast milk jaundice
   b. Hypothyroidism
   c. Hepatic enzyme deficiencies
   d. Inborn errors of metabolism
   e. Hepatitis from various causes

3. **Obstruction:**
   a. Atresia of intra- or extrahepatic bile ducts
   b. Congenital bile-duct cyst

Box 52.6

INDICATORS THAT JAUNDICE MAY BE PATHOLOGICAL

- Becomes apparent during the first day of life
- Rises faster than 75 µmol/l/day
- Exceeds 250 µmol/l
- Persists beyond 10 days of age
- Is associated with pale stools, dark urine or bilirubinuria

---

Box 52.7

INVESTIGATION OF SUSPECTED PATHOLOGICAL JAUNDICE

1. Mother's blood group, baby's blood group and Coombs' test – to look for rhesus or ABO incompatibility
2. Haemoglobin and blood film – to look for anaemia and signs of haemolysis
3. Unconjugated and conjugated serum bilirubin concentrations – to estimate the risk of encephalopathy and to look for signs of obstruction
4. Liver function tests – for evidence of liver disease
5. Test urine for reducing substances (? galactosaemia)
6. Check thyroid screening result and repeat if indicated

---

such as hypothyroidism or hepatitis, must be excluded before the diagnosis of breast milk jaundice can be safely accepted.

Obstructive jaundice

The diagnosis must be considered in any baby who is still jaundiced at 2 weeks of age and is an important diagnosis to make. The history of pale stools and dark urine should be sought and the urine tested for bilirubin. If obstructive jaundice is suspected, the biliary tree should be investigated using ultrasound, radioisotope scans and possibly liver biopsy. Most cases of biliary atresia can be treated, at least partially, by surgical anastomosis of the liver to the small bowel. Long-term, liver transplantation will be required by many survivors of neonatal surgery.

Jaundice due to haemolysis

Some of the pathological causes of neonatal jaundice can raise the serum concentration of unconjugated bilirubin to levels at which encephalopathy might occur. This is most likely with rhesus disease but occasionally happens with ABO incompatibility or other haemolytic disorders. The use of anti-D immunoglobulin to treat rhesus negative women after childbirth or obstetric procedures has made rhesus disease quite rare. ABO incompatibility usually exists when a group O mother has a group B or A baby (see Ch. 42).

Treatment of pathological jaundice

Above an age-specific bilirubin threshold, phototherapy is indicated. This involves the use of high-intensity light in the 450 nanometre wavelength to convert stable lipid-soluble unconjugated bilirubin into unstable water-soluble isomers which can be excreted in the bile without the need for conjugation (Fig. 42.1). It takes about 12–24 hours to have an effect on the rate of rise of the bilirubin. If the bilirubin rises above a further threshold despite phototherapy, an exchange transfusion is required.

Low-birth-weight infants

Although low-birth-weight (LBW) babies account for only 10% of all births in the UK they account for around 70% of the perinatal mortality rate. Approximately two-thirds of LBW babies are preterm (Fig. 52.4) and the rest are term but small-for-dates (SFD).

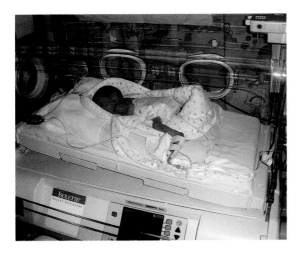

Fig. 52.4 **A 26-week preterm infant has immature lungs, skin, central nervous system, gastrointestinal system and genitourinary system, and is also more prone to infection.**

Prematurity-related problems

Survival increases from approximately 5% at 23 weeks' gestation to 95% at 31 weeks. About 25% of these survivors have some disability – including cerebral palsy, short stature, respiratory difficulties, visual impairment and poor school performance. It is now well established that corticosteroids given to mothers who subsequently deliver preterm are effective in reducing the incidence of respiratory distress syndrome by around 50% as well as the risk of periventricular haemorrhage. Whether or not to start resuscitation with an extremely premature infant (less than 24 weeks) can sometimes be a difficult question and, ideally, discussions with the prospective parents should have taken place beforehand in order to gauge their wishes.

The problems of prematurity are outlined in Table 52.5.

Problems with being small for dates

By definition, 10% of babies are small for dates, the majority for no pathological reason. Around a third, however, have fetal growth restriction as defined as 'a baby which has failed to reach its genetic growth potential', and are more at risk of peripartum hypoxia and neonatal hypoglycaemia. The implications of fetal growth restriction are discussed further on page 365.

Infection

Although the fetus is generally isolated from the external bacteriological environment, some pathogens are occasionally able to cross the placenta and infect the baby. This may sometimes lead to permanent damage and the details of some of these conditions are discussed on page 348.

Newborn babies are immunocompromised relative to older children for the reasons shown in Box 52.8 and are therefore at increased risk of infection. Neonatal

---

Box 52.8

IMMUNOLOGICAL DEFICIENCIES AMONG NORMAL INFANTS

1. Complete lack of IgM and IgA – only humoral activity is IgG from mother
2. Low numbers of neutrophils with poor chemotactic and killing powers
3. Poor local inflammatory response allows spread of organisms to circulation

Table 52.5
The problems of prematurity

Skin	Extremely preterm infants have a very high surface area to mass ratio and thin skin, and are extremely liable to hypothermia. This means that it is vitally important to deliver in a warm room with heated towels for drying and some method to keep the baby warm during resuscitation, e.g. an overhead heater. Survival is directly related to the temperature of the infant on admission to the neonatal intensive care unit
Lung	At 23–24 weeks the respiratory epithelial cells start to differentiate into type I (gas exchange) and type II (surfactant production) pneumocytes. Surfactant levels at this gestation are therefore very low but can be increased by antenatal glucocorticoids (see RDS, p. 471). Respiratory support is often by mechanical ventilation, either 'conventional' or with 'high-frequency oscillation', and exogenous prophylactic surfactant administration. A large proportion of extremely preterm infants develop chronic lung disease of prematurity (bronchopulmonary dysplasia), with continuing requirements for respiratory support
Central nervous system	The subependymal germinal matrix lies close to the ventricular space and contains the developing brain cells of the premature infant. Bleeding from this very vascular area may occur with preterm delivery, giving rise to periventricular haemorrhage. A major intraventricular haemorrhage may lead to hydrocephalus and cortical damage. The extremely preterm infant is also prone to ischaemic brain injury from low arterial oxygen tension, hypotension, or reduced cerebral blood flow. Subsequent periventricular cysts (periventricular leucomalacia) may form and, if this happens, long-term neurological sequelae are likely
	The location of brain injury in the white matter adjacent to the lateral ventricles means that the arising disability is mainly motor and often affects the lower limbs. This presents as a spastic diplegia with relative sparing of the intellect and affects about 10% of babies with birth weights below 1500 g
GI system	Structurally the bowel is well developed by the end of the second trimester but there is functional immaturity. Motility and food absorption are both reduced and early enteral feeding may not be tolerated. Parenteral nutrition may be needed during the early days and weeks, but this may lead to numerous problems, both from the need to maintain adequate venous access and the tolerability of the amino acid and lipid solutions
	Necrotizing enterocolitis (NEC) is not uncommon in premature infants, and is characterized by ischaemic bowel necrosis. Although the aetiology is unclear, it typically presents after the introduction of enteral feeds and is postulated to be an abnormal reaction to bowel colonization
Liver	There may be jaundice, poor clotting, poor glucose control and a limited ability to excrete waste products
Blood	There is reduced immunoglobulin and white cell function so that the risk of sepsis is increased. Furthermore, frequent use of multiple, broad-spectrum antibiotics renders the tiny baby more prone to infection with sub-pathogenic bacteria such as *Staphylococcus epidermidis*, and fungi, especially *Candida albicans*
Eye	Early vasoconstriction damage to the retina occurs as a result of high oxygen pressure and other factors. The incidence of this is reduced by using ventilation at lower Po_2 levels. Secondary proliferation of weaker, potentially haemorrhagic, vessels occurs, a condition referred to as retinopathy of prematurity. Regular ophthalmological review is vital as early laser or cryotherapy treatment of these new vessels can preserve vision

infections may be with organisms from the birth canal, such as group B β-haemolytic streptococci, or from the neonatal environment, for example *Escherichia coli*, *Proteus* species, *Staphylococcus aureus* and *Staph. epidermidis*. The risks are of pneumonia, meningitis, pyelonephritis and osteomyelitis and a low index of suspicion is important for these conditions.

Some common minor infections are considered below.

Conjunctivitis

'Sticky eyes' are common and most cases respond rapidly to topical antibacterial treatment. Infection with gonorrhoea and chlamydia, however, may be more serious.

- Gonococcal ophthalmia usually presents as a fulminant, unilateral or bilateral, purulent infection during the first few days of life. The maternal social history may give a clue. Prompt diagnosis and treatment with systemic and local penicillin is needed to prevent corneal damage and permanent visual impairment.
- Chlamydial eye infections usually present as sticky eyes which do not settle with conventional antibacterial agents. The diagnosis is best made from corneal brushings but can be made from an ordinary eye swab if the laboratory is asked to look specifically for the organism. Treatment is with tetracycline eye drops and systemic erythromycin to clear the organisms from the upper respiratory tract, from where they may go on to cause pneumonia.

Systemic tetracycline is never given to babies or young children because it stains dental enamel and interferes with its development.

Candida

'Thrush' infections are common in either the mouth or in the nappy area and are caused by a yeast, *Candida albicans*. In the mouth, the appearance is of adherent white patches of exudate. In the nappy area, inflammation may be confused with other causes of nappy rash, although satellite lesions around the main area of erythema are suggestive of candida. Treatment is with topical nystatin or one of the more modern antifungal agents, such as miconazole.

Skin sepsis

Skin sepsis is relatively common and usually due to staphylococci, although streptococci and other organisms may be involved. Paronychia, pustules and peri-umbilical infection are the most likely manifestations. Blistering and desquamation are seen with some strains of staphylococci. All suspected staphylococcal or streptococcal infections should be taken very seriously and a low threshold for systemic treatment is appropriate.

Urinary tract infection

Urinary tract infection in babies is more common in baby boys than in girls and is usually caused by *E. coli* and other Gram-negative organisms. Screening can be performed using bag specimens but diagnosis is best confirmed by suprapubic aspiration. Because of the association with congenital abnormalities of the urinary tract an ultrasound scan or other imaging techniques should be considered.

Meningitis

Neonatal meningitis is most commonly caused by group B streptococci or *E. coli* and has a very high morbidity and mortality. A very low threshold for investigation and treatment is appropriate.

Key points

- Good-quality neonatal care is extremely important, and may have key implications for the rest of a baby's life.

- Those born prematurely need skilled intensive support, and those born with presumed hypoxia need appropriate resuscitation.

- The early neonatal period is often the time when congenital abnormalities become apparent, and precise diagnosis and management can make a difference to the quality of life, or even influence whether the baby will live or die.

Bibliography

Gynaecology

Menorrhagia

Maresh MJ, Metcalfe MA et al 2002 The VALUE national hysterectomy study: description of the patients and their surgery. BJOG: an International Journal of Obstetrics & Gynaecology 109(3):302–12

Stewart A, Cummins C, Gold L, Jordan R, Phillips W 2001 The effectiveness of the levonorgestrel-releasing intrauterine system in menorrhagia: a systematic review. BJOG: an International Journal of Obstetrics and Gynaecology 108(l): 74–86

Polycystic Ovarian Syndrome

Costello MF, Eden JA 2003 A systematic review of the reproductive system effects of metformin in patients with polycystic ovary syndrome. Fertility and Sterility 79(l): 1–13

Hopkinson ZEC, Sattar N, Fleming R, Greer IE 1998 Polycystic ovarian syndrome: the metabolic syndrome comes to gynaecology. British Medical Journal 317: 329–332

Contraception

Beral V, Hermon C et al 1999 Mortality associated with oral contraceptive use: 25 year follow up of cohort of 46000 women from Royal College of General Practitioners' oral contraception study British Medical Journal 318: 96–100

von Hertzen H, Piaggio G et al 2002 WHO Research Group on Post-ovulatory Methods of Fertility Regulation. Low dose mifepristone and two regimens of levonorgestrel for emergency contraception: a WHO multicentre randomised trial. Lancet 360(9348): 1803–10

Miscarriage

Levine JS, Branch DW, Rauch J 2002 The antiphospholipid syndrome New England Journal of Medicine 346(10): 752–763

Rai R, Cohen H, Dave M, Regan L 1997 Randomised controlled trial of aspirin and aspirin plus heparin in pregnant women with recurrent miscarriage associated with phospholipid antibodies (or antiphospholipid antibodies) British Medical Journal 314: 253

Rai R, Backos M, Baxter N Chilott I, Regan L 2000 Recurrent miscarriage – an aspirin a day? Human Reproduction 15(10): 2220–2223

Ectopic Pregnancy

Stovall TG, Ling FW 1993 Single-dose methotrexate: an expanded clinical trial. American Journal of Obstetrics and Gynaecology:1759–1965

Tulandi T, Saleh A 1999 Surgical management of ectopic pregnancy. Clinical Obstetrics and Gynaecology 42(l):31–8

Premenstrual Syndrome

Johnson SR 1998 Premenstrual syndrome therapy. Clinical Obstetrics and Gynaecology 41: 405–421

HRT

Hulley S, Grady D et al 1998 Randomized trial of estrogen plus progestin for secondary prevention of coronary heart disease in postmenopausal women (HERS trial). Journal of the American Medical Association 280: 605–613

Troop P 2002 Risks and benefits of estrogen plus progestin in healthy postmenopausal women. (Women's Health Initiative) Journal of the American Medical Association 2882:321–333

Incontinence

Bo K, Talseth T, Holme I 1999 Single blind, randomised controlled trial of pelvic floor exercises, electrical stimulation, vaginal cones, and no treatment in management of genuine stress incontinence in women. British Medical Jornal 318(7182):487–93

Chancellor MB 2002 New frontiers in the treatment of overactive bladder and incontinence Urology 4 (suppl): 50–56

Reilly ETC et al 2002 Prevention of postpartum stress incontinence in primigravidae with increased bladder neck mobility: a randomised controlled trial of antenatal pelvic floor exercises; British Journal of Obstetrics and Gynaecology 109: 68–76

Ward K, Hilton P 2002 United Kingdom and Ireland Tension-free Vaginal Tape Trial Group. Prospective multicentre randomised trial of tension-free vaginal tape and colposuspension as primary treatment for stress incontinence. British Medical Journal 325(7355):67

Oncology

Kitchener H 2003 The value of HPV testing. The Obstetrician and Gynaecologist 5(l): 10–14

Trimbos JB, Parmar M, Vergote I et al 2003 International Collaborative Ovarian Neoplasm trial 1 and Adjuvant ChemoTherapy In Ovarian Neoplasm Trial: two parallel randomized phase III trials of adjuvant chemotherapy in patients with early-stage ovarian carcinoma. Journal of the National Cancer Institute 95(2):105–12

Obstetrics

Maternal Mortality

Drife J 2000 Maternal mortality: national and international perspectives. In: O'Brien S (ed). Yearbook of obstetrics and gynaecology, Vol 8, 86–96 RCOG Press, London

Ghosh MK 2001 Maternal mortality:a global perspective. Journal of Reproductive Medicine. 46(5): 427–33

Lewis G (Ed) 1997–1999 Confidential Enquiries into Maternal Deaths in the United Kingdom. Why mothers die. RCOG Press, London

Doppler

Lees C 2000 Uterine artery doppler: time to establish the ground rules. Ultrasound in Obstetrics and Gynaecology 16: 607–609

Bibliography

Papageorghiou AT, Yu CK, Bindra R, Pandis G, Nicolaides KH 2001 Multicenter screening for pre-eclampsia and fetal growth restriction by transvaginal uterine artery doppler at 23 weeks of gestation. Ultrasound in Obstetrics and Gynecology 18(5): 441–9

Prenatal diagnosis

Hyett J, Perdu M, Sharland G, Snijders R, Nicolaides KH 1999 Using fetal nuchal translucency to screen for major congenital cardiac defects at 10–14 weeks of gestation: population based cohort study. British Medical Journal 318: 81–85

Wald NJ, Watt HC, Hackshaw AK 1999. Integrated screening for Down's syndrome based on tests performed during the first and second trimesters. NEJM 342: 461–467

Preterm labour

Kenyon SL,Taylor DJ, Tarnow-Mordi W 2001 ORACLE Collaborative Group. Broad-spectrum antibiotics for preterm, prelabour rupture of fetal membranes: the ORACLE I randomised trial. Lancet 357(9261): 979-88

Kenyon SL, Taylor DJ, Tarnow-Mordi W 2001 ORACLE Collaborative Group. Broad-spectrum antibiotics for spontaneous preterm labour: the ORACLE II randomised trial. Lancet. 357(9261):989–94

The Worldwide Atosiban versus Beta-agonists Study Group 2001 Effectiveness and safety of the Oxytocin Antagonist Atosiban versus beta-adrenergic agonists in the treatment of preterm labour. BJOG: an International Journal of Obstetrics & Gynaecology 108;133–42

Pre-eclampsia/eclampsia

CLASP Collaborative Group 1994 A randomised trial of low-dose aspirin for the prevention and treatment of pre-eclampsia among 9364 pregnant women. Lancet 343: 619–929

Eclampsia Trial Collaborative Group 1995 Which anticonvulsant for women with eclampsia? Evidence from the Collaborative Eclampsia trial. Lancet 345: 1455–1463

Hall DR, Odendaal HJ, Kirsten GF, Smith J, Grové D 2000 Expectant Management of early onset, severe pre-eclampsia:perinatal outcome. BJOG:an International Journal of Obstetrics and Gynaecology 107: 1258–1264

The Magpie Trial Collaborative Group 2002 Do women with pre-eclampsia, and their babies, benefit from magnesium sulphate? The Magpie Trial: a randomised placebo-controlled trial. Lancet Vol 359 1877–1890

Multiple Pregnancy

Martin GJC, Umur A et al 2001 Twin-twin transfusion syndrome: etiology, severity and rational management Current Opinion in Obstetrics and Gynecology 13: 193–206

Breech presentation

Hannah ME, Hannah WJ et al 2000 Planned caesarean section versus planned vaginal birth for breech presentation at term: a randomised multicentre trial. Term Breech Trial Collaborative Group. Lancet 356(9239): 1375–83

Induction of Labour

Hannah ME, Ohlsson A et al 1996 Induction of labour compared with expectant management for prelabor rupture of the membranes at term; The New England Journal of Medicine 334: 1005–1010

Intrapartum care

Impey L, Reynolds M 2003 Admission cardiotocography: a randomised controlled trial. Lancet 361: 465–70

Johanson R, Newburn M et al 2002 Has the medicalisation of childbirth gone too far? British Medical Jurnal 324: 892-895

Murphy D, Liebling RE 2001 Early maternal and neonatal morbidity associated with operative delivery in second stage of labour: a cohort study. Lancet 358: 1203–07

Norén H, Amer-Wåhlin I 2003 Fetal electrocardiography in labour and neonatal outcome: Data from the Swedish randomised controlled trial on intrapartum fetal monitoring. American Journal of Obstetrics and Gynecology 188: 183–92

Intrapartum cerebral palsy

McLennan A 1999 A template for defining a causal relation between acute intrapartum events and cerebral palsy: international consensus statement. British Medical Journal 319: 1054–1059

General interest

Dawkins RT 1989 The selfish gene. Oxford Paperbacks

Godfrey KM, Parker DJ, Barker P 2000 Fetal Nutrition and adult disease. The American Journal of Clinical Nutrition, 71 (5) 1244S–13521S

International Human Genome Sequencing Consortium. 2001 Initial sequencing and analysis of the human genome. Nature 409: 860–921

O'Dowd M, Philipp E 2000 The history of obstetrics and gynaecology The Parthenon Publishing Group, London

Websites

The World Health Organisation: the United Nations specialised agency for health, for a global view of health: www.who.int/en/

FIGO - the International Federation of Gynecology and Obstetrics : a worldwide organisation supporting obstetricians and gynecologists: www.figo.org/

The Cochrane database: the definitive collection of randomised controlled trials: www.cochrane.org/

Royal College of Obstetricians and Gynaecologists, UK with useful obstetric guidelines, access to medline and links to other colleges worldwide: www.rcog.org.uk

The British Medical Journal: free access to full text at www.bmj.com/, with access to medline

Wellbeing: A charity supporting medical research into pregnancy, birth and the care of the new born babies, women's, menopause, osteoporosis and incontinence: http://www.wellbeing.org.uk/

NICE - The National Institute for Clinical Excellence: to provide patients, health professionals and the public with reliable guidance on current "best practice": www.nice.org.uk/

Scottish Intercollegiate Guidelines Network (SIGN): development and dissemination of national clinical guidelines: www.sign.ac.uk/

The Multiple Births Foundation provides support for multiple birth families and professionals http://www.multiplebirths.org.uk

The National Organization for Rare Disorders provides information about rare diseases for patients and clinicians: http://www.rarediseases.org/

Index

Page numbers in **bold** refer to figures, tables or boxes.

485

Index

Index

Index